2

Controversies in Neuro-Oncology

Best Evidence Medicine for Brain Tumor Surgery

Thieme

Controversies in Neuro-Oncology

Best Evidence Medicine for Brain Tumor Surgery

Alfredo Quiñones-Hinojosa, MD, FAANS, FACS
Professor of Neurological Surgery and Oncology
Neuroscience and Cellular and Molecular Medicine
Director, Brain Tumor Surgery Program
Johns Hopkins–Bayview
Director, Pituitary Surgery Program
The Johns Hopkins Hospital
Baltimore, Maryland

Shaan M. Raza, MD
Department of Neurosurgery
The Johns Hopkins Hospital
Baltimore, Maryland

Thieme
New York · Stuttgart

Thieme Medical Publishers, Inc.
333 Seventh Ave.
New York, NY 10001

Executive Editor: Kay Conerly
Managing Editor: Judith Tomat
Editorial Assistant: Genevieve Kim
Senior Vice President, Editorial and Electronic Product Development: Cornelia Schulze
Production Editor: Kenneth L. Chumbley
International Production Director: Andreas Schabert
Vice President, Finance and Accounts: Sarah Vanderbilt
President: Brian D. Scanlan
Compositor: Prairie Papers Inc.
Printer: Everbest Printing Co. Ltd.

Library of Congress Cataloging-in-Publication Data

Controversies in neuro-oncology : best-evidence medicine for brain tumor surgery / [edited by] Alfredo Quiñones-Hinojosa, Shaan M. Raza.
p. ; cm.
Includes bibliographical references and index.
ISBN 978-1-60406-755-2—ISBN 978-1-60406-756-9 (eISBN)
I. Quiñones-Hinojosa, Alfredo. II. Raza, Shaan M.
[DNLM: 1. Brain Neoplasms—surgery. 2. Brain Neoplasms—radiotherapy. 3. Evidence-Based Medicine—methods. 4. Neurosurgical Procedures. 5. Radiosurgery—methods. WL 358]
RC280.B7
616.99'481—dc23

2013013422

Important note: Medical knowledge is ever-changing. As new research and clinical experience broaden our knowledge, changes in treatment and drug therapy may be required. The authors and editors of the material herein have consulted sources believed to be reliable in their efforts to provide information that is complete and in accord with the standards accepted at the time of publication. However, in view of the possibility of human error by the authors, editors, or publisher of the work herein or changes in medical knowledge, neither the authors, editors, nor publisher, nor any other party who has been involved in the preparation of this work, warrants that the information contained herein is in every respect accurate or complete, and they are not responsible for any errors or omissions or for the results obtained from use of such information. Readers are encouraged to confirm the information contained herein with other sources. For example, readers are advised to check the product information sheet included in the package of each drug they plan to administer to be certain that the information contained in this publication is accurate and that changes have not been made in the recommended dose or in the contraindications for administration. This recommendation is of particular importance in connection with new or infrequently used drugs.

Printed in China

5 4 3 2 1

ISBN 978-1-60406-755-2

Also available as an e-book:
eISBN 978-1-60406-756-9

To our families for their love, devotion, inspiration, and endless support in our academic and clinical pursuits.

To our mentors for their patient guidance and mentorship and for instilling in us the importance and excitement of seeking answers and new knowledge.

Contents

Foreword

I am honored by my assignment to pen a Foreword to this unprecedented achievement by Drs. Quinones and Raza.

In their Preface, Quinones and Raza acknowledge the past, but the emphasis throughout is to address major surgical controversies in conjunction with each expert's recommendations and the critical supporting evidence. The authorship of each section is a literal "who's who" in the field.

Looking ahead, the authors emphasize the need for prospective clinical studies to generate higher levels of evidence to support our practice.

I envy the editors—who are also contributors—for a book that I had one day hoped to write. I came into the field before it acquired a name. I and others subscribed to the belief that there are no "benign" brain tumors. The distinction between benign and malignant was more time-related than biology-related. In effect, the difference had the same end-point (death), preceded by disability. Exceptions were rare, such as densely-calcified meningiomas, whose victims outlived the tumor. In the past, the life-cycle of these tumors reached a steady state in which cell-death met or exceeded the rate of mitotic cell birth. One such example is the time-scale of irradiated meningiomas.

In closing, I expose my insecurity as the sole author of a Foreword to an achievement so grand and comprehensive.

All neurosurgeons, medical and surgical generalists, and subspecialists need to have this volume in their library as they sit in front of each patient to provide an unbiased and evidence-based recommendation.

As neurosurgeons, we are pledged to give every patient the best-known advice: "doing unto others what you want done to you," devoid of personal prejudice and contrary personal experience.

Sincerely and with gratitude to the authors,

Charles B. Wilson, MD, DSc, MSHA
Professor Emeritus
Department of Neurological Surgery
University of California–San Francisco
San Francisco, California

Preface

> In these days when science is clearly in the saddle and when our knowledge of disease is advancing at a breathless pace, we are apt to forget that not all can ride and that he also serves who waits and who applies what the horseman discovers.
>
> *Harvey Cushing*

The field of neurosurgery is considered by some as relatively young, but in the last several decades its practice has undergone a tremendous metamorphosis. Within the specialty, neurooncology has perhaps experienced the greatest degree of expansion. With our improved anatomic understanding in parallel with technological advances, we've seen the innovation of new surgical techniques (e.g., endoscopy for skull base tumors) along with the adoption of new technologies into the operating room (e.g., intraoperative MRI, 5-aminolevulinic acid). Concurrently, our recognition of the fact that modern medical care demands multidisciplinary collaboration has placed the neurosurgical management of brain tumors in harmony with other surgical and nonsurgical specialists. This collaboration has also fostered innovation with the introduction of varying treatment options (e.g., radiosurgery) and protocols that are now part of our armamentarium. Furthermore, as any clinician who participates in the care of cancer patients recognizes, our search for a cure via research has also spurred the development of new biologic therapies, which we must now try to understand and incorporate if possible into our decision making while caring for patients.

As we sit in front of patients and attempt to present our best clinical recommendation, more often than we like, we still rely primarily on our experience and a limited understanding of the published evidence, which can often be based on flawed studies. These practical clinical issues are now magnified with the recent health care reform. With the need to improve spending and access to health care, physicians are now increasingly being asked to justify interventions and to provide better care at a more affordable cost. With the introduction of organizations such as Accountable Care Organizations , institutional practices are now linking provider reimbursements to quality metrics, while being liable for the appropriateness and efficiency of the health care provided. Consequently, any intervention must be justified by data. Hence, it is imperative that we not only have a mastery of the evidence but also have good quality evidence to guide and defend our clinical decision making, while providing the best care possible.

In light of these obstacles, we set out to create an up-to-date review by different world-experts that would address some of the major surgical controversies in the field of neurooncology in the context of evidence-based medicine. We asked the major leaders in the field to not only summarize and critique currently available evidence but also to provide their expert opinion regarding their assigned topic. The book will cover the major tumor types and their associated controversies. Each chapter will provide not only the relevant background but also discuss all the relevant literature on the subject. At the end of each chapter, you will find a table summarizing each expert's recommendations and their level of supporting evidence. In this process we intend not only to provide you with a guide to navigate some of the major decisions encountered while talking to patients with brain tumors, but also to understand the supporting evidence. This body of work is not intended to be final but a starting point from which one can further build evidence to support our management of patients that is based on best-evidence-medicine.

We hope that as you read this text you will appreciate the great amount of research that has been done thus far in the field by so many dedicated experts. Nonetheless, this volume should also highlight the need for prospective clinical studies to generate higher levels of evidence to support our practice. While the art of medicine lies in a practitioner's experience and clinical acumen, objective data is still necessary as a foundation. Hence, neurosurgeons need to remain intensely involved with basic, translational, and clinical research to help improve and innovate the care of patients, especially in the context of surrounding social and government changes. As you will see, major challenges and knowledge gaps still remain to which we hope future research will provide answers.

Alfredo Quiñones-Hinojosa

Shaan M. Raza

Acknowledgments

In the fall of 2010, we conceived an idea for a book that would highlight the current state of affairs, controversies, and underlying evidence around the management of brain tumors. Initially, due to the rapid evolution in science and medicine, we were apprehensive about whether or not such a book would be worthwhile; however, our concerns vanished as we discussed the concept with friends and colleagues around the world.

Assembling the material for this book has given us time to reflect on the things that matter most to us and the people who have shaped our training and current practices. We are humbled by the mentors and colleagues with whom we have had the privelege of working, and the new relationships we continue to form. We are extremely grateful to our mentors and colleagues who contributed to this project, all of whom are well published and innovative thinkers. We appreciate them taking the time to write thoughtful text addressing some of the more controversial topics in our field. Their reviews and expert insights into the evidence behind our practices have helped to make this book a unique addition to the neurosurgical library.

We are extraordinarily thankful for the support and encouragement that we have received from our Chairman, Dr. Henry Brem, and our Director of Neuro-oncology, Dr. Alessandro Olivi, as we initiated this project and throughout the entire process. We are also grateful to our colleagues in the Departments of Neurosurgery and Oncology at Johns Hopkins, as well as many other medical students, residents, and fellows, who have continued to work together to help us with the material over many nights, weekends, and holidays to ensure we produced a book that would make us all proud.

Profound gratitude goes to the tremendous efforts of the editorial staff at Thieme Publishers: Kay Conerly (Executive Editor), Judith Tomat (Managing Editor), Genevieve Kim (Editorial Assistant), and Kenny Chumbley (Production Editor), in addition to Colleen Hickson (Administrative Assistant at Johns Hopkins), for their patient support and commitment to excellence. Their tireless efforts made the process of putting together this project truly an enjoyable experience. Well-deserved thanks go out to our Physician Assistant, Jill Anderson, and Medical Office Coordinator, Tasha Leak, for their patience and continued care for our patients battling brain tumors.

Contributors

Manmeet S. Ahluwalia, MD, FACP
Section Head, Neuro-Oncology Outcomes
The Rose Ella Burkhardt Brain Tumor and Neuro-Oncology Center, Neurological Institute
Cleveland Clinic
Cleveland, Ohio

Isabel Arrillaga-Romany, MD, PhD
Center for Neuro-Oncology
Dana-Farber Cancer Institute
Brigham and Women's Cancer Center
Boston, Massachusetts

Ashok R. Asthagiri, MD
Assistant Clinical Investigator
Surgical Neurology Branch
National Institute of Health
Bethesda, Maryland

Javier Avendaño, MD
Neurosurgeon
Department of Neurosurgery
Médica Sur Hospital
Mexico City, Mexico

Garni Barkhoudarian, MD
Faculty Neurosurgeon
Brain Tumor Center and Pituitary Disorders Program
John Wayne Cancer Institute at St. John's Health Center
Santa Monica, California

D. David Beahm, MD
Assistant Professor
University of Kansas Medical Center
Department of Otolaryngology
Kansas City, Kansas

Kimon Bekelis, MD
Section of Neurosurgery
Dartmouth-Hitchcock Medical Center
Lebanon, New Hampshire

Lorenzo Bello, MD
Associate Professor of Neurosurgery
Università degli Studi di Milano
Director of Neurosurgical Oncology
Istituto Clinico Humanitas, IRCCS
Milano, Italy

Mitchel S. Berger, MD, FACS, FAANS
Kathleen M. Plant Distinguished Professor
Chairman, Department of Neurological Surgery
Director, Brain Tumor Research Center
University of California–San Francisco
San Francisco, California

Henry Brem, MD
Professor of Neurological Surgery and Oncology
Director, Department of Neurosurgery
Harvey Cushing Professor of Neurosurgery
Neurosurgeon-in-Chief
The Johns Hopkins Hospital
Director, Hunterian Neurosurgical Research Laboratory
Baltimore, Maryland

Jeffrey N. Bruce, MD
Edgar M. Housepian Professor of Neurological Surgery
Department of Neurological Surgery
Columbia University
New York, New York

Daniel P. Cahill III, MD, PhD
Laboratory Director
Department of Neurosurgery
Massachusetts General Hospital
Boston, Massachusetts

Bob S. Carter, MD, PhD
Professor and Chief of Neurosurgery
University of California–San Diego
La Jolla, California

Kaisorn L. Chaichana, MD
Department of Neurosurgery
Johns Hopkins University School of Medicine
Baltimore, Maryland

Roukoz Chamoun, MD
Department of Neurosurgery
University of Kansas Hospital
Kansas City, Kansas

Steven D. Chang, MD
Robert C. and Jeannette Powell Professor of Neurosurgery
Department of Neurosurgery
Stanford University School of Medicine
Stanford, California

Clark C. Chen, MD, PhD
Chief, Stereotactic and Neurosurgery
Department of Neurosurgery
University of California–San Diego
La Jolla, California

E. Antonio Chiocca, MD, PhD, FAANS
Professor of Surgery
Harvard Medical School
Neurosurgeon-in-Chief and Chairman
Department of Neurosurgery
Co-Director, Institute for the Neurosciences at the Brigham and Women's Faulkner Hospital
Surgical Director, Center for Neuro-Oncology
Dana-Farber Cancer Institute
Boston, Massachusetts

Osamah J. Choudhry, MD
Department of Neurosurgery
New York University Medical Center
New York, New York

Geoffrey P. Colby, MD, PhD
Department of Neurosurgery
Johns Hopkins University School of Medicine
Baltimore, Maryland

Juan Barges Coll, MD, MSc
Assistant Professor
Skull Base Surgery
Instituto Nacional de Neurología y Neurocirugía
Hospital Medica Sur Neurosurgical Department
Mexico City, Mexico

Alexander L. Coon, MD
Assistant Professor of Neurosurgery, Neurology, and Radiology
Director of Endovascular Neurosurgery
The Johns Hopkins Hospital
Baltimore, Maryland

William T. Couldwell, MD, PhD
Professor and Chairman
Department of Neurosurgery
University of Utah
Salt Lake City, Utah

Ramiro Del Valle, MD
Director
Gamma Knife Unit
Médica Sur Hospital
Mexico City, Mexico

Franco DeMonte, MD, FRCSC, FACS
Professor of Neurosurgery and Head and Neck Surgery
Mary Beth Pawelek Chair in Neurosurgery
Department of Neurosurgery
The University of Texas M. D. Anderson Cancer Center
Houston, Texas

Mahua Dey, MD
Department of Surgery, Neurosurgery
University of Chicago
Chicago, Illinois

Hugues Duffau, MD, PhD
Professor and Chairman
Department of Neurosurgery and INSERM 1051
Montpellier University Medical Center
Montpellier, France

Erin M. Dunbar, MD
Assistant Professor
Department of Neurosurgery
University of Florida
Gainesville, Florida

Victoria Ebiana, MD
Department of Neurological Surgery
The Neurological Institute
Columbia University
New York, New York

Jason C. Eck, DO, MS
Orthopedic Spine Surgeon
Center for Sports Medicine and Orthopedics
Chattanooga, Tennessee

J. Bradley Elder, MD
Assistant Professor
Department of Neurological Surgery
The Ohio State University College of Medicine
Columbus, Ohio

James J. Evans, MD
Director of Cranial Base and Pituitary Surgery
Associate Professor of Neurological Surgery and Otolaryngology
Thomas Jefferson University
Philadelphia, Pennsylvania

Christopher J. Farrell, MD
Assistant Professor
Department of Neurological Surgery
Thomas Jefferson University
Philadelphia, Pennsylvania

John C. Flickinger, MD
Professor
Departments of Neurological Surgery and Radiation Oncology
University of Pittsburgh School of Medicine
Pittsburgh, Pennsylvania

Howard Francis, MD, MBA
Associate Professor, Deputy Director
Department of Otolaryngology–Head and Neck Surgery
Johns Hopkins University School of Medicine
Baltimore, Maryland

Rohan Garje, MD
Department of Internal Medicine
Fairfiew Hospital, CCHS
Cleveland, Ohio

Anand V. Germanwala, MD
Assistant Professor
Department of Neurosurgery
Johns Hopkins University School of Medicine
Baltimore, Maryland

David Gonda, MD
Department of Neurosurgery
University of California–San Diego
LaJolla, California

Chad R. Gordon, DO
Assistant Professor
Department of Plastic and Reconstructive Surgery
Johns Hopkins University School of Medicine
Baltimore, Maryland

Mari L. Groves, MD
Department of Neurosurgery
The Johns Hopkins Hospital
Baltimore, Maryland

Costas G. Hadjipanayis, MD, PhD
Chief of Neurosurgery Service
Emory University Hospital Midtown
Department of Neurosurgery
Emory University School of Medicine
Atlanta, Georgia

Douglas A. Hardesty, MD
Department of Neurosurgery
Barrow Neurological Institute
Phoenix, Arizona

Sze Chun Ho, MD
Department of Neurological Surgery
National Institutes of Health
Bethesda, Maryland

Zain A. Husain, MD
Clinician
Department of Therapeutic Radiology
Yale Medical Group
Norwich, Connecticut

Brian Yu-Jin Hwang, MD
Department of Neurosurgery
The Johns Hopkins Hospital
Baltimore, Maryland

Christopher Jackson, BA
Medical Student, Research Fellow
Department of Neurosurgery
Johns Hopkins University School of Medicine
Baltimore, Maryland

George Jallo, MD
Professor of Neurosurgery, Pediatrics and Oncology
Department of Neurosurgery
Johns Hopkins University School of Medicine
Baltimore, Maryland

Hideyuki Kano, MD, PhD
Research Assistant Professor
Department of Neurological Surgery
University of Pittsburgh
Pittsburgh, Pennsylvania

Syed M. A. Karim, MD
Department of Surgery
Southeast Michigan Brain and Spine Surgery
Grand Blanc, Michigan

Tyler J. Kenning, MD
Assistant Professor
Department of Neurosurgery
Albany Medical Center
Albany, New York

Lawrence Kleinberg, MD
Associate Professor
Co-Director of Sterotactic Radiosurgery
Department of Radiation Oncology and Molecular Radiation Servies
Johns Hopkins University School of Medicine
Baltimore, Maryland

Douglas Kondziolka, MD, MSc, FRCSC, FACS
Professor of Neurosurgery Vice Chair
Clinical Research (Neurosurgery)
Professor of Radiation Oncology Director
Center for Advanced Radiosurgery
New York University Langone Medical Center
New York, New York

Carmen Kut, BS
Department of Biomedical Engineering
Johns Hopkins University School of Medicine
Baltimore, Maryland

Young Kwok, MD
Associate Professor
Department of Radiation Oncology
University of Maryland School of Medicine
Baltimore, Maryland

John Laterra, MD, PhD
Professor
Department of Neurology
Johns Hopkins University School of Medicine
Baltimore, Maryland

Edward R. Laws Jr., MD, FACS
Department of Neurosurgery
Brigham and Women's Hospital
Boston, Massachusetts

Maciej S. Lesniak, MD, MHCM, FACS
Professor of Neurosurgery, Neurology, and Cancer Biology
Director, Neurosurgical Oncology and the Neuro-Oncology Research Laboratories
The University of Chicago
Chicago, Illinois

Michael Lim, MD
Assistant Professor of Neurosurgery, Oncology and Institute of NanoBiotechnology
Director of the Brain Tumor Immunotherapy Program
Director of the Metastatic Brain Tumor Center
The Johns Hopkins Hospital
Baltimore, Maryland

Li-Mei Lin, MD
Department of Neurological Surgery
Johns Hopkins University School of Medicine
Baltimore, Maryland

James K. Liu, MD
Director, Center for Skull Base and Pituitary Surgery
Assistant Professor
Department of Neurological Surgery
Neurological Institute of New Jersey
Rutgers University–New Jersey Medical School
Newark, New Jersey

James K. C. Liu, MD
Department of Neurosurgery
Cleveland Clinic
Cleveland, Ohio

Bjorn Lobo, MD
Department of Neurosurgery
Cleveland Clinic
Cleveland, Ohio

Russell R. Lonser, MD
Professor and Chairman
Department of Neurological Surgery
The Ohio State University Wexner Medical Center
Columbus, Ohio

L. Dade Lunsford, MD, FACS
Lars Leksell Professor of Neurosurgery
Distinguished Professor
Director, Residency Training Program
Director, Center for Image Guided Neurosurgery
Department of Neurological Surgery
University of Pittsburgh
Pittsburgh, Pennsylvania

Neal Luther, MD
Neurosurgeon
Department of Neurosurgery and Spine Surgery
New Hampshire NeuroSpine Institute
Bedford, New Hampshire

Usama Mahmood, MD
Assistant Professor
Division of Radiation Oncology
The University of Texas M. D. Anderson Cancer Center
Houston, Texas

Hani R. Malone, MD
Department of Neurological Surgery
Columbia University
New York City, New York

Minesh Mehta, MD
Professor
Department of Radiation Oncology
Feinberg School of Medicine
Northestern University
Chicago, Illinois

Jacques Morcos, MD, FRCS (Eng), FRCS (Ed)
Professor of Clinical Neurosurgery and Otolaryngology
Department of Neurological Surgery
Lois Pope Life Center
University of Miami
Miami, Florida

Soriaya Motivala, MD
Department of Neurosurgery
Mt. Sinai Hospital
New York, New York

Mustafa Nadi, MD
Pediatric Neurosurgeon Fellow
Department of Neurosurgery
The Hospital for Sick Children
The Arthur and Sonia Labatt Brain Tumour Research Center
University of Toronto
Toronto, Canada

Peter Nakaji, MD
Professor of Neurosurgery
Director, Neurosurgery Residency Training Program
Division of Neurosurgery
Barrow Neurological Institute
Phoenix, Arizona

Edjah K. Nduom, MD
Department of Neurosurgery
Emory University School of Medicine
Atlanta, Georgia

Ajay Niranjan, MD, MBA
Director of Operations
UPMC Brain Mapping Center
Director of Radiosurgery Research
Associate Professor of Neurological Surgery
University of Pittsburgh Medical Center
Pittsburgh, Pennsylvania

Andrew Norden, MD, MPH
Assistant Professor of Neurology
Center for Neuro-Oncology
Dana-Farber Cancer Institute
Boston, Massachusetts

Smruti K. Patel, BA
Department of Neurological Surgery
University of Medicine and Dentistry of New Jersey, New Jersey Medical School
Newark, New Jersey

Chirag G. Patil, MD, MS
Assistant Professor, Neurosurgery
Director, Center for Neurosurgical Outcomes Research
Department of Neurosurgery
Cedars-Sinai Medical Center
Los Angeles, California

Gustavo Pradilla, MD
Skulk Base and Cerebrovascular Surgery Fellow
Department of Neurosurgery
University of Miami
Miami, Florida

Alfredo Quiñones-Hinojosa, MD, FAANS, FACS
Professor of Neurological Surgery and Oncology
Neuroscience and Cellular and Molecular Medicine
Director, Brain Tumor Surgery Program
Johns Hopkins–Bayview
Director, Pituitary Surgery Program
The Johns Hopkins Hospital
Baltimore, Maryland

Shaan M. Raza, MD
Department of Neurosurgery
The Johns Hopkins Hospital
Baltimore, Maryland

Pablo F. Recinos, MD
Department of Neurosurgery
Johns Hopkins University School of Medicine
Baltimore, Maryland

Kristin Janson Redmond, MD, MPH
Department of Radiation Oncology and Molecular Radiation Sciences
Johns Hopkins University School of Medicine
Baltimore, Maryland

William F. Regine, MD
Professor and Chair
Department of Radiation Oncology
University of Maryland School of Medicine
Baltimore, Maryland

Daniele Rigamonti, MD, FACS
Salisbury Family Professor
Professor of Neurosurgery, Radiology and Radiation Oncology, and Oncology
Director of Cerebrospinal Fluid Diseases Center
Director of Sterotactic Radiosurgery
Johns Hopkins University School of Medicine
Baltimore, Maryland

Marco Riva, MD
Universita degli Studi di Milano
Milano, Italy

David W. Roberts, MD
Professor of Surgery (Neurosurgery)
Chief, Section of Neurosurgery
Geisel School of Medicine at Dartmouth
Lebanon, New Hampshire

Marc R. Rosen, MD
Professor of Otolaryngology–Head and Neck Surgery and Neurological Surgery
Clinical Vice Chairman
Department of Otolaryngology–Head and Neck Surgery
Thomas Jefferson University
Philadelphia, Pennsylvania

James T. Rutka MD, PhD, FRCSC
R. S. McLaughlin Professor and Chair
Department of Surgery, Division of Neurosurgery
The Hospital for Sick Children
Toronto, Canada

Jacob Ruzevick, BS
Research Fellow
Department of Neurosurgery
Johns Hopkins University School of Medicine
Baltimore, Maryland

Nader Sanai, MD
Director, Division of Neurosurgical Oncology
Director, Barrow Brain Tumor Research Center
Division of Neurological Surgery
Barrow Neurological Institute
St. Joseph's Hospital and Medical Center
Phoenix, Arizona

Eric Sankey, BS
Medical Student
Johns Hopkins University School of Medicine
Baltimore, Maryland

Michael Schiraldi, MD, PhD
Department of Neurosurery
Cedars-Sinai Medical Center
Los Angeles, California

Theodore H. Schwartz, MD, FACS
Professor of Neurosurgery, Neurology, and Otolaryngology
Director, Pituitary and Epilepsy Surgery
Co-Director, Surgical Neuro-Oncology
Brain and Spine Center
Director, Epilepsy Research Laboratory
Brain and Mind Research Institute
Weill Cornell Medical College
New York Presbyterian Hospital
New York, New York

Ganesh M. Shankar, MD, PhD
Department of Neurosurgery
Massachusetts General Hospital
Boston, Massachusetts

Jason Sheehan, MD, PhD
Alumni Professor and Vice Chair
Department of Neurological Surgery
University of Virginia
Charlottesville, Virginia

Robert F. Spetzler, MD
Director, Barrow Neurological Institute
J. N. Harber Chairman and Professor of Neurological Surgery
Division of Neurological Surgery
Barrow Neurological Institute
St. Joseph's Hospital and Medical Center
Phoenix, Arizona

Edward W. Swanson, MD
Department of Plastic and Reconstructive Surgery
The Johns Hopkins Hospital
Baltimore, Maryland

Rafael J. Tamargo, MD, FAANS, FACS
Walter E. Dandy Professor of Neurosurgery
Director, Division of Cerebrovascular Neurosurgery
Professor of Neurosurgery and Otolaryngology
Vice-Chairman, Department of Neurosurgery
Neurosurgery Co-Director, Neurosciences Critical Care Unit
Department of Neurosurgery
Johns Hopkins University School of Medicine
Baltimore, Maryland

M. Özgür Taşkapilioglu, MD
Assistant Professor
Uludag University Medical School
Department of Neurosurgery
Bursa, Turkey

Jennie W. Taylor, MD
Neuro-Oncology Fellow
Department of Neurology
Massachusetts General Hospital Cancer Center
Dana-Farber Cancer Institute
Boston, Massachusetts

Alexander R. Vaccaro, MD, PhD
Professor
Attending Surgeon of Orthopaedics and Neurosurgery
Vice Chairman
Department of Orthopaedics
Thomas Jefferson University Hospital
Philadelphia, Pennsylvania

Anand Veeravagu, MD
Department of Neurosurgery
Stanford University School of Medicine
Stanford, California

J. Dawn Waters, MD
Division of Neurosurgery
University of California–San Diego
San Diego, California

Jon D. Weingart, MD
Professor of Neurosurgery and Oncology
Department of Neurosurgery
Johns Hopkins University School of Medicine
Baltimore, Maryland

David B. Weintraub, MD
Surgical Neurology Branch
National Institute of Neurological Disorders and Stroke
National Institutes of Health
Bethesda, Maryland

Patrick Y. Wen, MD
Professor of Neurology, Harvard Medical School
Director, Center For Neuro-Oncology
Dana-Farber Cancer Institute
Boston, Massachusetts

David A. Wilson, MD
Medical Director of Radiology Ambulatory Care Center
Vice Chairman
Department of Radiology
Saint Barnabas Medical Center
Livingston, New Jersey

Alex M. Witek, MD
Department of Neurosurgery
Cleveland Clinic
Cleveland, Ohio

David S. Wolf, MD, PhD
Department of Neurology
Johns Hopkins University School of Medicine
Baltimore, Maryland

Graeme F. Woodworth, MD
Assistant Professor
Department of Neurosurgery, Anatomy, and Neurobiology
University of Maryland School of Medicine
Baltimore, Maryland

David S. Xu, MD
Division of Neurological Surgery
Barrow Neurological Institute
St. Joseph's Hospital and Medical Center
Phoenix, Arizona

Zhiyuan Xu, MD, MSc
Clinical Instructor
Gamma Knife Center
University of Virginia
Charlottesville, Virginia

Tong Yang, MD, PhD
Department of Neurosurgery
University of Washington
Seattle, Washington

1

*Introduction to Best Evidence Medicine**

Alexander R. Vaccaro and Jason C. Eck

Throughout the past decade there has been an initiative to utilize sound scientific evidence in medical decision making, thereby to improve patient care. This concept is referred to as evidence-based medicine (EBM), and it has been advocated by physicians, epidemiologists, insurance payers, the media, and patients. In 2001, the *New York Times Magazine* selected it as one of the most important ideas for making a difference in our lives.[1] It has been applied to nearly every subspecialty in medicine, has been the topic of focus issues in peer-reviewed journals, and has been discussed in consensus statements of medical societies.[2–5]

Although EBM has been widely discussed, there remains an overall lack of understanding among many investigators and clinicians. Effective application of this concept to patient care requires a better understanding of the process, which involves five steps (**Fig. 1.1**). First, the question has to be defined. Although this may appear to be a straightforward task, it can be one of the most problematic issues related to EBM. For EBM to be effective, the question has to be well defined in terms of the patient population, confounding factors, specific treatments or interventions, and measured outcomes. The question being asked determines the most appropriate type of study with which to obtain the answer. Not every question is most appropriately addressed with a randomized, controlled trial (RCT). Fisher and Wood have summarized the common types of studies, along with their advantages and disadvantages (**Table 1.1**).[6]

The second component of EBM involves searching the evidence. This task has been simplified by the use of multiple search engines, which allow a comprehensive search of specific terms in multiple databases of English and foreign language journals.

The third step is to perform a critical appraisal of the literature. This step involves categorizing the current literature based on study type and level of evidence and applying grades of recommendation. There are various methods used to categorize levels of evidence. One of the most commonly utilized is that adopted by the American edition of the *Journal of Bone and Joint Surgery*, and which is outlined in

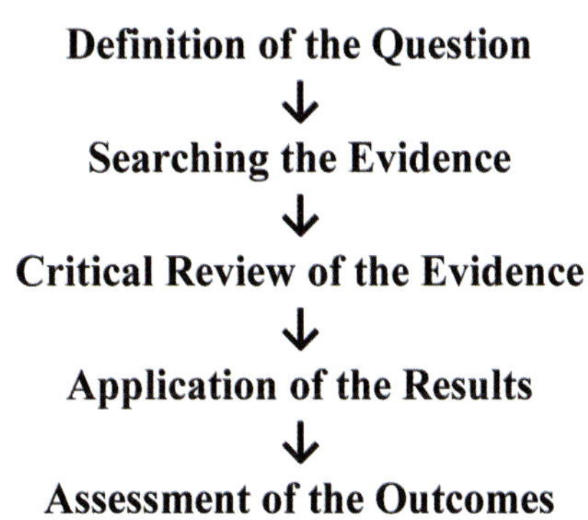

Fig. 1.1 Diagram of the five components of evidence-based medicine.

* Dr. Alfredo Quiñones-Hinojosa and Dr. Shaan M. Raza adapted this chapter with permission from *Controversies in Spine Surgery: Best Evidence Recommendations* by Alexander R. Vaccaro and Jason C. Eck. New York: Thieme Publishers, 2010.

Table 1.1 Types of study design, their advantages and disadvantages

Type of study	Type of design	Advantages	Disadvantages
Observational studies	Case report	Used for rare clinical events	No comparison group
	Case series	Experiences with new or complex treatments	No comparison group
	Cohort studies	Compare two treatments Resemble "real life" clinical situations	Prone to confounding
	Case-control studies	Small sample size Short duration	Prone to confounding and bias
Experimental studies	Randomized, controlled studies	Avoidance of confounding	Expensive Limited generalization Difficulties in study recruitment and conduct

Source: Fisher CG, Wood KB. Introduction to and techniques of evidence-based medicine. Spine 2007;32:S66–S72. Reprinted with permission.

Table 1.2.[7,8] As detailed in **Table 1.2**, studies are first categorized as therapeutic, prognostic, diagnostic, or economic studies. Once this is done, the study is assigned a level based on the type of study performed. Study designs that eliminate the most bias and control for the most confounding factors receive a higher ranking. RCTs are given the highest ranking, and case reports and expert opinions are given the lowest rankings. Grades of recommendation are then applied according to the criteria set forth by Guyatt et al.[9] As with applying levels of evidence, grades of recommendation provide a reproducible method for assigning a score to the study based on the strength of the article and a clear risk/benefit ratio for the described treatment. As **Table 1.3** describes, the better the grade of recommendation, the more clear the risk/benefit ratio and stronger recommendation to accept the proposed treatment described in the article.

The fourth component is to apply the literature results to patient care. This step takes the information gained in the previous steps and allows the clinician to develop appropriate treatment recommendations supported by the literature. In neuro-oncological surgery, there are a limited number of RCTs and highly graded studies. As a result, it can be more difficult for these clinicians to base their practice on clinical data. Unfortunately, in fields with few highly graded studies, clinicians often base their decisions on anecdotal evidence alone. The authors propose that, even in the absence of highly graded studies, the best available evidence should be identified and considered in clinical decision making. We refer to this as best evidence medicine. Even in the absence of high-level scientific studies, there is often a collection of lower-grade studies that can provide some guidance for clinical decision making.

The fifth and final step is to audit the outcome. To continue the process of EBM, it is crucial to continue to add to the available scientific information. By continuing to evaluate various treatment options, we develop an expanding database of information on which to base future clinical decisions.

RCTs have become the gold standard for clinical trials in the medical fields. Randomization in medical trials has a long history, dating back to 1948, when streptomycin was being tested for tuberculosis.[10] Unfortunately, there are several key issues that complicate the routine use of the RCT in surgical trials. The first of these is the preference of the patient. In general, patients are willing to accept randomization in pharmaceutical treatments if the various treatment options are felt to be similar. This is often not the case in surgical trials. Patients are much less likely to accept randomization into surgical versus nonsurgical treatment groups. An additional logistical problem with the surgical RCT is the difficulty in blinding either the patient or the primary investigator to the assigned treatment arm. A final difficulty is the often unacceptable crossover rate of patients from conservative to surgical treatment arms. This problem has been highlighted by several recent RCTs for spinal surgery.[11–13]

Many journals have begun to clearly state the level of evidence of each article to help readers determine the strength of the information presented. Unfortunately, determining a study's level of evidence is only part of determining the strength of the information presented. Readers must themselves critically analyze an article for potential weaknesses, bias, or statistical flaws. Several articles provide guidance for critically reviewing scientific studies.[5,14–17] A poorly conducted RCT may have a Level I ranking but provide less scientifically sound information than a

Table 1.2 Levels of evidence for primary research question

	Treatment	Disease	Test
I	1. Randomized, controlled trial a. Significant difference b. No significant difference but confidence intervals 2. Systematic review[b] of Level I randomized, controlled trials (studies were homogeneous)	1. Prospective study[a] 2. Systematic review[b] of Level I studies	1. Testing of previously developed diagnostic criteria in series of consecutive patients (with universally applied reference "gold" standard) 2. Systematic review[b] of Level I studies
II	1. Prospective cohort study[c] 2. Poor-quality randomized, controlled trial (e.g., < 80% follow-up) 3. Systematic review[b] a. Level II studies b. Nonhomogeneous Level I studies	1. Retrospective study[d] 2. Study of untreated controls from a previous randomized, controlled trial 3. Systematic review[b] of Level II studies	1. Development of diagnostic criteria on basis of consecutive patients (with universally applied reference gold standard) 2. Systematic review[b] of Level II studies
III	1. Case-control study[e] 2. Retrospective cohort study[d] 3. Systematic review[b] of Level III studies		1. Study of nonconsecutive patients (no consistently applied reference gold standard) 2. Systematic review[b] of Level III studies
IV	Case series (non-, or historical, control groups)	Case series	1. Case-control study 2. Poor reference standard
V	Expert opinion	Expert opinion	Expert opinion

Source: Fisher CG, Wood KB. Introduction to and techniques of evidence-based medicine. Spine 2007;32:S66–S72. Reprinted with permission.

[a] All patients were enrolled at the same point in their disease course (inception cohort) with ≥ 80% follow-up of enrolled patients.
[b] A study of results from two or more previous studies.
[c] Patients were compared with a control group of patients treated at the same time and institution.
[d] The study was initiated after treatment was performed.
[e] Patients with a particular outcome ("cases" with, for example, a failed arthroplasty) were compared with those who did not have the outcome ("controls" with, for example, a total hip arthroplasty that did not fail).

lower-ranked but well-conducted case series. When critically analyzing an article, the reader must ask various questions to determine the strength of the study, as detailed in **Table 1.4**. The overall strength of the study can be determined by considering the answers to these and other questions.

A common source of error in study design, which has been highlighted recently in multiple fields, is failure to include a sufficient number of subjects to make an accurate conclusion.[18–20] Readers and investigators are very familiar with the concept of the *p*-value in determining statistical significance. If the results are more than a given *p*-value (typically 0.05) there is no statistically significant difference between the two groups. What is less well understood is that, if the study's sample size is too small, there could be an actual difference that is not detected. This refers to the power of a study and the potential for a beta (type II) error. The beta error refers to the probability of the study results concluding that no statistically significant difference exists when there *is* an actual difference. The power of the study is the probability that it can detect a difference between two groups if it does actually exist, and it is calculated as (1 – beta). It is widely accepted that a beta error of 20% is acceptable, which gives a study a power of 80%.

Within the field of neuro-oncology, there are several landmark prospective studies that have assessed both oncological outcomes and surgical measures. Westphal et al reported one of the first such randomized studies involving the surgical resection of malignant astrocytomas followed by implantation of Gliadel wafers (Eisai, Woodcliff Lake, NJ).[21] Although it did not directly assess surgical outcomes, this study was one of the first to demonstrate the difficulties in performing a prospective study with surgical patients where surgical variables (e.g., technique, extent of resection) must be controlled and accounted for. Similar efforts were demonstrated by Stummer et al in their randomized phase 3 study measuring the clinical efficacy of 5-aminolevulinic acid in the surgical resection of high-grade astrocytomas.[22] Although this study was complicated by concerns over the appropriateness of the primary outcome measures assessed (i.e., 6-month progression-free survival and overall survival vs a direct surgical outcome such as extent of resection), the study design attempted to address the complexities of randomizing surgical

Table 1.3 Current approach to grades of recommendations

Grade of recommendation	Clarity of risk/benefit	Methodological strength of supporting evidence	Implications
1A	Clear	Randomized trials without important limitations	Strong recommendation; can apply to most patients in most circumstances without reservation
1B	Clear	Randomized trials with important limitations (inconsistent results, methodological flaws[a])	Strong recommendation; likely to apply to most patients
1C+	Clear	No randomized controlled trials (RCTs), but RCT results can be unequivocally extrapolated, or overwhelming evidence from observational studies	Strong recommendation; can apply to most patients in most circumstances
1C	Clear	Observational studies	Intermediate-strength recommendation; may change when stronger evidence available
2A	Unclear	Randomized trials without important limitations	Intermediate-strength recommendation; best action may differ depending on circumstances or patients' or societal values
2B	Unclear	Randomized trials with important limitations (inconsistent results, methodological flaws)	Weak recommendation; alternative approaches likely to be better for some patients under some circumstances
2C	Unclear	Observational studies	Very weak recommendations; other alternatives may be equally reasonable

Source: Fisher CG, Wood KB. Introduction to and techniques of evidence-based medicine. Spine 2007;32:S66–S72. Reprinted with permission.

Note: Because studies in categories B and C are flawed, it is likely that most recommendations in these classes will be Level 2. The following considerations will bear on whether the recommendation is Grade 1 or Grade 2: the magnitude and precision of the treatment effect, patients' risk of the target event being prevented, the nature of the benefit, the magnitude of the risk associated with treatment, variability in patient preferences, variability in regional resource availability and health care delivery practices, and cost considerations. Inevitably, weighing these considerations involves subjective judgment.

[a] These situations include randomized, controlled trials with both lack of blinding and subjective outcomes, where the risk of bias in measurement of outcomes is high, and with large loss to follow-up.

Table 1.4 Questions for critical appraisal of a scientific study

Why was the study performed?
What was the funding source for the study?
Are there clearly defined aims of the study?
How were patients randomized?
Was there a control group of similar patients?
Are there sufficient numbers to determine statistical significance?
Does statistical significance equal clinical significance?
Are the statistical methods appropriate?
Were all patients accounted for?
What was the dropout rate?
Was the power of the study calculated?
Are the conclusions supported by the results?

cohorts while accounting for surgeon technique and other variations.

One of the most compelling arguments against the need for prospective, randomized, placebo-controlled trials to support all clinical decision making was put forth by Smith and Pell.[23] These authors highlight the fact that there are no RCTs regarding the efficacy of a parachute for reducing the risk of major orthopedic injury or death associated with skydiving. They present two potential solutions for this problem. First, we could use common sense to support the risk/benefit ratio that the use of a parachute is justified to limit the potential for injury related to skydiving. The other alternative would be to invite those investigators who argue that an RCT is required for decision making to participate in an RCT on the use of a parachute for skydiving.

This book presents a concise review of the "best evidence medicine" for many of the most commonly disputed issues related to the practice of surgical care of neuro-oncology patients. Although several landmark prospective surgical studies exist within the field of neuro-oncology, unfortunately, relative to the importance of the field, there is a paucity of Level I evidence supporting decision making within the field. Moreover, a great deal of our decision making is based on randomized studies that vary greatly with regard to their study power (i.e., beta error). For the many reasons already discussed, there is often no Level I or II evidence available on some of these topics. As a result, it becomes more difficult for the clinician to make informed decisions based on the peer-reviewed literature. Yet, in the current climate of declining economic resources for health care, it is now increasingly important to assess the efficacy of our interventions and objectively determine the appropriate indications for surgical and nonsurgical intervention. Because a great deal of the "art of medicine" factors down to decision making individualized to the patient, which often cannot be derived from the perfect study, our decision making should be based on evidence as much as possible. This best evidence-based approach attempts to clarify and summarize the strongest evidence available and provide recommendations based on this information.

■ References

1. Hitt J. The year in ideas: A to Z. Evidence based medicine. New York Times Magazine December 9, 2001
2. Andersson GBK, Bridwell KH, Danielsson A, et al. Evidence-based medicine summary statement. Spine (Phila Pa 1976) 2007;32(19, Suppl):S64–S65
3. Bandopadhayay P, Goldschlager T, Rosenfeld JV. The role of evidence-based medicine in neurosurgery. J Clin Neurosci 2008;15(4):373–378
4. Haines SJ. Evidence-based neurosurgery. Neurosurgery 2003;52(1):36–47
5. Schünemann HJ, Bone L. Evidence-based orthopaedics: a primer. Clin Orthop Relat Res 2003;413:117–132
6. Fisher CG, Wood KB. Introduction to and techniques of evidence-based medicine. Spine (Phila Pa 1976) 2007;32(19, Suppl):S66–S72
7. Wright JG, Swiontkowski MF, Heckman JD. Introducing levels of evidence to the journal. J Bone Joint Surg Am 2003; 85-A(1):1–3
8. Obremskey WT, Pappas N, Attallah-Wasif E, Tornetta P III, Bhandari M. Level of evidence in orthopaedic journals. J Bone Joint Surg Am 2005;87(12):2632–2638
9. Guyatt G, Schuneman HG, Cook D, et al. Grades of recommendation for antithrombotic agents. Chest 2001;119(Suppl):3–7
10. Medical Research Council. Streptomycin treatment of pulmonary tuberculosis. BMJ 1948;2(4582):769–782
11. Tosteson AN, Skinner JS, Tosteson TD, et al. The cost effectiveness of surgical versus nonoperative treatment for lumbar disc herniation over two years: evidence from the Spine Patient Outcomes Research Trial (SPORT). Spine (Phila Pa 1976) 2008;33(19):2108–2115
12. Weinstein JN, Lurie JD, Tosteson TD, et al. Surgical versus nonoperative treatment for lumbar disc herniation: four-year results for the Spine Patient Outcomes Research Trial (SPORT). Spine (Phila Pa 1976) 2008;33(25):2789–2800
13. Weinstein JN, Tosteson TD, Lurie JD, et al; SPORT Investigators. Surgical versus nonsurgical therapy for lumbar spinal stenosis. N Engl J Med 2008;358(8):794–810
14. Bhandari M, Giannoudis PV. Evidence-based medicine: what it is and what it is not. Injury 2006;37(4):302–306
15. Greenhalgh T. How to read a paper: statistics for the non-statistician, I: Different types of data need different statistical tests. BMJ 1997;315(7104):364–366
16. Oxman AD, Sackett DL, Guyatt GH; The Evidence-Based Medicine Working Group. Users' guides to the medical literature, I: How to get started. JAMA 1993;270(17):2093–2095
17. Urschel JD. How to analyze an article. World J Surg 2005; 29(5):557–560
18. Bailey CS, Fisher CG, Dvorak MF. Type II error in the spine surgical literature. Spine (Phila Pa 1976) 2004;29(10): 1146–1149
19. Bernstein J, McGuire K, Freedman KB. Statistical sampling and hypothesis testing in orthopaedic research. Clin Orthop Relat Res 2003;413(413):55–62
20. Lochner HV, Bhandari M, Tornetta P III. Type-II error rates (beta errors) of randomized trials in orthopaedic trauma. J Bone Joint Surg Am 2001;83 A(11):1650 1655
21. Westphal M, Hilt DC, Bortey E, et al. A phase 3 trial of local chemotherapy with biodegradable carmustine (BCNU) wafers (Gliadel wafers) in patients with primary malignant glioma. Neuro-oncol 2003;5(2):79–88
22. Stummer W, Pichlmeier U, Meinel T, Wiestler OD, Zanella F, Reulen HJ; ALA-Glioma Study Group. Fluorescence-guided surgery with 5-aminolevulinic acid for resection of malignant glioma: a randomised controlled multicentre phase III trial. Lancet Oncol 2006;7(5):392–401
23. Smith GCS, Pell JP. Parachute use to prevent death and major trauma related to gravitational challenge: systematic review of randomised controlled trials. BMJ 2003;327(7429): 1459–1461

■ SECTION I ■

Astrocytomas

2

The Role of Gross Total Resection in Low-Grade Gliomas

Marco Riva and Lorenzo Bello

Gliomas are a heterogeneous group of intra-axial central nervous system (CNS) neoplasms of glial origin with differing histology, behavior, molecular characteristics, natural history, and, thus, prognosis.[1] Four distinct tumor grades have been identified, as reported in the World Health Organization (WHO) classification.[2] The term *low-grade gliomas* (LGGs)[3] commonly refers to grade II astrocytoma, grade II oligoastrocytoma, and grade II oligodendroglioma, and the term is used as such throughout this chapter. Compared with high-grade gliomas, LGGs differ in terms of epidemiology, clinical features, proliferation rate, mitotic activity, and angiogenesis phenomena. They thus require specific treatment protocols.[3–5]

■ General Clinical Features

LGGs are slow and continuously growing tumors, typically characterized by a radiologically determined diameter increase of 3.5 mm/y.[6–8] They gradually evolve into higher-grade gliomas, behaving aggressively, undergoing anaplastic transformation, and determining neurological disability and, ultimately, death.[8–10]

They typically affect young adults, around 40 years of age. The male-to-female ratio is 1.5. LGGs are definitely less common than other primary brain tumors, but they are not a rare entity, representing 15 to 30% of all primary brain tumors diagnosed annually,[1] thus accounting for 2,700 to 4,600 cases of CNS neoplasm each year in the United States.[3,11]

LGGs typically have a supratentorial location; interestingly, a tendency for these tumors to occur in eloquent areas or in their proximity has been reported.[12] Eloquent supratentorial brain sites are practically defined as areas relevant to basic neurological functions, such as the sensorimotor, language, and visuospatial cortical and subcortical structures.[12–15]

Clinically, LGGs frequently present with seizures (in up to 80 to 90% of cases).[16–18] Headache, personality changes, and focal neurological deficits are the other most common symptoms, though they are unusual or develop over many years. The neurological symptoms include motor/sensory deficits, dysphasia/aphasia, disinhibition, apathy, visuospatial disturbances, and others according to tumor location and size.[19]

LGGs are typically identified as a nonenhancing mass on conventional magnetic resonance imaging (MRI) scans, while they are identified as a hyperintense signal abnormality in T2-weighted or fluid-attenuated inversion recovery (FLAIR) sequences. In fact, these tumors can appear either as poorly circumscribed and invasive or as well-circumscribed lesions. The former are more suggestive of astrocytomas and the latter of oligodendrogliomas, which can occasionally contain calcifications and, also occasionally, contrast enhancement.[20]

The 5-year overall survival (OS) and progression-free survival (PFS) rates in randomized studies range from 58 to 72% and 37 to 55%, respectively.[1,3,5,21–27]

Using multivariate analysis, two phase III trials recognized the following as unfavorable prognostic factors: age greater than 40 years, astrocytoma histology, largest dimension of tumor > 6 cm, tumor crossing the midline, and the presence of neurological deficit before resection. Patients with up to two of these factors are placed in the low-risk group, whereas patients with three or more are identified as high risk. In addition, grade II oligodendrogliomas are known to have a better 5-year survival rate (70%) than mixed gliomas (56%) and astrocytomas (37%).[23–27]

Extensive and more detailed descriptions of the clinical features, diagnostic workup, and available treatment for LGGs are beyond the scope of this chapter, which instead focuses on the role of gross total surgical resection of LGGs in the adult population.

■ The Role of Surgery

Several investigations in the last two decades have been increasingly supportive of the role and oncological efficacy of surgical management[3,19,22,28] of LGGs (**Table 2.1**). Current neurosurgical treatment has several goals[19]: (1) to obtain adequate and representative tissue specimens with which to reach an effective histological diagnosis and proper genetic and molecular analysis (MGMT methylation status, 1p19q loss of heterozygosity, IDH-1 and -2 mutation); (2) to achieve the widest feasible cytoreduction and to avoid or slow eventual malignant transformation; (3) to relieve the patient's neurological signs and symptoms, including seizures; and (4) to minimize postoperative morbidity while preserving the best achievable quality of life.

Despite extensive study, controversy remains regarding the best treatment of these lesions. In particular, as acknowledged by US and European management guidelines,[5,29] the effect of surgery on OS and PFS is still uncertain. This chapter thus explores and critically analyzes the impact surgery can have on the natural history of LGGs. In particular, the chapter assesses the level of evidence favoring maximal tumor resection for improving outcome. The best evidence was thus gleaned from international study results published in the last two decades.

Table 2.1 Studies on the role of the extent of resection in low-grade glioma

First author	Publication date	Time period	Study type	Evidence level
Philippon JH[36]	1993	1978–87	Case series	IV
Berger MS[38]	1994	1977–90	Case series	IV
Rajan B[37]	1994	1974–90	Retrospective	III
Leighton C[39]	1997	1979–95	Retrospective	III
Van Veelen MLC[40]	1998	1975–89	Retrospective	III
Nakamura M[41]	2000	1983–96	Case series	IV
Shaw E[42]	2002	1986–94	Prospective	II
Johannesen TB[43]	2003	1970–93	Case series	IV
Yeh SA[44]	2005	1985–97	Case series	IV
Claus EB[45]	2005	1997–2003	Case series	IV
Smith JS[35]	2008	1989–2005	Retrospective	III
Rezvan A	2009	1985–2003	Retrospective	III
McGirt MJ[47]	2008	1996–2007	Retrospective	III
Ius T[48]	2012	1998–2011	Retrospective	III

Before the Evidence: Definition of Outcome and Extent of Resection

Prior to the actual evidence analysis, a few crucial questions must be answered to properly address this issue. In particular, the definitions of *outcome* and the *extent of resection* (EoR) are critical.

Defining the outcome and determining what is properly considered outcome is not easy. Parameters can include the following: the OS, the PFS, the rate of malignant transformation, the functional status of the patient and the improvement of preoperative neurological deficits or disturbances, such as seizure control, or the neuropsychological long-term outcome. Which of these are really indicative of, or should be considered as, a true clinical benefit? Are there studies properly addressing these issues in relation to surgical treatment? A high degree of heterogeneity regarding the definition of *outcome* is present in the studies, which hampers a precise, broad analysis.

The definition of the EoR has evolved[30] in the last two decades from a surgeon-based macroscopic judgment to an MRI-based evaluation weighted on the preoperative volumetric computation of the tumor's burden; occasionally, the postoperative remnant per se was also considered for EoR analysis. For LGGs, the lesion extent is evaluated as the hyperintense signal abnormality on T2-weighted or, more recently, on FLAIR MRI sequences. In addition, a volumetric analysis is currently recommended over the one-[31] or two-dimesional[32] volume calculation: the type of analysis used was shown to dramatically affect the data.[22,33] A recent recommendation[34] has called for the following method of assessment of the EoR[35]: EoR (%) = [(Preoperative volume − Postoperative volume)/Preoperative volume] × 100%. However, the authors stress that this method bears further testing. Ideally, the postoperative MRI scan should be obtained within 48 hours of surgery or 2–3 months after surgery. If the EoR is expressed as a percentage, there is no consensus on the qualitative definition of gross total, subtotal, or partial resection. Nevertheless, an EoR greater than 90% is generally but not unambiguously accepted and defined as gross total resection. Given the paucity of studies addressing this issue, no definitive conclusion can be drawn on the best evidence supporting any methodological analysis of the EoR. However, the most recent literature and recommendations advocate for expressing the EoR as a percentage, using volumetric analysis to assess pre- and postoperative volumes on FLAIR images.

Recommendations for Assessment of the Extent of Resection (EoR) in Low-Grade Gliomas (LGGs)

1. The extent of resection should be calculated using volumetric analysis of pre- and postoperative (obtained within 24 to 48 hours postsurgery) conventional MRI scans, using FLAIR sequence, as follows:

   EoR (%) = [(Preoperative volume – Postoperative volume)/Preoperative volume] × 100%

   (Grade 2C Recommendation, Level II–V Evidence)
2. The definition of ***gross* total resection** varies among studies, but an EoR greater than 90% can be accepted as gross total (Grade 2C, Level II–V Evidence).

Extent of Resection Studies

A few studies[23,28,35–48] do meet the criteria of ensuring robust reliability and reproducibility of data regarding the impact of EoR on the outcome of LGGs, particularly regarding the effect of gross total resection on survival, tumor progression, or upgrading.

Limitations of the Studies

As also previously considered, the main discrepancies among the studies are the assessment of tumor features, the preoperative workup and neuroradiological evaluation, the employment of adjuvant postoperative treatments, the selection criteria, the applied statistical methods, and the definition of the EoR and of the outcome.

No randomized clinical trials were conducted on this topic. The studies are all retrospective or case-series investigations (Level of evidence III through IV). In particular, no randomization was made regarding extent of surgical resection. Outcome measures also differed among studies, but the majority used the 5-year OS.

In addition, a minority of the analyses reported a volumetric assessment of the EoR, whereas the majority were based on the surgeon's evaluation at the end of surgery. Also, some of the analyses lacked a consistent MRI preoperative evaluation of tumor extent. When an EoR threshold was used for defining the extent of the resection (i.e., gross total vs subtotal), distinct cutoffs were chosen. In addition, the analyses could also be biased by interobserver variability rates, which are rarely declared in this type of study.

When LGGs in eloquent areas are specifically considered, it should be noted that intraoperative mapping and monitoring techniques are not standardized among the institutions that employ them. This fact weakens the robustness of any comparison among reported studies. Although a thorough evaluation of this particular issue is reported in a following chapter, it is worth mentioning a recent meta-analysis[49] that showed, in spite of the limitations, that intraoperative neurophysiological monitoring did improve surgical performance in terms of both the extent of resection and the functional outcome.

Both univariate and multivariate statistical analyses were conducted, but their application varied among studies.

Evidence on the Extent of Resection

With these limitations acknowledged, it is fair to recognize that an increasingly strong body of evidence points toward a greater EoR as a reproducible factor influencing outcome (**Table 2.2**), especially in more recent analyses employing volumetric analysis. Over all, mean survival changed from 61.1 to 90.5 months with subtotal and gross total resection, respectively. A relevant study conducted by Smith and coauthors,[35] performed with volumetric EoR assessment, demonstrated a survival benefit for patients with the greatest EoR, even 10 years postsurgery, with a relative decreasing benefit for patients with a lower EoR.

These data suggest a different approach toward LGGs, shifting the treatment paradigm toward a more aggressive approach, aiming at maximal surgical resection (**Fig. 2.1**). Recent evidence seems to confirm this change, even for incidentally discovered, presumed LGGs.[8,9] Indeed, more recent analysis reported a better outcome, probably due to increased surgical skill, increased awareness of the issue, and systematic MRI assessment of the EoR.

A more aggressive surgical approach, initially planned for maximal achievable EoR, was also recently demonstrated in a particular subset of patients—those harboring a temporal lesion—to yield better seizure control than obtained with subtotal resection.[16–18]

At particular brain locations, such as the insular region, initially encouraging results[50–52] have also been reported by Level III and IV studies. The 5-year OS ranged from 92 to 100% in patients with an EoR greater then 90%, and the 5-year PFS was up to 88%, compared with 69%, in patients with greater and less than 90% EoR, respectively. These resection results are paired with acceptable morbidity and mortality profiles.

In addition, an increasing number of studies analyzed the impact of supportive technologies, such as intraoperative stimulation mapping (ISM), in

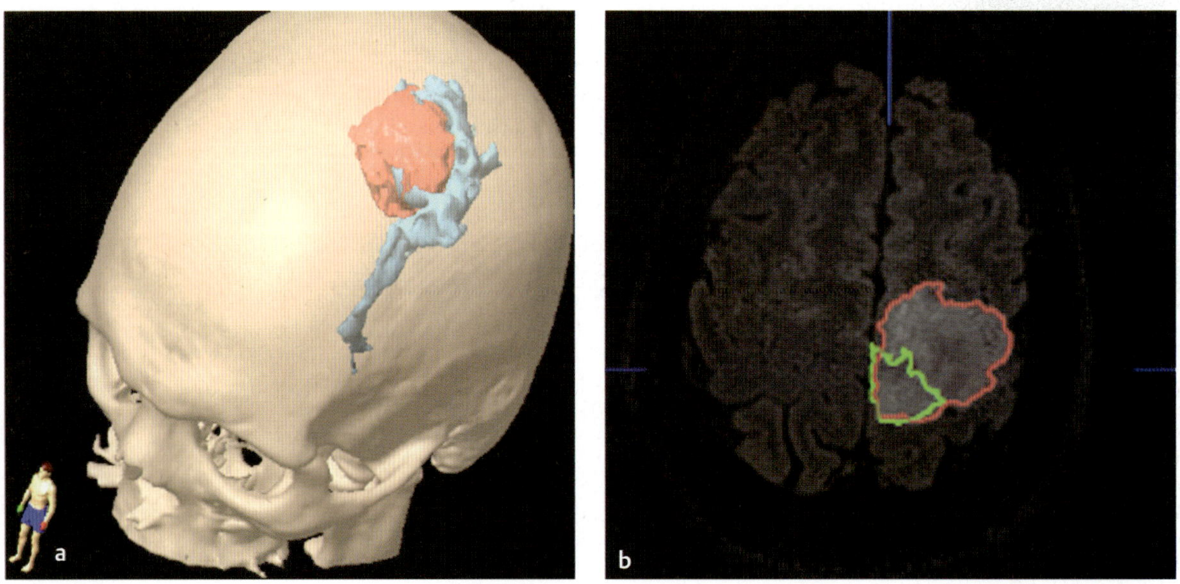

Fig. 2.1a,b A 42-year-old man harbored a left frontal WHO grade II astrocytoma (IDH-1 and MGTM methylation positive), affected by partial seizures with secondary generalization. **(a)** The lesion grew cortically and subcortically within the motor system, disrupting the anatomy of the left corticospinal tract (CST), as depicted in **(d)** fiber tractography, where the CST is depicted in white and superimposed on the T1-weighted morphological scan. **(b)** Preoperative volume, contoured in red, was volumetrically analyzed (iPlan Cranial Software, Brainlab, Fieldkirchen, Germany) and was determined to be 23.7 cm^3.

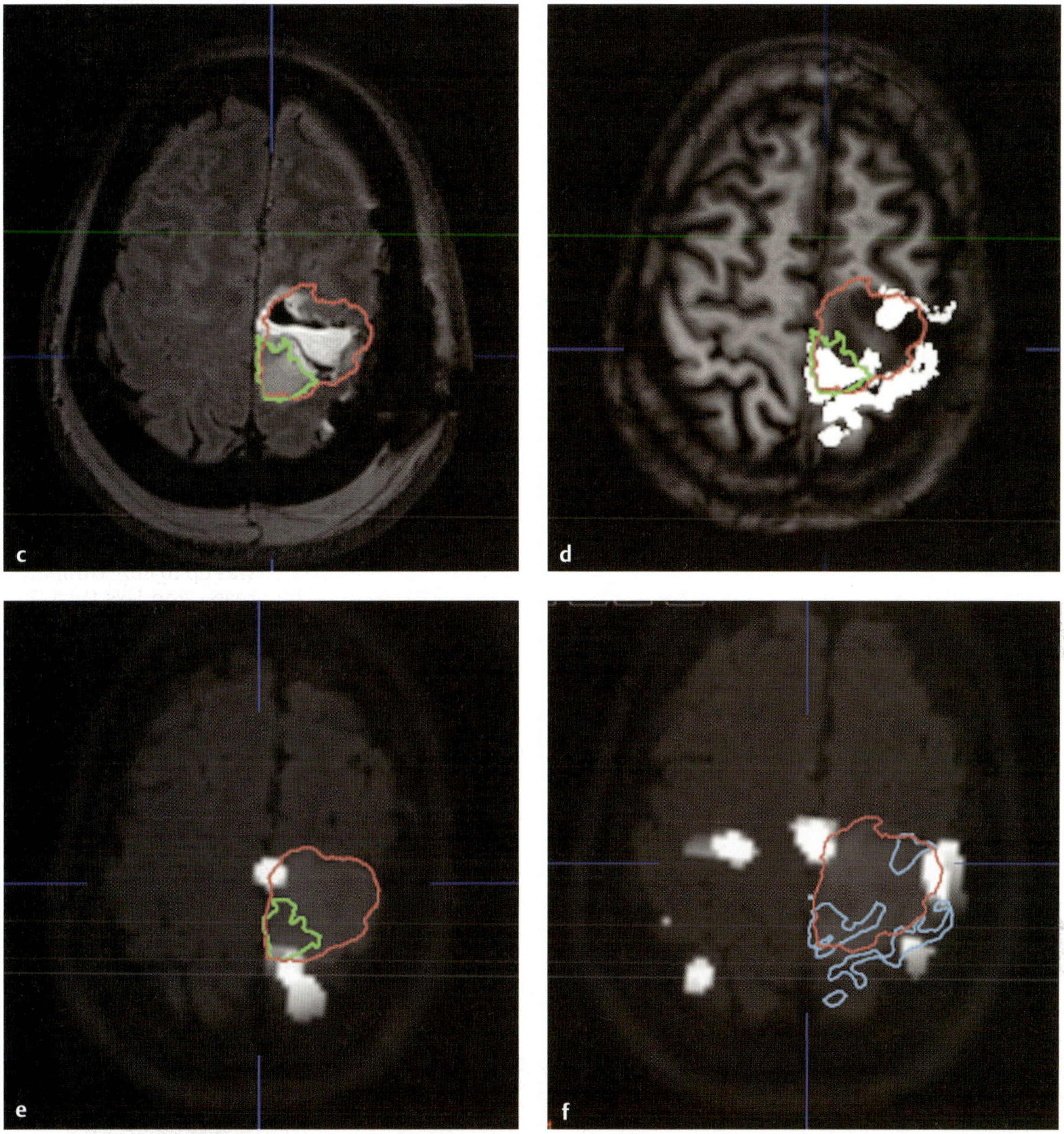

Fig. 2.1c–f *(Continued)* **(c)** Postoperative volume, contoured in green, was 8.7 cm^3. Extent of resection can thus be worked out as: (23.7 – 8.7)/23.7 = 0.63 = 63%. After registering all the available preoperative and postoperative MRI scans, lesion, residue, and CST contour can be superimposed along with preoperative functional MRI (fMRI) foot and hand motor tasks **(e,f)** on the MRI morphological scan. It has to be noted that the lesion residue corresponded to CST because resection stopped where direct motor potentials were subcortically evoked by intraoperative direct electrical stimulation; thus the resection was performed according to functional boundaries. The two types of information, in particular the FT CST depiction and the intraoperative neurophysiologic finding, matched. After transient postoperative right leg motor impairment, the patient recovered well, and at 3-month follow-up evaluation he displayed neither neurological nor neuropsychological deficits. Although under AEDs, no new seizures occurred. This case exemplifies the paradigm shift in surgical management of these lesions, where an aggressive attitude, aimed at maximal feasible resection, is balanced by the preservation of the patient's functional status, as assessed by imaging and neurophysiologic technologies.

Table 2.2 Analytic view of the studies on the role of the extent of resection in low-grade glioma

Study #	No. of patients	Histology	Preoperative	EoR assesment	EoR subgroup		5-year OS (%)	5-year PFS (%)
1	179	AA	CT/MRI	Macroscopic	Gross total	45	80	
				Nonvolumetric	Subtotal	95	50	
					Biopsy	39	45	
2	53	AA, ODG, OA	CT/MRI	Volumetric	< 50%	8	+	+
				CT/MRI	50–89%	18		
					90–99%	14		
					100%	13		
3	82	AA, ODG, OA	CT/MRI	Macroscopic	Total	11	90	
				Nonvolumetric	Subtotal	30	36	
				CT	Partial/biopsy	22/19	31/28	
4	166	AA, ODG, OA	CT/MRI	Macroscopic	Gross total[a]	84	82	53
				Nonvolumetric	Subtotal	82	64	46
5	90	AA, ODG, OA	CT	Macroscopic	Gross total[c]	13	62	46
				Nonvolumetric	Subtotal/biopsy	59/18	18/33	18/23
6	88	AA	CT	Macroscopic	Radical[a]	43		
				Nonvolumetric	Nonradical	45		
7	203	AA, ODG, OA	CT/MRI	Macroscopic	Gross total	29	88	+
				Nonvolumetric	Subtotal	71	56	
					Biopsy	103	71	
8	993	AA, ODG, OA	CT	Macroscopic	Gross total	173	N.S.	
		Pilocytic A		Nonvolumetric	Subtotal	689		
					Biopsy	131		
9	93	AA, ODG, OA	CT	Macroscopic	Gross total[b]	13	92	84
				Nonvolumetric	Subtotal/biopsy	71/9	52	41
10	156	AA, ODG, OA	MRI	Volumetric	Gross total[d]	56	N.S.	
				MRI	Subtotal	100		
11	216	AA, ODG, OA	MRI	Volumetric	0–40%	10		
				MRI	41–69%	18		
					70–89%	25		
					90–99%	12	97	75
					100%	35	98	78
12	130	AA, ODG, OA	None/MRI	Nonvolumetric	Gross total[a]	91	+	+
				MRI	Subtotal	39		
13	170	AA, ODG, OA	MRI	Nonvolumetric	Gross total	65	95	+
				MRI	Near total	39	80	
					Subtotal	66	70	
14	190	AA, ODG, OA	MRI	Volumetric	> 90%	91	93	> 75
				MRI	70–89%	69	84	50–75
					< 70%	30	41	< 25

Abbreviations: AA, anaplastic astrocytoma; CT, computed tomography; MRI, magnetic resonance imaging; OA, oligoastrocytoma; ODG, oligodendroglioma.

[a] Gross total/radical: > 90%. Subtotal/nonradical: < 90%
[b] Gross total: > 80%. Subtotal: 20–80%, biopsy < 20%
[c] Gross total: > 75%. Subtotal/biopsy: < 75%
[d] Gross total: no signal abnormalities on postresective MRI
[e] Benefit present

achieving a greater EoR with none or few late severe neurological deficits.[15,16,49,53–55] ISM is acknowledged as the gold standard for brain mapping. ISM in fact enhanced the EoR while preserving the patient's functional integrity, simultaneously providing the patient with a greater EoR and improved survival and functional outcome. An increased rate of early postoperative deficits is present in series using ISM, but deficits usually fully resolve within a few weeks up to 3 months; they are probably due to EoR in close proximity to functional boundaries, or due to transient postoperative sequelae, such as perilesional contusion, edema, and hypoperfusion. Nevertheless, improved long-term neurological outcome is reported in observational retrospective studies, especially in eloquent brain locations, which are often involved by LGGs. In these areas, a more extensive surgical resection is achieved when ISM is employed because ISM enables a consistent intraoperative recognition of true eloquent brain, eventually leading to a better neuro-oncological outcome, as measured by OS and PFS.

Expert Recommendations

1. No Level I study is available on the surgical treatment of LGGs. No Grade 1 recommendations can thus be drawn.
2. Surgical resection to maximally resect the tumor is the first treatment option for patients harboring an LGG (Grade 2C Recommendation, Level II–IV Evidence).

■ Summary and Conclusions

A critical issue in planning the surgical resection of an LGG is preservation of the patient's functional integrity. This requires the identification of eloquent brain structures. Therefore, mapping and monitoring techniques are recommended for this type of surgery. The awake craniotomy and adjuvant technologies, such as functional MRI, diffusion-tensor imaging with fiber tractography (DTI-FT), and intraoperative stimulation mapping, are critically relevant and are further explored in the following chapters.

Given the paucity of investigations based on robust evidence level, new studies are expected to further increase and improve the evidence supporting a more extensive surgical resection to yield better outcomes, independently of other clinical and molecular variables.[56] However, systematic description and the application of measured parameters and outcome definitions that also include quality of life and the malignant degeneration rate are needed.

Randomized trials specifically focused on the role of EoR are unlikely to be accomplished for several reasons; thus, retrospective studies or prospective trials could constitute a reliable and more feasible approach.

■ References

1. Zouaoui S, Rigau V, Mathieu-Daudé H, et al; Société française de neurochirurgie (SFNC) et le Club de neuro-oncologie de la SFNC; Société française de neuropathologie (SFNP); Association des neuro-oncologues d'expression française (ANOCEF). French brain tumor database: general results on 40,000 cases, main current applications and future prospects. Neurochirurgie 2012;58(1):4–13
2. Kleihues P, Louis DN, Scheithauer BW, et al. The WHO classification of tumors of the nervous system. J Neuropathol Exp Neurol 2002;61(3):215–225
3. Sanai N, Chang S, Berger MS. Low-grade gliomas in adults. J Neurosurg 2011;115(5):948–965
4. Schiff D, Brown PD, Giannini C. Outcome in adult low-grade glioma: the impact of prognostic factors and treatment. Neurology 2007;69(13):1366–1373
5. Soffietti R, Baumert BG, Bello L, et al; European Federation of Neurological Societies. Guidelines on management of low-grade gliomas: report of an EFNS-EANO Task Force. Eur J Neurol 2010;17(9):1124–1133
6. Mandonnet E, Delattre JY, Tanguy ML, et al. Continuous growth of mean tumor diameter in a subset of grade II gliomas. Ann Neurol 2003;53(4):524–528
7. Pallud J, Mandonnet E, Duffau H, et al. Prognostic value of initial magnetic resonance imaging growth rates for World Health Organization grade II gliomas. Ann Neurol 2006; 60(3):380–383
8. Pallud J, Fontaine D, Duffau H, et al. Natural history of incidental World Health Organization grade II gliomas. Ann Neurol 2010;68(5):727–733
9. Potts MB, Smith JS, Molinaro AM, Berger MS. Natural history and surgical management of incidentally discovered low-grade gliomas. J Neurosurg 2012;116(2):365–372
10. Chaichana KL, McGirt MJ, Laterra J, Olivi A, Quiñones-Hinojosa A. Recurrence and malignant degeneration after resection of adult hemispheric low-grade gliomas. J Neurosurg 2010; 112(1):10–17
11. Bondy ML, Scheurer ME, Malmer B, et al; Brain Tumor Epidemiology Consortium. Brain tumor epidemiology: consensus from the Brain Tumor Epidemiology Consortium. Cancer 2008;113(7, Suppl):1953–1968
12. Duffau H, Capelle L. Preferential brain locations of low-grade gliomas. Cancer 2004;100(12):2622–2626
13. Wu JS, Zhou LF, Tang WJ, et al. Clinical evaluation and follow-up outcome of diffusion tensor imaging-based functional neuronavigation: a prospective, controlled study in patients with gliomas involving pyramidal tracts. Neurosurgery 2007; 61(5):935–948
14. Sanai N, Mirzadeh Z, Berger MS. Functional outcome after language mapping for glioma resection. N Engl J Med 2008; 358(1):18–27

15. Chang EF, Clark A, Smith JS, et al. Functional mapping-guided resection of low-grade gliomas in eloquent areas of the brain: improvement of long-term survival. Clinical article. J Neurosurg 2011;114(3):566–573
16. Chang EF, Potts MB, Keles GE, et al. Seizure characteristics and control following resection in 332 patients with low-grade gliomas. J Neurosurg 2008;108(2):227–235
17. Lee JW, Wen PY, Hurwitz S, et al. Morphological characteristics of brain tumors causing seizures. Arch Neurol 2010; 67(3):336–342
18. Englot DJ, Han SJ, Berger MS, Barbaro NM, Chang EF. Extent of surgical resection predicts seizure freedom in low-grade temporal lobe brain tumors. Neurosurgery 2012;70(4): 921–928
19. Bello L, Dimeco F, Casaceli G, Gaini SM. Surgical management of low-grade gliomas. In: Schmidek & Sweet Operative Neurosurgical Techniques. 6th ed. New York, NY: Elsevier; 2012: in press
20. Henson JW, Gaviani P, Gonzalez RG. MRI in treatment of adult gliomas. Lancet Oncol 2005;6(3):167–175
21. Claus EB, Black PM. Survival rates and patterns of care for patients diagnosed with supratentorial low-grade gliomas: data from the SEER program, 1973-2001. Cancer 2006;106(6): 1358–1363
22. Sanai N, Berger MS. Glioma extent of resection and its impact on patient outcome. Neurosurgery 2008;62(4):753–764
23. Schomas DA, Laack NN, Rao RD, et al. Intracranial low-grade gliomas in adults: 30-year experience with long-term follow-up at Mayo Clinic. Neuro-oncol 2009;11(4):437–445
24. Pignatti F, van den Bent M, Curran D, et al; European Organization for Research and Treatment of Cancer Brain Tumor Cooperative Group; European Organization for Research and Treatment of Cancer Radiotherapy Cooperative Group. Prognostic factors for survival in adult patients with cerebral low-grade glioma. J Clin Oncol 2002;20(8):2076–2084
25. van den Bent MJ, Afra D, de Witte O, et al; EORTC Radiotherapy and Brain Tumor Groups and the UK Medical Research Council. Long-term efficacy of early versus delayed radiotherapy for low-grade astrocytoma and oligodendroglioma in adults: the EORTC 22845 randomised trial. Lancet 2005;356(9490):985–990. Erratum in: Lancet 2006;367(9525):1818 54:1442–1448
26. Shaw EG, Wang M, Coons SW, et al. Final report of Radiation Therapy Oncology Group (RTOG) protocol 9802: radiation therapy (RT) versus RT+procarbazine, CCNU and vincristine (PCV) chemotherapy for adult low grade gliomas (LGG). J Clin Oncol 2008;26:90S
27. Chang EF, Clark A, Jensen RL, et al. Multiinstitutional validation of the University of California at San Francisco Low-Grade Glioma Prognostic Scoring System. Clinical article. J Neurosurg 2009;111(2):203–210
28. Keles GE, Lamborn KR, Berger MS. Low-grade hemispheric gliomas in adults: a critical review of extent of resection as a factor influencing outcome. J Neurosurg 2001;95(5):735–745
29. National Comprehensive Cancer Network Guidelines Version 1. 2012, Central Nervous System Cancers. www.nccn.org
30. Jaffe CC. Measures of response: RECIST, WHO, and new alternatives. J Clin Oncol 2006;24(20):3245–3251
31. Therasse P, Arbuck SG, Eisenhauer EA, et al. New guidelines to evaluate the response to treatment in solid tumors. European Organization for Research and Treatment of Cancer, National Cancer Institute of the United States, National Cancer Institute of Canada. J Natl Cancer Inst 2000;92(3):205–216
32. Macdonald DR, Cascino TL, Schold SC Jr, Cairncross JG. Response criteria for phase II studies of supratentorial malignant glioma. J Clin Oncol 1990;8(7):1277–1280
33. Dempsey MF, Condon BR, Hadley DM. Measurement of tumor "size" in recurrent malignant glioma: 1D, 2D, or 3D? AJNR Am J Neuroradiol 2005;26(4):770–776
34. van den Bent MJ, Wefel JS, Schiff D, et al. Response assessment in neuro-oncology (a report of the RANO group): assessment of outcome in trials of diffuse low-grade gliomas. Lancet Oncol 2011;12(6):583–593
35. Smith JS, Chang EF, Lamborn KR, et al. Role of extent of resection in the long-term outcome of low-grade hemispheric gliomas. J Clin Oncol 2008;26(8):1338–1345
36. Philippon JH, Clemenceau SH, Fauchon FH, Foncin JF. Supratentorial low-grade astrocytomas in adults. Neurosurgery 1993;32(4):554–559
37. Rajan B, Pickuth D, Ashley S, et al. The management of histologically unverified presumed cerebral gliomas with radiotherapy. Int J Radiat Oncol Biol Phys 1994;28(2):405–413
38. Berger MS, Deliganis AV, Dobbins J, Keles GE. The effect of extent of resection on recurrence in patients with low grade cerebral hemisphere gliomas. Cancer 1994;74(6):1784–1791
39. Leighton C, Fisher B, Bauman G, et al. Supratentorial low-grade glioma in adults: an analysis of prognostic factors and timing of radiation. J Clin Oncol 1997;15(4):1294–1301
40. van Veelen MLC, Avezaat CJJ, Kros JM, van Putten W, Vecht Ch. Supratentorial low grade astrocytoma: prognostic factors, dedifferentiation, and the issue of early versus late surgery. J Neurol Neurosurg Psychiatry 1998;64(5):581–587
41. Nakamura M, Konishi N, Tsunoda S, et al. Analysis of prognostic and survival factors related to treatment of low-grade astrocytomas in adults. Oncology 2000;58(2):108–116
42. Shaw E, Arusell R, Scheithauer B, et al. Prospective randomized trial of low- versus high-dose radiation therapy in adults with supratentorial low-grade glioma: initial report of a North Central Cancer Treatment Group/Radiation Therapy Oncology Group/Eastern Cooperative Oncology Group study. J Clin Oncol 2002;20(9):2267–2276
43. Johannesen TB, Langmark F, Lote K. Progress in long-term survival in adult patients with supratentorial low-grade gliomas: a population-based study of 993 patients in whom tumors were diagnosed between 1970 and 1993. J Neurosurg 2003;99(5):854–862
44. Yeh SA, Ho JT, Lui CC, Huang YJ, Hsiung CY, Huang EY. Treatment outcomes and prognostic factors in patients with supratentorial low-grade gliomas. Br J Radiol 2005;78(927): 230–235
45. Claus EB, Horlacher A, Hsu L, et al. Survival rates in patients with low-grade glioma after intraoperative magnetic resonance image guidance. Cancer 2005;103(6):1227–1233
46. Ahmadi R, Dictus C, Hartmann C, et al. Long-term outcome and survival of surgically treated supratentorial low-grade glioma in adult patients. Acta Neurochir (Wien) 2009;151(11): 1359–1365
47. McGirt MJ, Chaichana KL, Attenello FJ, et al. Extent of surgical resection is independently associated with survival in patients with hemispheric infiltrating low-grade gliomas. Neurosurgery 2008;63(4):700–707, author reply 707–708
48. Ius T, Isola M, Budai R, et al. Low-grade glioma surgery in eloquent areas: volumetric analysis of extent of resection and its impact on overall survival. A single-institution experience in 190 patients. J Neurosurg 2012;117(6):1039–1052
49. Duffau H, Capelle L, Denvil D, et al. Usefulness of intraoperative electrical subcortical mapping during surgery for low-grade gliomas located within eloquent brain regions: functional results in a consecutive series of 103 patients. J Neurosurg 2003;98(4):764–778
50. Simon M, Neuloh G, von Lehe M, Meyer B, Schramm J. Insular gliomas: the case for surgical management. J Neurosurg 2009;110(4):685–695
51. Sanai N, Polley MY, Berger MS. Insular glioma resection: assessment of patient morbidity, survival, and tumor progression. J Neurosurg 2010;112(1):1–9

52. Skrap M, Mondani M, Tomasino B, et al. Surgery of insular nonenhancing gliomas: volumetric analysis of tumoral resection, clinical outcome, and survival in a consecutive series of 66 cases. Neurosurgery 2012;70(5):1081–1093
53. Duffau H, Capelle L, Sichez N, et al. Intraoperative mapping of the subcortical language pathways using direct stimulations. An anatomo-functional study. Brain 2002;125(Pt 1): 199–214
54. De Witt Hamer PC, Robles SG, Zwinderman AH, Duffau H, Berger MS. Impact of intraoperative stimulation brain mapping on glioma surgery outcome: a meta-analysis. J Clin Oncol 2012;30(20):2559–2565
55. Bello L, Gambini A, Castellano A, et al. Motor and language DTI Fiber Tracking combined with intraoperative subcortical mapping for surgical removal of gliomas. Neuroimage 2008; 39(1):369–382
56. Sankar T, Moore NZ, Johnson J, et al. Magnetic resonance imaging volumetric assessment of the extent of contrast enhancement and resection in oligodendroglial tumors. J Neurosurg 2012;116(6):1172–1181

3

The Role of Surgery in the Management of High-Grade Gliomas (Newly Diagnosed, Recurrent, and Multifocal High-Grade Gliomas)

Brian Yu-Jin Hwang, Kaisorn L. Chaichana, and Alfredo Quiñones-Hinojosa

Gliomas are the most common primary malignant brain tumor in adults, accounting for ~ 70% of the 22,500 newly diagnosed cerebral malignancies every year.[1,2] Glioblastoma multiforme (GBM) is classified as World Health Organization (WHO) grade IV. These tumors represent 60 to 70% of malignant gliomas and are associated with high rates of morbidity and mortality.[1,3] In fact, without treatment, a majority of patients will die within 3 months of diagnosis. Despite best medical and surgical treatments, the median survival rate of GBM patients remains under 16 months, with fewer than 25% of patients surviving up to 2 years.[4,5]

GBMs commonly affect adults, with a peak incidence at 45 to 70 years and a slight male preponderance.[6] Most cases are considered sporadic, but exposure to ionizing radiation and a history of neurocutaneous syndromes, such as tuberous sclerosis and neurofibromatosis 1 and 2, have been associated with higher incidences.[1,5,7] GBM can develop from low-grade (WHO grade II) and anaplastic (WHO grade III) astrocytomas, but, in a majority of cases, they arise de novo without evidence of a preexisting lesion.[2] Gliomas typically involve the white matter of cerebral hemispheres but may occur in the gray matter and other regions of the central nervous system, including the brainstem and spinal cord.[2,8] Their infiltrative nature makes them particularly recalcitrant to currently available treatments.[3,5]

As with any neurological lesion, clinical manifestation of GBM is dependent on the anatomical location and extent of invasion. According to the Glioma Outcomes Project, 53 to 57% of patients initially presented with headaches, whereas 56% of grade III and 23% of grade IV lesions were associated with seizures. Other symptoms commonly seen at diagnosis include psychocognitive changes, visual deficits, weakness, and language problems.[9]

Surgery, though not curative, remains a critical component in the management of high-grade gliomas.[3] Goals of surgery are generally (1) to establish pathological diagnosis, (2) to relieve mass effect and clinical symptoms, and (3) to facilitate adjuvant therapies through maximal possible resection. Stereotactic mapping and intraoperative magnetic resonance imaging (MRI) guidance have led to improved surgical safety and extent of resection, which in turn have translated to near doubling of survival rates from 3–4 to 7–12 months.[10,11] Nevertheless, the impact of surgery on GBM needs to be better defined, particularly for recurrent and multifocal tumors. This chapter reviews the role of surgery in the management of GBMs using an evidence-based approach.

■ Literature Review[12]

Does Gross Total Resection Improve Outcome in Patients with a Newly Diagnosed GBM?

Level I Evidence

No Level I study of this subject could be found.

Level II to Level III Evidence

Extensive resection of GBMs is challenging because the tumors are invasive, infiltrative, and frequently involve eloquent areas.[13] Safe extensive resection has become possible with the aid of cortical mapping, tumor fluorescence techniques, and intraoperative MRI guidance.[14–17] Extensive resection has been theorized to improve outcome by minimizing tumor burden and facilitating response to adjuvant therapies.[9,18–20] Nevertheless, with no Level I data currently available, it remains unclear whether the extent of tumor resection is associated with prolonged overall survival.[21–23] To date, only a few studies with Level II evidence have demonstrated that gross total resection (GTR) of GBMs improves outcome (**Table 3.1**).[8,45] In a prospective study of 124 patients with newly diagnosed glioblastomas, Brown et al reported that gross total surgical resection was associated with significantly longer survival and improved quality of life at up to 4-month follow-up.[24] In a small prospective study, Schneider et al showed that complete resection of GBMs more than doubled the mean survival seen with incomplete resection (537 days vs 237 days), without a significant increase in surgical morbidity.[25]

Several retrospective studies have reported that extensive tumor resection is associated with improved survival in GBM patients (**Table 3.1**). In an analysis of a 949 patient cohort, McGirt et al showed that the extent of primary resection was independently associated with longer survival for GBM patients.[26] Maximal benefit was seen in patients who underwent GTR. Survival benefit was also seen in patients who received near total resection (NTR), defined as rim enhancement of the resection cavity only, and to a lesser degree after subtotal resection (STR), defined as residual nodular enhancement.[26] The result was independent of age, functional status, and subsequent treatment modalities. Based on these findings, the authors recommended that one should aim for maximal possible resection within the margin of safety. Other, smaller retrospective studies have also shown that increased extent of resection may lead to improved survival for patients with malignant gliomas.[10,27]

Several studies have compared the survival benefits of surgery versus biopsy. Laws et al conducted a retrospective analysis of the prospective, multicenter Glioma Outcomes Project database and concluded that the positive prognostic value of resection compared with biopsy was maintained even after controlling for high-risk patients potentially overrepresented in the biopsy group.[28] Buckner also supported that GTR is associated significantly prolonged survival compared with biopsy alone.[29]

Table 3.1 Extent of surgery and its impact on survival in patients with newly diagnosed high-grade gliomas

Study	Level of evidence[51]	Patients (*N*)	GTR (%)	NTR (%)	STR (%)	Biopsy (%)	GTR median survival (months)	STR median survival (months)	Biopsy median survival (months)	Significance ($P < 0.05$)
Brown et al 2005[24]	II	124	49 (40)	–	22 (18)	22 (18)	–	–	–	Y
Schneider et al 2005[25]	III/IV	27	10 (37)	–	17 (63)	–	18	8	–	–
Lacroix et al 2001[10 a]	III/IV	233	107 (46)	–	126 (54)	–	13	–	1.4	Y
Bucci et al 2004[27 b]	III/IV	39	12 (31)	18 (46)	9 (23)	–	122	14.1	–	Y
McGirt et al 2009[26]	III/IV	949	330 (35)	388 (41)	231 (24)	–	13	11	8	Y

Abbreviations: GTR, gross total resection; NTR, near total resction; STR, subtotal resection; –, not available; Y, yes.

[a] Extent of resection was dichotomized to ≥ 98% and < 98%

[b] Pediatric series with median age of 12.3 years. Patients who underwent were included in the STR group for survival analysis.

Does Surgery Improve Outcome in Patients with Multifocal or Multicentric GBM?

Level I Evidence

No Level I study on this subject could be found.

Level II to Level III Evidence

GBMs present as multiple synchronous lesions in 0.5 to 20% of cases.[30] Lesions with an established pattern of dissemination either through local extension or via commissural or cerebrospinal fluid pathways are considered multifocal,[31] whereas multicentric GBMs consist of distinct foci that are widely separated without evidence of dissemination.[31,32] Multifocal and multicentric GBMs are thought to represent a more migratory and invasive group of tumors and have been associated with less favorable outcomes.[32] The clinical significance of distinguishing multifocal and multicentric disease is undetermined.[32,33] There are as yet no clear management guidelines for these challenging tumors. Furthermore, the role of surgery in the treatment of multifocal and multicentric GBMs remains controversial.

Some authors have supported surgical resection, particularly of a single dominant focus, followed by chemotherapy and radiation for improved survival.[30,34] Others have recommended biopsy over surgery because of significant perioperative risk and potentially minimal survival benefit.[35] Recent studies have shown that surgical resection of multifocal or multicentric GBMs may in fact have a positive impact on survival. In a retrospective analysis of 25 cases of multicentric GBM, Salvati et al found that patients who underwent surgery for any accessible lesions had longer mean survival than those who underwent biopsy (9.5 months vs 2.8 months).[36] The study was underpowered and, importantly, those who underwent biopsy had either surgically inaccessible or eloquent lesions and were less likely to receive adjuvant radiotherapy. Based on the results, the authors recommend surgical treatment for multicentric GBMs whenever possible and reserve stereotactic biopsy for high-risk cases.[36]

Hassaneen et al employed an aggressive surgical approach by performing in a single session multiple craniotomies for resection of multifocal and multicentric GBMs.[32] The authors showed that these patients had survival duration and complication risk comparable with those who underwent surgery for a solitary GBM when matched for preoperative Karnofsky performance scale (KPS) score, tumor functional grade, extent of resection, age at time of surgery, and year of surgery.[32] The study was limited by its small cohort size and the fact that the analysis included only patients with multifocal or multicentric GBMs who underwent resection of all lesions. Nevertheless, the study provided evidence that aggressive surgical treatment can be safely undertaken in a select group of multifocal or multicentric GBM patients with possible survival benefit.

Does Surgery Improve Outcome in Patients with Recurrent GBM?

Level I Evidence

No Level I study on this subject could be found.

Level II to Level III Evidence

GBMs nearly always recur despite treatment with maximal safe resection, radiation, and chemotherapy.[3,37,38] Recurrence is frequently seen at a median survival time of 34 to 36 weeks.[39,40] No standard therapy exists for recurrent lesions, but repeat surgery and adjuvant therapies are often considered.[37] However, the role of surgery in recurrent GBMs and guidelines for risk stratification remain undetermined. Associated surgical risks and generally poor survival have often led to a limited role for surgery in the management of recurrent GBMs.[26] Nevertheless, mounting evidence has indicated that repeat surgery can be performed with acceptable risks and can potentially lead to a higher level of function and prolonged survival (**Table 3.2**).[39,41–43] Studies have identified preoperative KPS score, extent of resection, age, time interval between the first and second surgeries, and presence of an oligodendroglial component as significant predictors of outcome after repeat surgery.[22,26,28,39,41–43]

Park et al analyzed a cohort of recurrent GBM patients who underwent repeat surgery and found that tumor involvement of eloquent/critical brain location, preoperative KPS score, and tumor volume independently predicted postoperative survival.[38] The authors identified preoperative KPS score of 80 and tumor volume of 50 cm^3 as critical thresholds in predicting survival. In the study, patients without the three risk factors had a median survival of 10.8 months, whereas those with all three survived a median duration of 1.0 month. These findings were validated in an independent cohort of recurrent GBM patients.[38] Although the study failed to account for postsurgical adjuvant therapies, it strongly suggested that careful patient selection could lead to acceptable survival in a select group of these high-risk patients.[38]

A number of studies have shown that repeated resection of recurrent GBMs may improve seizure

Table 3.2 Outcomes after repeat surgery in patients with recurrent high-grade gliomas

Study	Level of evidence[51]	Patients (N)	Median interval between first and second surgeries (months)	Surgery (%)	No surgery (%)	Post-operative adjuvant therapy (%)	Median survival after surgery (months)	Median survival after no surgery (months)	Significance ($P < 0.05$)
Ammirati et al 1987[39]	III/IV	35	10.8	35 (100)	–	41 (75)	9	–	–
Harsh et al 1987[43]	III/IV	39	–	39 (100)	–	–	9	–	–
Dirks et al 1993[42]	III/IV	43	10	43 (100)	–	43 (100)	4.8	–	–
Barker et al 1998[41]	III/IV	176	6.6[a]	46 (26)	130 (74)	39 (85)	9	5.8	Y
Park et al 2010[38]	III/IV	34	11.1[b]	34 (100)	–	–	7.4	–	–
Hong et al 2012[37]	III/IV	42	–[c]	42 (100)	–	18 (43)	19	–	–

Abbreviations: –, not available; Y, yes.

[a] Median interval between initial diagnosis and reoperation

[b] Median interval between initial diagnosis and recurrence

[c] 35 (83%) of patients had 6-month progression-free survival after initial surgery

control and neurological status as well as survival.[44] Hong et al performed multiple repeated resections (up to six surgeries) for recurrent GBM and found that such an aggressive surgical approach followed by chemoradiation was associated with significantly improved survival time and long-term survival rate compared with nonsurgical management.[37] The authors also reported that a progression-free interval greater than 3 months significantly predicted prolonged survival after surgery.

Does Surgery Improve Outcomes in Elderly Patients?

Level I Evidence

No Level I study on this subject could be found.

Level II to Level III Evidence

Age is one of the most important predictors of outcome for GBM patients.[23,45,46] GBM patients older than 64 have a nearly threefold shorter 1-year survival compared with younger age groups.[47] Unfavorable outcomes observed in elderly patients have been attributed to inherently high surgical risks, reduced tolerance of and sensitivity to therapies, and neurodegeneration.[48,49] Presumed poor prognosis for elderly patients has often led to less aggressive treatments in this population. However, in this population the impact of surgery on outcome remains controversial (**Table 3.3**). Older series reported only modest survival benefit from surgery in GBM patients aged ≥ 65 years and questioned its value.[50] On the contrary, Stark et al sought aggressive surgical treatments, including reoperation in recurrent cases, and found that total tumor resection was significantly associated with prolonged survival (median of 64 weeks) in patients aged ≥ 60 years.[51]

Recently, Ewelt et al retrospectively analyzed a large cohort of elderly GBM patients in an attempt to better define the risk stratification for patients aged > 65 years.[47] In the study, the authors showed that age < 75 years and preoperative KPS score ≥ 70 were associated with significant survival benefit, and that, in their series, the decision for resection was strongly affected by KPS but not by age. Furthermore, the extent of resection (biopsy, partial, complete) was a good predictor of outcome in patients treated with radiation and chemotherapy, with median survival of 2.2, 7.0, and 13.9 months, respectively.[47] Complete resection also conferred significantly longer progression-free survival compared with partial resection.

In one of the largest series to date, Chaichana et al analyzed 205 GBM patients aged > 65 years and also

Table 3.3 Outcomes after surgery in elderly patients with high-grade gliomas

Study	Level of evidence[51]	Patients (*N*)	Age cut-off (yrs)	Surgery (%)	Biopsy (%)	No surgery (%)	Median survival after surgery (months)	Median survival after biopsy (months)	Median survival after no surgery (months)	Significance ($P < 0.05$)
Kelly et al 1994 [50]	III/IV	128	65	40 (31)	88 (69)	–	6.75	3.9	–	N
Stark et al 2007 [51]	III/IV	185	60	185 (100)	–	–	16	–	–	–
Chaichana et al 2011 [52]	III/IV	205	65	133 (65)	72 (35)	–	5.7	4.0	–	Y
Chaichana et al 2011 [53]	III/IV	129	65	129 (100)	–	–	7.9	–	–	–

Abbreviations: –, not available; Y, yes.

demonstrated that surgical resection was associated with improved survival without added morbidity or mortality compared with biopsy. In this study, age > 70 years was also shown to be associated with significantly reduced survival benefit when compared with the younger age group.[52] Chaichana et al further investigated the surgical cohort in a separate study and identified preoperative KPS score < 80, history of chronic obstructive pulmonary disease, and tumor size larger than 4 cm as independent negative prognostic factors.[53] In all, the authors concluded that aggressive surgical resection should be considered in older patients, and careful patient selection may lead to prolonged survival without increased surgical risk.[52,53]

Expert Recommendations[51]

1. Extent of surgery is associated with prolonged survival in patients with high-grade glioma (Grade 1C Recommendation, Level II/III Evidence).
2. Surgical resection may have survival benefit in patients with multifocal or multicentric high-grade glioma. Aggressive surgical management may be considered in this select group of patients (Grade 2C Recommendation, Level II/III Evidence).
3. Surgical resection may have survival benefit in patients with recurrent high-grade glioma. Careful patient selection is important for optimizing outcome (Grade 1C Recommendation, Level II/III Evidence).
4. Surgical resection can be performed in elderly patients with high-grade glioma with acceptable complication risks and may lead to improved outcome (Grade 1C Recommendation, Level II/III Evidence).

■ Summary and Conclusions

GBM is the most common malignant primary brain tumor of adulthood. The management of GBM remains challenging, and the median survival remains less than 2 years despite advances in medical and surgical therapies. Currently, the standard treatment consists of maximal surgical resection, radiation, and chemotherapy. Surgery is critical in GBM management because it establishes diagnosis, relieves mass effect, and facilitates adjuvant therapies by reducing the residual tumor burden. Maximal surgical resection has consistently been shown to prolong survival and improve quality of life in newly diagnosed GBM patients with solitary lesions. Importantly, extent of resection is associated with maximal survival benefit; therefore, GTR should always be attempted without causing new neurological deficits. However, the role of surgery in high-risk patients such as the elderly and in those with recurrent or multifocal/multicentric GBMs remains controversial. Nevertheless, continued advances in surgical and multimodal therapies and refined patient selection and risk stratification will likely lead to improved outcome even in these challenging subsets of patients.

■ References

1. Fisher JL, Schwartzbaum JA, Wrensch M, Wiemels JL. Epidemiology of brain tumors. Neurol Clin 2007;25(4):867–890, vii
2. Louis DN, Ohgaki H, Wiestler OD, et al. The 2007 WHO classification of tumours of the central nervous system. Acta Neuropathol 2007;114(2):97–109
3. Wen PY, Kesari S. Malignant gliomas in adults. N Engl J Med 2008;359(5):492–507

4. Chaichana KL, Parker SL, Olivi A, Quiñones-Hinojosa A. Long-term seizure outcomes in adult patients undergoing primary resection of malignant brain astrocytomas. Clinical article. J Neurosurg 2009;111(2):282–292
5. Schwartzbaum JA, Fisher JL, Aldape KD, Wrensch M. Epidemiology and molecular pathology of glioma. Nat Clin Pract Neurol 2006;2(9):494–503, quiz 1, 516
6. Ohgaki H, Kleihues P. Population-based studies on incidence, survival rates, and genetic alterations in astrocytic and oligodendroglial gliomas. J Neuropathol Exp Neurol 2005;64(6): 479–489
7. Farrell CJ, Plotkin SR. Genetic causes of brain tumors: neurofibromatosis, tuberous sclerosis, von Hippel-Lindau, and other syndromes. Neurol Clin 2007;25(4):925–946, viii
8. McGirt MJ, Goldstein IM, Chaichana KL, Tobias ME, Kothbauer KF, Jallo GI. Extent of surgical resection of malignant astrocytomas of the spinal cord: outcome analysis of 35 patients. Neurosurgery 2008;63(1):55–60
9. Chang SM, Parney IF, Huang W, et al; Glioma Outcomes Project Investigators. Patterns of care for adults with newly diagnosed malignant glioma. JAMA 2005;293(5):557–564
10. Lacroix M, Abi-Said D, Fourney DR, et al. A multivariate analysis of 416 patients with glioblastoma multiforme: prognosis, extent of resection, and survival. J Neurosurg 2001;95(2): 190–198
11. Walker MD, Alexander E Jr, Hunt WE, et al. Evaluation of BCNU and/or radiotherapy in the treatment of anaplastic gliomas. A cooperative clinical trial. J Neurosurg 1978;49(3):333–343
12. U.S. Preventive Services Task Force. The Guide to Clinical Preventive Services: Recommendations of the U.S. Preventive Services Tack Force. Washington, DC: Agency for Healthcare Research and Quality; 2006
13. Claes A, Idema AJ, Wesseling P. Diffuse glioma growth: a guerilla war. Acta Neuropathol 2007;114(5):443–458
14. Muragaki Y, Iseki H, Maruyama T, et al. Usefulness of intraoperative magnetic resonance imaging for glioma surgery. Acta Neurochir Suppl (Wien) 2006;98:67–75
15. Schiffbauer H, Berger MS, Ferrari P, Freudenstein D, Rowley HA, Roberts TP. Preoperative magnetic source imaging for brain tumor surgery: a quantitative comparison with intraoperative sensory and motor mapping. J Neurosurg 2002;97(6): 1333–1342
16. Senft C, Bink A, Franz K, Vatter H, Gasser T, Seifert V. Intraoperative MRI guidance and extent of resection in glioma surgery: a randomised, controlled trial. Lancet Oncol 2011; 12(11):997–1003
17. Stummer W, Pichlmeier U, Meinel T, Wiestler OD, Zanella F, Reulen HJ; ALA-Glioma Study Group. Fluorescence-guided surgery with 5-aminolevulinic acid for resection of malignant glioma: a randomised controlled multicentre phase III trial. Lancet Oncol 2006;7(5):392–401
18. Barker FG II, Prados MD, Chang SM, et al. Radiation response and survival time in patients with glioblastoma multiforme. J Neurosurg 1996;84(3):442–448
19. Butowski N, Lamborn KR, Berger MS, Prados MD, Chang SM. Historical controls for phase II surgically based trials requiring gross total resection of glioblastoma multiforme. J Neurooncol 2007;85(1):87–94
20. Keles GE, Chang EF, Lamborn KR, et al. Volumetric extent of resection and residual contrast enhancement on initial surgery as predictors of outcome in adult patients with hemispheric anaplastic astrocytoma. J Neurosurg 2006;105(1):34–40
21. Hess KR. Extent of resection as a prognostic variable in the treatment of gliomas. J Neurooncol 1999;42(3):227–231
22. McGirt MJ, Chaichana KL, Attenello FJ, et al. Extent of surgical resection is independently associated with survival in patients with hemispheric infiltrating low-grade gliomas. Neurosurgery 2008;63(4):700–707, author reply 707–708
23. Nazzaro JM, Neuwelt EA. The role of surgery in the management of supratentorial intermediate and high-grade astrocytomas in adults. J Neurosurg 1990;73(3):331–344
24. Brown PD, Maurer MJ, Rummans TA, et al. A prospective study of quality of life in adults with newly diagnosed high-grade gliomas: the impact of the extent of resection on quality of life and survival. Neurosurgery 2005;57(3):495–504
25. Schneider JP, Trantakis C, Rubach M, et al. Intraoperative MRI to guide the resection of primary supratentorial glioblastoma multiforme—a quantitative radiological analysis. Neuroradiology 2005;47(7):489–500
26. McGirt MJ, Chaichana KL, Gathinji M, et al. Independent association of extent of resection with survival in patients with malignant brain astrocytoma. J Neurosurg 2009;110(1): 156–162
27. Bucci MK, Maity A, Janss AJ, et al. Near complete surgical resection predicts a favorable outcome in pediatric patients with nonbrainstem, malignant gliomas: results from a single center in the magnetic resonance imaging era. Cancer 2004;101(4):817–824
28. Laws ER, Parney IF, Huang W, et al; Glioma Outcomes Investigators. Survival following surgery and prognostic factors for recently diagnosed malignant glioma: data from the Glioma Outcomes Project. J Neurosurg 2003;99(3):467–473
29. Buckner JC. Factors influencing survival in high-grade gliomas. Semin Oncol 2003;30(6, Suppl 19):10–14
30. Salvati M, Cervoni L, Celli P, Caruso R, Gagliardi FM. Multicentric and multifocal primary cerebral tumours: methods of diagnosis and treatment. Ital J Neurol Sci 1997;18(1):17–20
31. Batzdorf U, Malamud N. The problem of multicentric gliomas. J Neurosurg 1963;20:122–136
32. Hassaneen W, Levine NB, Suki D, et al. Multiple craniotomies in the management of multifocal and multicentric glioblastoma. Clinical article. J Neurosurg 2011;114(3):576–584
33. Kyritsis AP, Levin VA, Yung WK, Leeds NE. Imaging patterns of multifocal gliomas. Eur J Radiol 1993;16(3):163–170
34. Showalter TN, Andrel J, Andrews DW, Curran WJ Jr, Daskalakis C, Werner-Wasik M. Multifocal glioblastoma multiforme: prognostic factors and patterns of progression. Int J Radiat Oncol Biol Phys 2007;69(3):820–824
35. Chadduck WM, Roycroft D, Brown MW. Multicentric glioma as a cause of multiple cerebral lesions. Neurosurgery 1983; 13(2):170–175
36. Salvati M, Caroli E, Orlando ER, Frati A, Artizzu S, Ferrante L. Multicentric glioma: our experience in 25 patients and critical review of the literature. Neurosurg Rev 2003;26(4): 275–279
37. Hong B, Wiese B, Bremer M, et al. Multiple microsurgical resections for repeated recurrence of glioblastoma multiforme. Am J Clin Oncol 2012 Apr 6. [Epub ahead of print]
38. Park JK, Hodges T, Arko L, et al. Scale to predict survival after surgery for recurrent glioblastoma multiforme. J Clin Oncol 2010;28(24):3838–3843
39. Ammirati M, Galicich JH, Arbit E, Liao Y. Reoperation in the treatment of recurrent intracranial malignant gliomas. Neurosurgery 1987;21(5):607–614
40. Choucair AK, Levin VA, Gutin PH, et al. Development of multiple lesions during radiation therapy and chemotherapy in patients with gliomas. J Neurosurg 1986;65(5):654–658
41. Barker FG II, Chang SM, Gutin PH, et al. Survival and functional status after resection of recurrent glioblastoma multiforme. Neurosurgery 1998;42(4):709–720
42. Dirks P, Bernstein M, Muller PJ, Tucker WS. The value of reoperation for recurrent glioblastoma. Can J Surg 1993;36(3): 271–275
43. Harsh GR IV, Levin VA, Gutin PH, Seager M, Silver P, Wilson CB. Reoperation for recurrent glioblastoma and anaplastic astrocytoma. Neurosurgery 1987;21(5):615–621
44. Hou LC, Veeravagu A, Hsu AR, Tse VC. Recurrent glioblastoma multiforme: a review of natural history and management options. Neurosurg Focus 2006;20(4):E5
45. Barker FG II, Chang SM, Larson DA, et al. Age and radiation response in glioblastoma multiforme. Neurosurgery 2001; 49(6):1288–1297

46. Pierga JY, Hoang-Xuan K, Feuvret L, et al. Treatment of malignant gliomas in the elderly. J Neurooncol 1999;43(2): 187–193
47. Ewelt C, Goeppert M, Rapp M, Steiger HJ, Stummer W, Sabel M. Glioblastoma multiforme of the elderly: the prognostic effect of resection on survival. J Neurooncol 2011;103(3):611–618
48. Basso U, Tosoni A, Vastola F, Brandes AA. Guidelines for the treatment of malignant gliomas in elderly patients. Forum (Genova) 2003;13(1):46–60
49. Brandes AA, Monfardini S. The treatment of elderly patients with high-grade gliomas. Semin Oncol 2003;30(6, Suppl 19): 58–62
50. Kelly PJ, Hunt C. The limited value of cytoreductive surgery in elderly patients with malignant gliomas. Neurosurgery 1994;34(1):62–66
51. Stark AM, Hedderich J, Held-Feindt J, Mehdorn HM. Glioblastoma—the consequences of advanced patient age on treatment and survival. Neurosurg Rev 2007;30(1):56–61
52. Chaichana KL, Garzon-Muvdi T, Parker S, et al. Supratentorial glioblastoma multiforme: the role of surgical resection versus biopsy among older patients. Ann Surg Oncol 2011; 18(1):239–245
53. Chaichana KL, Chaichana KK, Olivi A, et al. Surgical outcomes for older patients with glioblastoma multiforme: preoperative factors associated with decreased survival. Clinical article. J Neurosurg 2011;114(3):587–594

4

Adjuvants in the Surgical Resection of Astrocytomas (Intraoperative MRI and 5-ALA)

Kimon Bekelis and David W. Roberts

■ Intraoperative Magnetic Resonance Imaging in the Resection of Astrocytomas

Intraoperative magnetic resonance imaging (iMRI) was introduced more than a decade ago to maximize intraoperative resection control.[1,2] Intraoperative MRI has been used to update neuronavigation information and to detect residual tumor, potentially eliminating the need for a return to the operating room.[3] Image-guidance technologies (variably labeled frameless stereotaxy, neuronavigation, or image-guided surgery) based upon co-registration of the surgical field with preoperative imaging datasets, such as those from computed tomography (CT), MRI, and positron-emission tomography (PET), had developed in a similar attempt to assist surgical interventions but are limited because noncontemporaneous imaging is subject to inaccuracy deriving from brain displacement (shift) and deformation associated with tissue removal, cerebrospinal fluid loss, and retraction, particularly at the later stages of resection. Glial neoplasms, both high and low grade, have been the most common tumors where iMRI has been used as an adjunct, but others, including metastasis, meningioma, and pituitary tumors, have also been resected utilizing this technology. Especially in the case of astrocytoma and malignant glioma, the extent of resection has been associated with prolonged progression-free survival, making the use of iMRI very appealing.

iMRI implementations have incorporated both low- and high-field-strength magnets. Low-field-strength iMRI refers to systems of less than 0.5 T, whereas high-field-strength systems start at 1.5 T.[1] The choice of system depends on the desired image quality, available imaging modalities, integration into the existing workflow, and cost.

Despite the widespread use of iMRI and the multiple systems being developed for better integration of this modality into the operating room workflow, the evidence for its use remains limited. Because iMRI-guided surgery requires expensive equipment and prolongs surgery time, justification for its widespread use is required.

Evidence for iMRI Use in the Resection of Low- and High-Grade Gliomas

No randomized, controlled trials have been published to date investigating the utility of iMRI in comparison with standard neuronavigation techniques. On the other hand, there are significant limitations in the published literature on iMRI (**Table 4.1**). Most studies have offered descriptive statistics of a heterogeneous population with mixed pathology. Extent of resection has been measured in different ways among the available studies, with a few studies not providing

Table 4.1 Level of evidence for the use of intraoperative MRI (iMRI) for astrocytoma resection

Level of evidence	Study	Topic
I	No studies	
II	Kubben et al 2011[1]	Systematic review of all studies on iMRI for gliomas
III	Senft et al 2010[5]	Case-control study comparing extent of resection and median survival in patients with GBM with and without iMRI (retrospective)
	Hirschberg et al 2005[6]	Case-control study with matched control on median survival for GBM with and without iMRI (retrospective)
IV	Knauth et al 1999[7]	Case series comparing contrast enhancement in intraoperative and postoperative MRI in high-grade glioma (retrospective)
	Wirtz et al 2000[8]	Case series demonstrating the extent of resection for primary and recurrent glioma with the use of iMRI (retrospective)
	Bohinski et al 2001[9]	Case series demonstrating the extent of resection for supratentorial glioma with the use of iMRI (prospective)
	Nimsky et al 2003[10]	Case series demonstrating the extent of resection for supratentorial glioma with the use of iMRI (retrospective)
	Schneider et al 2005[12]	Extent of resection for supratentorial GBM (retrospective)
	Muragaki et al 2006[13]	Case series demonstrating the extent of resection for supratentorial GBM with the use of iMRI (retrospective)
	Nimsky et al 2006[11]	Case series demonstrating the extent of resection for supratentorial GBM with the use of iMRI (retrospective)
	Hatiboglu et al 2009[14]	Case series demonstrating the extent of resection for supratentorial glioma with the use of iMRI (retrospective)
	Lenaburg et al 2009[15]	Case series demonstrating the extent of resection for supratentorial glioma with the use of iMRI (retrospective)
	Kuhnt et al 2011[16]	Case series demonstrating the extent of resection for supratentorial glioma with the use of iMRI (prospective)

a definition of gross total resection (GTR). Outcome parameters have often been mentioned without stratification for the various pathological diagnoses. Survival data have been available in a minority of the studies, comparing GTR with subtotal resection or iMRI-guided surgery with conventional neuronavigation-assisted surgery. In addition, control groups, when present, have not always been equivalent to the study groups, mainly with regard to tumor location and type of navigation system. No studies with overlapping data were included in the analysis.

Level I Evidence

There are no Level I studies comparing length of survival or extent of resection in cases of iMRI with cases of conventional neuronavigation.

Level II Evidence

There is one systematic review[1] of the available evidence on the added value of iMRI-guided resection of glial tumors compared with conventional neuronavigation-assisted resection, with respect to extent of resection, quality of life, and survival. Kubben et al[1] identified 12 studies fulfilling their selection criteria. Several limitations and sources of bias were apparent, and these may have affected the conclusions drawn, including overestimation of the added value of iMRI-guided surgery, as the authors recognize. Their conclusion was that, based on the available literature, there is at best Level II evidence supporting the use of iMRI in increasing the extent of resection, prolonging survival, and improving quality of life after the resection of astrocytomas.

In another single-center study, Senft et al[5] retrospectively analyzed their experience with glioblastoma multiforme resection in 41 patients. Surgery was guided by low-field-strength iMRI in 10 cases and by conventional neuronavigation in the rest. Postoperative MRI within 72 hours of surgery showed GTR in all iMRI cases and in 19 of 31 patients undergoing neuronavigation-assisted resection. Although median survival according to extent of resection was better in the GTR group (74 vs 44 weeks, $p < 0.001$), median survival according to treatment groups, despite the favorable trend, did not reach statistical significance (88 weeks for the iMRI group vs 68 weeks for the conventional neuronavigation group, $p = 0.07$). This study is associated with obvious selection bias, given the nonrandomization of patients into the two treatment groups.

Level III Evidence

In a retrospective analysis of their series of 32 patients, Hirschberg et al[6] demonstrated that GTR was achieved in only 5 of the 27 patients on initial iMRI imaging during surgery. They did not provide data on the extent of resection after the last iMRI scan. Postoperatively, 16% of the patients demonstrated improved functional status, 55% remained unchanged, and 29% were functionally worse. Subsequently, they compared this group of patients with matched controls, but, despite the favorable trend, they failed to demonstrate a difference in survival (14.5 vs 12.1, $p = 0.14$). The lack of equivalence among the compared groups is a major limitation of the study, restricting the value of the conclusions. Extrapolation from residual tumor evident on first imaging to risk of residual tumor when iMRI is not available is difficult given the surgeon's subjective decision-making threshold to acquire imaging.

Level IV Evidence

There are multiple studies providing no better than Level IV evidence on the utility of iMRI during the resection of gliomas. The authors mainly attempt to demonstrate the contribution of iMRI in more extensive tumor resection in retrospective series, without control groups. Knauth et al[7] retrospectively analyzed their experience with iMRI in 41 patients where GTR was intended. GTR was achieved in 76% of the cases in the early postoperative MRI in comparison with 37% of cases during the first iMRI. Wirtz et al[8] in a similar study of 68 cases demonstrated that in 66% of the patients the resection was continued based on the data provided by the iMRI scan. Patients with GTR had improved survival in comparison to patients with subtotal resection (13.3 months vs 9.2 months, $p = 0.035$). Bohinski et al[9] prospectively reached the same conclusions, with 57% of their 30 patients with high-grade gliomas undergoing additional resections because of the results of iMRI. There was no mention of postoperative performance scores.

Nimsky et al[10,11] compared the performance of 0.2 T and 1.5 T iMRI scanners. GTR was achieved after the last scan in 7 out of 32 cases with 0.2 T iMRI, and in 23 out of 57 cases with 1.5 T iMRI. The authors do not mention the intended GTR in the 0.2 T iMRI cases, whereas GTR was not intended in 25 out of the 57 1.5 T iMRI cases. By using manual segmentation they reported a mean additional resection of 12% in intended subtotal resection cases, and a mean additional resection of 20% in intended GTR cases.

Schneider et al[12] demonstrated that GTR was achieved on the last iMRI scan in 11 of 31 retrospective analyzed glioma patients, in comparison with 2 of the 31 on the first iMRI scan. In agreement with prior studies, the median survival was significantly better for patients with GTR. Muragaki et al[13] demonstrated 90% extent of resection in their group of 30 patients with glioblastoma multiforme, with the use of a 0.3-T iMRI scanner. In a prospective cohort of 27 patients with GBM near eloquent areas, Hatiboglu et al[14] achieved GTR in 24 patients after the last iMRI scan on a 1.5-T iMRI scanner. Similarly, Lenaburg et al[15] demonstrated that in 72% of their cases further resection was pursued based on the results of a 0.2-T iMRI scan, resulting in greater than 95% resection in 27 of their 35 cases. Finally, Kuhnt et al[16] demonstrated that in 135 patients with GBM, greater resection was achieved with the use of iMRI. Patients with a resection greater than 98% demonstrated a survival benefit.

Recommendations for the Use of Intraoperative MRI in Glioma Resection

1. The use of iMRI is recommended during glioma resection when available in the provider's institution. It is associated with greater extent of resection in comparison to conventional neuronavigational techniques. There is a trend toward improved survival in glioma patients undergoing iMRI-assisted resections, in comparison with conventional neuronavigation techniques (Grade 1C Recommendation, Levels II/III Evidence).
2. No clear difference in clinical performance has been detected between low- and high-field iMRI. Therefore, system selection should be based on a balance between the imaging capabilities needed (e.g., fiber tracking available with high-field iMRI) and the cost (Grade 2C Recommendation, Level IV Evidence).

■ 5-ALA in the Resection of Astrocytomas

Despite the added value of intraoperative navigation techniques, there is still a need for better in situ visualization of gliomas, given the infiltrative nature of the disease.[17,18] This need is even greater considering the increasing body of evidence supporting more extensive resections.[19] 5-Aminolevulinic acid (5-ALA)-induced fluorescence has been used as a tumor-specific biomarker that allows more accurate discrimination of pathological from normal tissue.[20] ALA is a natural precursor in the heme biosynthetic pathway. Exogenous administration of ALA leads to significant accumulation of the fluorescent compound, protoporphyrin IX (PpIX), one step prior to conversion of PpIX to heme by the enzyme ferrochelatase. PpIX selectively accumulates in malignant cells as a result of several incompletely understood mechanisms, including reduced activity of ferrochelatase, elevated intracellular 5-ALA uptake, and delayed PpIX secretion from the cell.[20] Previous studies have shown that PpIX accumulates with high specificity and in sufficient concentrations in high-grade glioma to allow visual fluorescence detection of tumor tissue.[21] The use of a modified microscope with a light source that can alternate between conventional white and fluorophore-exciting blue light facilitates user-friendly implementation of this technology.

Evidence for 5-ALA Use in the Resection of Astrocytomas

There are limited but high-quality data supporting the use of 5-ALA as a biomarker during the resection of gliomas (**Table 4.2**). Most of the evidence supports its use in high-grade gliomas, although most recent results support its applicability in lower-grade tumors too. The initial studies were based on the detection of visible fluorescence. However, the field is rapidly expanding with the development of intraoperative probes allowing the quantitation of fluorescence, even in areas where visible fluorescence is lacking. No studies with overlapping data were included in the analysis.

Level I Evidence

In a phase 3 randomized, controlled, multicenter trial, Stummer et al[22] compared 139 patients who underwent fluorescent tumor resection with 131 patients who underwent conventional microsurgery with white light. Patients with tumors located in the midline, bas-

Table 4.2 Level of evidence for the use of intraoperative fluorescence for astrocytoma resection

Level of evidence	Study	Topic
I	Stummer et al 2006[22]	Randomized, controlled, multicenter phase 3 trial comparing extent of resection and median survival in patients with GBM with and without intraoperative fluorescence
II	Nabavi et al 2009[24]	Multicenter, noncontrolled phase 2 study demonstrating the positive predictive value of intraoperative fluorescence during the resection of GBM
	Stummer et al 2011[23]	Multicenter, noncontrolled phase 2 study demonstrating the safety profile of intraoperative fluorescence during the resection of GBM in elderly patients
III	Panciani et al 2005	Case-control study with use of the same patients as controls comparing the sensitivity and specificity of intraoperative fluorescence with standard navigation techniques (prospective)
IV	Stummer et al 2000[20]	Case series demonstrating the extent of resection for supratentorial GBM with the use of intraoperative fluorescence (prospective)
	Hefti et al 2008[26]	Case series demonstrating the sensitivity and specificity of the use of intraoperative fluorescence for high-grade gliomas (prospective)
	Feigl et al 2010[28]	Case series demonstrating the extent of resection with the use of intraoperative fluorescence in combination with intraoperative monitoring for high-grade gliomas (prospective)
	Díez Valle et al 2011[27]	Case series demonstrating the extent of resection and positive predictive value of intraoperative fluorescence for high-grade gliomas (prospective)
	Valdés et al 2011[29]	Case series comparing the performance of intraoperative qualitative and quantitative fluorescence in the same patients with benign tumors and low- and high-grade gliomas (prospective)

al ganglia, cerebellum, or brainstem as well as those with multifocal tumors, substantial non-contrast-enhancing tumor areas, medical contraindications to the receipt of 5-ALA, and Karnofsky performance scores lower than 60, were excluded from the trial. The study was terminated early, with a median patient follow-up of 35.4 months. GTR was achieved in 65% of the patients assigned to the 5-ALA arm, in comparison with 36% in patients assigned to white light ($p < 0.0001$). In addition, patients randomized to 5-ALA had a longer 6-month progression-free survival than did those randomized to white light (41% vs 21.1%). The use of 5-ALA was not associated with an increase in severe adverse events. The authors also identified a lower incidence of repeat surgery in patients assigned to 5-ALA ($p = 0.03$). Conventional neuronavigation was not controlled for, and no conclusions can be drawn about its relative value in comparison with 5-ALA.

Level II Evidence

In a multicenter, noncontrolled phase 2 study, Stummer et al[23] attempted to gather additional safety data in a more general unselected cohort. The safety profile of 5-ALA was proven to be very favorable in the elderly population. In addition, post hoc analysis showed overall medial survival to be longest in patients receiving 5-ALA and treated by concomitant radiation and temozolomide, a benefit that was maintained in the elderly.

In another multicenter, noncontrolled phase 2 study, Nabavi et al[24] demonstrated the value of fluorescence in recurrent gliomas primarily resected based on neuronavigation information. The positive predictive value of all biopsies taken from the resection cavity was found to be 91.7% in areas of strong fluorescence and 82.4% in areas of weak fluorescence. Prior treatment modalities do not seem to alter the value of 5-ALA guidance.

Level III Evidence

Panciani et al[25] compared the performance of 5-ALA and image guidance applied in the same patients in a prospective study of 23 cases of suspected high-grade glioma. Decision-making based on 5-ALA showed a sensitivity of 91.1% and a specificity of 89.4% ($p < 0.001$), whereas conventional neuronavigation demonstrated a significantly lower sensitivity (57.8%) and specificity (57.4%).

Level IV Evidence

Several prospective or retrospective case series have supported the feasibility of the use of 5-ALA in the resection of high-grade gliomas. Stummer et al,[20] in their initial experience, demonstrated a 63% complete resection of contrast-enhancing tumors in 52 prospectively studied consecutive patients. Residual fluorescent tissue, which was left unresected in eloquent areas, correlated with residual contrast enhancement in magnetic resonance imaging (MRI) scans. Hefti et al[26] underscored the limitations of the technique, pointing out that strong fluorescence was associated with 98% sensitivity and 100% specificity, whereas weak fluorescence reduced the sensitivity to 76% and the specificity to 85%. Similar results were reported by Díez Valle et al,[27] who demonstrated a positive predictive value of 100% for strong fluorescence. In addition, 5-ALA has been combined with intraoperative monitoring in the resection of tumors of eloquent areas by Feigl et al,[28] achieving a 64% GTR.

Valdés et al[29] have explored the added value of quantitative fluorescence as detected by a specially designed probe. They demonstrated that the results of quantitative fluorescence (measuring PpIX concentration) were superior to visible fluorescence in their series of 14 patients harboring various pathologies, from benign tumors and low-grade gliomas to high-grade gliomas. These findings were clinically profound because they demonstrated that ALA-induced PpIX is a targeting biomarker for a variety of intracranial tumors beyond high-grade gliomas.

Expert Recommendations

1. The use of qualitative fluorescence for intraoperative guidance in patients with GBM is recommended for all patients that fit the inclusion criteria of the Stummer study. It is associated with more complete resection of contrast-enhancing tumors, leading to improved progression-free survival in comparison to standard microsurgical techniques (Grade 1B Recommendation, Level I Evidence).
2. The addition of quantitative fluorescence appears to be superior to qualitative methods alone. Although further studies are needed to establish the value of this technique, its use is recommended in centers that have this capacity (Grade 2C Recommendation, Level IV Evidence).
3. The use of qualitative and quantitative fluorescence for intraoperative guidance in patients with low-grade gliomas could be employed as an adjunct (Grade 2C Recommendation, Level IV Evidence.)
4. The use of qualitative fluorescence appears to demonstrate higher sensitivity and specificity than standard neuronavigational techniques (Grade 2C Recommendation, Level III Evidence).

■ References

1. Kubben PL, ter Meulen KJ, Schijns OE, ter Laak-Poort MP, van Overbeeke JJ, van Santbrink H. Intraoperative MRI-guided resection of glioblastoma multiforme: a systematic review. Lancet Oncol 2011;12(11):1062–1070
2. Black PM, Moriarty T, Alexander E III, et al. Development and implementation of intraoperative magnetic resonance imaging and its neurosurgical applications. Neurosurgery 1997;41(4):831–842
3. Black PM, Alexander E III, Martin C, et al. Craniotomy for tumor treatment in an intraoperative magnetic resonance imaging unit. Neurosurgery 1999;45(3):423–431
4. Nimsky C, Ganslandt O, Tomandl B, Buchfelder M, Fahlbusch R. Low-field magnetic resonance imaging for intraoperative use in neurosurgery: a 5-year experience. Eur Radiol 2002;12(11):2690–2703
5. Senft C, Franz K, Blasel S, et al. Influence of iMRI-guidance on the extent of resection and survival of patients with glioblastoma multiforme. Technol Cancer Res Treat 2010;9(4): 339–346
6. Hirschberg H, Samset E, Hol PK, Tillung T, Lote K. Impact of intraoperative MRI on the surgical results for high-grade gliomas. Minim Invasive Neurosurg 2005;48(2):77–84
7. Knauth M, Wirtz CR, Tronnier VM, Aras N, Kunze S, Sartor K. Intraoperative MR imaging increases the extent of tumor resection in patients with high-grade gliomas. AJNR Am J Neuroradiol 1999;20(9):1642–1646
8. Wirtz CR, Knauth M, Staubert A, et al. Clinical evaluation and follow-up results for intraoperative magnetic resonance imaging in neurosurgery. Neurosurgery 2000;46(5): 1112–1120
9. Bohinski RJ, Kokkino AK, Warnick RE, et al. Glioma resection in a shared-resource magnetic resonance operating room after optimal image-guided frameless stereotactic resection. Neurosurgery 2001;48(4):731–742
10. Nimsky C, Ganslandt O, Buchfelder M, Fahlbusch R. Glioma surgery evaluated by intraoperative low-field magnetic resonance imaging. Acta Neurochir Suppl (Wien) 2003;85: 55–63
11. Nimsky C, Ganslandt O, Buchfelder M, Fahlbusch R. Intraoperative visualization for resection of gliomas: the role of functional neuronavigation and intraoperative 1.5 T MRI. Neurol Res 2006;28(5):482–487
12. Schneider JP, Trantakis C, Rubach M, et al. Intraoperative MRI to guide the resection of primary supratentorial glioblastoma multiforme—a quantitative radiological analysis. Neuroradiology 2005;47(7):489–500
13. Muragaki Y, Iseki H, Maruyama T, et al. Usefulness of intraoperative magnetic resonance imaging for glioma surgery. Acta Neurochir Suppl (Wien) 2006;98:67–75
14. Hatiboglu MA, Weinberg JS, Suki D, et al. Impact of intraoperative high-field magnetic resonance imaging guidance on glioma surgery: a prospective volumetric analysis. Neurosurgery 2009;64(6):1073–1081
15. Lenaburg HJ, Inkabi KE, Vitaz TW. The use of intraoperative MRI for the treatment of glioblastoma multiforme. Technol Cancer Res Treat 2009;8(2):159–162
16. Kuhnt D, Becker A, Ganslandt O, Bauer M, Buchfelder M, Nimsky C. Correlation of the extent of tumor volume resection and patient survival in surgery of glioblastoma multiforme with high-field intraoperative MRI guidance. Neuro-oncol 2011; 13(12):1339–1348
17. Sherman JH, Hoes K, Marcus J, Komotar RJ, Brennan CW, Gutin PH. Neurosurgery for brain tumors: update on recent technical advances. Curr Neurol Neurosci Rep 2011;11(3): 313–319
18. Stummer W, Kamp MA. The importance of surgical resection in malignant glioma. Curr Opin Neurol 2009;22(6): 645–649
19. Stummer W, Reulen HJ, Meinel T, et al; ALA-Glioma Study Group. Extent of resection and survival in glioblastoma multiforme: identification of and adjustment for bias. Neurosurgery 2008;62(3):564–576
20. Stummer W, Novotny A, Stepp H, Goetz C, Bise K, Reulen HJ. Fluorescence-guided resection of glioblastoma multiforme by using 5-aminolevulinic acid-induced porphyrins: a prospective study in 52 consecutive patients. J Neurosurg 2000;93(6):1003–1013
21. Roberts DW, Valdés PA, Harris BT, et al. Coregistered fluorescence-enhanced tumor resection of malignant glioma: relationships between D-aminolevulinic acid-induced protoporphyrin IX fluorescence, magnetic resonance imaging enhancement, and neuropathological parameters. Clinical article. J Neurosurg 2011;114(3):595–603
22. Stummer W, Pichlmeier U, Meinel T, Wiestler OD, Zanella F, Reulen HJ; ALA-Glioma Study Group. Fluorescence-guided surgery with 5-aminolevulinic acid for resection of malignant glioma: a randomised controlled multicentre phase III trial. Lancet Oncol 2006;7(5):392–401
23. Stummer W, Nestler U, Stockhammer F, et al. Favorable outcome in the elderly cohort treated by concomitant temozolomide radiochemotherapy in a multicentric phase II safety study of 5-ALA. J Neurooncol 2011;103(2):361–370
24. Nabavi A, Thurm H, Zountsas B, et al; 5-ALA Recurrent Glioma Study Group. Five-aminolevulinic acid for fluorescence-guided resection of recurrent malignant gliomas: a phase II study. Neurosurgery 2009;65(6):1070–1076
25. Panciani PP, Fontanella M, Schatlo B, et al. Fluorescence and image guided resection in high grade glioma. Clin Neurol Neurosurg 2012;114(1):37–41
26. Hefti M, von Campe G, Moschopulos M, Siegner A, Looser H, Landolt H. 5-aminolevulinic acid induced protoporphyrin IX fluorescence in high-grade glioma surgery: a one-year experience at a single institution. Swiss Med Wkly 2008;138(11-12): 180–185
27. Díez Valle R, Tejada Solis S, Idoate Gastearena MA, García de Eulate R, Domínguez Echávarri P, Aristu Mendiroz J. Surgery guided by 5-aminolevulinic fluorescence in glioblastoma: volumetric analysis of extent of resection in single-center experience. J Neurooncol 2011;102(1):105–113
28. Feigl GC, Ritz R, Moraes M, et al. Resection of malignant brain tumors in eloquent cortical areas: a new multimodal approach combining 5-aminolevulinic acid and intraoperative monitoring. J Neurosurg 2010;113(2):352–357
29. Valdés PA, Leblond F, Kim A, et al. Quantitative fluorescence in intracranial tumor: implications for ALA-induced PpIX as an intraoperative biomarker. J Neurosurg 2011;115(1): 11–17

5

The Role of Intraoperative Mapping in the Resection of Low-Grade Gliomas

Hugues Duffau

In the past decade, improved understanding of the natural history of World Health Organization grade II glioma, that is, diffuse low-grade glioma (LGG), led to a renewed interest in surgery. It is now well known that LGG is a premalignant primary brain tumor, characterized by a slow but continuous growth (linear evolution of the mean diameter ~ 4 mm/y, even in incidental LGG), migration along the white matter pathways, and unavoidable anaplastic transformation.[1–3] All the recent and rigorous studies based on objective evaluation of the extent of resection (EoR) on postoperative MRI have shown that surgery had a significant impact on both malignant degeneration and overall survival in patients with LGG.[4,5] Consequently, after many years of controversy, guidelines now recommend maximal surgical resection as the first therapeutic option—see for instance the European Federation of Neurological Societies guidelines.[6] This paradigmatic shift should lead neurosurgeons to move from performing a single "tumorectomy" (i.e., removing only what is visible on imaging) toward an extensive resection (i.e., subtotal, total, or even supratotal resection) of a chronic and diffuse tumoral cerebral disease.

On the other hand, most patients with LGG experience no or only slight neurological deficit at the time of the first magnetic resonance imaging (MRI) scan, usually performed because of inaugural seizures or even for an independent reason with incidental discovery.[7] Thus, in addition to the optimization of EoR, preservation of the quality of life (QoL) is currently a priority in (precocious) surgery for LGG[8]—despite the fact that, for a long time, the vast majority of studies focused on overall survival but did not accurately investigate the QoL. Due to the frequent location of LGGs near or within the so-called eloquent areas[9,10] and due to their infiltrative nature (poorly demarcated), it was traditionally considered nearly impossible to perform extensive glioma resection, and the risk of generating permanent postoperative sequelae was high. Indeed, numerous surgical series have reported a postoperative rate of permanent and severe deficit between 13 and 27.5%.[11]

To solve this dilemma, namely to optimize the benefit-to-risk ratio of surgery, brain surgeons should change their thinking as well as their technique on the basis of a new concept; that is, they should perform surgical resection according to corticosubcortical functional boundaries and not according to oncological limits. *The underlying principle is to shift from imaging-guided surgery to mapping-guided surgery.*[12] To this end, it is mandatory to understand the cerebral anatomofunctional organization at the individual level, given the interindividual variability already demonstrated in healthy volunteers[13] as well as in epileptic patients.[14] Moreover, this variability is increased in cases of LGG due to mechanisms of brain redistribution induced by the slow growth of the tumor.[15] Therefore, many arguments support the unpredictability of functional eloquence based on anatomical features alone and the fact that patients should not be considered ineligible for surgery on the basis of anatomical considerations alone.[16] Rather, neurosurgeons need to take advantage of modern technology and mapping methods to create individualized maps and management plans. The ultimate aim is to remove a part of the brain invaded by tumoral cells, on the condition that this part of the central nervous system can be functionally compensated—that there will be no impact on the QoL.

This chapter reviews how, in addition to functional neuroimaging, the method of intraoperative electrostimulation mapping (IEM), especially in awake patients, has allowed significantly improved results with LGG surgery, with (1) an increase in the surgical indications for tumor located within eloquent areas classically considered inoperable, (2) optimization of the EoR, with an impact on malignant transformation and overall survival, and (3) preservation, or even improvement of, the QoL—control of epilepsy and cognitive status. The aim is to revisit conceptual and technical aspects of LGG surgery in light of these new ideas in the fields of neuro-oncology and cognitive neurosciences, ideas that recently emerged from translational research.[17]

■ Preoperative Cognitive Assessment: Not a Luxury, but a Crucial Baseline

It is amazing to observe a low rate of neurological deficits in LGG patients, even though these tumors often involve the so-called eloquent areas. This is due to cerebral plasticity: because the LGG is a slow-growing tumor, it gives the brain many years for functional remapping, with a recruitment of perilesional or remote areas within the ipsilesional or contralateral hemisphere.[18] The recent integration of these concepts into the therapeutic strategy has resulted in dramatic changes in the surgical management of LGGs, with an increase in surgical indications in functional areas that were for a long time considered unresectable.[19]

Nonetheless, one must be aware of a high rate of cognitive deficits at the time of diagnosis, especially with regard to high-order functions, such as executive functions, attention, concentration, working memory, or emotion[20,21]*—in spite of a normal social and professional life in most LGG patients.* Thus, a systematic preoperative assessment of higher functions and health-related QoL is now recommended[21] (1) to search for a possible neuropsychological deficit not detected by a standard neurological examination, (2) to adapt the strategy according to these individual results (e.g., decision for surgery first vs neoadjuvant chemotherapy in cases of very diffuse LGGs generating important cognitive deficits), (3) to adapt the surgical methodology itself to the results of this assessment, for example, to perform functional mapping under local anesthesia even in the right hemisphere in right-handers in cases of a preoperative, slight language deficit,[22] (4) to benefit from a presurgical baseline allowing a comparison with the postsurgical evaluation, and (5) to plan a specific functional rehabilitation program following the surgery, notably if it induced transient neurological deficits. Interestingly, in series that performed objective neuropsychological and health-related QoL assessment after surgery, postoperative visuospatial, memory, attention, planning, learning, emotional, motivational, and behavioral deficits have regularly been observed.[21] For instance, a recent study showed that increased reaction time during a naming task performed immediately after resection was significantly correlated to return to work.[23] Therefore, it is likely that more patients experienced this kind of disturbance than is described in the literature. This underestimation by neurosurgeons is due to the fact that the identification of such "subtle" deficits is not possible using a single standard clinical examination. Unfortunately, extensive neurocognitive evaluation was scarcely achieved before and after LGG surgery, especially when the lesion was located outside the so-called language areas. To improve this clinical practice, a standardized examination of neurocognitive outcome has recently been proposed.[21]

In the same line of thinking, and beyond the objective neuropsychological scores, it is crucial to define the QoL for each patient on the basis of the individual's job, habits, hobbies, and projects. The aim is to prioritize the brain functions that should be preserved throughout the resection, and to tailor the intraoperative tasks based on this preparatory discussion with patients and their family. In other words, the intraoperative mapping should be personalized (discussion follows).[24]

■ Preoperative Neuroimaging Should Be Interpreted with Caution

Although progress in oncological neuroimaging enabled a better knowledge of the natural course of LGG, and whereas advances in functional neuroimaging have raised the question of more extensive glioma surgery, paradoxically, these have also led to several conceptual limitations.

From an oncological point of view, one should be aware of the fact that conventional MRI, including T2/fluid-attenuated inversion recovery (FLAIR)-weighted MRI, does not show the whole disease. Indeed, LGG invades the brain beyond the abnormalities visible on imaging, with tumor cells present at a distance of 10 to 20 mm from the tumor boundaries defined by MRI.[25] This recently led to broader glioma removal, at least in nonfunctional areas. Such so-called supracomplete resection dramatically changed the natural history of LGG (even if it cannot cure it), by delaying the recurrence and above all the malignant transformation.[26] Therefore, when LGG is distant from eloquent structures, in essence, image-guided resection is not useful because in these cases it could be possible to remove more tumor cells while preserving function if the resection is constrained by functional boundaries rather than by the T2/FLAIR-weighted MRI. Unfortunately, the integration of preoperative MRI into neuronavigation or the wider use of intraoperative MRI is based on a reductionist concept (i.e., the exclusive removal of the signal abnormality) with no attempt to increase the resection beyond these landmarks—even if they do not reflect the entirety of the glioma. In other words, image-guided resection may represent a lost opportunity for patients with diffuse low-grade gliomas (DLGGs) outside eloquent brain areas.[27]

From a functional point of view, advances in functional neuroimaging, such as functional MRI (fMRI), magnetoencephalography, diffusion tensor imaging (DTI), and transcranial magnetic stimulation have enabled noninvasive mapping of the whole brain. Functional imaging gives an estimation of the location of regions involved in sensorimotor, language, visual, and even higher cognitive functions in relation to the glioma, and allows the calculation of a lateralization index for language. As a consequence, according to several articles in the recent literature,[28] these methods might be useful for (1) surgical indications, partly depending on the LGG location and its relationships with eloquent areas detected by functional imaging (allowing an estimation of the tumor resectability); (2) surgical planning, namely the selection of the surgical approach and the delineation of the limits of resection; and (3) selection of the surgical technique, especially the decision to awaken the patient intraoperatively if the glioma is close to somatosensory, language, or cognitive areas.[28] Therefore, neurosurgeons seem to believe that the data provided by fMRI and DTI are a direct reflection of the neural foundations of the brain. Indeed, many studies are based on the exclusive use of fMRI/DTI for the surgical indications and planning, as well as on the exclusive use of functional imaging directly in the operating room (preoperative data incorporated in a neuronavigational system or intraoperative fMRI/DTI).[29]

Nevertheless, it is crucial to underscore that functional neuroimaging methods are not yet reliable enough at the individual scale, mainly because they are based on biomathematical reconstruction, and their results may change according to the model used. Correlations with intraoperative electrophysiology have clearly demonstrated that the sensitivity of fMRI was only ~ 71% for movement,[30] and from 59 to 100% for language (specificity from 0 to 97%).[31] Such discrepancies can be explained by a neurovascular decoupling in cases of glioma (blood oxygen level dependent [BOLD] imaging response in the vicinity of gliomas does not reflect the neuronal signal as accurately as it does in healthy tissue), by inadequate tasks (not adapted to the location of the glioma or to the neurological status of the patient), or by methodological problems (e.g., selection of the threshold). As a consequence, there is a risk of false-negative results. This could lead to operation on a patient without the use of IEM, although the glioma is actually located in critical areas not detected by preoperative fMRI. Therefore, there is a high risk of inducing a permanent deficit. According to the same principle, the calculation of the lateralization index may be dangerous in patients with atypical distribution of language. Indeed, in patients with a right-sided tumor, even if the lateralization index shows a majority of language activations in the left hemisphere, it does not mean that the minority of language sites activated in the right hemisphere do not correspond to crucial epicenters.[22] Consequently, if there is any doubt, awake language mapping should be performed intraoperatively because *fMRI is not able to differentiate essential regions from areas that can be functionally compensated and thus removed.*[27] Moreover, an erroneous interpretation of brain reshaping (pseudoreorganization) can be made.[32]

DTI allows tractography of the main white matter fibers as well as their location in relation to the glioma. This new method needs to be validated, especially by IEM, before it can be used routinely for surgical planning. Indeed, comparison of distinct fiber tracking software tools has found differing results, indicating that DTI results have to be applied with caution intraoperatively, especially in the case of an abnormal or distorted fiber tract anatomy.[33] Moreover, comparison between DTI and intrasurgical subcortical stimulation mapping demonstrated that DTI was not yet optimal for mapping language tracts in patients. A recent study found only an 82% positive correlation, showing that negative tractography did not rule out the persistence of a fiber tract, especially when invaded by a glioma.[34] Moreover, it is worth noting that DTI enables the study of the anatomy but not the function of the subcortical pathways.

Consequently, several negative impacts of functional imaging must be emphasized. The first risk is in selecting a patient for glioma surgery based on the close proximity between fMRI activation and the tumor when in fact this "eloquent area" did not actually represent a crucial epicenter in the functional network and could have been removed with no permanent deficit. This would result in a lost chance from an oncological standpoint because of a false-positive finding on fMRI. For instance, this issue was described for LGGs invading the so-called Broca area, which were removed with favorable outcomes, although this region was a priori thought to be critical on the basis of functional neuroimaging.[18,35] Furthermore, in the operating room, beyond the risk of damage to functional structures not identified by fMRI/DTI due to their actual lack of sensitivity and due to the increasing brain shift throughout the resection of a voluminous glioma (which decreases the reliability of the data provided by DTI), the dogmatic rule that emerged given the poor accuracy of these techniques is to take 5 to 10 mm of margin around the presumed functional regions according to neuroimaging.[36] Again, such a strategy is at odds with the oncological goal, which is to optimize the EoR. It was shown in more than 100 consecutive patients with LGGs in language areas that the resection could be pursued with no margin without increasing the permanent morbidity.[36,37] Finally, a recent study to assess the utility of DTI in the surgical treatment of motor eloquent tumors demonstrated that tractography of pyramidal pathways did not influence the surgical planning or the intraoperative course.[38] In summary, there is a double risk of (1) not selecting a patient for surgery even though the tumor was operable, or (2) prematurely stopping resection resulting in a lower impact on the natural course of the LGG. This point is essential because it has never been discussed in the literature. *Indeed, there is no series about fMRI/DTI that reported both the long-term functional and oncological outcomes; that is, there is no series actually demonstrating the real impact on QoL and overall survival (conversely to IEM)* (to be discussed).

With the goal being to overcome these pitfalls, one can currently consider performing longitudinal studies based on pre-, intra-, and postoperative mapping, rather than being content with static information based on a unique presurgical functional neuroimaging analysis.[12] In other words, the real interest of functional imaging, due to the fact that it is noninvasive, is that it can be repeated over time to analyze the patterns of brain reorganization in the patient.[39] This information is very important for envisioning reoperation in LGGs (discussed in the following paragraph). However, because of the current limitations of fMRI/DTI, even if neurosurgeons can take into account the data provided by neuroimaging (at least partly), they should also integrate invasive IEM in their surgical strategy, especially (but not exclusively) for surgery in eloquent structures, to optimize the "oncofunctional ratio" of the resection.[17]

■ Awake Intraoperative Electrostimulation Mapping Combined with Cognitive Monitoring: Toward a Function-Guided Resection

As mentioned, intraoperatively, the integration of multimodal imaging into frameless stereotactic surgery was extensively used in the past decade and is referred to as functional neuronavigation.[29] Nonetheless, the sole randomized trial failed to demonstrate a significant impact of navigation on postoperative outcomes.[40] This can be explained by the limitations of fMRI and DTI already detailed, as well as by the high risk of intraoperative brain shift due to surgical retraction, mass effect, gravity, EoR (especially for voluminous tumors), and cerebrospinal fluid leakage. Several technical improvements have been proposed to reduce the effects of this shift: combination with intraoperative ultrasonography, producing real-time imaging; use of mathematical models based on data from ultrasonography or digital images that track cortical displacement; and intraoperative MRI.[29,41] However, the reliability of the improvements has yet to be optimized. Indeed, their actual impact on the malignant transformation simultaneously with preservation of QoL remains to be demonstrated in LGGs.

Methodological Issues: Cortical Intraoperative Electrostimulation Mapping

As a consequence, *IEM remains the gold standard in LGG surgery*.[42] Although intraoperative electrostimulation mapping (IEM) can be performed under general anesthesia for tumors invading motor areas, there is now evidence supporting the use of awake mapping with active participation of the patient, even near the central region.[24] Indeed, movements and action are more complex than a single muscle contraction. It was recently shown that IEM could generate more subtle motor disturbances in awake patients, such as arrest or acceleration of movement, due to the disruption of the network involved in cognitive control of movement.[43] Beyond motor mapping, IEM has been extensively demonstrated to be an easy, reliable, reproducible, safe, and comparatively inexpensive method for identifying structures crucial for brain functions.[44,45] The main goal is to perform online anatomofunctional correlations by way of ongoing interactions between the anesthesiologist, speech therapist/neuropsychologist/neurologist, neurosurgeon, and patient. IEM is used to mimic a focal and transitory virtual lesion to obtain individual functional mapping at both the cortical and subcortical levels, and to test whether a structure involved by a lesion is still crucial for neurologic function—in 15 to 20% of cases in LGG.[18] Therefore, it is possible to decide whether the brain area tested can be removed, according to the induction of transitory functional disturbances (or lack thereof) during its stimulation. Indeed, if IEM of an essential area generates a transient disruption of the task performed by the patient, then this area should be preserved. Thus individualized cortical mapping is obtained before the resection, which can be tailored according to the results of the functional map.[12,17,19,27]

In practice, bipolar electrode tips spaced 5 mm apart and delivering a biphasic current (pulse frequency 60 Hz, single-pulse phase duration 1 msec) is applied to the brain. The current intensity adapted to each patient is determined by progressively increasing the amplitude in 1 mA increments from a baseline of 1 mA until a functional response is elicited, with 4 mA as the upper limit under local anesthesia to avoid the generation of seizures. The patient is never informed when the brain is stimulated. To prevent seizures, no site is stimulated twice in succession. Each cortical site of the entire cortex exposed by the bone flap is tested three times to ensure that the site is crucial for brain function as demonstrated by generation of disturbances during its three stimulations and with normalization of function as soon as the stimulation is stopped.[44,45]

Interestingly, recent series showed that the surgical procedure could be simplified by avoiding the use of intraoperative electrocorticography, despite a reliability equivalent to that of IEM, and without increasing the rate of seizures.[11,37] However, in cases of stimulation-induced seizures, the use of cold Ringer's lactate is recommended to abrogate the seizure activity. In addition, some authors have emphasized the value of "negative mapping" (no identification of eloquent sites) in the setting of a tailored cortical exposure.[46–48] It is worth noting that negative mapping can be dangerous in LGG surgery, especially in nonexpert hands. Indeed, due to the fact that LGG is poorly delineated, the limit of the resection will be essentially guided according to functional criteria. Because negative mapping can be due to false-negative results for methodological reasons, it does not guarantee the absence of eloquent sites. In the experience reported by Sanai et al, 4 of 243 (1.6%) patients who experienced permanent postoperative language deficits had no positive sites detected prior to their resections.[46] In another series with 309 patients who underwent surgeries with IEM, mapping was found to be negative in 109 cases, and 9% of these patients developed a long-term deficit.[47] Taylor and Bernstein previously reported negative mapping in 70% of patients, but 3.6% of them experienced a permanent neurological deficit.[48] Thus negative mapping cannot prevent persistent postsurgical deficit in all cases. For this reason, other authors advocate a wider bone flap to obtain systematic functional responses before the resection.[37,44,45] It is especially recommended to expose the ventral premotor cortex (i.e., the lateral part of the precentral gyrus) in all cases, whatever the location of the tumor. Indeed, by having the patient perform a simple automatic task such as counting, it is possible to systematically induce speech arrest over this area (and thus to identify the optimal threshold of intensity).[37] In other words, "minimally invasive neurosurgery" means "minimal morbidity" and not "minimal bone flap size." *Moreover, positive mapping might also allow optimization of the EoR, given that tumor removal can be pursued until eloquent areas are encountered, that is, with no margin around the functional structures.* A recent study demonstrated that, in a consecutive and homogeneous series of 115 LGGs in the left dominant hemisphere, the rate of permanent deficit remained lower than 2% despite the absence of margin around the language sites.[37] Indeed, Gil-Robles and Duffau showed that the EoR could be dramatically increased by avoiding the preservation of 5 to 10 mm around the functional areas, as usually proposed in the classical literature (**Fig. 5.1**).[36] Interestingly, the authors also showed that it was not logical to leave a small amount of tumor involving the cortex when the resection was performed into areas of contact with white matter pathways at the subcortical level (to be discussed) because the cortical area not removed was in fact disconnected and thus no longer functional.

One of the major advantages of IEM for brain mapping in adult patients is that it *intrinsically* does not cause any false-negatives—if the methodology is rigorously applied as already detailed. Indeed, IEM is highly sensitive for detecting the cortical and axonal eloquent structures, and it also provides a unique opportunity to study brain connectivity because each area responsive to stimulation is in fact an input gate into a large-scale network rather than an isolated discrete functional site.[49]

Intraoperative Functional Monitoring and Test Selection

As mentioned, the selection of intrasurgical tasks to be administrated to the patient is crucial to preserving maximal QoL.[12,17,24,27] Indeed, IEM allows the mapping of many brain functions, such as motor function (by inducing involuntary motor response or disturbance of movement), somatosensory function (by eliciting dysesthesias described by the patient), visual function (by eliciting phosphenes and/or visual field deficits described by the patient), audiovestibular function (by inducing vertigo), language (spontaneous speech, counting, object naming, comprehension, writing, reading, bilingualism, switching from one language to another, etc.), and also the mapping of higher-order functions, such as calculation, memory, spatial cognition, cross-modal judgment, or emotional processing. Therefore, due to the limitation of time (because the patient can be tired at the end of the procedure), intraoperative testing should be adapted to each patient according to several individual parameters (job, hobby, handedness, results of the preoperative neuropsychological examination, location of the tumor, results of the

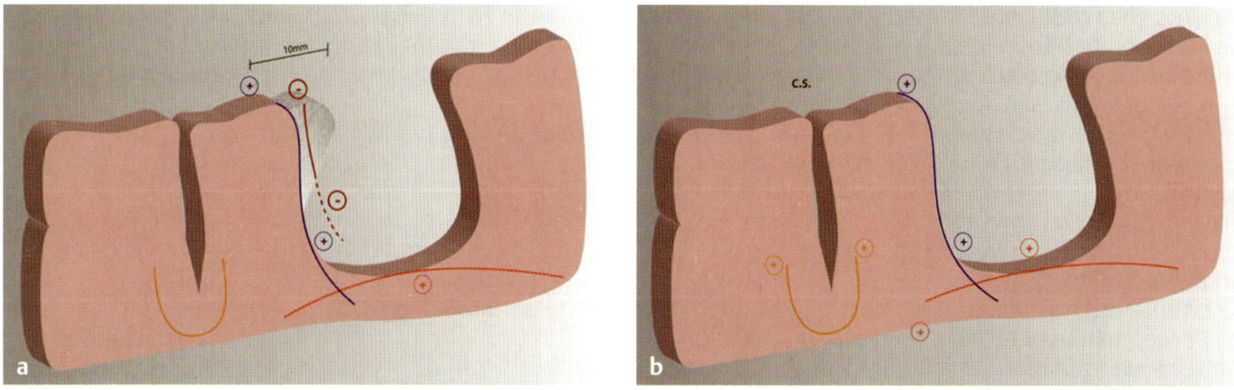

Fig. 5.1 **(a)** Schematic showing a classical resection of a tumor involving eloquent areas, by leaving a 10 mm security margin from the positive cortical stimulation site (*blue +*). If subcortical stimulation is performed, the projection fibers' "vertical connectivity" will be identified at the bottom of the sulcus (*blue +*, e.g., pyramidal tracts). In the depth of the cavity, the "horizontal connectivity" or long-distance association fibers (e.g., arcuate fasciculus) will represent the deep functional subcortical boundary (*red +*). Interestingly, the cortex invaded by the tumor (*in gray*) is functionally useless given that the resection has been pursued until the subcortical pathways have been encountered (*blue and red +*). Thus the fibers arising from this cortex have been disrupted because they do not respond to stimulation (*brown –*). As a consequence, this cortex was disconnected and can therefore be removed with no functional risk. **(b)** Schematic showing the removal of a tumor involving eloquent areas without leaving any margin and using subcortical functional boundaries. Using dissection, the fibers coming from the cortex are found subcortically (the projection fibers, i.e., vertical connectivity, *in blue +*), where the resection is stopped. Again, the horizontal connectivity, namely the long-distance association fibers, represents the other subcortical functional boundaries in the depth of the cavity (e.g., arcuate fasciculus, *red +*). Using this "functional map-guided surgery," the resection is improved in comparison with the classical concept of a 10 mm security margin without eliciting permanent deficit because the eloquent networks have been preserved. (From Teixidor P, Gatignol P, Leroy M, Masuet-Aumatell C, Capelle L, Duffau H. Assessment of verbal working memory before and after surgery for low-grade glioma. J Neurooncol 2007;81(3):305–313. Reprinted with permission.)

preoperative functional neuroimaging), with the goal of mapping the networks underlying the functions that have to be preserved intraoperatively—and to serve as boundaries of the resection.[12,17,24,27] For instance, it can be important to test different languages as well as language switching intrasurgically in multilingual patients, or to map calculation in a school teacher, or spatial cognition in a dancer, or working memory in a manager, or syntax in a writer, or judgment in a lawyer, and so on.[50–54] It means that, in addition to standard tasks, such as counting to induce speech arrest over the ventral premotor cortex (and thus to identify the optimal threshold of intensity), picture naming for lesions located within the "dominant hemisphere," or line bisection task when the glioma involves the right "nondominant" parietal lobe, intraoperative mapping should be personalized.

To this end, it is crucial that a speech therapist/neuropsychologist/neurologist be present in the operating room to interpret accurately the kind of disorders induced by IEM. For example, during a classical naming task, an untrained observer will detect only anomia, whereas an expert in the field of language will detail speech arrest, anarthria, speech apraxia, phonological disturbances, semantic paraphasia, anomia, syntactic errors, or even perseveration due to disturbances of executive control.[55] *In other words, beyond IEM, online cognitive monitoring throughout the resection is essential to optimize the benefit-to-risk ratio of surgery.*

Intraoperative Subcortical Stimulation Mapping: Detection and Preservation of the "Connectome"

In addition to cortical mapping before lesion removal, another major issue is the use of subcortical IEM throughout the resection.[37,44,45,55] Indeed, even if identification of eloquent cortex is crucial, it is definitely not enough in glioma surgery. On the one hand, LGG is known to migrate along white matter tracts, in particular along the long-distance association pathways.[1] Thus, maximization of EoR means that glioma removal should not be stopped prior to contact with these bundles, with no margin.[36,37] On the other hand, unlike the major potential for brain reorganization at the cortical level, subcortical plasticity is very limited.[56] Recently, a probabilistic atlas of functional resectability of LGG was devised based on residual tumor left due to invasion of critical areas, as determined by IEM. Interestingly, a "minimal common brain" was evidenced, that is, a common core among patients that could not be removed, mainly including white matter connectivity and supporting the essential role of these subcortical networks in cerebral processing.[57] This is in agreement with previous brain lesion studies,[56] which have taught that damage of the subcortical tracts generated more severe deficit than cortical injury. Indeed, lesions restricted to white matter can cause dysfunction of large-scale cognitive networks. Therefore, the neurosurgeon should know precisely the fibers that cannot be cut and should be able to identify as well as preserve them in all cases. These include (1) the input and output networks (i.e., the pyramidal, thalamocortical, and optic tracts subserving motor, somatosensory, and visual functions, respectively), (2) the oral and written language networks in the "dominant hemisphere," and (3) the spatial network, generating disturbances of spatial cognition (e.g., hemineglect or vestibular responses) during stimulation (to be discussed in detail later in the chapter).

Interestingly, according to the same principle as already described at the cortical level, IEM can also identify eloquent subcortical structures. It allows the study of the anatomofunctional connectivity by directly and regularly stimulating the white matter tracts and deep gray nuclei throughout the resection, and by eliciting transitory functional disruption when deep crucial areas are being approached. Furthermore, IEM has enabled a better understanding of the "connectome," showing that dynamic cerebral processing was underlain by parallel distributed and interactive networks, the so-called hodotopy (from the Greek *topos* = place and *hodos* = road or path).[58] This connectionist view also opens the door to the concept of cerebral plasticity, which is crucial in LGG surgery.

Yet it is puzzling to note that intrasurgical subcortical mapping was very rarely reported in glioma surgery, and that neurosurgeons began to demonstrate some interest in white matter pathways only after the recent development of DTI, which is not sufficiently reliable, as already discussed. Consequently, different tracts participating in distinct neural functions must be extensively detailed; it is crucial for surgeons to have a good three-dimensional representation of the subcortical bundles in their mental imaging before they operate on the brain (with or without functional neuroimaging). To this end, even if DTI represents an excellent didactic tool with which to learn this complex architecture, neurosurgeons should return to dissection of cadavers, especially the white matter tracts, using the Klinger method.[59,60] Indeed, these bundles can now be dissected in light of the data provided by IEM, especially with regard to the cortical terminations of the subcortical pathways, which are still poorly known.[61,62] Knowledge of relationships between brain structure and function can be successfully applied for a better understanding of the surgical anatomy, as discussed in the following sections.

Motor Pathways

In precentral LGG, after detection and preservation of the primary motor cortex using cortical stimulation, the corresponding descending motor pathways and their somatotopy (i.e., the fibers in the corona radiata, with, from medial to lateral, the pyramidal tracts of the lower limb, upper limb, and face) should be identified using subcortical IEM and should be spared.[63] The pyramidal pathways may also be detected within the posterior limb of the internal capsule, representing the deep boundaries for temporal or (fronto-)temporoinsular paralimbic gliomas.[64] Interestingly, the existence of a "motor negative network" eliciting movement arrest when stimulated, and involved in motor control, has recently been evidenced.[43]

Somatosensory Tracts

In retrocentral LGGs, the thalamocortical somatosensory pathways and their somatotopy must be detected by IEM, which generates dysesthesias or tingling in awake patients.[63,65] Of note, stimulation of the white matter under the retrocentral gyrus may also induce disturbances in movement control, likely due to transient inhibition of U fibers within the rolandic region.[43]

Optic Radiations

Visual pathways should be mapped in awake patients operated on for a temporo-(occipito)-parietal glioma. Their stimulation may generate a "shadow" (negative effect) or phosphenes (positive effect) in the contralateral visual field, sometimes associated with metamorphopsia (i.e., visual illusion).[66] However, due to the subjectivity of the response, it was recently proposed to use a picture-naming task, with presentation of two objects situated diagonally on a screen divided into four quadrants. An image was presented in the quadrant to save and another image was presented in the opposite quadrant. Using this specific test, in a consecutive series of 14 patients (including 12 LGGs), visual symptoms were elicited in all cases during IEM. These disturbances led the surgeon to stop the tumor resection at this level. Postoperatively, one patient had a permanent hemianopsia, despite an expected quadrantanopsia in 12 cases, with a mean EoR of 93.6%. These original findings showed that online identification of optic radiations is a reliable and effective method by which to avoid hemianopsia in surgery for LGGs involving visual pathways. Patients can be left with only a residual quadrantanopsia without consequence to the QoL, especially for driving.[67]

Language Pathways

In precentral LGGs within the dominant hemisphere, after identification of the motor and language cortical sites in the ventral premotor cortex and eventually in the (middle and inferior) frontal gyri, IEM may allow the detection of the language pathways (**Fig. 5.2**). Medially, subcortical mapping can identify the fasciculus subcallosal medialis (running from the supplementary motor area and cingulate gyrus to the head of the caudate nucleus), which induces a transient transcortical motor aphasia during its stimulation because this tract is involved in the initiation of language.[68] It seems that this fascicle could correspond to the indirect pathway of the frontal aslant tract.[69] Posteriorly, the tract coming from the premotor ventral cortex must be detected and spared because it is crucial for speech production: its stimulation generates dysarthria or complete anarthria with a high level of reproducibility.[70] More laterally, the operculoinsular connections should also be identified by eliciting a complete speech arrest during IEM: these connections are involved in speech planning.[71]

In addition to these locoregional language pathways, subcortical IEM also enables the detection of long-distance association pathways, first with the deep part of the superior longitudinal fasciculus—the so-called arcuate fasciculus (AF).[68] In patients with an LGG involving the dominant insula or inferior frontal gyrus, subcortical IEM can identify the anterior part of AF, running within the anterior floor of the external capsule (under the superior part of the insula) to go to the posterior portion of the inferior and middle frontal gyri.[65,68] IEM generates transitory symptoms observed in conduction aphasia, that is, phonemic paraphasia and repetition disturbances. AF must also be detected at the level of its posterosuperior loop, located under the supramarginal gyrus, in patients operated on for a parietal LGG within the dominant hemisphere.[65] The same symptoms combining phonemic paraphasias and repetition disorders are elicited with reproducibility, without any semantic paraphasia.[72] In the same vein, AF should constitute the deep limit of resection in temporal LGGs within the dominant side because the inferior and middle temporal gyri correspond to the posterior cortical terminations of the long segment of AF. Thus, the posterior part of its posterior funiculus should represent the anterior functional limit of resection in posterior temporal LGGs, and the anterior part of the anterior funiculus of AF should be used as

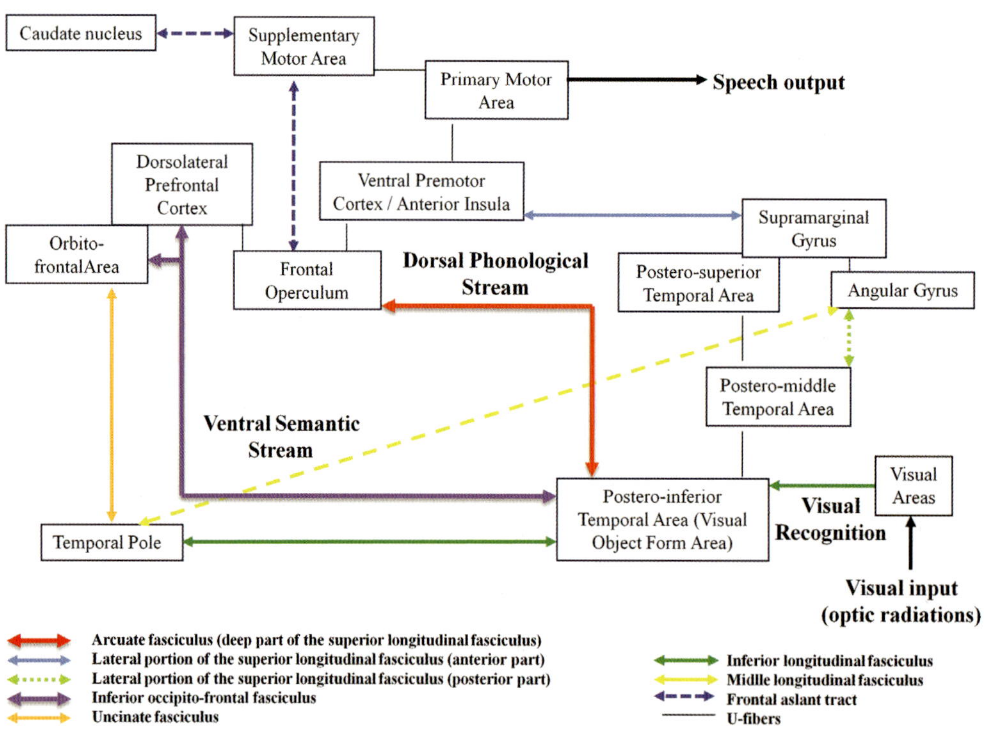

Fig. 5.2 Proposal of a hodotopical model of language, with incorporation of anatomical constraints, elaborated on the basis of structural–functional correlations provided by intraoperative corticosubcortical electrostimulation mapping. (From Duffau H, ed. Brain Mapping: From Neural Basis of Cognition to Surgical Applications. New York, NY: Springer; 2011. Modified with permission.)

the posterior functional boundary in anterior and midtemporal LGGs. Interestingly, dominant AF also appears to subserve a wide network involved in language switching (from a native language to another language or vice versa). Its IEM may disrupt such function, which is important to detect and to spare in bilingual patients.[50,73] More recently, grammatical gender errors were induced by axonal stimulation of the dominant AF, supporting the possible role of this pathway (connecting the middle temporal gyrus and the inferior frontal gyrus, themselves inducing the same grammatical disturbances when stimulated) in syntactic processing.[54]

In addition to the AF, the lateral part of the superior longitudinal fasciculus is important to preserve. In retrocentral suprasylvian LGGs involving the dominant hemisphere, after detection of the language cortical sites over the ventral premotor cortex (in front of the tumor) and over the supramarginal gyrus and/or angular gyrus (behind the tumor), IEM of the corresponding frontoparietal subcortical network generates speech apraxia.[65] This operculo-opercular loop, called "the lateral part of the superior longitudinal fasciculus, part III," constitutes the anterior segment of the indirect pathway of the dorsal phonological stream, which runs parallel and lateral to the AF, by connecting the Broca area with the inferior parietal lobe Geschwind territory, as recently shown by DTI as well as by anatomical dissection.[62,74] This subcomponent of the superior longitudinal fasciculus should be preserved during surgery because it seems to represent the neural basis of verbal working memory.[62]

In parallel, subcortical IEM also demonstrated the crucial role of the inferior fronto-occipital fasciculus (IFOF) in the "ventral semantic route," by eliciting reproducible semantic paraphasia when stimulated.[55] In frontal LGGs involving the dominant hemisphere, especially in tumors located within the pars orbitaris of the inferior frontal gyrus and the dorsolateral prefrontal area, the anterior part of the IFOF should be detected and should represent the deep boundaries. Indeed, a recent anatomical study combining dissection and DTI showed that IFOF had five anterior cortical terminations: the inferior frontal gyrus, middle frontal gyrus, dorsolateral prefrontal cortex, orbitofrontal cortex, and frontal pole.[61] IFOF must also be identified throughout resection for insular DLGGs in the dominant side by inducing the same symptoms (semantic paraphasias) during IEM of its intermediate part located in the anterior floor of the external capsule (in front and inferior to the AF, and behind and superior to the uncinate fasciculus), that is, in the temporal stem.[59] Again, the IFOF should be detected in temporal LGGs (semantic disorders when stimulated) because it represents the deep limit of the resection (above the roof of the temporal horn of the ventricle).[55] Of note, the IFOF seems also to be involved in visual-verbal incongruence judgment.[53]

A recent series specifically dedicated to the study of occipital LGGs showed that, at least in the dominant hemisphere, both the AF and the IFOF may represent the deep and anterior boundaries of the resection when an extensive occipital lobectomy has been decided.[75]

Interestingly, IEM of the anterior part of the inferior longitudinal fasciculus, in front of the visual object form area (i.e., the basal part of the temporo-occipital junction, involved in high-level visual processing such as reading),[76] as well as IEM of the uncinate fasciculus,[77] never generated language disturbances, at least during the picture-naming test—even if the uncinate fasciculus was, as recently described, likely involved in proper name retrieval.[78] In the same way, IEM of the anterior part of the middle longitudinal fasciculus (i.e., a pathway connecting the angular gyrus to the temporal pole and running under the superior temporal sulcus) seems not to generate language disturbances.[79] In practice, it means that these fasciculi can be removed without aphasia in temporal LGGs involving the dominant hemisphere. This indirect pathway from the temporo-occipital areas to the prefrontal region, with a relay in the temporal pole (temporo-occipital area, inferior longitudinal fasciculus, temporal pole, uncinate fasciculus, orbitofrontal, and prefrontal areas) might be compensated by the direct pathway constituted by the IFOF.[76] However, the posterior part of the inferior longitudinal fasciculus should be preserved in temporo-occipital LGGs because it plays a crucial role in reading, as demonstrated by IEM, which elicited reproducible visual paraphasia and dyslexia.[80]

Of note, beyond the stimulation of the white matter, IEM of the deep gray nuclei is important when they are involved by an LGG. Stimulation of the head of the dominant caudate in a frontomesial glioma in contact with the deep striatum generates perseverations, namely the repetition of the previous item when the next item is presented to the patient. These data support an inhibitory role of the caudate in the control of cognition.[81] Furthermore, at the end of the resection of insular LGGs on the dominant side, IEM of the lateral part of the lentiform nucleus induces anarthria,[82] supporting the likely role of this structure in the planning of articulation, in association with the insula and ventral premotor cortex.[70,71]

Finally, it is crucial to underline the need for intraoperative cortical and subcortical language mapping for patients with LGGs in the right hemisphere when they are left-handed or ambidextrous.[83] Due to bilateral mirror representation of speech in both hemispheres, this should also be considered in a small fraction of right-handed patients.[22]

Pathways Underlying Spatial Cognition

In LGGs involving the right ("nondominant") parietotemporal junction, IEM must also map the white matter tracts implied in spatial awareness to avoid postoperative left-sided neglect. To this end, it is possible to use a line-bisection task in awake patients. During the stimulation of the lateral part (part II) of the superior longitudinal fasciculus, a significant rightward deviation is observed.[52] IEM of the right superior longitudinal fasciculus may also induce vertigo by disrupting a large network between the parietoinsular vestibular cortex and the visual and sensorimotor areas.[84]

Interestingly, although mapping of the commissural white matter pathways has been performed, no functional responses were elicited by IEM of the corpus callosum. Such results have allowed resection of LGGs involving this structure without any consequence to the QoL, whatever the location of the "callosectomy."[85]

In all cases except with regard to the corpus callosum, these functional bundles should constitute the subcortical functional limits of the resection. However, this list of tracts is not exhaustive. Indeed, the functional connectivity underlying emotional and behavioral processing is currently poorly known. Furthermore, the role of some pathways is still unclear, as for instance the role of the middle longitudinal fasciculus.[23]

In summary, it is mandatory to map both horizontal corticocortical connectivity (long-distance association fibers) as well as vertical corticosubcortical connectivity (projection fibers), with the aim to preserve the networks underlying the "minimal common core" of the brain. Consequently, from a practical point of view, removal of voluminous LGGs infiltrating several subcortical bundles can be performed without the use of a microscope. Indeed, the main risk in this kind of surgery, except for vascular injury, is to cut the connectome. Therefore, it is important in the depth of the resection to have a global three-dimensional view of the surgical field, and not to focus on a specific point, in order to anticipate when the subcortical IEM must be begun. It may also be recommended to systematically use the same lateral position for each patient, whatever the location of the glioma (given that it is possible to access frontal, parietal, temporal, insular, and even occipital tumors in this position), in order for the neurosurgeon to keep the same mental reconstruction of the different fibers from one patient to the next without introducing any confounding factor, such as head rotation. Interestingly, the Cavitron Ultrasonic Surgical Aspirator (CUSA, Integra Life Sciences, Plainsboro, NJ) may represent an additional mapping tool within the white matter because it can induce transient functional disturbances that are confirmed afterward by stimulation. This interference with mapping might be interpreted as a transitory inhibition of axonal conduction due to a mechanical distortion of fibers.[86] This important point means that, when the patient is awake and performs continuously the tasks throughout the tumor removal, it is not mandatory to stimulate regularly, but instead, only when the resection arrives close to the functional pathways (information that is given online thanks to cognitive feedback from the patient, the transient disturbances induced by the CUSA, and knowledge of the white matter anatomy). In other words, it is possible to avoid wasting time by using subcortical IEM to find the deep eloquent structures only at the end of the procedure. Time is precious in awake surgery because the patient can be tired after 1 to 2 hours of resection. In the same way, with a voluminous glioma (e.g., a frontotemporoinsular tumor), time can be saved by first identifying the cortical boundaries, then performing a subpial dissection to the point of contact with the eloquent structures until reaching the depth of the sulci, and finally, upon arriving within the white matter pathways, continuing tumor removal until functional fibers have been identified. If this technique is applied all around the glioma, once the area of the brain invaded by the tumor has been "disconnected," it is possible to put the patient under general anesthesia and to take all the time needed to finish the resection (especially when vessels, such as the sylvian fissure, are encountered, which do not require the participation of the patient). Using this method, the patient is awake only to provide the surgeon with the functional boundaries of the resection. This implies that surgeons should no longer begin tumor removal in "noneloquent" areas and progress toward functional areas; they should instead begin resection near the critical structures.[27]

Finally, it is worth noting that, for deep LGGs, a shorter trajectory is not always the safer approach. In some cases, it can be preferable to select a more complex surgical approach to avoid cutting functional pathways, based on the results of intrasurgical cortical and subcortical IEM.

■ Functional and Oncological Outcomes: The Significant Contribution of Intraoperative Electrostimulation Mapping

In the past decade, IEM has led to impressive improvements in functional and oncological results for LGG surgery.

First, patients who were classically not selected for surgery on the basis of pure anatomical criteria (e.g., gliomas involving the precentral gyrus or the pars opercularis of the left inferior frontal gyrus) can now benefit from resection regardless of the tumor location. In particular, it has been demonstrated that IEM allows significantly increased surgical indications for LGGs involving so-called eloquent areas, based on comparison with a control group of patients who underwent resection under general anesthesia with no mapping.[11] For example, surgical resection is possible with no permanent neurological worsening for LGGs located within the Broca area, Wernicke area, insula, left dominant inferior parietal lobule, retrocentral area, and even the precentral gyrus.[18,19,35,64,65,71,87] In practice, it means that LGG resection is contraindicated in cases of very diffuse glioma ("gliomatosis-like"), especially when the tumor has invaded both hemispheres through the corpus callosum. In these cases, neoadjuvant chemotherapy can be proposed to induce tumor shrinkage and thereby allow consideration of subsequent surgical resection.[88]

Second, despite an increased number of surgeries in critical regions, the rate of permanent neurological deficits was shown to be significantly lower thanks to awake mapping (i.e., less than 2% in the recent series using IEM). Interestingly, this rate of less than 2% of permanent deficits is very reproducible among the teams using awake mapping worldwide.[37,46] In comparison, in series that did not use awake mapping, the rate of sequelae ranged from 13 to 27.5%, with a mean around 19%.[11] In other words, despite a frequent transitory neurological worsening in the immediate postoperative period (due to maximal tumor removal according to corticosubcortical functional limits using IEM, leading to a specific functional rehabilitation), *more than 98% of patients recovered their presurgical status after LGG resection within eloquent brain areas guided by IEM and returned to normal social and professional lives.*[37] Furthermore, beyond the fact that surgery is able to *preserve* brain functions, a new concept is to emphasize its possibility to *increase* the QoL by removing an LGG, as demonstrated by extensive neurocognitive assessment performed after surgical resection.[20,21,88] This can be explained by a relief of seizures after resection in at least 80% of patients who suffered from preoperative intractable epilepsy. In particular, with the aim of optimizing the control of seizures in intractable epilepsy due to paralimbic LGGs, it was recently suggested to systematically remove the mesiotemporal structures, even if not invaded by the tumor.[89] In addition, an objective improvement in high-order functions, such as working memory, was observed in more than 30% of patients, especially following a personalized cognitive rehabilitation.[20]

Third, it could be argued that the use of IEM, even if it enables preservation of, or improvement in, the QoL, might prevent optimal removal of an LGG. In fact, a comparative study between LGG resection performed without or with intrasurgical stimulation showed that the EoR was significantly increased thanks to IEM, with better functional results following resection within eloquent areas.[11] Interestingly, a recent study reported for the first time a series of patients who underwent two consecutive surgeries without and with awake mapping. Nine patients underwent surgery for an LGG in functional sites under general anesthesia in other institutions. The resection was subtotal in three cases and partial in six cases. There was a postoperative worsening in three cases. A second surgery was then performed in the awake condition with IEM (resection according to functional boundaries at cortical and subcortical levels). Postoperative MRI showed that the resection was complete in five cases and subtotal in four cases (no partial removal) and that EoR was significantly improved in all cases in comparison with the first surgery. There was no permanent neurological worsening. Three patients improved compared with the presurgical status. All patients returned to normal professional and social lives. These original results demonstrate that awake surgery with IEM, known to preserve the QoL in patients with LGG, is also able to significantly improve the EoR for lesions located in functional regions.[90] Recently, because it is now well known that isolated tumoral cells exist beyond the signal abnormality visible on FLAIR-weighted MRI scans of LGGs, it was proposed to remove not only the FLAIR hypersignal but also an additional margin according to functional boundaries, to achieve a "supratotal" resection.[26] For example, in a frontopolar LGG involving the left "dominant hemisphere," a supratotal resection consists of performing a left lobectomy until—but not before—functional cortical and subcortical structures have been encountered (**Fig. 5.3**). Interestingly, the rate of anaplastic transformation was significantly lower in a series of supratotal resections of LGGs when compared with a control group of patients who underwent "only" a complete resection (i.e., removal of only the FLAIR-weighted MRI abnormality).[26]

Last but not least, the group at the University of California–San Francisco demonstrated for the first time in a series of 281 patients that the use of functional mapping–guided resection of LGGs in presumed eloquent areas, thanks to a reliable intraoperative delineation of true functional and nonfunctional regions, allowed not only a maximization of tumor resection but also a significant improvement of long-term survival.[91] This is in agreement with the literature on LGG resection, which shows a direct relationship between the EoR and median survival in all series with accurate calculation of the volume of residual tumor using objective postoperative FLAIR-weighted MRI.[4]

Interestingly, reoperation was also demonstrated to have a significant impact on overall survival in LGG resection, without a higher risk of permanent deficits, including tumors resected within eloquent areas,[92] thanks to mechanisms of brain plasticity that can occur between two surgeries.[18,39]

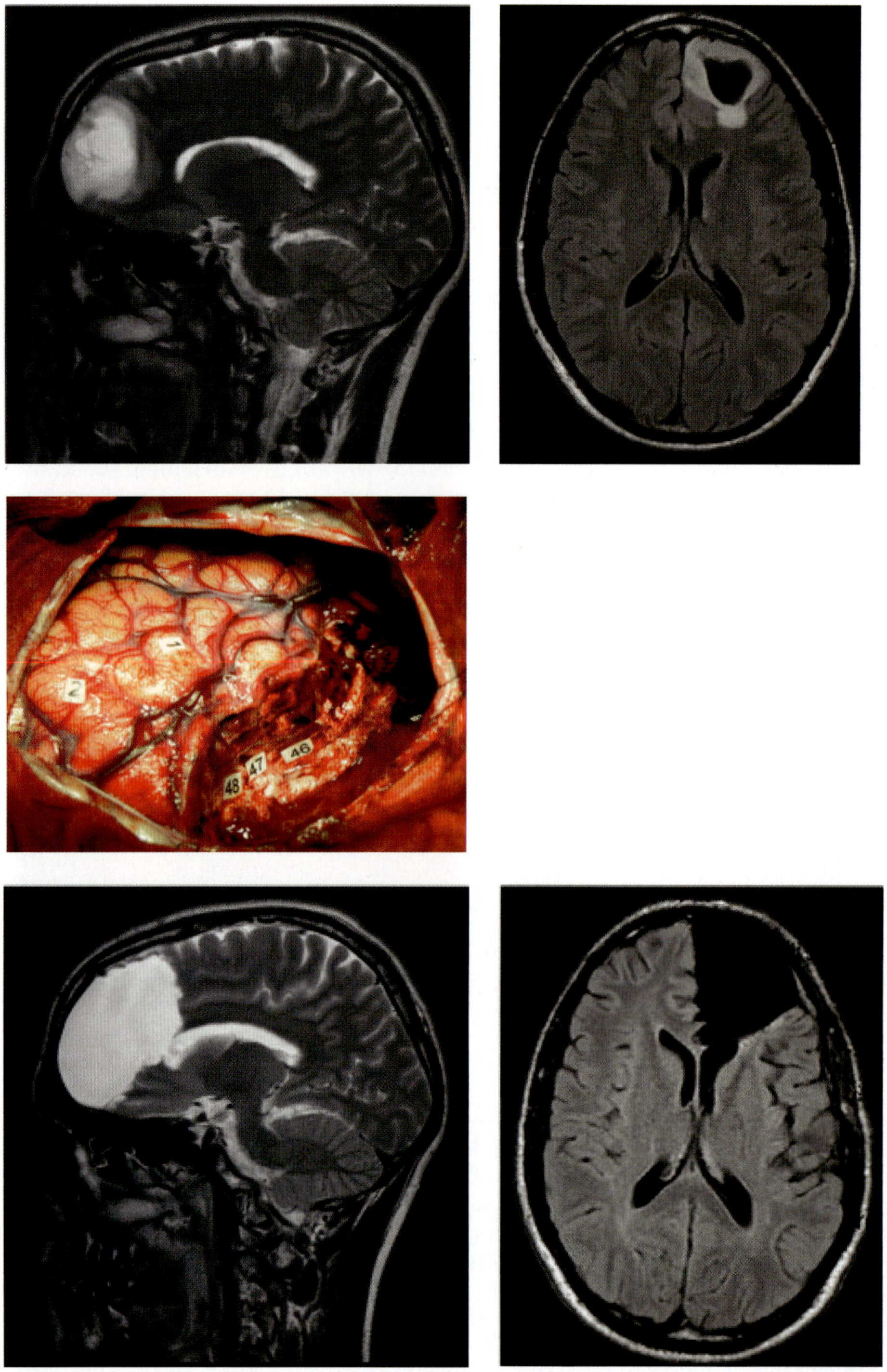

Fig. 5.3 **(a)** Preoperative sagittal T2-weighted and axial fluid-attenuated inversion recovery (FLAIR)-weighted magnetic resonance imaging (MRI) showing a diffuse low-grade glioma located in a “nonfunctional” area (i.e., the left frontal pole) in a patient with no neurological deficit except very mild disturbances of the verbal episodic memory detected by an extensive neuropsychological assessment. It should be noted that the tumor was far from the ventricle. **(b)** Intraoperative photograph after resection performed under local anesthesia. The resection was performed according to functional boundaries identified using intraoperative electrostimulation mapping (IEM) at the cortical (1: ventral premotor cortex inducing speech arrest when stimulated; 2: primary motor cortex of the face) and the subcortical levels (46: phonemic paraphasia due to the stimulation of the anterior part of the superior longitudinal fasciculus; 47: perseveration during stimulation of the head of the caudate nucleus; 48: fibers coming from the ventral premotor cortex eliciting speech arrest during stimulation). **(c)** Postoperative sagittal T2-weighted and axial FLAIR-weighted MRI showing a supratotal resection of the glioma. Note the large opening of the ventricle, demonstrating that a margin was taken around the MRI-defined abnormalities. The patient returned to a normal social and professional life, with no deficit and no seizures. (From Yordanova Y, Moritz-Gasser S, Duffau H. Awake surgery for WHO grade II gliomas within “noneloquent” areas in the left dominant hemisphere: toward a “supratotal” resection. J Neurosurg 2011;115(2):232–239.)

■ The Next Step: Individual Functional Brain Remapping after Initial Resection

In the past decade, numerous observations of dramatic recovery following massive resection of brain regions invaded by LGGs have been reported.[18,19,93] Such functional compensation was attributed to cerebral plasticity, namely, the continuous process allowing short-, middle-, and long-term remodeling of the neuronosynaptic maps to optimize the functionality of brain networks.[15,94] Beyond the evidence of intraoperative acute remapping using repeated electrostimulation throughout the resection (likely due to the unmasking of redundancies), noninvasive functional neuroimaging allows the additional study of mechanisms of reshaping before and after surgical resection.[95] Preoperatively, different patterns of redistribution have been described in LGGs, with (1) activations within the tumor, due to the infiltrative feature of DLGGs; (2) perilesional reorganization; (3) recruitment of remote areas within the ipsilesional hemisphere; (4) recruitment of homologous regions in the contralateral hemisphere; and (5) association of these different mechanisms.[18,93,94] Interestingly, longitudinal studies based on serial functional imaging after the surgery showed new degrees of reshaping, as a probable consequence of tumor removal as well as adapted postoperative individualized functional rehabilitation. For example, functional neuroimaging performed following the recovery of a transient postsurgical supplementary motor area syndrome showed the compensatory recruitment of the contralesional supplementary motor area and premotor area.[95] A "jump" of perilesional activation was also reported following LGG resection, for instance from the precentral sulcus to the central sulcus in tumors involving the premotor region.[39]

This improved knowledge of plasticity phenomena has led to proposed reoperation(s) when, due to the involvement of eloquent areas, the resection was not complete at the end of the previous surgery. Thanks to functional reshaping (verified using IEM), it was possible to increase the EoR during a second and even during a third surgery, while preserving brain functions (**Fig. 5.4**).[92] Therefore, a multistage surgical approach made possible maximal LGG removal in critical regions traditionally considered unresectable, such as the central area, Broca area, Wernicke area, and insular lobe (even in the left "dominant" hemisphere).[18,19,35,64,65,71,93,94]

However, it is important to again insist on the fact that extensive resections with no neurological consequences can be achieved only when the essential subcortical connectivity is preserved—in a "hodotopical," rather than a "localizational," view of brain organization.[17,58,96]

Expert Recommendations

1. Image-guided surgery based on T2/fluid-attenuated inversion recovery (FLAIR) signal change or contrast enhancement is based on a reductionist concept; active tumor exists beyond this signal change and should be included as part of the resection without incurring any neurological deficit (Grade 2C Recommendation, Level III/IV Evidence).
2. Functional neuroimaging methods are not reliable enough to ensure safe surgical resection of eloquent cortex lesions (Grade 1C Recommendation, Level III/IV Evidence).
3. Contrary to traditional beliefs, low-grade gliomas can still involve eloquent cortical structures and white fiber tracts as opposed to displacing them—highlighting the importance of intraoperative mapping (Grade 1 Recommendation, Level III/IV Evidence).
4. Intraoperative mapping can permit "supratotal" resection as opposed to gross total resection based on functional limitations (Grade 1C Recommendation, Level III/IV Evidence).
5. Intraoperative mapping has now rendered patients with eloquent cortex low-grade gliomas candidates for surgery with acceptable neurological and oncological results (Grade 1C Recommendation, Level III/IV Evidence).
6. Extremely infiltrative, "gliomatosis-like," low-grade gliomas are still not candidates for surgical resection despite the growing role of intraoperative mapping (Grade 1C Recommendation, Level III Evidence).
7. Studies demonstrate improved extent of resection (EoR), neurological function, and quality of life for eloquent cortex low-grade gliomas resected with intraoperative mapping versus those resected without such techniques. In these patients, improved EoR has also been linked with improved long-term survival (Grade 1C+ Recommendation, Level II/III Evidence).

■ Summary and Conclusions

In summary, recent technological and conceptual advances have enabled early surgical resection of LGGs according to functional (rather than oncological) boundaries provided by pre- and intraoperative methods of individual mapping at cortical and subcortical levels, in a hodotopical and plastic view of brain processing. This has allowed a dramatic improvement in the benefit-to-risk ratio of surgery. A recent meta-analysis of IEM's impact on glioma surgery outcome in a population of 8,091 adult patients demonstrated that glioma resections using IEM were

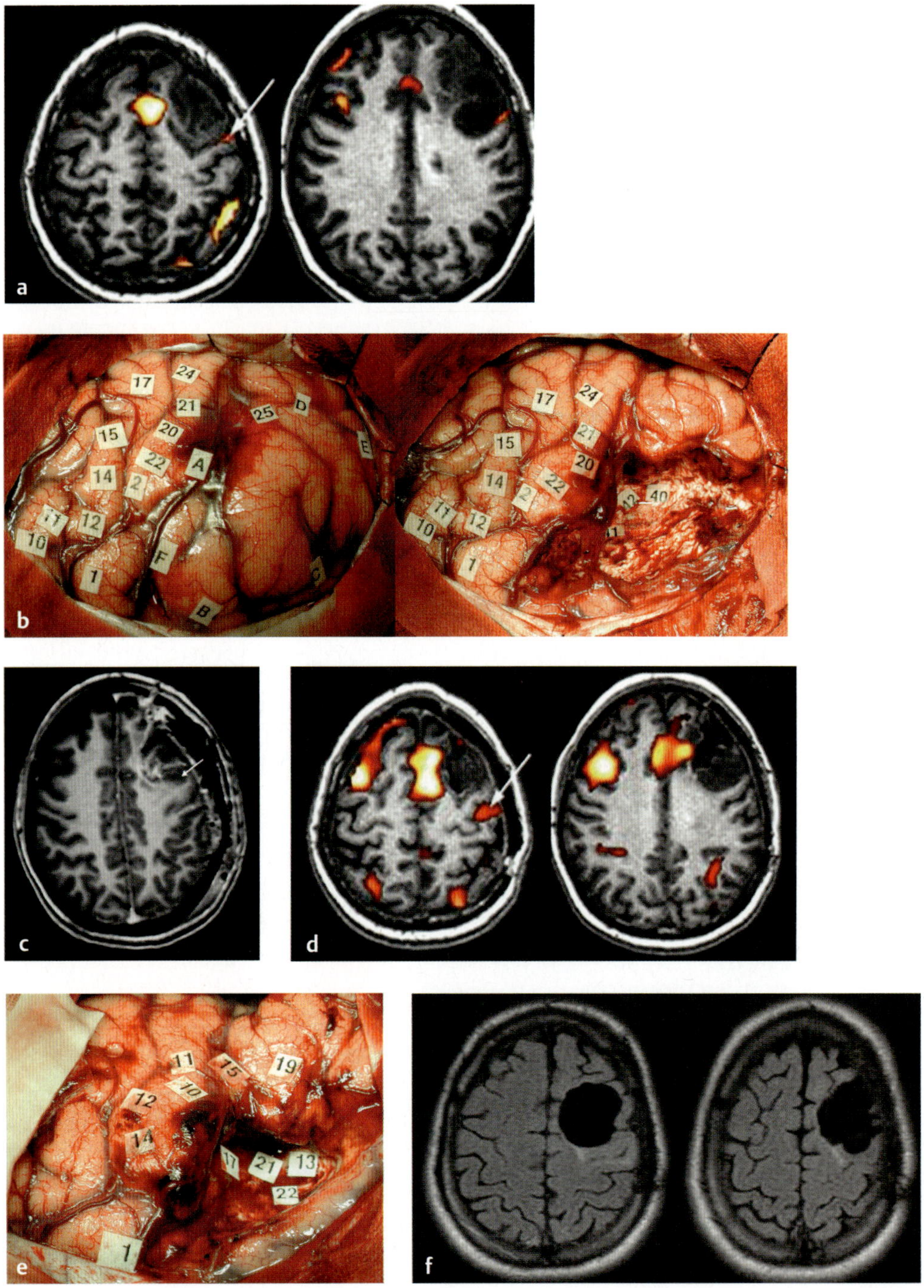

Fig. 5.4 Illustration of the multiple-stage surgical approach. **(a)** Preoperative language functional magnetic resonance imaging (fMRI) scan in a patient without deficit, bearing a low-grade glioma involving the left premotor area. Language activation was very close to the posterior part of the tumor (*arrow*). **(b)** Intraoperative views before (*left*) and after (*right*) resection of the glioma, delineated by letter tags. Intraoperative electrostimulation mapping (IEM) shows a reshaping of the eloquent maps, with a recruitment of perilesional language sites, allowing a subtotal resection with, nevertheless, a posterior residue due to invasion of crucial areas (number tags). **(c)** Immediate postoperative enhanced T1-weighted MRI showing the residue (*arrow*). **(d)** Postoperative language fMRI 4 years after the first fMRI, showing a recruitment of the contralateral hemisphere, and the posterior displacement of activation previously located at the posterior border of the tumor (*arrow*). **(e)** Intraoperative view during the second surgery, confirming the remapping and allowing a more extensive tumor resection with no permanent deficit. **(f)** Postoperative axial fluid-attenuated inversion recovery (FLAIR)-weighted MRI showing the improvement of the extent of resection thanks to functional reshaping, in a patient with a normal neurological examination and enjoying a normal life. (From Duffau H, ed. Brain Mapping: From Neural Basis of Cognition to Surgical Applications. New York, NY: Springer; 2011. Modified with permission.)

significantly associated with fewer late severe neurological deficits and more extensive resection, even while more frequently involving eloquent locations.[42] *This indicates that IEM should be universally implemented as the standard of care for glioma surgery.*[42]

It is time to move toward functional neuro-oncology and prophylactic neurosurgery in cases of LGG. Indeed, on the basis of these optimized results of LGG surgery, it was recently proposed to perform resection in asymptomatic patients in whom LGG has been incidentally discovered.[97,98] To this end, stronger interaction with the fundamental neurosciences should be developed to (1) build updated models of cognition and brain plasticity, (2) elaborate biomathematical models of LGG growth and migration, and (3) study the dynamic interactions between the natural course of a disease (LGG) and the adaptive behavior of its host (the brain), with the goal being the best individualized therapeutic strategy for each patient. Such a link between cognitive/behavioral neurosciences (studying the neural basis of cerebral functions resulting from a combination of anatomy, functional mapping, and cognitive models) and oncological neurosurgery would begin to address the classical dilemma—survival versus brain functions—by enabling more ambitious resection that increases the overall survival and preserves (or even improves) the QoL of patients with LGGs. However, this evolution requires brain surgeons to reorient their thinking from operating on a tumor mass within the brain to operating on a nervous system that is involved by a chronic tumoral disease. In other words, neurosurgeons should see first the brain, and not the glioma, to adapt the surgical procedure to the anatomofunctional organization of each patient. This implies that brain surgeons must also change to a surgical technique within, rather than outside of, the central nervous system.

Therefore, in all cases, the purpose of brain surgery should be to achieve the optimal EoR associated with the best QoL by preserving both basic and higher neurological functions (i.e., emotional and executive functions). To this end, awake surgery with IEM should be systematically used, even in presumed noneloquent areas. This seems to be the most effective route toward a modern and personalized functional surgical neuro-oncology.

■ References

1. Mandonnet E, Capelle L, Duffau H. Extension of paralimbic low grade gliomas: toward an anatomical classification based on white matter invasion patterns. J Neurooncol 2006;78(2):179–185
2. Mandonnet E, Pallud J, Clatz O, et al. Computational modeling of the WHO grade II glioma dynamics: principles and applications to management paradigm. Neurosurg Rev 2008;31(3):263–269
3. Pallud J, Mandonnet E, Duffau H, et al. Prognostic value of initial magnetic resonance imaging growth rates for World Health Organization grade II gliomas. Ann Neurol 2006;60(3):380–383
4. Duffau H. Surgery of low-grade gliomas: towards a 'functional neurooncology'. Curr Opin Oncol 2009;21(6):543–549
5. Smith JS, Chang EF, Lamborn KR, et al. Role of extent of resection in the long-term outcome of low-grade hemispheric gliomas. J Clin Oncol 2008;26(8):1338–1345
6. Soffietti R, Baumert BG, Bello L, et al; European Federation of Neurological Societies. Guidelines on management of low-grade gliomas: report of an EFNS-EANO Task Force. Eur J Neurol 2010;17(9):1124–1133
7. Pallud J, Fontaine D, Duffau H, et al. Natural history of incidental World Health Organization grade II gliomas. Ann Neurol 2010;68(5):727–733
8. Mandonnet E, Duffau H, Bauchet L. A new tool for grade II glioma studies: plotting cumulative time with quality of life versus time to malignant transformation. J Neurooncol 2012;106(1):213–215
9. Duffau H, Capelle L. Preferential brain locations of low-grade gliomas. Cancer 2004;100(12):2622–2626
10. Parisot S, Duffau H, Chemouny S, Paragios N. Graph based spatial position mapping of low-grade gliomas. Med Image Comput Comput Assist Interv 2011;14(Pt 2):508–515
11. Duffau H, Lopes M, Arthuis F, et al. Contribution of intraoperative electrical stimulations in surgery of low grade gliomas: a comparative study between two series without (1985-96) and with (1996-2003) functional mapping in the same institution. J Neurol Neurosurg Psychiatry 2005;76(6):845–851
12. Duffau H. The challenge to remove diffuse low-grade gliomas while preserving brain functions. Acta Neurochir (Wien) 2012;154(4):569–574
13. Vigneau M, Beaucousin V, Hervé PY, et al. Meta-analyzing left hemisphere language areas: phonology, semantics, and sentence processing. Neuroimage 2006;30(4):1414–1432
14. Ojemann G, Ojemann J, Lettich E, Berger MS. Cortical language localization in left, dominant hemisphere: an electrical stimulation mapping investigation in 117 patients. J Neurosurg 1989;71(3):316–326
15. Desmurget M, Bonnetblanc F, Duffau H. Contrasting acute and slow-growing lesions: a new door to brain plasticity. Brain 2007;130(Pt 4):898–914
16. Pouratian N, Bookheimer SY. The reliability of neuroanatomy as a predictor of eloquence: a review. Neurosurg Focus 2010;28(2):E3
17. Duffau H, ed. Brain Mapping: From Neural Basis of Cognition to Surgical Applications. New York, NY: Springer; 2011
18. Duffau H. Lessons from brain mapping in surgery for low-grade glioma: insights into associations between tumour and brain plasticity. Lancet Neurol 2005;4(8):476–486
19. Duffau H. New concepts in surgery of WHO grade II gliomas: functional brain mapping, connectionism and plasticity—a review. J Neurooncol 2006;79(1):77–115
20. Teixidor P, Gatignol P, Leroy M, Masuet-Aumatell C, Capelle L, Duffau H. Assessment of verbal working memory before and after surgery for low-grade glioma. J Neurooncol 2007;81(3):305–313
21. Klein M, Duffau H, De Witt Hamer PC. Cognition and resective surgery for diffuse infiltrative glioma: an overview. J Neurooncol 2012;108(2):309–318
22. Vassal M, Le Bars E, Moritz-Gasser S, Menjot N, Duffau H. Crossed aphasia elicited by intraoperative cortical and subcortical stimulation in awake patients. J Neurosurg 2010;113(6):1251–1258
23. Moritz-Gasser S, Herbet G, Maldonado IL, Duffau H. Lexical access speed is significantly correlated with the return to professional activities after awake surgery for low-grade gliomas. J Neurooncol 2012;107(3):633–641
24. Duffau H. Awake surgery for nonlanguage mapping. Neurosurgery 2010;66(3):523–528

25. Pallud J, Varlet P, Devaux B, et al. Diffuse low-grade oligodendrogliomas extend beyond MRI-defined abnormalities. Neurology 2010;74(21):1724–1731
26. Yordanova YN, Moritz-Gasser S, Duffau H. Awake surgery for WHO grade II gliomas within "noneloquent" areas in the left dominant hemisphere: toward a "supratotal" resection. Clinical article. J Neurosurg 2011;115(2):232–239
27. Duffau H. A new concept of diffuse (low-grade) glioma surgery. Adv Tech Stand Neurosurg 2012;38:3–27
28. Pillai JJ. The evolution of clinical functional imaging during the past 2 decades and its current impact on neurosurgical planning. AJNR Am J Neuroradiol 2010;31(2):219–225
29. Ganslandt O, Grummich P, Nimsky C. Multimodal functional neuronavigation and intraoperative imaging. In: Duffau H, ed. Brain Mapping: From Neural Basis of Cognition to Surgical Applications. New York, NY: Springer; 2011:277–286
30. Bartos R, Jech R, Vymazal J, et al. Validity of primary motor area localization with fMRI versus electric cortical stimulation: a comparative study. Acta Neurochir (Wien) 2009;151(9):1071–1080
31. Giussani C, Roux FE, Ojemann J, Sganzerla EP, Pirillo D, Papagno C. Is preoperative functional magnetic resonance imaging reliable for language areas mapping in brain tumor surgery? Review of language functional magnetic resonance imaging and direct cortical stimulation correlation studies. Neurosurgery 2010;66(1):113–120
32. Ulmer JL, Krouwer HG, Mueller WM, Ugurel MS, Kocak M, Mark LP. Pseudo-reorganization of language cortical function at fMR imaging: a consequence of tumor-induced neurovascular uncoupling. AJNR Am J Neuroradiol 2003;24(2):213–217
33. Bürgel U, Mädler B, Honey CR, Thron A, Gilsbach J, Coenen VA. Fiber tracking with distinct software tools results in a clear diversity in anatomical fiber tract portrayal. Cent Eur Neurosurg 2009;70(1):27–35
34. Leclercq D, Duffau H, Delmaire C, et al. Comparison of diffusion tensor imaging tractography of language tracts and intraoperative subcortical stimulations. J Neurosurg 2010;112(3):503–511
35. Benzagmout M, Gatignol P, Duffau H. Resection of World Health Organization grade II gliomas involving Broca's area: methodological and functional considerations. Neurosurgery 2007;61(4):741–752
36. Gil-Robles S, Duffau H. Surgical management of World Health Organization grade II gliomas in eloquent areas: the necessity of preserving a margin around functional structures. Neurosurg Focus 2010;28(2):E8
37. Duffau H, Peggy Gatignol ST, Mandonnet E, Capelle L, Taillandier L. Intraoperative subcortical stimulation mapping of language pathways in a consecutive series of 115 patients with grade II glioma in the left dominant hemisphere. J Neurosurg 2008;109(3):461–471
38. Buchmann N, Gempt J, Stoffel M, Foerschler A, Meyer B, Ringel F. Utility of diffusion tensor-imaged (DTI) motor fiber tracking for the resection of intracranial tumors near the corticospinal tract. Acta Neurochir (Wien) 2011;153(1):68–74
39. Robles SG, Gatignol P, Lehéricy S, Duffau H. Long-term brain plasticity allowing a multistage surgical approach to World Health Organization grade II gliomas in eloquent areas. J Neurosurg 2008;109(4):615–624
40. Willems PW, Taphoorn MJ, Burger H, Berkelbach van der Sprenkel JW, Tulleken CA. Effectiveness of neuronavigation in resecting solitary intracerebral contrast-enhancing tumors: a randomized controlled trial. J Neurosurg 2006;104(3):360–368
41. Gasser T, Ganslandt O, Sandalcioglu E, Stolke D, Fahlbusch R, Nimsky C. Intraoperative functional MRI: implementation and preliminary experience. Neuroimage 2005;26(3):685–693
42. De Witt Hamer PC, Robles SG, Zwinderman AH, Duffau H, Berger MS. Impact of intraoperative stimulation brain mapping on glioma surgery outcome: a meta-analysis. J Clin Oncol 2012;30(20):2559–2565
43. Schucht P, Moritz-Gasser S, Herbet G, Raabe A, Duffau H. Subcortical electrostimulation to identify network subserving motor control. Hum Brain Mapp 2012 Jun 19. doi: 10.1002/hbm.22122. [Epub ahead of print]
44. Duffau H. Intraoperative cortico-subcortical stimulations in surgery of low-grade gliomas. Expert Rev Neurother 2005;5(4):473–485
45. Duffau H. Contribution of cortical and subcortical electrostimulation in brain glioma surgery: methodological and functional considerations. Neurophysiol Clin 2007;37(6):373–382
46. Sanai N, Mirzadeh Z, Berger MS. Functional outcome after language mapping for glioma resection. N Engl J Med 2008;358(1):18–27
47. Kim SS, McCutcheon IE, Suki D, et al. Awake craniotomy for brain tumors near eloquent cortex: correlation of intraoperative cortical mapping with neurological outcomes in 309 consecutive patients. Neurosurgery 2009;64(5):836–845
48. Taylor MD, Bernstein M. Awake craniotomy with brain mapping as the routine surgical approach to treating patients with supratentorial intraaxial tumors: a prospective trial of 200 cases. J Neurosurg 1999;90(1):35–41
49. Mandonnet E, Winkler PA, Duffau H. Direct electrical stimulation as an input gate into brain functional networks: principles, advantages and limitations. Acta Neurochir (Wien) 2010;152(2):185–193
50. Moritz-Gasser S, Duffau H. Evidence of a large-scale network underlying language switching: a brain stimulation study. J Neurosurg 2009;111(4):729–732
51. Duffau H, Denvil D, Lopes M, et al. Intraoperative mapping of the cortical areas involved in multiplication and subtraction: an electrostimulation study in a patient with a left parietal glioma. J Neurol Neurosurg Psychiatry 2002;73(6):733–738
52. Thiebaut de Schotten M, Urbanski M, Duffau H, et al. Direct evidence for a parietal-frontal pathway subserving spatial awareness in humans. Science 2005;309(5744):2226–2228
53. Plaza M, Gatignol P, Cohen H, Berger B, Duffau H. A discrete area within the left dorsolateral prefrontal cortex involved in visual-verbal incongruence judgment. Cereb Cortex 2008;18(6):1253–1259
54. Vidorreta JG, Garcia R, Moritz-Gasser S, Duffau H. Double dissociation between syntactic gender and picture naming processing: a brain stimulation mapping study. Hum Brain Mapp 2011;32(3):331–340
55. Duffau H, Gatignol P, Mandonnet E, Peruzzi P, Tzourio-Mazoyer N, Capelle L. New insights into the anatomo-functional connectivity of the semantic system: a study using cortico-subcortical electrostimulations. Brain 2005;128(Pt 4):797–810
56. Duffau H. Does post-lesional subcortical plasticity exist in the human brain? Neurosci Res 2009;65(2):131–135
57. Ius T, Angelini E, Thiebaut de Schotten M, Mandonnet E, Duffau H. Evidence for potentials and limitations of brain plasticity using an atlas of functional resectability of WHO grade II gliomas: towards a "minimal common brain." Neuroimage 2011;56(3):992–1000
58. De Benedictis A, Duffau H. Brain hodotopy: from esoteric concept to practical surgical applications. Neurosurgery 2011;68(6):1709–1723
59. Martino J, Vergani F, Robles SG, Duffau H. New insights into the anatomic dissection of the temporal stem with special emphasis on the inferior fronto-occipital fasciculus: implications in surgical approach to left mesiotemporal and temporoinsular structures. Neurosurgery 2010;66(3, Suppl Operative):4–12
60. Martino J, De Witt Hamer PC, Vergani F, et al. Cortex-sparing fiber dissection: an improved method for the study of white matter anatomy in the human brain. J Anat 2011;219(4):531–541

61. Sarubbo S, de Benedictis A, Maldonado IL, Basso G, Duffau H. Frontal terminations for the inferior fronto-occipital fascicle: anatomical dissection, DTI study and functional considerations on a multi-component bundle. Struct Brain Funct, In press
62. Martino J, De Witt Hamer PC, Berger MS, et al. Analysis of the subcomponents and cortical terminations of the perisylvian superior longitudinal fasciculus: a fiber dissection and DTI tractography study. Brain Struct Funct 2013;218(1):105–121
63. Duffau H, Capelle L, Denvil D, et al. Usefulness of intraoperative electrical subcortical mapping during surgery for low-grade gliomas located within eloquent brain regions: functional results in a consecutive series of 103 patients. J Neurosurg 2003;98(4):764–778
64. Duffau H. A personal consecutive series of surgically treated 51 cases of insular WHO grade II glioma: advances and limitations. J Neurosurg 2009;110(4):696–708
65. Maldonado IL, Moritz-Gasser S, de Champfleur NM, Bertram L, Moulinié G, Duffau H. Surgery for gliomas involving the left inferior parietal lobule: new insights into the functional anatomy provided by stimulation mapping in awake patients. J Neurosurg 2011;115(4):770–779
66. Duffau H, Velut S, Mitchell MC, Gatignol P, Capelle L. Intraoperative mapping of the subcortical visual pathways using direct electrical stimulations. Acta Neurochir (Wien) 2004;146(3):265–269
67. Gras-Combe G, Moritz-Gasser S, Herbet G, Duffau H. Intraoperative subcortical electrical mapping of optic radiations in awake surgery for glioma involving visual pathways. J Neurosurg 2012;117(3):466–473
68. Duffau H, Capelle L, Sichez N, et al. Intraoperative mapping of the subcortical language pathways using direct stimulations: an anatomo-functional study. Brain 2002;125(Pt 1): 199–214
69. Thiebaut de Schotten M, Dell'Acqua F, Valabregue R, Catani M. Monkey to human comparative anatomy of the frontal lobe association tracts. Cortex 2012;48(1):82–96
70. Duffau H, Capelle L, Denvil D, et al. The role of dominant premotor cortex in language: a study using intraoperative functional mapping in awake patients. Neuroimage 2003; 20(4):1903–1914
71. Duffau H, Moritz-Gasser S, Gatignol P. Functional outcome after language mapping for insular World Health Organization grade II gliomas in the dominant hemisphere: experience with 24 patients. Neurosurg Focus 2009;27(2):E7
72. Maldonado IL, Moritz-Gasser S, Duffau H. Does the left superior longitudinal fascicle subserve language semantics? A brain electrostimulation study. Brain Struct Funct 2011; 216(3):263–274
73. Moritz-Gasser S, Duffau H. Cognitive processes and neural basis of language switching: proposal of a new model. Neuroreport 2009;20(18):1577–1580
74. Catani M, Jones DK, ffytche DH. Perisylvian language networks of the human brain. Ann Neurol 2005;57(1):8–16
75. Viegas C, Moritz-Gasser S, Rigau V, Duffau H. Occipital WHO grade II gliomas: oncological, surgical and functional considerations. Acta Neurochir (Wien) 2011;153(10):1907–1917
76. Mandonnet E, Nouet A, Gatignol P, Capelle L, Duffau H. Does the left inferior longitudinal fasciculus play a role in language? A brain stimulation study. Brain 2007;130(Pt 3): 623–629
77. Duffau H, Gatignol P, Moritz-Gasser S, Mandonnet E. Is the left uncinate fasciculus essential for language? A cerebral stimulation study. J Neurol 2009;256(3):382–389
78. Papagno C, Miracapillo C, Casarotti A, et al. What is the role of the uncinate fasciculus? Surgical removal and proper name retrieval. Brain 2011;134(Pt 2):405–414
79. De Witt Hamer PC, Moritz-Gasser S, Gatignol P, Duffau H. Is the human left middle longitudinal fascicle essential for language? A brain electrostimulation study. Hum Brain Mapp 2011;32(6):962–973
80. Mandonnet E, Gatignol P, Duffau H. Evidence for an occipito-temporal tract underlying visual recognition in picture naming. Clin Neurol Neurosurg 2009;111(7):601–605
81. Duffau H. The "frontal syndrome" revisited: lessons from electrostimulation mapping studies. Cortex 2012;48(1): 120–131
82. Gil Robles S, Gatignol P, Capelle L, Mitchell MC, Duffau H. The role of dominant striatum in language: a study using intraoperative electrical stimulations. J Neurol Neurosurg Psychiatry 2005;76(7):940–946
83. Duffau H, Leroy M, Gatignol P. Cortico-subcortical organization of language networks in the right hemisphere: an electrostimulation study in left-handers. Neuropsychologia 2008; 46(14):3197–3209
84. Spena G, Gatignol P, Capelle L, Duffau H. Superior longitudinal fasciculus subserves vestibular network in humans. Neuroreport 2006;17(13):1403–1406
85. Duffau H, Khalil I, Gatignol P, Denvil D, Capelle L. Surgical removal of corpus callosum infiltrated by low-grade glioma: functional outcome and oncological considerations. J Neurosurg 2004;100(3):431–437
86. Carrabba G, Mandonnet E, Fava E, et al. Transient inhibition of motor function induced by the Cavitron ultrasonic surgical aspirator during brain mapping. Neurosurgery 2008;63(1): E178–E179
87. Sarubbo S, Le Bars E, Moritz-Gasser S, Duffau H. Complete recovery after surgical resection of left Wernicke's area in awake patient: a brain stimulation and functional MRI study. Neurosurg Rev 2012;35(2):287–292
88. Blonski M, Taillandier L, Herbet G, et al. Combination of neoadjuvant chemotherapy followed by surgical resection as a new strategy for WHO grade II gliomas: a study of cognitive status and quality of life. J Neurooncol 2012;106(2):353–366
89. Ghareeb F, Duffau H. Intractable epilepsy in paralimbic Word Health Organization grade II gliomas: should the hippocampus be resected when not invaded by the tumor? J Neurosurg 2012;116(6):1226–1234
90. De Benedictis A, Moritz-Gasser S, Duffau H. Awake mapping optimizes the extent of resection for low-grade gliomas in eloquent areas. Neurosurgery 2010;66(6):1074–1084
91. Chang EF, Clark A, Smith JS, et al. Functional mapping-guided resection of low-grade gliomas in eloquent areas of the brain: improvement of long-term survival. Clinical article. J Neurosurg 2011;114(3):566–573
92. Martino J, Taillandier L, Moritz-Gasser S, Gatignol P, Duffau H. Re-operation is a safe and effective therapeutic strategy in recurrent WHO grade II gliomas within eloquent areas. Acta Neurochir (Wien) 2009;151(5):427–436
93. Duffau H. Brain plasticity and tumors. Adv Tech Stand Neurosurg 2008;33:3–33
94. Duffau H. Brain plasticity: from pathophysiological mechanisms to therapeutic applications. J Clin Neurosci 2006;13(9): 885–897
95. Krainik A, Duffau H, Capelle L, et al. Role of the healthy hemisphere in recovery after resection of the supplementary motor area. Neurology 2004;62(8):1323–1332
96. Duffau H. The anatomo-functional connectivity of language revisited: new insights provided by electrostimulation and tractography. Neuropsychologia 2008;46(4):927–934
97. Potts MB, Smith JS, Molinaro AM, Berger MS. Natural history and surgical management of incidentally discovered low-grade gliomas. J Neurosurg 2012;116(2):365–372
98. Duffau H. Awake surgery for incidental WHO grade II gliomas involving eloquent areas. Acta Neurochir (Wien) 2012; 154(4):575–584

6

The Role of Awake Craniotomy in the Resection of Astrocytomas

Nader Sanai, Douglas A. Hardesty, and Mitchel S. Berger

Although a primary tenet of neurosurgical oncology is that survival can improve with greater tumor resection, this principle must be tempered by the potential for functional loss following a radical removal. Current neurosurgical innovations aim to improve our anatomical, physiological, and functional understanding of the surgical region of interest to prevent potential neurological morbidity during resection. Emerging imaging technologies, as well as state-of-the-art intraoperative techniques, can facilitate extent of resection while minimizing the associated morbidity profile. Specifically, the value of mapping motor and language pathways is well established for the safe resection of intrinsic tumors.

Interestingly, controversy persists regarding prognostic factors and treatment options for both low- and high-grade hemispheric gliomas. Among the various tumor- and treatment-related parameters, including tumor volume, neurological status, timing of surgical intervention, and the use of adjuvant therapy, age and tumor histology have been identified as primary predictors of patient prognosis. However, tumor eloquence has recently emerged as another critical factor affecting outcome, particularly as it relates to tumor extent of resection.[1] Importantly, despite significant advances in operative technique and preoperative planning, the effect of glioma extent of resection in prolonging tumor-free progression and survival remains unclear. Although the value of glioma resection in obtaining tissue diagnosis and decompressing mass effect is unquestionable, a lack of Level I evidence prevents similar certainty in assessing the influence of extent of resection. Even though low-grade and high-grade gliomas are distinct in their biologies, clinical behaviors, and outcomes, understanding the effect of surgery remains equally important for both. This is also true for lesions in areas of eloquence, where the close proximity of critical pathways, often related to language and motor function, can present a significant challenge to standard operative strategies.

Development of Cortical Mapping Strategies

Direct cortical stimulation has been employed in neurosurgery since 1930, first by Foerster,[2] and then by Penfield.[3–5] In recent years, the technique of intraoperative cortical stimulation has been adopted for the identification and preservation of language function and motor pathways. Stimulation depolarizes a very focal area of cortex, which, in turn, evokes certain responses. Although the mechanisms of stimulation effects on language are poorly understood, the principle is based upon the depolarization of local neurons and also of passing pathways, inducing local excitation or inhibition, as well as possible diffusion to more distant areas by way of orthodromic or antidromic propagation.[6] Studies employing optical imaging of bipolar cortical stimulation in monkey and human cortex have shown precise local changes, within 2 to 3 mm, after the activation of cortical tissue.[7,8] With the advent of the bipolar probe, avoidance of local diffusion and more precise mapping have been enabled with an accuracy estimated to be ~ 5 mm.[7]

Language mapping techniques were historically developed in the context of epilepsy surgery, where large craniotomies exposed the brain well beyond the region of surgical interest to localize multiple cortical regions containing stimulation-induced language and motor function (i.e., "positive" sites) prior to resection. Until recently, it has been thought that such positive-site controls must be established during language mapping before any other cortical area could be safely resected. Using this tactic, awake craniotomies traditionally identify positive language sites in 95 to 100% of the operative exposures. Brain tumor surgeons, however, are now evolving toward a different standard of language mapping, where smaller, tailored craniotomies often expose no positive sites, and tumor resection is therefore directed by the localization of cortical regions that contained no stimulation-induced language or motor function (i.e., "negative" sites). This "negative mapping" strategy represents a paradigm shift in language mapping technique by eliminating the neurosurgeon's reliance on the positive-site control in the operative exposure, thereby allowing for minimal cortical exposure overlying the tumor, less extensive intraoperative mapping, and a more time-efficient neurosurgical procedure.

Unreliability of Anatomical Localization

Prediction of cortical language sites through classic anatomical criteria is inadequate in light of the significant individual variability of cortical organization,[9–12] the distortion of cerebral topography from tumor mass effect, and the possibility of functional reorganization through plasticity mechanisms.[13–15] A consistent finding of language stimulation studies has been the identification of significant individual variability among patients.[10] Speech arrest is variably located and can go well beyond the classic anatomical boundaries of the Broca area for motor speech. It typically involves an area contiguous with the face-motor cortex and, yet, in some cases is seen several centimeters from the sylvian fissure. This variability has also been suggested by studies designed to preoperatively predict the location of speech arrest based upon the type of frontal opercular anatomy[16] or by using functional neuroimaging.[17–23] Similarly, for temporal lobe language sites, one study of temporal lobe resections assisted by subdural grids demonstrated that the distance from the temporal pole to the area of language function varied from 3 to 9 cm.[24] Functional imaging studies have also corroborated such variability.[25] Furthermore, because functional tissue can be located within the tumor nidus,[26] the standard surgical principle of debulking tumor from within to avoid neurological deficits is not always safe. Consequently, the use of intraoperative cortical and subcortical stimulation to accurately detect functional regions and pathways is essential for safely removing dominant hemisphere gliomas to the greatest extent possible.

Localization of Speech and Motor Function

Anatomical criteria are inadequate to determine speech and motor cortical organization in patients with brain tumors (Grade 1A Recommendation).

■ Current Intraoperative Language and Motor Mapping Techniques

In general, a limited craniotomy should expose the tumor and up to 2 cm of surrounding brain. Using bipolar electrodes, cortical mapping is started at a low stimulus (1.5 mA) and increased to a maximum of 6 mA, if necessary. A constant-current generator delivers biphasic square-wave pulses (each phase, 1.25 msec) in 4-second trains at 60 Hz across 1-mm bipolar electrodes separated by 5 mm. Stimulation sites (~ 10 to 20 per subject) can be marked with sterile numbered tickets. Throughout motor and language mapping, continuous electrocorticography should be used to monitor afterdischarge potentials and, therefore, eliminate the chance that speech or naming errors are caused by subclinical seizure activity.

Awake Cortical Stimulation and Impact of Language Mapping

Speech arrest is based upon blocking number counting without simultaneous motor response in the mouth or pharynx. Dysarthria can be distinguished from speech arrest by the absence of perceived or visible involuntary muscle contraction affecting speech. For naming or reading sites, cortical stimulation is applied for 3 seconds at sequential cortical sites during a slide presentation of line drawings or words, respectively. All tested language sites should be repeatedly stimulated at least three times. A positive essential site can be defined as an inability to name objects or read words in 66% or greater of the testing per site. In all cases, a 1-cm margin of tissue should be measured and preserved around each positive language site to protect functional tissue from the resection.[27] The extent of resection is directed by targeting contrast-enhancing regions for high-grade lesions and T2-hyperintense areas for low-grade lesions. Some groups advocate the use of language mapping along subcortical white matter pathways as well.[28,29]

Despite the considerable evidence supporting the use of intraoperative cortical stimulation mapping of language function, the efficacy of this technique in preserving functional outcome following aggressive glioma resection remains poorly understood. Nevertheless, the long-term neurological effects after using this technique for large, dominant-hemisphere gliomas are important to define to accurately advocate its use.[30]

No Level I, randomized trial exists for language mapping. Our experience with 250 consecutive patients with dominant-hemisphere gliomas (WHO grades II through IV) suggests that functional language outcome following awake mapping can be favorable, even in the setting of an aggressive resection[31] (**Table 6.1**). Over all, 159 of 250 patients (63.6%) had intact speech preoperatively. At 1 week postoperatively, 194 (77.6%) remained at their baseline language function, whereas 21 (8.4%) had worsened and 35 (14.0%) had new speech deficits. However, by 6 months, 52 (92.8%) of 56 patients with new or worsened language deficits had returned to baseline or better, and the remaining 4 (7.1%) were left with a permanent deficit. Interestingly, among these patients, any additional language deficit incurred as a result of the surgery improved by 3 months or not all. Thus, with the use of language mapping, only 1.6% (4 of 243 surviving patients) of all glioma patients developed a permanent postoperative language deficit. One explanation for this favorable postoperative language profile may be our strict adherence to the "1-centimeter rule," first described by Haglund et al, which demonstrated that, for temporal lobe tumors, a resection margin of 1 cm or more from a language site significantly reduces postoperative language deficits.[32]

Awake Cortical Stimulation and Intraoperative Speech Mapping in Glioma

1. Awake language mapping in dominant-hemisphere glioma is associated with a low incidence of permanent speech deficit and should be utilized whenever possible (Grade 1C Recommendation, Level II/III Evidence).
2. Transient speech deficits are not uncommon after awake craniotomy with language mapping, but resolve by 3 months.
3. A resection margin of 1 cm from positive language sites is recommended in temporal tumors to reduce postoperative deficits. postoperatively.

Cortical and Subcortical Motor Mapping Techniques

For patients with gliomas that are located within or adjacent to the rolandic cortex and thus the descending motor tracts, awake or asleep stimulation mapping of cortical and subcortical motor pathways enables the surgeon to identify the descending motor pathways during tumor removal and achieve an acceptable rate of permanent morbidity in high-risk functional areas.[33–35] Akin to speech mapping techniques, no randomized trial exists for motor mapping. The best evidence published comes from several retrospective studies over the last 15 years; all studies lack long-term survival data. In one recent study, new immediate postoperative motor deficits were documented in 59.3% of patients in whom a subcortical motor tract was identified intraoperatively and in 14.5% of those in whom subcortical tracts were not observed; permanent deficits were observed in 6.5% and 3.5% of patients (a nonsignificant difference), respectively.[33] In a study of subcortical motor pathways in 294 patients who underwent surgery for

Table 6.1 Recent studies of awake cortical stimulation and language mapping in glioma

Study (level of evidence)	No. patients	GTR	Overall PFS	Overall survival	New transient speech deficit	New permanent speech deficit
Sanai et al 2008[31] (III)	250	59.6%	NR	97%	22.4%	1.6%

Abbreviations: GTR, gross total resection; NR, not reported; PFS, progression-free survival.

hemispheric gliomas, 14 patients (4.8%) had a persistent motor deficit after 3 months. Interestingly, in this study, patients whose subcortical pathways were identified intraoperatively were statistically significantly more prone to develop an additional transient or permanent motor deficit (27.5% vs 13.1%).[35] In another study consisting of 60 patients (44 with glioma) with an 87% gross total or subtotal (< 10 cm^3 residual) resection rate, the overall neurological morbidity was 5% after the use of cortical motor mapping.[34] Thus, collectively, the recent literature suggests that intraoperative cortical and subcortical motor mapping can safely identify corridors for resection, as well as define the limits of tumor resection (**Table 6.2**).

Cortical Stimulation and Intraoperative Motor Mapping in Glioma

1. Awake or asleep motor mapping is associated with a low incidence, ~ 5%, of permanent motor deficit in patients with rolandic or perirolandic tumors and should be utilized whenever possible (Grade 1C Recommendation, Level II/III Evidence).
2. Transient motor deficits following motor mapping are common, but the majority of deficits resolve quickly.
3. The identification of subcortical motor tracts during intraoperative stimulation is associated with increased immediate postoperative deficits.
4. There is mixed evidence that the identification of subcortical motor tracts during intraoperative stimulation is associated with increased permanent postoperative deficits.

Tailored Craniotomies and the Value of Negative Mapping

In contrast to the classic mapping principles practiced in epilepsy surgery, where 95 to 100% of operative fields contain a positive language site, a paradigm shift is emerging in brain tumor language mapping, where positive language sites are not always found prior to resection. In our practice, because of our use of tailored cortical exposures, less than 58% of patients have essential language sites localized within the operative field. Our experience suggests that it is safe to employ a minimal exposure of the tumor and resect based upon a negative language map, rather than rely upon a wide craniotomy to find positive language sites well beyond the lesion. However, language mapping techniques like this are generally more successful and safer at high-volume neurosurgical centers.

Negative language mapping, however, does not necessarily guarantee the absence of eloquent sites. Despite negative brain mapping, permanent postoperative neurological deficits have been reported.[36] In our experience with 250 consecutive patients with dominant-hemisphere gliomas, all 4 of our patients with permanent postoperative neurological deficits had no positive sites detected prior to their resections. Other cases of unexpected postoperative deficits have also been attributed to progressive tumor infiltration into functional areas.[37] Furthermore, both intraoperative stimulation and functional imaging techniques have provided evidence for redistribution of functional neural networks in cases of stroke,[14,38,39] congenital malformations,[40,41] brain injury,[42] and tumor progression.[14,15,43] Not surprisingly, it has been

Table 6.2 Recent studies of cortical stimulation and motor mapping

Study (level of evidence)	No. patients	GTR	Overall PFS	Overall survival	New transient motor deficit	New permanent motor deficit
Carrabba et al 2007[33] (III)	146	59.6%	NR	NR	42%	5.4%
Keles et al 2004[35] (III)	294	NR	NR	NR	20.4%	4.8%
Duffau et al 1999[34] (III)	60	51%	NR	NR	27%	5%

Abbreviations: GTR, gross total resection; NR, not reported; PFS, progression-free survival.

hypothesized that brain infiltration by gliomas leads to reshaping or local reorganization of functional networks as well as neosynaptogenesis.[44,46] This would explain the frequent lack of clinical deficit despite glioma growth into eloquent brain areas,[14,43,46] as well as the transient nature of many postoperative deficits. In the case of language function located in the dominant insula, the brain's capacity for compensation of functional loss has also been associated with recruitment of the left superior temporal gyrus and left putamen.[46]

■ Literature Review

Assessing the Value of Intraoperative Stimulation Mapping

In the recent literature, ~ 90 publications examine the utility of intraoperative stimulation mapping techniques in achieving greater extent of resection for gliomas while minimizing morbidity. Within these studies, cohorts varied between 20 and 648 patients, with a median of 50 patients per study. Nearly all the reports provide Level III evidence in support of this microsurgical adjunct, with the exception of two randomized studies[47,48] that examined anesthetic or fluorescence-guided techniques to maximize extent of resection.

A recent meta-analysis of this growing literature included 8,091 patients and identified intraoperative cortical stimulation mapping as predictive of a twofold reduction (3.4% vs 8.2%) in late severe neurological deficits in adult patients with supratentorial infiltrative gliomas.[49] Importantly, the additional benefit did not come at the expense of extent of resection (75% gross total resection with mapping versus 58% without mapping), even though lesions were more often located in eloquent locations (99.9% vs 95.8%). Typically, the observed transient neurological deficits usually subsided within a few weeks to 3 months after resection and were due to the proximity of critical brain structures adjacent to the resection cavity. Ultimately, a randomized, controlled trial to determine the impact of awake craniotomies and stimulation mappings will be necessary to control for all known and unknown confounders inherent to the existing observational studies.

Expert Recommendations

1. Speech and motor mapping techniques are associated with a low incidence of permanent neurological deficit and should be utilized whenever possible to minimize the permanent morbidity associated with tumors arising from eloquent cortex (Grade 1C Recommendation, Level II/III Evidence).
2. A high percentage of patients undergoing resection with intraoperative mapping will experience perioperative transient speech or motor symptoms, but the majority of these deficits resolve within 3 months.
3. Intraoperative mapping techniques do not reduce the incidence of gross total resections in patients with eloquent gliomas.
4. There is insufficient long-term follow-up data on the role of stimulation mapping resections and overall or progression-free survival in patients with gliomas.

■ Summary and Conclusions

Glioma resections using awake craniotomy and intraoperative stimulation mapping techniques are associated with fewer neurological deficits and more extensive resection. Unlike motor function, speech and language are variably distributed and widely represented, thus emphasizing the utility of language mapping in this particular patient population. Using this approach, and in conjunction with standardized neuroanesthesia and neuromonitoring, the postoperative motor and language resolution profiles following glioma resection may be predictable. Specifically, in our experience, any additional language deficit incurred as a result of the surgery will improve by 3 months or not all. Our experience also emphasizes the value of negative language mapping in the setting of a tailored cortical exposure. Although the value of extent of resection remains less clear, the available literature for both low-grade and high-grade hemispheric gliomas demonstrates mounting evidence that a more extensive surgical resection is associated with a more favorable life expectancy for both low-grade and high-grade glioma patients. This objective should be cautiously pursued for all gliomas, even in the setting of eloquent location.

■ References

1. Chang EF, Smith JS, Chang SM, et al. Preoperative prognostic classification system for hemispheric low-grade gliomas in adults. J Neurosurg 2008;109(5):817–824
2. Foerster O. The cerebral cortex of man. Lancet 1931;2:309–312
3. Penfield W, Bolchey E. Somatic motor and sensory representation in the cerebral cortex of man as studied by electrical stimulation. Brain 1937;60:389–443
4. Penfield W, Frickson TC. Epilepsy and Cerebral Localization. A Study of the Mechanism, Treatment, and Prevention of Epileptic Seizures. Springfield, IL: Charles C Thomas; 1941
5. Penfield W, Rasmussen T. Secondary Sensory and Motor Representation. New York, NY: Macmillan; 1950
6. Ranck JB Jr. Which elements are excited in electrical stimulation of mammalian central nervous system: a review. Brain Res 1975;98(3):417–440
7. Haglund MM, Ojemann GA, Blasdel GG. Optical imaging of bipolar cortical stimulation. J Neurosurg 1993;78(5):785–793
8. Haglund MM, Ojemann GA, Hochman DW. Optical imaging of epileptiform and functional activity in human cerebral cortex. Nature 1992;358(6388):668–671
9. Herholz K, Thiel A, Wienhard K, et al. Individual functional anatomy of verb generation. Neuroimage 1996;3(3 Pt 1): 185–194
10. Ojemann G, Ojemann J, Lettich E, Berger M. Cortical language localization in left, dominant hemisphere: an electrical stimulation mapping investigation in 117 patients. J Neurosurg 1989;71(3):316–326
11. Ojemann GA. Individual variability in cortical localization of language. J Neurosurg 1979;50(2):164–169
12. Ojemann GA, Whitaker HA. Language localization and variability. Brain Lang 1978;6(2):239–260
13. Ojemann JG, Miller JW, Silbergeld DL. Preserved function in brain invaded by tumor. Neurosurgery 1996;39(2): 253–258
14. Seitz RJ, Huang Y, Knorr U, Tellmann L, Herzog H, Freund HJ. Large-scale plasticity of the human motor cortex. Neuroreport 1995;6(5):742–744
15. Wunderlich G, Knorr U, Herzog H, Kiwit JC, Freund HJ, Seitz RJ. Precentral glioma location determines the displacement of cortical hand representation. Neurosurgery 1998;42(1): 18–26
16. Quiñones-Hinojosa A, Ojemann SG, Sanai N, Dillon WP, Berger MS. Preoperative correlation of intraoperative cortical mapping with magnetic resonance imaging landmarks to predict localization of the Broca area. J Neurosurg 2003;99(2): 311–318
17. Dehaene S, Dupoux E, Mehler J, et al. Anatomical variability in the cortical representation of first and second language. Neuroreport 1997;8(17):3809–3815
18. Josse G, Hervé PY, Crivello F, Mazoyer B, Tzourio-Mazoyer N. Hemispheric specialization for language: brain volume matters. Brain Res 2006;1068(1):184–193
19. Seghier ML, Lazeyras F, Pegna AJ, et al. Variability of fMRI activation during a phonological and semantic language task in healthy subjects. Hum Brain Mapp 2004;23(3):140–155
20. Steinmetz H, Seitz RJ. Functional anatomy of language processing: neuroimaging and the problem of individual variability. Neuropsychologia 1991;29(12):1149–1161
21. Turkeltaub PE, Eden GF, Jones KM, Zeffiro TA. Meta-analysis of the functional neuroanatomy of single-word reading: method and validation. Neuroimage 2002;16(3 Pt 1):765–780
22. Tzourio-Mazoyer N, Josse G, Crivello F, Mazoyer B. Interindividual variability in the hemispheric organization for speech. Neuroimage 2004;21(1):422–435
23. Tzourio N, Crivello F, Mellet E, Nkanga-Ngila B, Mazoyer B. Functional anatomy of dominance for speech comprehension in left handers vs right handers. Neuroimage 1998;8(1):1–16
24. Davies KG, Maxwell RE, Jennum P, et al. Language function following subdural grid-directed temporal lobectomy. Acta Neurol Scand 1994;90(3):201–206
25. FitzGerald DB, Cosgrove GR, Ronner S, et al. Location of language in the cortex: a comparison between functional MR imaging and electrocortical stimulation. AJNR Am J Neuroradiol 1997;18(8):1529–1539
26. Skirboll SS, Ojemann GA, Berger MS, Lettich E, Winn HR. Functional cortex and subcortical white matter located within gliomas. Neurosurgery 1996;38(4):678–684
27. Lacroix M, Abi-Said D, Fourney DR, et al. A multivariate analysis of 416 patients with glioblastoma multiforme: prognosis, extent of resection, and survival. J Neurosurg 2001;95(2): 190–198
28. Duffau H, Capelle L, Denvil D, et al. Usefulness of intraoperative electrical subcortical mapping during surgery for low-grade gliomas located within eloquent brain regions: functional results in a consecutive series of 103 patients. J Neurosurg 2003;98(4):764–778
29. Duffau H, Capelle L, Sichez N, et al. Intraoperative mapping of the subcortical language pathways using direct stimulations: an anatomo-functional study. Brain 2002;125(Pt 1): 199–214
30. Sanai N, Berger MS. Mapping the horizon: techniques to optimize tumor resection before and during surgery. Clin Neurosurg 2008;55:14–19
31. Sanai N, Mirzadeh Z, Berger MS. Functional outcome after language mapping for glioma resection. N Engl J Med 2008;358(1):18–27
32. Haglund MM, Berger MS, Shamseldin M, Lettich E, Ojemann GA. Cortical localization of temporal lobe language sites in patients with gliomas. Neurosurgery 1994;34(4):567–576
33. Carrabba G, Fava E, Giussani C, et al. Cortical and subcortical motor mapping in rolandic and perirolandic glioma surgery: impact on postoperative morbidity and extent of resection. J Neurosurg Sci 2007;51(2):45–51
34. Duffau H, Capelle L, Sichez J, et al. Intra-operative direct electrical stimulations of the central nervous system: the Salpêtrière experience with 60 patients. Acta Neurochir (Wien) 1999;141(11):1157–1167
35. Keles GE, Lundin DA, Lamborn KR, Chang EF, Ojemann G, Berger MS. Intraoperative subcortical stimulation mapping for hemispherical perirolandic gliomas located within or adjacent to the descending motor pathways: evaluation of morbidity and assessment of functional outcome in 294 patients. J Neurosurg 2004;100(3):369–375
36. Taylor MD, Bernstein M. Awake craniotomy with brain mapping as the routine surgical approach to treating patients with supratentorial intraaxial tumors: a prospective trial of 200 cases. J Neurosurg 1999;90(1):35–41
37. Berger MS. Lesions in functional ("eloquent") cortex and subcortical white matter. Clin Neurosurg 1994;41:444–463
38. Chollet F, DiPiero V, Wise RJ, Brooks DJ, Dolan RJ, Frackowiak RS. The functional anatomy of motor recovery after stroke in humans: a study with positron emission tomography. Ann Neurol 1991;29(1):63–71
39. Weder B, Seitz RJ. Deficient cerebral activation pattern in stroke recovery. Neuroreport 1994;5(4):457–460
40. Lewine JD, Astur RS, Davis LE, Knight JE, Maclin EL, Orrison WW Jr. Cortical organization in adulthood is modified by neonatal infarct: a case study. Radiology 1994;190(1):93–96
41. Maldjian J, Atlas SW, Howard RS II, et al. Functional magnetic resonance imaging of regional brain activity in patients with intracerebral arteriovenous malformations before surgical or endovascular therapy. J Neurosurg 1996;84(3):477–483
42. Grady MS, Jane JA, Steward O. Synaptic reorganization within the human central nervous system following injury. J Neurosurg 1989;71(4):534–537
43. Fandino J, Kollias SS, Wieser HG, Valavanis A, Yonekawa Y. Intraoperative validation of functional magnetic resonance

imaging and cortical reorganization patterns in patients with brain tumors involving the primary motor cortex. J Neurosurg 1999;91(2):238–250
44. Duffau H, Capelle L, Denvil D, et al. Functional recovery after surgical resection of low grade gliomas in eloquent brain: hypothesis of brain compensation. J Neurol Neurosurg Psychiatry 2003;74(7):901–907
45. Thiel A, Herholz K, Koyuncu A, et al. Plasticity of language networks in patients with brain tumors: a positron emission tomography activation study. Ann Neurol 2001;50(5):620–629
46. Duffau H, Bauchet L, Lehéricy S, Capelle L. Functional compensation of the left dominant insula for language. Neuroreport 2001;12(10):2159–2163
47. Gupta DK, Chandra PS, Ojha BK, Sharma BS, Mahapatra AK, Mehta VS. Awake craniotomy versus surgery under general anesthesia for resection of intrinsic lesions of eloquent cortex—a prospective randomised study. Clin Neurol Neurosurg 2007; 109(4):335–343
48. Stummer W, Pichlmeier U, Meinel T, Wiestler OD, Zanella F, Reulen HJ; ALA-Glioma Study Group. Fluorescence-guided surgery with 5-aminolevulinic acid for resection of malignant glioma: a randomised controlled multicentre phase III trial. Lancet Oncol 2006;7(5):392–401
49. De Witt Hamer PC, Robles SG, Zwinderman AH, Duffau H, Berger MS. Impact of intraoperative stimulation brain mapping on glioma surgery outcome: a meta-analysis. J Clin Oncol 2012;30(20):2559–2565

7

The Role of Surgery versus Biopsy in the Management of Gliomas in the Elderly (Patients over 65)

Nader Sanai and Douglas A. Hardesty

Glioblastoma multiforme (GBM) is the most common primary brain malignancy, and the prognosis remains dismal despite decades of clinical and molecular research. The current standard of care for newly diagnosed GBM is a combination of aggressive microsurgical resection, fractionated radiotherapy, and adjuvant temozolomide chemotherapy.[1] Predictive factors for increased overall survival include high preoperative functional status, methylation status of O-6-methylguanine-DNA-methyltransferase (MGMT-methylation status), and young age at diagnosis.[2–6] A growing body of literature also identifies greater extent of resection (EoR) as predictive of improved overall survival among newly diagnosed glioblastoma patients.[7] Glioblastoma, however, remains a disease that primarily afflicts older patient populations, and the incidence of GBM in the elderly (as well as the average age at diagnosis) continues to rise.[8,9] Given the increasing incidence of GBM in older patients, and its relatively poorer clinical course, a critical question is whether aggressive therapy improves overall survival and quality of life for this patient population. Several of the clinical trials that have established the modern standard of care for GBM have excluded elderly patients; among other clinical trials without an exclusionary age criterion, the average patient age remains a decade or more younger than the average age at which GBM is diagnosed in population-based studies.[1,8,9] This raises the question whether similar treatment paradigms can be applied to older patients. Elderly GBM patients may have medical comorbidities, such as heart disease, pulmonary disease, diabetes, or dementia, that may increase their risk of perioperative morbidity and mortality from aggressive surgical resection. Alternatively, elderly GBM patients may be treated less aggressively by providers despite modest perioperative risk profiles due to a perceived (perhaps anecdotal) lack of benefit in the aged population.[5,10] Lastly, some authors have proposed that GBM in the elderly may be more resistant to radiation, more locally infiltrative, or more biologically aggressive than GBM in younger patients.[8] Currently, the standard of care for elderly patients with GBM is not well established and is inconsistent.[5] This chapter reviews the published English language literature to examine the role of aggressive microsurgical resection versus biopsy in elderly patients with glioblastoma.

■ Identifying the "Elderly" Population

Historically the term *elderly* in English neurosurgical literature has referred to patients over age 65. However, there is significant variation in reports, with cutoffs at 60, 65, 70, and even 80 years of age.[10] Admittedly, these limits are arbitrary, and population-based studies of patients with GBM demonstrate a decrease in estimated survival as the age at diagnosis increases.[5,8,11,12] To maintain internal consistency and allow fair comparison of the literature, we will specify the age group defined as elderly within each cited manuscript.

■ Modern Treatment Patterns for Glioblastoma Patients in the United States

The standard of care for management of GBM has evolved over the last decade in the United States. At present, a combination of aggressive microsurgical resection, fractionated radiation therapy, and concomitant chemotherapy is utilized for newly diagnosed glioblastoma patients, not infrequently in the setting of a clinical trial. However, numerous epidemiological surveys have shown that elderly patients less frequently undergo such multimodal therapy. Analysis of the Medicare Surveillance, Epidemiology, and End Results (SEER) database demonstrated that patients over the age of 75 were less likely to undergo surgical resection or radiation therapy compared with patients between ages 65 and 74.[12] Additional examination of this epidemiological database showed patient age to be the strongest single predictor of resection, radiation, and chemotherapy.[13] An increase in medical comorbidities was also associated with a decrease in radiation and chemotherapy utilization. Functional status was not captured by the SEER database, and so the magnitude of a potential selection bias for aggressive therapies could not be determined in these analyses. A study of patients treated at one high-volume brain tumor center did significantly associate higher preoperative Karnofsky performance scale (KPS) scores with the selection of radiation and chemotherapy.[14] However, despite the apparent underutilization of multimodal therapy for elderly patients with GBM, evidence exists that elderly patients not only tolerate radiation and chemotherapy but that these therapies also increase their survival.[14–22] As seen in other patient cohorts, MGMT-methylation status and preoperative functional status (according to the KPS score) are also prognostically significant among elderly patients with GBM.[16,17,23–25] Older age, however, has been inconsistently identified as a poor prognostic factor, but such analyses may be confounded by the relationship between functional status and age.[16,17,24–28]

■ Literature Review

Surgical Resection versus Biopsy for Malignant Glioma

Level I Evidence

A single prospective, randomized trial exists comparing surgical resection and biopsy in elderly patients (> 65 years) with malignant glioma (**Table 7.1**).[29] Prior to surgery, 13 patients were randomized to diagnostic biopsy and 10 to maximal surgical debulking. Four of the 13 patients undergoing stereotactic biopsy had anaplastic astrocytomas and the other nine GBMs. Preoperative functional scores and medical comorbidities were similar in the two groups, as were perioperative complications. Postoperative functional scores were not significantly altered from preoperative scores in either group. Most patients in both groups underwent further radiation and chemotherapy. Despite the small number of patients, surgical debulking demonstrated a strong survival benefit. Patients undergoing debulking had an average survival of 171 days, compared with 85 days in the stereotactic biopsy group. The authors concluded that maximal surgical debulking in the elderly is warranted and yields improved survival without increased surgical morbidity.

Level II Evidence

No recent Level II studies of note address the role of surgical resection versus biopsy in elderly patients with GBM.

Level III Evidence

Numerous retrospective series comparing the role of surgical resection versus biopsy for malignant glioma have been published (**Table 7.2**). Initial reports comparing surgical modalities were equivocal, whereas the majority of literature published since 2000 has demonstrated value to maximal extent of resection.

Whittle et al (1991) were one of the first groups to examine the role of resection versus biopsy in elderly patients (> 60 years) with malignant glioma.[30] The retrospective series consisted of 80 patients treated between 1983 and 1989, 63 of whom had pathologi-

Table 7.1 Review of Level I evidence

Study	Age limit	N (patients)	Overall survival	Complications
Vuorinen et al 2003[29]	> 65	23	Favors resection	No difference

Table 7.2 Review of Level III evidence

Study	Age limit	N (patients)	Overall survival	Complications
Whittle et al 1991[30]	> 60	63	Favors resection	Favors biopsy
Kelly and Hunt 1994[32]	> 65	128	Favors resection	No difference
Whittle et al 2002[31]	> 60	80	Favors resection	No difference
Patwardhan et al 2004[20]	> 59	13	No difference	No difference
Piccirilli et al 2006[33]	> 80	22	Favors resection	No difference
Stark et al 2007[34]	> 60	185	Favors resection	No difference
Barnholtz-Sloan et al 2008[12]	> 65	1753	Favors resection	Not reported
Combs et al 2008[35]	> 65	43	Favors resection	Not reported
Mukerji et al 2008[36]	> 65	34	Favors resection	No difference
Iwamoto et al 2009[14]	> 65	394	Favors resection	Not reported
Chaichana et al 2011[37]	> 65	80	Favors resection	No difference
Ewelt et al 2011[38]	> 65	103	Favors resection	Not reported
Scott et al 2011[28]	> 70	206	Favors resection	Not reported

cally confirmed Level III or IV supratentorial lesions. Aggressive resection yielded a small but significant survival benefit (15 vs 7 weeks) compared with biopsy alone. The addition of radiation therapy improved survival in both groups, yet debulking remained superior to biopsy. A high rate of perioperative complication, defined as iatrogenic neurological deficit or postoperative intracerebral hematoma, was seen in the resection group (21%). No perioperative complications were seen in the biopsy group. However, the effects of these specific complications upon reoperation, over all survival, and patient quality of life were not examined, and, over all, the authors did not endorse aggressive surgical management for elderly patients. Interestingly, in 2002 Whittle et al examined patients treated between 1989 and 1996 and demonstrated a persistent, significant survival advantage favoring resection versus biopsy.[31] In this follow-up series, a substantially lower rate of perioperative complications was reported among patients undergoing resection when compared with the authors' initial experience. In this updated series, the authors concluded that age alone should not influence surgical decision making.

Kelly and Hunt (1994) retrospectively examined 128 patients over 65 years of age undergoing biopsy or resection of GBM.[32] There were no differences in age or preoperative functional status between the two groups. The majority of patients underwent postoperative radiation, and rates of perioperative morbidity and mortality were similar. Over all, debulking surgery was associated with prolonged survival (27 weeks vs 15.4 weeks), although the authors noted this to be only a "modest" gain.

Patwardhan et al (2004) reviewed their experience with 30 GBM patients age 59 years or older.[20] A stepwise increase in survival was seen as patients underwent additional treatment modalities; the combination of maximal resection, radiation, and chemotherapy yielded the longest survival. Importantly, however, no patients underwent biopsy with radiation and chemotherapy. A small subset of patients underwent either biopsy only (n = 6), or resection only (n = 7) with no additional treatments. No significant difference was seen in the (altogether poor) survival between these two groups of patients (3.2 months for biopsy only vs 2.2 months for resection only).

Piccirilli et al (2006) examined 22 patients age > 80 years with good functional status (KPS > 70) undergoing treatment for GBM.[33] Again, a survival benefit was observed (16.7 vs 5.8 months) in favor of attempted gross total resection plus adjuvant therapy when compared with biopsy plus adjuvant therapy.

Stark et al (2007) reported a series of 185 patients over age 60 undergoing treatment for GBM.[34] The age of 60 was chosen following a univariate Kaplan-Meier survival analysis that demonstrated the greatest difference between patients above and below this threshold. In a subsequent multivariate analysis, GTR was highly associated with increased elderly patient survival when compared with subtotal resection or biopsy alone. KPS was improved or unchanged postoperatively in 81% of patients. Perioperative mortality was higher in the elderly group (4.8%) when compared with patients under age 60 (2.5%), but this difference was not statistically significant.

Barnholtz-Sloan et al (2008) queried the SEER database of Medicare patients over age 65 to identify 1,753 patients with GBM and 205 patients with anaplastic astrocytoma.[12] As already mentioned, older patients were less likely to undergo multimodal therapy. The use of debulking surgery and radiation therapy, however, was associated with increased survival for elderly patients with GBM when compared with biopsy and radiation therapy. Because functional status was not recorded in the SEER database, a potential selection bias for patients undergoing resection could not be ruled out.

Combs et al (2008) retrospectively reviewed 43 patients with GBM age 65 or older undergoing multimodal therapy at a single institution.[35] Sixty-seven percent of patients had either gross total or subtotal resections, whereas 33% had biopsy only. All patients received radiation therapy and temozolomide chemotherapy postoperatively. A statistically significant survival advantage was observed in the resection group compared with the biopsy-only group. Differences in functional status between patients undergoing resection versus biopsy were not reported, although the majority of patients (60%) had KPS ≥ 70.

Mukerji et al (2008) retrospectively reviewed 34 consecutive patients over age 65 with malignant glioma.[36] Most patients had preoperative KPS ≥ 70. Maximal surgical resection, with or without adjuvant radiation therapy, yielded significantly longer survival (median 7 vs 3 months) than did biopsy with or without radiation. No patient in either group had worsening postoperative neurological deficit, nor did any patient return to the operating room for additional surgery.

Iwamoto et al (2009) retrospectively reviewed their institutional experience with the management of elderly (> 65 years of age) patients with GBM.[14] Over all, 394 patients underwent treatment over the years 1997 to 2007. The majority of patients had either partial (53.8%) or gross total resections (27.7%); biopsy alone was used for 18.5% of patients. Multivariate analysis for overall survival favored greater resection when compared with biopsy in this cohort of patients. Furthermore, gross total resection yielded longer survival than did partial resection.

Chaichana et al (2011) retrospectively selected, from a consecutive cohort of 205 elderly (> 65 years) patients with GBM, 40 patients who underwent maximal tumor resection and 40 patients who had stereotactic biopsy.[37] These cohorts were matched for age, KPS, eloquent cortex involvement, and use of radiation/chemotherapy. The median survival was improved for patients who underwent resection versus those who had biopsy (5.7 months compared with 4.0 months). Perioperative complications did not differ between the groups.

Ewelt et al (2011) retrospectively reviewed 103 elderly (> 65 years) patients with GBM treated at a single institution.[38] A graded increase in overall and progression-free survival was seen in comparisons of biopsy, partial resection, and gross total resection. Multivariate analysis demonstrated extent of resection to be the most significant prognostic factor for these elderly patients with GBM, as compared with age or KPS.

Scott et al (2011) reviewed 206 patients over age 70 with GBM, and found a significant benefit in overall survival for any resection (gross total or subtotal) beyond biopsy.[28] Differences in pre- or postoperative functional status between patients undergoing resection versus biopsy were not reported, nor were perioperative complications. Patients with multifocal disease were less likely to receive surgical resection; nevertheless, debulking surgery remained a significant prognostic factor in a multivariate analysis.

Level IV Evidence

No recent Level IV studies of note address the role of surgical resection versus biopsy in elderly patients with GBM.

Expert Recommendations

1. Maximal surgical resection should be attempted in high-functioning (KPS ≥ 70) elderly patients with GBM to improve overall survival (Grade 1C+ Recommendation, Level I–III Evidence).
2. Standard adjuvant chemoradiation therapy is well tolerated after resection in elderly patients with GBM and should be used whenever possible to improve overall survival (Grade 2C Recommendation, Level III Evidence).
3. The role of surgical resection versus stereotactic biopsy in elderly patients with GBM with poor functional status is unclear, and treatment options should be individualized.

■ Summary and Conclusions

Although most of the available evidence is in the form of retrospective studies, the current neurosurgical literature for elderly patients with glioblastoma strongly favors maximal microsurgical resection as compared with biopsy. Importantly, perioperative complications associated with microsurgical resection are similar to those of biopsy in modern literature. The lone randomized trial in the field, although small, also favored resection over biopsy. Most of the available evidence comes from epidemiological registry queries, single- and multi-institutional case series, and case-control studies. Unfortunately, few studies to date examine quality of life metrics beyond pre- and postoperative KPS for patients undergoing resection versus biopsy. This remains a critical gap in the literature. Additionally, patient populations with poor baseline functional status have not been well studied, and the value of aggressive surgical resection in this subset remains unclear. In summary, advanced age is not a contraindication for aggressive, multimodal therapy in patients with GBM.

■ References

1. Stupp R, Hegi ME, Mason WP, et al; European Organisation for Research and Treatment of Cancer Brain Tumour and Radiation Oncology Groups; National Cancer Institute of Canada Clinical Trials Group. Effects of radiotherapy with concomitant and adjuvant temozolomide versus radiotherapy alone on survival in glioblastoma in a randomised phase III study: 5-year analysis of the EORTC-NCIC trial. Lancet Oncol 2009;10(5): 459–466
2. Siker ML, Wang M, Porter K, et al. Age as an independent prognostic factor in patients with glioblastoma: a Radiation Therapy Oncology Group and American College of Surgeons National Cancer Data Base comparison. J Neurooncol 2011; 104(1):351–356
3. Mirimanoff RO, Gorlia T, Mason W, et al. Radiotherapy and temozolomide for newly diagnosed glioblastoma: recursive partitioning analysis of the EORTC 26981/22981-NCIC CE3 phase III randomized trial. J Clin Oncol 2006;24(16):2563–2569
4. Paravati AJ, Heron DE, Landsittel D, et al. Radiotherapy and temozolomide for newly diagnosed glioblastoma and anaplastic astrocytoma: validation of Radiation Therapy Oncology Group-Recursive Partitioning Analysis in the IMRT and temozolomide era. J Neurooncol 2011;104(1):339–349
5. Chang SM, Parney IF, Huang W, et al; Glioma Outcomes Project Investigators. Patterns of care for adults with newly diagnosed malignant glioma. JAMA 2005;293(5):557–564
6. Hegi ME, Diserens AC, Gorlia T, et al. MGMT gene silencing and benefit from temozolomide in glioblastoma. N Engl J Med 2005;352(10):997–1003
7. Sanai N, Berger MS. Glioma extent of resection and its impact on patient outcome. Neurosurgery 2008;62(4):753–764
8. Brandes A, Fiorentino MV. Treatment of high-grade gliomas in the elderly. Oncology 1998;55(1):1–6
9. Davis FG, Freels S, Grutsch J, Barlas S, Brem S. Survival rates in patients with primary malignant brain tumors stratified by patient age and tumor histological type: an analysis based on Surveillance, Epidemiology, and End Results (SEER) data, 1973-1991. J Neurosurg 1998;88(1):1–10
10. Yovino S, Grossman SA. Treatment of glioblastoma in "elderly" patients. Curr Treat Options Oncol 2011;12(3):253–262
11. Barnholtz-Sloan JS, Maldonado JL, Williams VL, et al. Racial/ethnic differences in survival among elderly patients with a primary glioblastoma. J Neurooncol 2007;85(2):171–180
12. Barnholtz-Sloan JS, Williams VL, Maldonado JL, et al. Patterns of care and outcomes among elderly individuals with primary malignant astrocytoma. J Neurosurg 2008;108(4):642–648
13. Iwamoto FM, Reiner AS, Panageas KS, Elkin EB, Abrey LE. Patterns of care in elderly glioblastoma patients. Ann Neurol 2008;64(6):628–634
14. Iwamoto FM, Cooper AR, Reiner AS, Nayak L, Abrey LE. Glioblastoma in the elderly: The Memorial Sloan-Kettering Cancer Center experience (1997–2007). Cancer 2009;115(16): 3758–3766
15. Brandes AA, Vastola F, Basso U, et al. A prospective study on glioblastoma in the elderly. Cancer 2003;97(3):657–662
16. Fiorica F, Berretta M, Colosimo C, et al. Glioblastoma in elderly patients: safety and efficacy of adjuvant radiotherapy with concomitant temozolomide. Arch Gerontol Geriatr 2010; 51(1):31–35
17. Minniti G, De Sanctis V, Muni R, et al. Radiotherapy plus concomitant and adjuvant temozolomide for glioblastoma in elderly patients. J Neurooncol 2008;88(1):97–103
18. Minniti G, De Sanctis V, Muni R, et al. Hypofractionated radiotherapy followed by adjuvant chemotherapy with temozolomide in elderly patients with glioblastoma. J Neurooncol 2009;91(1):95–100
19. Mangiola A, Maira G, De Bonis P, et al. Glioblastoma multiforme in the elderly: a therapeutic challenge. J Neurooncol 2006;76(2):159–163
20. Patwardhan RV, Shorter C, Willis BK, et al. Survival trends in elderly patients with glioblastoma multiforme: resective surgery, radiation, and chemotherapy. Surg Neurol 2004;62(3): 207–213
21. Roa W, Brasher PM, Bauman G, et al. Abbreviated course of radiation therapy in older patients with glioblastoma multiforme: a prospective randomized clinical trial. J Clin Oncol 2004;22(9):1583–1588
22. Scott J, Tsai YY, Chinnaiyan P, Yu HH. Effectiveness of radiotherapy for elderly patients with glioblastoma. Int J Radiat Oncol Biol Phys 2011;81(1):206–210
23. Brandes AA, Franceschi E, Tosoni A, et al. Temozolomide concomitant and adjuvant to radiotherapy in elderly patients with glioblastoma: correlation with MGMT promoter methylation status. Cancer 2009;115(15):3512–3518
24. Donato V, Papaleo A, Castrichino A, et al. Prognostic implication of clinical and pathologic features in patients with glioblastoma multiforme treated with concomitant radiation plus temozolomide. Tumori 2007;93(3):248–256
25. Pierga JY, Hoang-Xuan K, Feuvret L, et al. Treatment of malignant gliomas in the elderly. J Neurooncol 1999;43(2): 187–193
26. Burger PC, Green SB. Patient age, histologic features, and length of survival in patients with glioblastoma multiforme. Cancer 1987;59(9):1617–1625
27. Kreth FW, Warnke PC, Scheremet R, Ostertag CB. Surgical resection and radiation therapy versus biopsy and radiation therapy in the treatment of glioblastoma multiforme. J Neurosurg 1993;78(5):762–766
28. Scott JG, Suh JH, Elson P, et al. Aggressive treatment is appropriate for glioblastoma multiforme patients 70 years old or older: a retrospective review of 206 cases. Neuro-oncol 2011; 13(4):428–436
29. Vuorinen V, Hinkka S, Färkkilä M, Jääskeläinen J. Debulking or biopsy of malignant glioma in elderly people—a randomised study. Acta Neurochir (Wien) 2003;145(1):5–10
30. Whittle IR, Denholm SW, Gregor A. Management of patients aged over 60 years with supratentorial glioma: lessons from an audit. Surg Neurol 1991;36(2):106–111
31. Whittle IR, Basu N, Grant R, Walker M, Gregor A. Management of patients aged >60 years with malignant glioma: good clinical status and radiotherapy determine outcome. Br J Neurosurg 2002;16(4):343–347
32. Kelly PJ, Hunt C. The limited value of cytoreductive surgery in elderly patients with malignant gliomas. Neurosurgery 1994;34(1):62–66
33. Piccirilli M, Bistazzoni S, Gagliardi FM, et al. Treatment of glioblastoma multiforme in elderly patients. Clinico-ther-

apeutic remarks in 22 patients older than 80 years. Tumori 2006;92(2):98–103
34. Stark AM, Hedderich J, Held-Feindt J, Mehdorn HM. Glioblastoma—the consequences of advanced patient age on treatment and survival. Neurosurg Rev 2007;30(1):56–61
35. Combs SE, Wagner J, Bischof M, et al. Postoperative treatment of primary glioblastoma multiforme with radiation and concomitant temozolomide in elderly patients. Int J Radiat Oncol Biol Phys 2008;70(4):987–992
36. Mukerji N, Rodrigues D, Hendry G, Dunlop PR, Warburton F, Kane PJ. Treating high grade gliomas in the elderly: the end of ageism? J Neurooncol 2008;86(3):329–336
37. Chaichana KL, Garzon-Muvdi T, Parker S, et al. Supratentorial glioblastoma multiforme: the role of surgical resection versus biopsy among older patients. Ann Surg Oncol 2011;18(1):239–245
38. Ewelt C, Goeppert M, Rapp M, Steiger HJ, Stummer W, Sabel M. Glioblastoma multiforme of the elderly: the prognostic effect of resection on survival. J Neurooncol 2011;103(3):611–618

8

The Role of Surgery in Brainstem Gliomas (Pediatric and Adult)

Mari L. Groves, Pablo F. Recinos, and George Jallo

Tumors occurring within the brainstem encompass 10 to 20% of all central nervous system tumors in the pediatric population. Although they can occur at any age, they typically present in childhood, with a mean age of diagnosis of 7 to 9 years.[1,2] In the United States, there are 150 to 300 cases each year.[3,4] There is no gender predilection. In adults, brainstem tumors are more rare, representing only ~ 2% of all brain tumors,[5] with a wider diversity of pathology.

The brainstem, or mesencephalon, is composed of the midbrain, pons, and medulla. Prior to modern imaging techniques the term *brainstem tumor* referred to a heterogeneous group of tumors that were all thought to arise from a single pathological entity. It is now understood that the behavior of these tumors depends on their anatomical location, whether they are diffuse or focal, and histopathology. The early 1980s saw the emergence of favorable neurosurgical outcomes for the resection of certain brainstem gliomas, although the overwhelming reports in the literature come from retrospective case series from a single institution (**Table 8.1**). Given their experience, however, neurosurgeons produced classification systems that attempted to identify tumors that would benefit from surgery and thus defined a management algorithm for these tumors. The development of magnetic resonance imaging (MRI) has been the cornerstone of modern treatment for these lesions because it has allowed tumor location to be clearly defined and tumor behavior to be more accurately predicted.

The initial classification schemes were based on computed tomography (CT)[4–8] and have been supplemented by MRI-based classifications.[9–11] MRI provides the most precise information regarding the tumor origin and most likely diagnosis, which can then predict its biological behavior. Additional imaging studies, such as angiography, MRI spectroscopy, or diffusion-weighted MRI sequences, may be utilized if there is uncertainty in the diagnosis. The most recent radiographic classification system proposed by Choux and colleagues divides brainstem tumors into four types: diffuse (type I), intrinsic focal (type II), focal exophytic (type III), and cervicomedullary (type IV).[12]

For the purposes of this discussion we will consider type I lesions separately from type II through IV lesions. Type I tumors are diffuse brainstem gliomas and account for 75% of all brainstem tumors.[11,13] Diffuse lesions are typically hypointense on T1-weighted MRI sequences, are noncontrast enhancing, and are moderately hyperintense on T2-weighted images.[10] These lesions most commonly occur within the pons and are malignant fibrillary astrocytomas (World Health Organization [WHO] grade III or IV) (**Fig. 8.1**). Retrospective case series have not shown a survival or functional improvement in patients undergoing surgical resection. The need for biopsy of these lesions is controversial and will be addressed further.

Type II lesions are focal, intrinsic tumors that can be cystic or solid (**Fig. 8.2**). These lesions are characterized by their well-demarcated appearance within

Table 8.1 Summary of biopsy data for diffuse brainstem tumors

Study	No. patients	Location	Pathology
Level III			
Kaplan et al 1996[19]	45 (24 stereotactic biopsy; 21 craniotomy all P)	Stereotatic biopsy: 14 diffuse, 9 pons, 1 midbrain Open sx: diffuse—8 biopsy, 2 partial, 4 STR, 1 GTR; pons—2 biopsy, 1 partial; midbrain 1 STR	13 LGA, 20 AA, 2 HGA
Schumacher et al 2007[39]	78	48 pons, mesencephalon 16, medulla/CM 14, extension of tumor in 14	68 LGA, 46 HGA, 10 E
Level IV			
Coffey, Lunsford 1985[33]	12 (1P, 11A)	4 pons/midbrain; 8 midbrain	2 HGA, 4 met, 6 others
Epstein, McCleary 1986[71]	34 (P)	22 pontomedullary diffuse; 4 focal; 8 CM	23 HGA, 11 LGA
Hood et al 1986[61]	12 (2P, 10A)	6 midbrain, 3 pons, 2 midbrain-pons, 1 medulla	6 HGA, 5 LGA, 1 vascular malformation
Mathisen et al 1987[62]	29 (12P, 17A)	–	14 glioma, 4 acoustic neuromas
Frank et al 1988[35]	33	–	15 HGA, 7 LGA, 2 mets
Franzini et al 1988[36]	45 (21P, 24A)	17 midbrain, 11 pons, 6 medulla, 10 midbrain-pons	19 LGA, 14 HGA, 3 hematoma
Epstein, Wisoff 1987[58]	20 (15P, 5A)	20 CM	11 LGA, 4 HGA, 3 GG, 2 E
Thomas et al 1988[38]	12 (11A, 1P)	8 pons, 2 pontomesencephalic, 1 medulla/pons, 1 cerebellar peduncle	5 LGA
Guthrie et al 1989[63]	4 (2P, 2A)	3 pontine, 1 cerebellum	1 PNET, 2 LGA
Abernathey et al 1989[64]	26 (6P, 20A)	NR	6 LGA, 8 LGA
Ryken et al 1992[65]	11 (1P, 10A)	7 pons, 3 midbrain, 1 cerebellum, 11 midbrain	4 HGA, 2 LGA,
Kratimenos et al 1992[37]	34	5 mid-pons, 8 pons, 10 pontomedullary	16 LGA, 7 HGA, 3 met
Kratimenos, Thomas 1993[66]	72	15 midbrain, 24 pontine, 4 medulla, 10 midbrain-pontine junction; 11 pontomedullary junction, 5 lateral pons, 2 diffuse pontine	20 LGA, 13 HGA, 6 met carcinomas
Steck, Friedman 1995[44]	24 (6P, 18A)	16 pons, 7 midbrain, 1 medullar	5 HGA, 11 LGA
Rajshekhar, Chandy 1995[67]	71	22 pontomedullary, p/m 15 pons and midbrain, 34 diffuse brainstem	51 LGA, 7 HGA
Kondziolka, Lunsford 1995[42]	40	20 midbrain, 18 pontine, 2 medullary	17 HGA, 9 LGA
Behnke et al 1997[15]	30 (P)	Open biopsy: 5 CM; 11 focal, 14 diffuse	16 LGA, 6 HGA, 4 PNET
Massager et al 2000[68]	30 (5P, 25A)	14 pons, 12 midbrain, 4 medulla	14 HGA, 4 LGA, 3 mets
Gonçalves-Ferreira et al 2003[69]	30 (3P, 27A)	Focal (19 pons, 10 midbrain). 11 lesions approached through transfrontal, all others SOC	14 astrocytomas
Samadani, Judy 2003[40]	293	–	–
Pincus et al 2006[43]	10	6 midbrain, 4 pons	6 LGA, 2 HGA
Roujeau et al 2007[41]	24 (P)	Diffuse pontine	2 LGA, 22 HGA
Rajshekhar, Moorthy 2010[70]	106 (P)	81 diffuse, 21 focal, 4 exophytic	12 JPA, 64 LGA, 19 HGA, 1 E

Abbreviations: –, not reported; AA, anaplastic astrocytoma; ADIM, acute disseminated encephalomyelitis; CM, cervicomedullary: CPP, choroid plexus papilloma; CSF, cerebrospinal fluid; E, ependymomas; GG, ganglioglioma; GTR, gross total resection ~ 100%; HGA, high-grade astrocytoma; JPA, juvenile pilocytic astrocytoma; LGA, low-grade astrocytoma; met, metastatic lesion; NR, not recorded; oligo, oligodendroglioma; PML, progressive multifocal leukoencephalopathy; PNET, primitive neuroectodermal tumor; near total resection > 90; SOC, suboccipital; STR, subtotal resection 50–90%; partial resection < 50%; TB, tuberculosis.

% Diagnosis made	Unusual disease	Morbidity	Mortality
97% (35/36)	–	11% (5)	0
94% (119/126)	Oligodendroglioma, GG, CPP, schwannoma, venous anomaly	3.2% (4)	0
100	Lymphoma, neuroepithelial cysts, chronic inflammation, hematoma	0	0
100	–	17% (6)	11% (4)
100	–	8% (1)	0
100	Pinealoma, medulloblastoma, ependymoma, AVM, CSF cyst ependymoma, meningioma, lymphoma, arachnoid cyst, cavernous malformation ependymoma, PNET, lymphoma, metastatic, neurinoma, arachnoid cyst, cholesteoma	3% (1)	0
100	Pinealoma, medulloblastoma, ependymoma, AVM, CSF cyst ependymoma, meningioma, lymphoma, arachnoid cyst, cavernous malformation ependymoma, PNET, lymphoma, metastatic, neurinoma, arachnoid cyst, cholesteoma	21% (7)	3% (1)
100	Pinealoma, medulloblastoma, ependymoma, AVM, CSF cyst ependymoma, meningioma, lymphoma, arachnoid cyst, cavernous malformation ependymoma, PNET, lymphoma, metastatic, neurinoma, arachnoid cyst, cholesteoma	4% (2)	0
100	–	0	0
92% (11/12)	4 hematoma, 2 granuloma	0	0
100	1 radionecrosis demyelinating, infarction, radionecrosis, abscess, oligo, ependymoma	0	0
100	1 radionecrosis demyelinating, infarction, radionecrosis, abscess, oligo, ependymoma	0	0
91% (10/11)	Adenocarcinoma, ependymoma, hematoma	0	0
94% (32/34)	Lymphoma, neuroblastoma, 4 nonneoplastic	6%	0
97% (70/72)	Lymphoma, neuroblastoma, neuroectodermal, 8 nonneoplastic conditions	3% (2)	0
96% (23/24)	Lymphoma, germinoma, chordoma, PML	8% (2)	4%
98.5% (68/69)	Ependymoma, TB, cysts, abscess, encephalitis	7%	0
95%	Carcinoma, lymphoma, radiation necrosis, angiitis, storage disease, neuroepithelial cyst	2.5% (1)	0
100%	Oligo, ependymoma	NR	NR
100	Gangliocytoma, lymphoma, vasculitis, ependymoma, leukemia, infection	7% (2)	0
93% (26/28)	Lymphoma, GG, infection, ADIM, PML, *Aspergillus*	7%	0
94% in 1st biopsy, 96% in 2nd biopsy		4% transient, 1% perm	0.30%
100	Demyelination, medulloblastoma	10% (1)	0
100		8% (2)	0
99% (105/106)	Necrosis, 6 TB, 1 toxoplasmosis, 1 encephalitis, 1 cyst	10% (11)	0

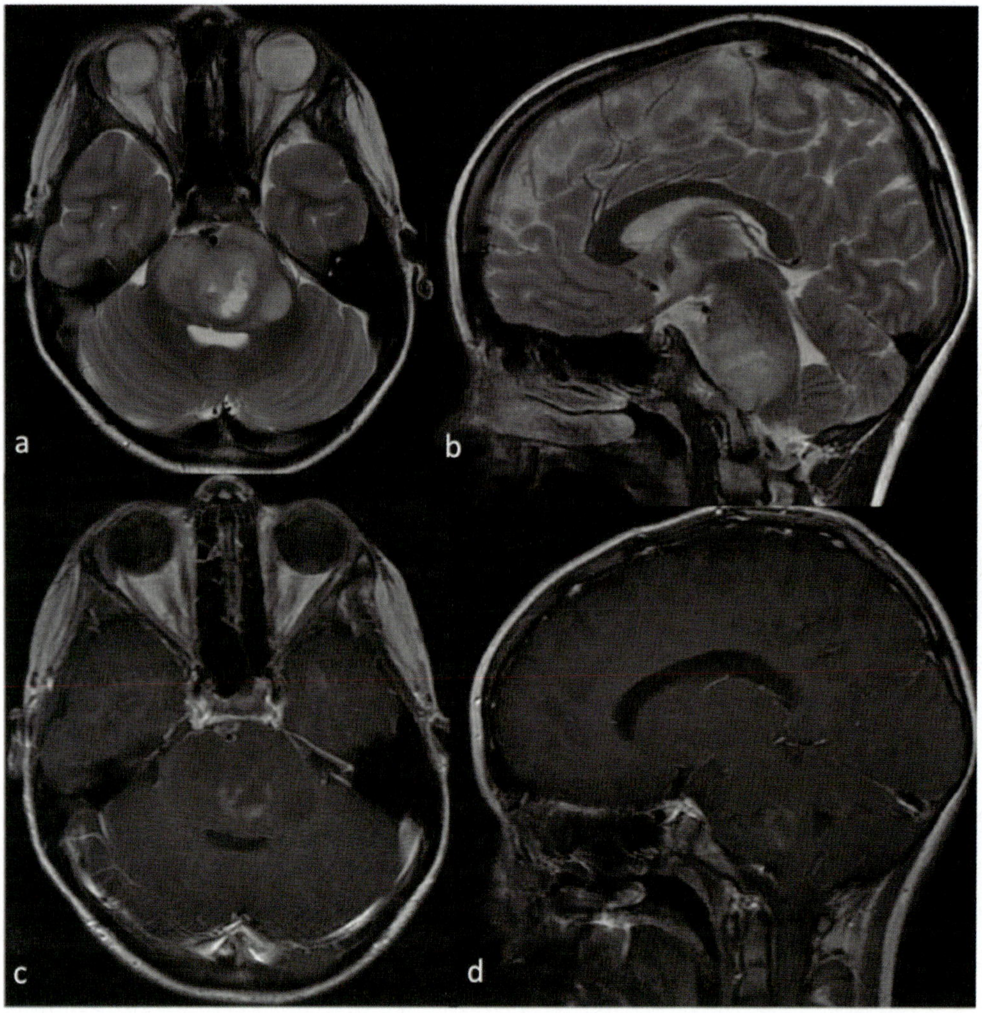

Fig. 8.1 Diffuse pontine glioma as seen on **(a)** axial and **(b)** sagittal T2 and **(c)** axial and **(d)** sagittal T1 gadolinium-enhanced magnetic resonance imaging sequences. Typical imaging characteristics are seen, including heterogeneous tumor mass, poorly demarcated borders, and global expansion of the pons. Diffuse tumors are the most common type of brainstem lesion and are invasive tumors that involve the pontine parenchyma.

the surrounding tissue and typically produce minimal brainstem edema.[12] These lesions are most commonly low-grade gliomas (WHO I or II). There is variable contrast enhancement on T1-weighted MRI; however, uniform enhancement is more characteristic of pilocytic astrocytomas.[14] Type III lesions are defined as dorsal exophytic tumors that arise from the subependymal glial tissue of the fourth ventricle and grow both dorsally and laterally[12,15] (**Fig. 8.3**). There are reports that exophytic brainstem tumors which have a lateral and ventral growth pattern tend to be higher grade than those exophytic lesions that extend dorsally.[14,16,17] Type IV lesions are cervicomedullary tumors that present and behave similarly to intramedullary spinal cord gliomas[8,12] (**Fig. 8.4**). These lesions are typically low-grade and noninfiltrative, with growth that is confined by the white matter of the corticospinal tract and medial lemniscus.[16]

■ Presentation

As is the case for other neuraxis lesions, patient presentation is dependent on the location of the brainstem tumor. A complete clinical picture is necessary for workup and should include a thorough history and physical examination. Old school pictures may be necessary to track the emergence of cranial neuropathies. Declining school performance can be related

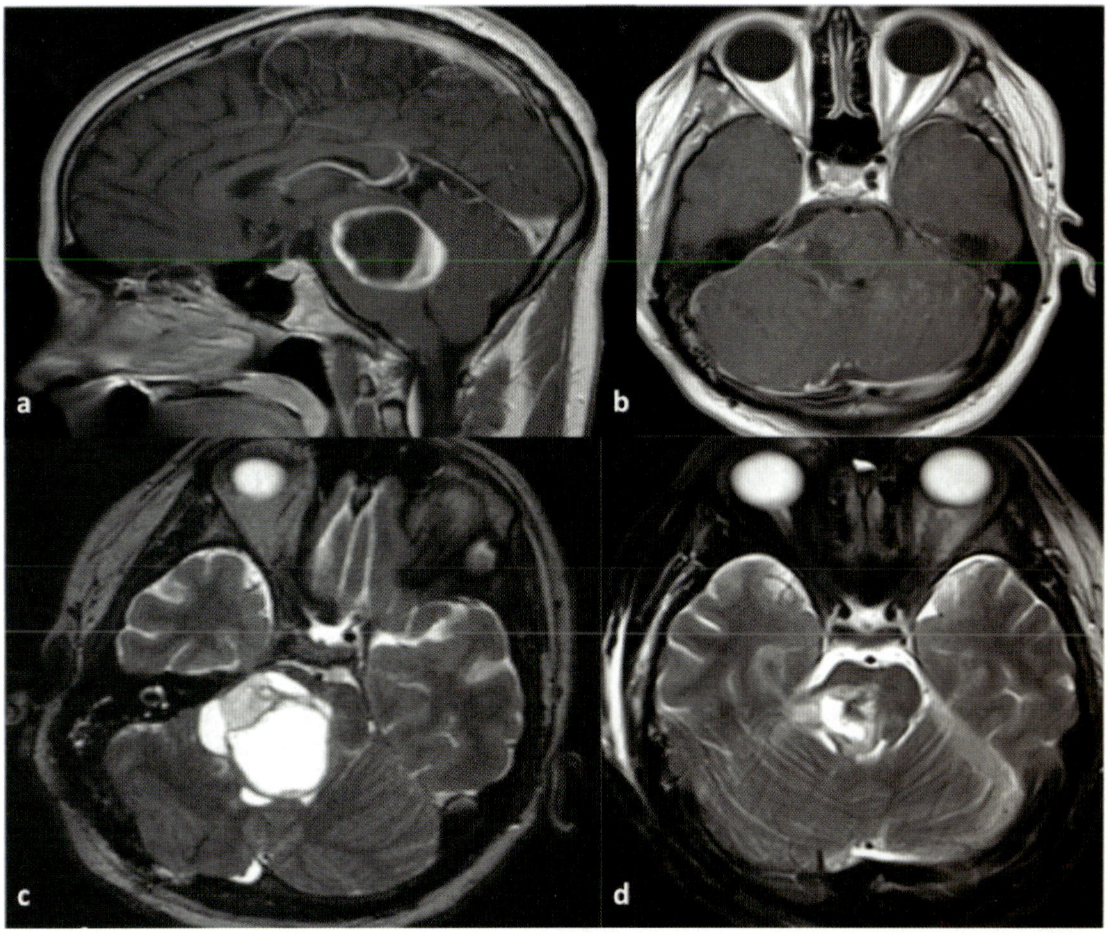

Fig. 8.2 Focal intrinsic pontine tumor as seen on preoperative **(a)** sagittal T1 gadolinium-enhanced and **(c)** axial T2 magnetic resonance imaging sequences. The tumor is seen fully within the pons but has well-demarcated borders and a large cystic component. Focal tumors can also be completely solid without an associated cyst. This patient was diagnosed with a juvenile pilocytic astrocytoma. Following surgery, elimination of the gadolinium enhancement **(b)** and collapse of the cystic space **(d)** are seen.

to visual disturbances or symptoms of hydrocephalus. There may also be a history of upper respiratory tract infections, pneumonias, or changes in voice.[18] Three important components should be ascertained during the workup: signs and symptoms related to the intra-axial component, signs and symptoms of hydrocephalus, and symptom onset.

Type I tumors are diffuse and typically more malignant lesions. They progress rapidly (weeks to months) and will present acutely with multiple cranial neuropathies, ataxia, long tract signs, and/or cerebellar signs.[19] Interruption of the corticospinal tract fibers results in upper motor neuron signs that include loss of fine motor skills, spasticity, initial hyporeflexia followed by hyperreflexia, and an upgoing extensor plantar reflex.[19] Cranial neuropathies are most commonly sixth- and seventh-nerve weakness.[15,20] Cerebellar dysfunction can manifest as both appendicular and axial ataxia.[20]

Type II lesions are focal, intrinsic tumors that are generally low-grade gliomas. They have a longer prodrome (months to years) than the diffuse lesions. Clinical symptoms depend on location. Midbrain gliomas are low-grade lesions.[21] Tectal lesions primarily compress the sylvian aqueduct, causing obstructive hydrocephalus and oculomotor paresis. Focal pontine lesions have a poorer prognosis and present with facial paresis, hearing loss, or long tract findings.[11,16] Focal medullary lesions can present with lower cranial nerve deficits that can manifest as voice changes, swallowing difficulty, or pneumonias due to microaspirations. Preoperative medullary dysfunction portends a challenging perioperative course and often carries a high surgical

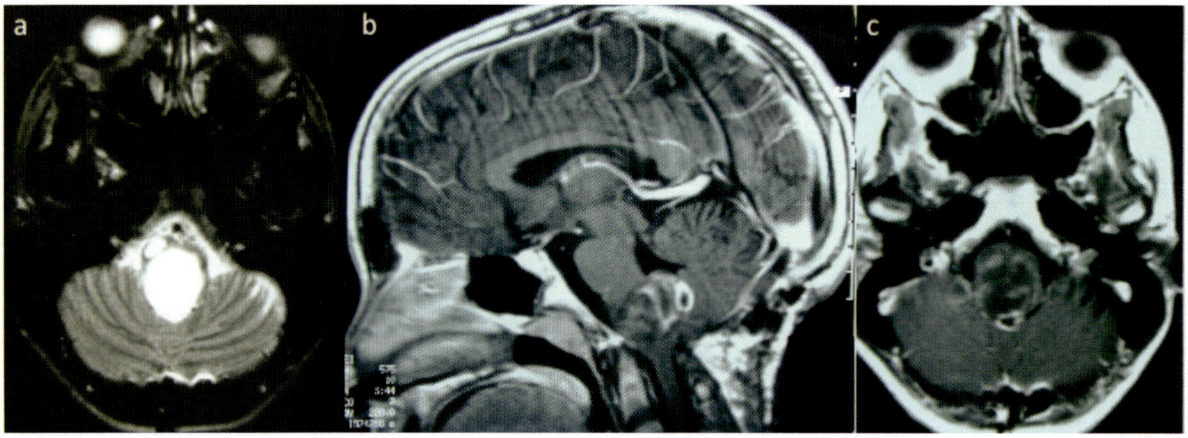

Fig. 8.3 Dorsal exophytic tumor as seen on **(a)** axial T2 image and **(b)** sagittal and **(c)** axial T1 gadolinium-enhanced magnetic resonance imaging sequences. The tumor is arising from the dorsal pontine surface along the floor of the fourth ventricle. The tumor has well-demarcated borders and focal contrast enhancement. Typically, the tumor exerts mass effect on the brainstem without parenchymal invasion.

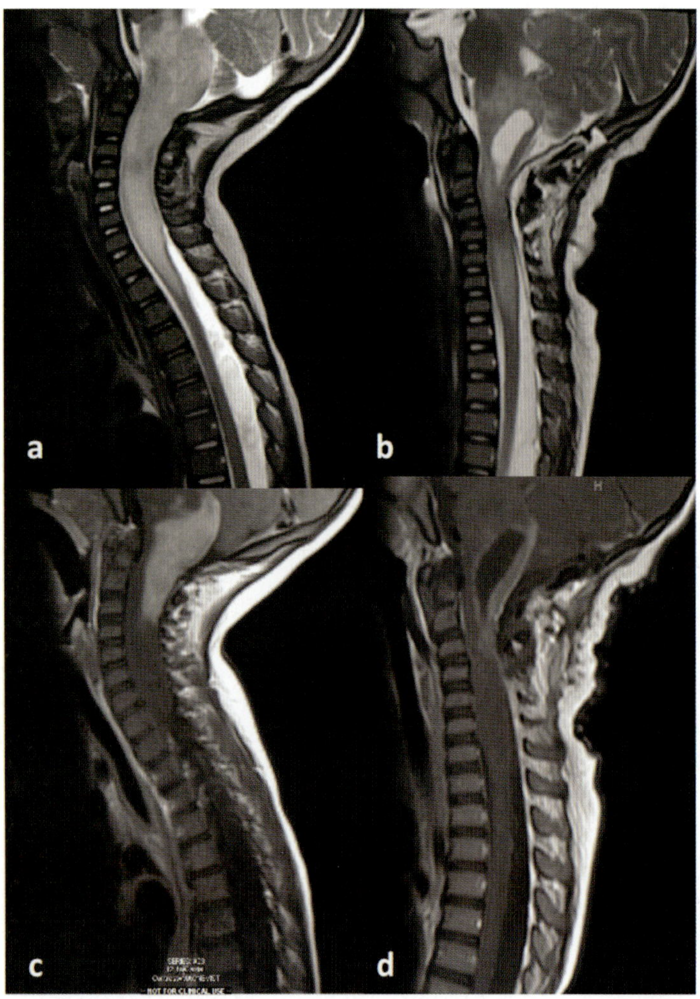

Fig. 8.4 Cervicomedullary tumor as seen on sagittal **(a)** T2 and **(c)** T1 gadolinium magnetic resonance imaging (MRI) sequences. Diffuse enhancement along with cord expansion is seen into the upper cervical cord. Surgically, the gadolinium-enhanced area is targeted for resection, and any associated syrinx or cysts are left in place unless there is significant mass effect. Postoperative images demonstrate significant resection of the mass in **(b)** T2 and **(d)** T1 gadolinium-enhanced MRI sequences.

morbidity.[18] Atypical tumors are more common in adults than children and should be considered if a patient presents with a focal, nonenhancing tumor and rapid progression. An excisional biopsy should be considered when atypical features are present to rule out a primitive neuroectodermal tumor or other aggressive neoplasm.

The dorsal exophytic component that defines type III tumors may produce symptoms due to direct compression of the underlying brainstem or with elevated intracranial pressure (ICP) secondary to obstructive hydrocephalus. This manifests as headaches, ataxia, intractable vomiting, blurry vision secondary to papilledema, and torticollis.

Type IV tumors are also associated with an indolent course. Medullary dysfunction can be present as described previously. Cervical cord dysfunction will also manifest as chronic neck pain and progressive cervical myelopathy with associated weakness and spasticity. Aggressive surgical resection with an attempt at gross total resection has been associated with improved long-term control and overall survival.[15,22–25]

■ Treatment

It is clear that brainstem tumors do not all exhibit the same behavior. Classification of these lesions based on location and focality parse out the more surgically favorable type II to IV lesions from diffuse type I tumors.[26] Type I tumors are malignant lesions with a rapidly progressive course and poor prognosis. There is no role for radical surgery, and biopsy is reserved for cases that are indeterminate on MRI or with unusual presentations. Proponents of brainstem biopsy argue that a histopathological diagnosis provides prognostic information, guides therapeutic decisions, and avoids misdiagnosis of low-grade lesions that mimic high-grade lesions.[15,27–29] Focal tumors (type II through IV) are generally amenable to surgical resection. The goal of surgical treatment of these tumors is to maximize tumor resection while minimizing neurological sequelae. However, given the close proximity of critical areas of the brainstem, surgical morbidity is significantly higher than in tumor resections supratentorially.[16,20,30]

Evidence-Based Indications for Brainstem Biopsy

Brainstem lesion biopsy has come in and out of favor in the workup of these lesions since image guidance became available in 1975. Biopsy of brainstem lesions was popularized over the following decade with various retrospective case series from single institutions showing high diagnostic yields with low morbidity and mortality in both children and adults.[31–38] However, as MRI emerged as a diagnostic tool, many argued that sampling tissue was unnecessary in patients with diffuse brainstem tumors, given that diagnosis could be made with clinical presentation and imaging characteristics.[12,19] However, Epstein was critical that a small biopsy specimen did not provide useful information and that the risk associated with the procedure outweighed the clinical benefit.[23,26] Stroink and colleagues further reinforced the argument against biopsy when they showed that biopsy of these brainstem lesions had a poor diagnostic yield and was not representative of the tumor as a whole.[6] The majority of this early work was the result of retrospective analysis of a single center (**Table 8.1**). Diagnostic criteria then shifted from a combination of histological and radiological characteristics to exclusively radiological criteria based on several brainstem tumor classification systems.[9,11,12,23,26]

Level I and Level II Evidence

There is no Level I or II evidence comparing biopsy followed by adjuvant therapy to adjuvant therapy alone.

Level III Evidence

As part of the Children's Cancer Group study, Kaplan and colleagues extrapolated data regarding the need for biopsy in patients with brainstem gliomas.[19] The study was conducted as a cooperative phase 1/2 clinical trial to determine the toxicity of hyperfractionated radiotherapy and to estimate the potential efficacy of two total doses of hyperfractionated radiotherapy in children with brainstem gliomas. However, as part of their study they collected prospective data on the surgical treatment for diagnosis and treatment. The treating neurosurgeon determined whether the patients underwent biopsy or a more formal resection; however, they found tissue diagnosis did not alter the adjuvant therapy in children with brainstem gliomas. A total of 119 children were recruited, and, of those, 45 (38%) underwent a tumor operation. Stereotactic biopsy was performed in 24 patients, and 21 patients underwent surgical resection. Biopsies confirmed the MRI diagnosis of brainstem gliomas in every patient who underwent surgery. Because there was no difference between the radiographic and pathological diagnosis, the authors concluded that biopsies and tissue diagnosis were rarely needed to confirm the diagnosis or to alter treatment. They concluded that there are three reasons to offer surgery for brainstem tumors: for type II through IV tumors, if there is a questionable diagnosis, or if the biopsy results will alter treatment for a patient in a prospective clinical trial.[19]

The German Pediatric Oncology and Hematology group reviewed 142 cases of brainstem tumors, comparing MRI data with histological diagnosis from multiple centers.[39] Three blinded observers were able to correctly identify tumors and nonneoplastic lesions, reaching a sensitivity of 94%. However, the ability to correctly establish WHO grading varied between 12 and 74%. The authors concluded that, based on 14 imaging criteria together with the patient's history and symptoms, the diagnosis of a brainstem tumor as opposed to a nonmalignant cause could be made.[39] They then concluded that the need for biopsy is rare and should be assessed on a case-by-case basis.

Level IV Evidence

There has been a resurgence of interest in biopsy with the publication of several studies advocating that biopsy can alter management of patients with diffuse pontine lesions and that MRI may be inadequate. Samadani and Judy collected a meta-analysis of 293 brainstem biopsies in both adults and children.[40] They found that a diagnosis was made in 94% of patients after the first biopsy and over 96% of the time for second biopsy cases. In addition, 4% of patients had a transient neurological deficit, with 1% having a permanent neurological deficit, with a mortality rate of 0.3%.[40] Given that, in the adult population, the differential diagnosis for nonenhancing brainstem lesions is more varied, biopsy of this population may be indicated. In children, the overwhelming majority of diffuse pontine lesions are high-grade gliomas.[40]

Roujeau and colleagues also published a series of 24 stereotactic brainstem tumor biopsies in which a histological diagnosis was obtained in all patients.[41] Twenty-two were either grade III or IV, one was a grade II, and one was a pilocytic astrocytoma. Two patients suffered a transient neurological deficit, but both resolved at 2 months. In the patients with low-grade lesions, the pathology altered the management, and radiotherapy was delayed. Upon progression, the patient with the grade I tumor underwent surgery to attempt resection, whereas the patient with the grade II tumor was treated with radiation therapy.[41]

Behnke and colleagues also reported a series of 30 patients with intra-axial, endophytic tumors of the pons and medulla undergoing open surgery for excision. In five cases, the tumor had a focal appearance.[15] There were nine patients with a diffuse pattern of growth on MRI that included three grade I and six grade II astrocytomas. In this case, histopathologically benign tumors can mimic malignant tumors radiographically.[15,29] Kumar and colleagues also reported a series of 100 patients with intracranial grade I astrocytomas that had features mimicking high-grade gliomas on MRI.[29] Within their series, 76 were pediatric patients and 24 had brainstem tumors.

In the modern era, stereotactic biopsy is a relatively safe procedure with morbidity rates between 2.5 and 11%[30,39,40,42–44] and mortality rates of 0.05 to 2.6%.[39] Diagnostic yields range from 87 to 100%.[40,42–44] There is also growing consensus that biopsy-proven diagnosis will be an enrollment criterion for ongoing clinical trials.[12,41] This potential need for tissue diagnosis in the setting of a safe surgical procedure will drive some toward biopsy of these diffuse lesions.

Conclusion

Level III and IV evidence has shown that a diagnosis can be obtained from a brainstem biopsy with relatively low morbidity and mortality. In the pediatric population, diffuse brainstem lesions are almost uniformly gliomas that lead to a rapidly progressive course and poor prognosis. In the adult population, the rate of more unusual, noncancerous lesions is slightly higher and can warrant biopsy dependent on the clinical presentation. Biopsy is at times necessary to obtain a histopathological diagnosis and to guide therapeutic interventions and can be done in a safe manner. Several groups in Europe have implemented image-guided stereotactic biopsy of brainstem gliomas at diagnosis as a way to obtain biologically informative tumor material (**Table 8.1**).

Recommendations for Biopsy of Diffuse Pontine Tumors

1. With current technology, stereotactic biopsy of brainstem lesions provides a diagnosis 94 to 100% of the time. Morbidity associated with the procedure ranges from 2.5 to 11% and an associated mortality of 0.05 to 2.6% (Grade 1C Recommendation, Level III/IV Evidence).
2. Indications for biopsy include an atypical appearance on MRI or an unusual clinical presentation. Biopsy is also indicated when entry into a clinical trial mandates a formal histological diagnosis (Grade 2C Recommendation, Level III/IV Evidence).

Evidence-Based Indications for Surgical Resection

Improved imaging has helped distinguish lesions that are more amenable to surgical intervention, including types II through IV of brainstem tumors. These tumors are typically managed similarly to low-grade tumors found in other accessible areas, with aggressive surgical resection being used as the primary therapeutic modality. For deep-seated brainstem lesions that may not be amenable to aggressive resection, conformal radiation therapy or chemotherapy has been typically considered.

Level I Evidence

There are no Level I data regarding surgical treatment of brainstem tumors versus surgery with radiation and chemotherapy.

Level II Evidence

In a recent report, Wisoff and colleagues showed that the factor most strongly associated with outcome in all low-grade gliomas is the extent of surgical removal.[45] A prospective cohort study (CCG 9891/POG8930) found that histological type, extent of residual tumor, and disease site were significantly associated with progression-free survival (PFS) and overall survival. Of the 518 patients enrolled, 74 patients had midline tumors, which included thalamic–basal ganglia and dorsal exophytic brainstem tumors.[45] They showed that children who underwent a gross total resection of their low-grade gliomas in all locations had greater than 90% 5-year PFS. Children with less extensive tumor removal had a 56% PFS at 5 years. The 5- and 8-year PFSs were 61% and 51% for midline and chiasmatic tumors.[45]

Level III Evidence

Fisher and colleagues also aimed to determine the long-term natural history of low-grade astrocytomas through a retrospective cohort study.[46] They assessed 278 children, of whom 40 had brainstem lesions. Overall survival at 5 and 10 years was 87% and 83%, respectively, with a PFS of 55% and 42%. Patients with residual tumor after surgery had a 5-year PFS of 48% with observation alone. This result was no different from that for patients who had radiotherapy following resection.[46] Of the 40 patients with brainstem lesions, one patient had gross total resection, 21 had a subtotal resection, and 18 had a partial resection or biopsy. Of the brainstem tumors, 55% were juvenile pilocytic astrocytomas (JPAs), 33% being diffuse astrocytomas or unclassifiable low-grade astrocytoma, and 12% without an available specimen. The patients diagnosed with JPAs had an improved survival versus the patients who were diagnosed with diffuse astrocytoma.[46]

Lesniak and colleagues reported a series of 89 patients from 1985 to 2000 who underwent surgery or radiation and chemotherapy.[47] JPA was diagnosed in 52.6% of patients, with an additional 17.6% diagnosed with fibrillary astrocytoma. Patients diagnosed with high-grade lesions (21.1%) all underwent both chemotherapy and radiotherapy, whereas those who presented with a local recurrence also underwent revision surgery followed by radiation treatment. The survival rates for patients undergoing surgical treatment related to tumor pathology.[47] The authors also found that patients with a rapid onset of symptoms (< 6 mo) had a poorer prognosis than those with a prolonged clinical presentation (> 6 mo). A contrast-enhancing tumor was also associated with improved survival. They also showed that, for the cohort treated with either radiation, chemotherapy, or both, radiation was the only form of therapy that showed any survival benefit. They demonstrated no additional progression-free or overall survival benefit for patients treated with chemotherapy.[47]

Level IV Evidence

Focal intrinsic, dorsal exophytic, and cervicomedullary lesions present less controversy for treatment. Over the last two decades, an increasing number of case series have shown that these subgroups of brainstem gliomas have significantly longer survival rates than diffuse pontine gliomas. The subsets of brainstem tumors that are not diffuse are more often associated with low-grade pathologies and offer a better prognosis (**Tables 8.2, 8.3, 8.4**). These tumors share four characteristics associated with good prognosis: long duration of symptoms before diagnosis, low-grade histology, amenability to surgical resection, and long-term survival.[48]

Early surgery is favored as a first-line intervention with the hope of operating prior to neurological decline or adjuvant therapy. The goal of surgery is to decrease the tumor burden while avoiding neurological complications. Gross total resection is not the gold standard; significant morbidities can be associated with damage to cranial nerve nuclei, including tracheostomy and ventilator dependence as well as a feeding gastrostomy.[11,16,48]

Focal Intrinsic Brainstem Tumors

Vandertop and colleagues described 12 focal midbrain tumors in children.[49] Nearly 50% of the patients presented with signs consistent with obstructive hydrocephalus, and the other 50% presented with long-tract signs. The lesions the authors describe were confined to the tectal plate or tegmentum and

Table 8.2 Summary of Level IV evidence for surgical resection of focal brainstem tumors

Study	No. patients	Histology	Surgery	Adjuvant therapy	Outcome
Vandertop et al 1992[49]	12	12 LGA	9 near total, 3 partial	6 XRT, 2 XRT + chemotherapy	12 alive, mean 30 m
Pierre-Kahn et al 1993[50]	75	47 LGA, 22 HGA, 1 GG, 2 ependymoma, 2 PNET, 1 other	10 GTR, 22 STR, 43 partial	12 perioperative radiation; 64 postop rads	55% survival at 5 y (mean follow-up 31 m), 49% at 10 y; 74% at 3 y in benign tumors, 22% at 3 y in malignant tumors
Farmer et al 2001[51]	13	10 LGA, 3 GG	13 STR		11 alive, 92% 5 y survival; 83% PFS at 5 y (median survival 38 m)
Lesniak et al 2003[47]	57	40 LGA, 3 GG, 12 HGA, 1 oligo, 1 PNET	29 GTR, 8 near total, 15 STR, 5 partial	16 XRT, 12 XRT and/or chemotherapy	60% alive at 5 y (median follow-up > 120 m)
Kestle et al 2004[52]	25	25 LGA (JPA)	12 GTR, 13 STR	6 postop XRT, 1 chemotherapy; 1 preop chemotherapy/XRT	28 alive 100 alive at 5 y, 51% PFS at 5 y, 44% at 10 (mean follow-up of 70 m)
Sandri et al 2006[53]	17	12 LGA, 2 GG, 3 HGA	4 near total (> 80%), 7 STR, 6 partial	6 XRT, 2 XRT + chemotherapy	14 alive, 87% alive at 5 y, 59% PFS 5 y (median follow-up 25 m)
Teo, Siu 2008[54]	34	7 GBM, 4 AA, 12 low-grade astrocytoma grade II, 8 JPA, 3 GG	12 GTR, 19 near total (> 90%), 3 STR (> 50%, < 90%)	10 radiation	26 alive, 75% alive at 5 y, 66% PFS 5 y (median follow-up 46 m)

Abbreviations: AA, anaplastic astrocytoma; GG, ganglioglioma; GTR, gross total resection ~ 100%; HGA, high-grade astrocytoma; JPA, juvenile pilocytic astrocytoma; LGA, low-grade astrocytoma; oligo, oligodendroglioma; PFS, progression-free survival; PNET, primitive neuroectodermal tumor; TNR, near total resection > 90%; STR, subtotal resection 50–90%; partial resection < 50%; XRT, radiation therapy.

Table 8.3 Summary of Level IV evidence for surgical resection of dorsal exophytic brainstem tumors

Study	No. patients	Histology	Surgery	Adjuvant therapy	Outcome	Progression
Stroink et al 1987[58]	16	13 LGA, 2 GG, 1 HGA	16 STR	7 XRT	Median follow-up 7 y	94% 5-year PFS
Pollack et al 1993[56]	18	16 LGA grade I or II, 1 astrocytoma grade III, 1 GG	–	2	17 alive (median 113 m)	4
Khatib et al 1994[57]	12	11 JPA, 1 LGA	6 NTR; 6 STR	2	11 alive (median 26 m)	3
Fischbein et al 1996[10]	10	–	–	–	7 alive (mean 35 m)	–

Abbreviations: GG, ganglioglioma; HGA, high-grade astrocytoma; JPA, juvenile pilocytic astrocytoma; LGA, low-grade astrocytoma; NTR, near total resection > 90%; PFS, progression-free survival; STR, subtotal resection 50–90%; XRT, radiation therapy.

Table 8.4 Summary of Level IV evidence for surgical resection of cervicomedullary brainstem tumors

Study	No. patients	Histology	Surgery	Adjuvant therapy	Outcome	Progression
Epstein, Wisoff 1987[58]	20	11 LGA, 4 AA, 3 GG, 2 E	–	4	16 alive median 24 m	4/4 of high-grade tumors, 1/16 of low-grade tumors
Robertson et al 1994[24]	17	10 LGA, 6 GG, 1 mixed astrocytoma	2 GTR, 15 STR	2	15 alive, median 48 m	6
Behnke et al 1997[15]	4	3 JPA, 1 E	–	–	–	–
Weiner et al 1997[25]	39	15 LGA, 9 E, 7 GG, 3 JPA, 3 AA, 2 mixed gliomas	12 GTR, 7 NTR, 15 STR, 5 PR	None	39 alive, mean 48 m	3/4 of high-grade tumors, 12/35 of low-grade tumors; 89% alive at 5 years, 60% 5-year PFS
Di Maio et al 2009[59]	9	2 JPA, 2 GG, 5 LGA	Following adjuvant therapy: 3 NTR; 1 30%; before adjuvant therapy: 1 biopsy; 4 < 25%; 3 STR	3 XRT + chemotherapy, 2 XRT, 1 chemotherapy	5 alive, median 114 m	75% OS at 5 y, 50% OS at 10 y

Abbreviations: AA, anaplastic astrocytoma; E, ependymomas; GG, ganglioglioma; GTR, gross total resection ~ 100%; JPA, juvenile pilocytic astrocytoma; LGA, low-grade astrocytoma; OS, overall survival; PFS, progression-free survival; STR, subtotal resection 50–90%; NTR, near total resection > 90%; PR, partial resection < 50%.

cerebral peduncle. These tumors had well-defined edges with a solid consistency and homogeneous enhancement. A significant reduction in tumor mass was obtained in 75% of the patients, with minimal surgical morbidity and improvement in 33%.[49] All tumors were nonpilocytic, low-grade astrocytomas. Six of these patients underwent adjuvant radiotherapy due to partial resection or progressive enlargement in the residual tumor. Their follow-up was relatively short and ranged from 1 month to 5 years, but all 12 patients were alive at the conclusion of the study, with a mean follow-up of 30 months.[49]

In 1993 Pierre-Kahn and colleagues published a retrospective analysis of patients treated at their institution between 1970 and 1990.[50] The patients presented with exophytic or surface brainstem tumors and underwent partial, subtotal, or total removal of their tumors. The authors showed that the patients with malignant tumors had a poor prognosis that was not significantly impacted by surgery. However, the survival rate for low-grade tumors was impacted by the surgeon's ability to perform a subtotal or total resection.[50] Benign tumors had a survival rate of 74% at 3 years versus malignant tumors with a survival rate of 22% at 4 years. For low-grade lesions, the 3- and 5-year survival rates were also significantly higher after total or subtotal removal than after partial removal (94% vs 52%).[50] There were no recurrences noted in patients with low-grade tumors who had total or subtotal resections and were not postoperatively radiated.

Farmer and colleagues reported on their case series of 22 patients who had focal brainstem gliomas in comparison with 15 patients with diffuse pontine gliomas.[51] They found that PFS and overall survival were significantly worse in the patients with diffuse pontine gliomas. The patients who underwent surgical resection had either low-grade astrocytomas or gangliogliomas. At the conclusion of their study, the authors found that the patients who underwent subtotal resection without radiation therapy had a 92% survival rate at 5 years as well as an 83% PFS at 5 years.[51]

Kestle and colleagues described a case series of 28 patients with JPA of the brainstem.[52] The study comprised 25 patients who underwent resection, and of those patients a gross or near total resection was obtained in 12 patients. Of the 12 patients, seven were observed, with one tumor recurrence noted during follow-up. In the 10 patients with solid residual tumor who were observed, progression was seen in five over the course of the follow-up. The 5- and

10-year PFS was 74 and 62% for those patients who achieved a gross or near total resection. When there was residual solid tumor, the PFS fell to 19% at 5 and 10 years.[52] All patients were alive at the last follow-up, with a mean follow-up period of 5.8 years.

Sandri and colleagues compared diffuse brainstem tumors with focal brainstem tumors in 31 patients. Those with diffuse brainstem tumors were treated with radiotherapy and chemotherapy. For the patients with focal lesions, adjuvant therapy was considered only in cases of progression.[53] Although patients with diffuse brainstem tumors did have some improvement in symptoms, the median time from diagnosis to progression and subsequent death was 8 months and 13 months, respectively. Their 2-year overall survival rate was only 12.3%. In the patients with focal lesions, the 4-year overall survival and disease-free survival were 87.4% and 58.8%, respectively. The patients who showed recurrence were treated with radiation or radiation plus chemotherapy. At the conclusion of the series, 14 of 17 patients were still alive, with a median follow-up of 46 months.[53]

Teo and Siu also reported a series of 34 patients who underwent resection of focal brainstem lesions between 1999 and 2005.[54] They were able to achieve gross or near total resection in 31 patients. They also showed a significant difference in 5-year survival rates between those with high-grade gliomas and those with low-grade gliomas, 33% versus 100%. However, their data did not show that the degree of tumor resection was associated with improved outcomes at 6 months. At the conclusion of their study, a total of 26 patients were alive, with an overall survival at 5 years of 75% and PFS at 5 years of 66%, with a median follow-up of 46 months.[54] Additionally, 10 of their patients underwent postoperative radiation and were among those still alive at the conclusion of the study.

Dorsal Exophytic Brainstem Tumors

Dorsal exophytic tumors are the most amenable to gross total resection. A standard midline suboccipital craniotomy with possible extension to C1 is the standard approach. The telovelar approach is used to expose the fourth ventricle because it avoids injury to the vermis and cerebellar tonsils. These tumors arise from the ependymal cells of the fourth ventricular floor[55]; thus, care should be taken when these tumors are followed into brainstem parenchyma. These patients also have obstructive hydrocephalus and should be monitored postoperatively if their hydrocephalus persists despite resection. They should be treated with cerebrospinal fluid diversion[13,55,56] (**Table 8.3**).

Stroink and colleagues reported a series of 16 patients with dorsal exophytic transependymal brainstem gliomas from 1949 to 1985.[6] They showed that these patients had a longer history of symptoms compared with patients with a more malignant type of brain tumor. All patients underwent subtotal resection, and seven went on to have further radiotherapy. The authors documented a 94% overall survival at 5 years, with a median follow-up of 7 years.[6] One patient died of shunt malfunction, but otherwise all patients were still alive at the conclusion of the study. Stroink et al compared this current group to 25 patients who had tumors that were purely intrinsic and solid, who had no survivors beyond 23 months.[6]

Pollack and colleagues also published their series of 18 dorsal exophytic brainstem gliomas that underwent resection of the exophytic portion.[56] There was no attempt to remove any intrinsic component of the tumor. There were 16 low-grade lesions. At the conclusion of the study, 17 patients were alive, and only four patients had had a demonstrated recurrence. Of those four, three patients underwent further resection, and two of those patients proceeded with a third tumor-debulking surgery. Overall survival was 94%, with an 83% PFS at 5 years.[56]

Khatib and colleagues reported a series of 12 patients with dorsal exophytic brainstem gliomas.[57] They found that these patients were younger than children with other types of brainstem tumors. They also had a relatively long duration of symptoms. In the 11 patients with JPA, tumor resection ranged from 50 to 100%. At the conclusion of the study, 11 patients were still alive, with one patient succumbing to secondary leukemia from chemotherapy. Three patients who did not undergo postoperative adjuvant therapy presented with recurrences leading to a PFS at 2 years of 67%. Overall survival at 2 years was 100%.

Cervicomedullary Junction Tumors

Type IV tumors include medullary tumors, and those at the cervicomedullary junction are typically approached through a combined suboccipital craniotomy and removal of the dorsal lateral rim of the foramen magnum, with the addition of a cervical laminectomy or laminotomy for caudally extending tumors. These tumors have characteristics similar to those of intramedullary spinal cord tumors; thus aggressive surgical resection has been favored given several case series (**Table 8.4**).

Epstein and Wisoff presented their management of 20 cervicomedullary junction tumors.[58] The patients presented with indolent findings, and radical excision was performed in all patients. In their series, there was no surgical mortality, and postoperative neurological recovery was related to preoperative neurological status. All patients with malignant astrocytomas died within 6 to 9 months of surgery. At the conclusion of the study, 15 patients were alive, with a median follow-up of 24 months.[58]

Robertson and colleagues reported a series of 17 children; 11 patients were newly diagnosed, and 6 patients had tumor progression following prior radiotherapy.[24] The majority of patients underwent a subtotal resection. At 4 years, overall survival for newly diagnosed patients was 100%, and PFS was 70%. For patients presenting after recurrence, overall survival at 4 years was only 62%, and PFS was 41%.[24]

Behnke and colleagues reported a series of 25 children with 2-year follow-up who presented with intrinsic pontine/medullary tumors.[15] The authors described a more acute decline for their patients, with an overall survival of only 32% at 2 years and a median survival time of only 9 months. There were 10 patients still alive after 2 years, with a mean follow-up of 75 months. All patients with high-grade lesions died within the follow-up period despite radiation treatment. Behnke et al describe the holocord-type tumors as similar to the cervicomedullary tumors.[15] These patients had an improved prognosis, with only two patients not surviving the follow-up period. Those that did survive had been followed for a mean of 75 months and were in good clinical condition during this time. The remaining tumor mass has remained stable, without recurrence or clinical progression on imaging.[15]

Weiner and colleagues reviewed their experience in a case series consisting of 39 patients with intra-axial cervicomedullary tumors.[25] Of the 23 patients who had had a previous biopsy or subtotal resection, 13 had received previous radiation therapy, and six had received previous chemotherapy. The authors found that a higher proportion of patients with high-grade lesions experienced tumor progression compared with patients with low-grade tumors (75% vs 30%). The 5-year PFS was 60%, and overall survival was 89%.[25]

In a recent retrospective case review, Di Maio and colleagues reported on nine patients with cervicomedullary tumors who underwent surgical resection.[59] They found that five patients were alive with a median follow-up at 9.5 years. The overall survival at 5 and 10 years was 75% and 50%, respectively. Interestingly, the authors noted that surgery following adjuvant therapy improved the definition of the brainstem–tumor interface in four patients. In those cases, they were able to obtain more extensive resections without neurological worsening. They advocated for a less aggressive initial surgical approach supplemented by postoperative chemotherapy that was designed to preserve brainstem function.[59]

Expert Recommendations

1. There is an improved survival benefit with a more complete resection for focal, dorsal, exophytic, and cervicomedullary brainstem lesions (Grade 1C+ Recommendations, Level II/IV Evidence).
2. Low-grade lesions that typically occur in the brainstem have an improved survival and outcome following surgery regardless of whether adjuvant therapy is given (Grade 1C Recommendations, Level IV Evidence).
3. High-grade lesions are more often diffuse in appearance and occur in the pons. These tumors have a poor prognosis even with surgical resection and adjuvant therapy (Grade 1C, Level IV Evidence).
4. Multiple clinical trials of multiple chemotherapeutic agents have not shown any benefit in progression-free survival as a form of therapy for brainstem gliomas (Grade 1C+ Recommendation, Level II–IV Evidence).

■ Summary and Conclusions

There is currently no Level I evidence comparing surgical resection alone with surgical resection plus adjuvant therapy. One Level II study of a prospective cohort trial examining all pediatric brain tumors shows an improved survival benefit with a more complete resection. Several Level IV retrospective cohort studies support this finding as well and also find that low-grade pathologies are associated with an improved outcome even without adjuvant therapy. Multiple retrospective case series have supported these findings for focal intrinsic, dorsal exophytic, and cervicomedullary brainstem lesions. These types of brainstem tumors often have an improved outcome in comparison with the type I diffuse pontine tumors. The patients with diffuse, high-grade lesions uniformly have a poor prognosis despite surgical resection or adjuvant radiation and chemotherapy. Future prospective, randomized studies will be difficult to carry out given the relatively rare nature of the disease and the evidence now for surgical resection. Currently there are no data suggesting improved outcomes for patients receiving treatment at tertiary care centers. However, patients should receive care from a comprehensive hospital with microsurgical capabilities and access to reliable neuromonitoring.[45] Finally, multiple clinical trials have studied the effects of chemotherapeutic agents for brainstem gliomas, and almost all have shown no improvement in overall survival or PFS.[60] Future studies to help optimize adjuvant treatment will be necessary in treatment of brainstem tumors.

■ References

1. Littman P, Jarrett P, Bilaniuk LT, et al. Pediatric brain stem gliomas. Cancer 1980;45(11):2787–2792
2. Berger MS, Edwards MS, LaMasters D, Davis RL, Wilson CB. Pediatric brain stem tumors: radiographic, pathological, and clinical correlations. Neurosurgery 1983;12(3):298–302
3. Allen J. Brain stem glioma. Neurol Neurosurg 1983;4:2–7
4. Walker DA, Punt JA, Sokal M. Clinical management of brain stem glioma. Arch Dis Child 1999;80(6):558–564
5. White HH. Brain stem tumors occurring in adults. Neurology 1963;13:292–300
6. Stroink AR, Hoffman HJ, Hendrick EB, Humphreys RP, Davidson G. Transependymal benign dorsally exophytic brain stem gliomas in childhood: diagnosis and treatment recommendations. Neurosurgery 1987;20(3):439–444
7. Alvisi C, Cerisoli M, Maccheroni ME. Long-term results of surgically treated brainstem gliomas. Acta Neurochir (Wien) 1985;76(1-2):12–17
8. Epstein F, McCleary EL. Intrinsic brain-stem tumors of childhood: surgical indications. J Neurosurg 1986;64(1):11–15
9. Barkovich AJ, Krischer J, Kun LE, et al. Brain stem gliomas: a classification system based on magnetic resonance imaging. Pediatr Neurosurg 1990-1991;16(2):73–83
10. Fischbein NJ, Prados MD, Wara W, Russo C, Edwards MS, Barkovich AJ. Radiologic classification of brain stem tumors: correlation of magnetic resonance imaging appearance with clinical outcome. Pediatr Neurosurg 1996;24(1):9–23
11. Albright AL. Brain stem gliomas. In: Winn HR, ed. Youmans Neurological Surgery. Philadelphia, PA: Saunders; 1996:2603–2611
12. Choux M, Lena G, Do L. Brainstem tumors. In: Choux M, Di Rocco C, Hockley A, eds. Pediatric Neurosurgery. New York, NY: Churchill Livingstone; 2000:471–491
13. Epstein F, Wisoff JH. Intrinsic brainstem tumors in childhood: surgical indications. J Neurooncol 1988;6(4):309–317
14. Recinos PF, Sciubba DM, Jallo GI. Brainstem tumors: where are we today? Pediatr Neurosurg 2007;43(3):192–201
15. Behnke J, Christen HJ, Brück W, Markakis E. Intra-axial endophytic tumors in the pons and/or medulla oblongata, I: Symptoms, neuroradiological findings, and histopathology in 30 children. Childs Nerv Syst 1997;13(3):122–134
16. Jallo GI, Biser-Rohrbaugh A, Freed D. Brainstem gliomas. Childs Nerv Syst 2004;20(3):143–153
17. Epstein FJ, Farmer JP. Brain-stem glioma growth patterns. J Neurosurg 1993,78(3).408–412
18. Abbott R, Shiminski-Maher T, Epstein FJ. Intrinsic tumors of the medulla: predicting outcome after surgery. Pediatr Neurosurg 1996;25(1):41–44
19. Kaplan AM, Albright AL, Zimmerman RA, et al. Brainstem gliomas in children: a Children's Cancer Group review of 119 cases. Pediatr Neurosurg 1996;24(4):185–192
20. Albright AL, Pollack IF. Brainstem gliomas. In: Winn HR, ed. Youmans Neurological Surgery. Philadelphia, PA: Saunders; 2003:3663–3670
21. Bowers DC, Georgiades C, Aronson LJ, et al. Tectal gliomas: natural history of an indolent lesion in pediatric patients. Pediatr Neurosurg 2000;32(1):24–29
22. Abbott R, Shiminski-Maher T, Wisoff JH, Epstein FJ. Intrinsic tumors of the medulla: surgical complications. Pediatr Neurosurg 1991-1992–1992;17(5):239–244
23. Epstein FJ. Prognosis in pediatric brain-stem gliomas. J Neurosurg 1987;67(2):323–324
24. Robertson PL, Allen JC, Abbott IR, Miller DC, Fidel J, Epstein FJ. Cervicomedullary tumors in children: a distinct subset of brainstem gliomas. Neurology 1994;44(10):1798–1803
25. Weiner HL, Freed D, Woo HH, Rezai AR, Kim R, Epstein FJ. Intra-axial tumors of the cervicomedullary junction: surgical results and long-term outcome. Pediatr Neurosurg 1997;27(1):12–18
26. Epstein F. A staging system for brain stem gliomas. Cancer 1985;56(7, Suppl):1804–1806
27. Albright AL, Price RA, Guthkelch AN. Brain stem gliomas of children: a clinicopathological study. Cancer 1983;52(12):2313–2319
28. Reigel DH, Scarff TB, Woodford JE. Biopsy of pediatric brain stem tumors. Childs Brain 1979;5(3):329–340
29. Kumar AJ, Leeds NE, Kumar VA, et al. Magnetic resonance imaging features of pilocytic astrocytoma of the brain mimicking high-grade gliomas. J Comput Assist Tomogr 2010;34(4):601–611
30. Albright AL, Guthkelch AN, Packer RJ, Price RA, Rourke LB. Prognostic factors in pediatric brain-stem gliomas. J Neurosurg 1986;65(6):751–755
31. Artigas J, Ferszt R, Brock M, Kazner E, Cervós-Navarro J. The relevance of pathological diagnosis for therapy and outcome of brain stem gliomas. Acta Neurochir Suppl (Wien) 1988;42:166–169
32. Broggi G, Franzini A, Migliavacca F, Allegranza A. Stereotactic biopsy of deep brain tumors in infancy and childhood. Childs Brain 1983;10(2):92–98
33. Coffey RJ, Lunsford LD. Diagnosis and treatment of brainstem mass lesions by CT-guided stereotactic surgery. Appl Neurophysiol 1985;48(1-6):467–471
34. Coffey RJ, Lunsford LD. Stereotactic surgery for mass lesions of the midbrain and pons. Neurosurgery 1985;17(1):12–18
35. Frank F, Fabrizi AP, Frank-Ricci R, Gaist G, Sédan R, Peragut JC. Stereotactic biopsy and treatment of brain stem lesions: combined study of 33 cases (Bologna-Marseille). Acta Neurochir Suppl (Wien) 1988;42:177–181
36. Franzini A, Allegranza A, Melcarne A, Giorgi C, Ferraresi S, Broggi G. Serial stereotactic biopsy of brain stem expanding lesions. Considerations on 45 consecutive cases. Acta Neurochir Suppl (Wien) 1988;42:170–176
37. Kratimenos GP, Nouby RM, Bradford R, Pell MF, Thomas DG. Image directed stereotactic surgery for brain stem lesions. Acta Neurochir (Wien) 1992;116(2-4):164–170
38. Thomas DG, Bradford R, Gill S, Davis CH. Computer-directed stereotactic biopsy of intrinsic brain stem lesions. Br J Neurosurg 1988;2(2):235–240
39. Schumacher M, Schulte-Mönting J, Stoeter P, Warmuth-Metz M, Solymosi L. Magnetic resonance imaging compared with biopsy in the diagnosis of brainstem diseases of childhood: a multicenter review. J Neurosurg 2007;106(2, Suppl):111–119
40. Samadani U, Judy KD. Stereotactic brainstem biopsy is indicated for the diagnosis of a vast array of brainstem pathology. Stereotact Funct Neurosurg 2003;81(1-4):5–9
41. Roujeau T, Machado G, Garnett MR, et al. Stereotactic biopsy of diffuse pontine lesions in children. J Neurosurg 2007;107(1, Suppl):1–4
42. Kondziolka D, Lunsford LD. Results and expectations with image-integrated brainstem stereotactic biopsy. Surg Neurol 1995;43(6):558–562
43. Pincus DW, Richter EO, Yachnis AT, Bennett J, Bhatti MT, Smith A. Brainstem stereotactic biopsy sampling in children. J Neurosurg 2006;104(2, Suppl):108–114
44. Steck J, Friedman WA. Stereotactic biopsy of brainstem mass lesions. Surg Neurol 1995;43(6):563–567
45. Wisoff JH, Sanford RA, Heier LA, et al. Primary neurosurgery for pediatric low-grade gliomas: a prospective multi-institutional study from the Children's Oncology Group. Neurosurgery 2011;68(6):1548–1554
46. Fisher PG, Tihan T, Goldthwaite PT, et al. Outcome analysis of childhood low-grade astrocytomas. Pediatr Blood Cancer 2008;51(2):245–250

47. Lesniak MS, Klem JM, Weingart J, Carson BS Sr. Surgical outcome following resection of contrast-enhanced pediatric brainstem gliomas. Pediatr Neurosurg 2003;39(6):314–322
48. Bricolo A, Turazzi S. Surgery for gliomas and other mass lesions of the brainstem. Adv Tech Stand Neurosurg 1995;22: 261–341 Review
49. Vandertop WP, Hoffman HJ, Drake JM, et al. Focal midbrain tumors in children. Neurosurgery 1992;31(2):186–194
50. Pierre-Kahn A, Hirsch JF, Vinchon M, et al. Surgical management of brain-stem tumors in children: results and statistical analysis of 75 cases. J Neurosurg 1993;79(6):845–852
51. Farmer JP, Montes JL, Freeman CR, Meagher-Villemure K, Bond MC, O'Gorman AM. Brainstem gliomas: a 10-year institutional review. Pediatr Neurosurg 2001;34(4):206–214
52. Kestle J, Townsend JJ, Brockmeyer DL, Walker ML. Juvenile pilocytic astrocytoma of the brainstem in children. J Neurosurg 2004;101(1, Suppl):1–6
53. Sandri A, Sardi N, Genitori L, et al. Diffuse and focal brain stem tumors in childhood: prognostic factors and surgical outcome: experience in a single institution. Childs Nerv Syst 2006;22(9):1127–1135
54. Teo C, Siu TL. Radical resection of focal brainstem gliomas: is it worth doing? Childs Nerv Syst 2008;24(11):1307–1314
55. Jallo GI, Freed D, Roonprapunt C, Epstein F. Current management of brainstem gliomas. Annals of Neurosurgery 2003;3:1–17
56. Pollack IF, Hoffman HJ, Humphreys RP, Becker L. The long-term outcome after surgical treatment of dorsally exophytic brain-stem gliomas. J Neurosurg 1993;78(6):859–863
57. Khatib ZA, Heideman RL, Kovnar EH, et al. Predominance of pilocytic histology in dorsally exophytic brain stem tumors. Pediatr Neurosurg 1994;20(1):2–10
58. Epstein F, Wisoff J. Intra-axial tumors of the cervicomedullary junction. J Neurosurg 1987;67(4):483–487
59. Di Maio S, Gul SM, Cochrane DD, Hendson G, Sargent MA, Steinbok P. Clinical, radiologic and pathologic features and outcome following surgery for cervicomedullary gliomas in children. Childs Nerv Syst 2009;25(11):1401–1410
60. Frazier JL, Lee J, Thomale UW, Noggle JC, Cohen KJ, Jallo GI. Treatment of diffuse intrinsic brainstem gliomas: failed approaches and future strategies. J Neurosurg Pediatr 2009;3(4):259–269
61. Hood TW, Gebarski SS, McKeever PE, Venes JL. Stereotaxic biopsy of intrinsic lesions of the brain stem. J Neurosurg 1986; 65(2):172–176
62. Mathisen JR, Giunta F, Marini G, Backlund EO. Transcerebellar biopsy in the posterior fossa: 12 years experience. Surg Neurol 1987;28(2):100–104
63. Guthrie BL, Steinberg GK, Adler JR. Posterior fossa stereotaxic biopsy using the Brown-Roberts-Wells stereotaxic system. Technical note. J Neurosurg 1989;70(4):649–652
64. Abernathey CD, Camacho A, Kelly PJ. Stereotaxic suboccipital transcerebellar biopsy of pontine mass lesions. J Neurosurg 1989;70(2):195–200
65. Ryken TC, Hitchon PW, Roach RM, Traynelis VC. Infratentorial stereotactic biopsy: a review of 11 cases. Stereotact Funct Neurosurg 1992;59(1-4):111–114
66. Kratimenos GP, Thomas DG. The role of image-directed biopsy in the diagnosis and management of brainstem lesions. Br J Neurosurg 1993;7(2):155–164
67. Rajshekhar V, Chandy MJ. Computerized tomography-guided stereotactic surgery for brainstem masses: a risk-benefit analysis in 71 patients. J Neurosurg 1995;82(6):976–981
68. Massager N, David P, Goldman S, et al. Combined magnetic resonance imaging- and positron emission tomography-guided stereotactic biopsy in brainstem mass lesions: diagnostic yield in a series of 30 patients. J Neurosurg 2000;93(6):951–957
69. Gonçalves-Ferreira AJ, Herculano-Carvalho M, Pimentel J. Stereotactic biopsies of focal brainstem lesions. Surg Neurol 2003;60(4):311–320
70. Rajshekhar V, Moorthy RK. Status of stereotactic biopsy in children with brain stem masses: insights from a series of 106 patients. Stereotact Funct Neurosurg 2010;88(6):360–366
71. Epstein F, McCleary EL. Intrinsic brain-stem tumors of childhood: surgical indications. J Neurosurg 1986;64(1):11–15

9

The Role of Local Drug Delivery in Management of Newly Diagnosed and Recurrent High-Grade Gliomas

Mahua Dey, Henry Brem, and Maciej S. Lesniak

With the average lifespan of 14.6 months after best available therapy, patients with malignant glioma (MG), a heterogeneous group of malignancies derived from glial cells, are in desperate need for better therapeutic options.[1] Current standard of care involves a multidisciplinary approach with gross total resection when possible, followed by single-agent adjuvant therapy with temozolomide (TMZ) and radiation therapy (XRT). However, the failure rate of this therapeutic regimen is 100%, with local recurrence within 2 cm of the original lesion in 90% of the cases.[2] Cumulative local and systemic toxicity over a short period of time limits the use of these treatment modalities for recurrent disease. Because local recurrence is the failure pattern of the current strategy, local drug delivery has emerged as an alternative or adjunct to systemic drug delivery with a potential for maximizing therapeutic abilities while minimizing systemic toxicity.

■ Limitations of Systemic Chemotherapy

Traditional intravenous (IV) systemic chemotherapeutic agents have had minor success in the treatment of several solid tumors; however, their use in this setting is limited by dose-dependent systemic toxicities. Most systemically administered drugs do not reach the brain. Even in the best situations, where a small fraction of administered drug actually reaches the brain, it is at concentrations where the systemic toxicity becomes the dose-limiting factor. More importantly, when it comes to intracranial malignancies, systemic chemotherapy is not only limited by systemic toxicity, it is also limited by drug penetration of the blood–brain barrier (BBB), blood–cerebrospinal fluid (CSF) barrier (BCB), and blood–tumor barrier (BTB). BBB is a physiological and pharmacological barrier to the influx of molecules from the bloodstream to the brain formed by capillary endothelial tight junctions. BCB is formed by choroid epithelial tight junctions and regulates penetration of molecules within the interstitial fluid and CSF, and BTB is the pathological BBB of the MG's microvasculature. BCB is further fortified by an active organic acid transport system that actively removes chemotherapeutic agents from CSF and prevents their diffusion into the brain parenchyma. To overcome all these pharmacological barriers, very high doses of toxic antineoplastic agents are necessary. These high doses are usually accompanied by serious side effects such as pulmonary fibrosis, myelosuppression, and hepatic and renal failure.[3]

Efficacy of systemic chemotherapy in the setting of MGs has been tested over the last several decades, and the types of chemotherapeutic agents used are limited to small, electrically neutral, lipid-soluble compounds. Most common compounds tested in clinical trials are antiproliferative drugs (e.g., nitrosoureas) and alkylation agents (e.g., TMZ) that have some ability to cross the BBB. A systematic review and meta-analysis of all available randomized trials comparing radiotherapy alone with radiotherapy plus chemotherapy with nitrosoureas concluded that there is a small but clear improvement in survival resulting from the addition of chemotherapy.[4] The alkylating agent TMZ was tested by Stupp et al in phase 2 and phase 3 clinical trials for newly diagnosed glioblastoma multiforme (GBM) with concomitant administration of 75 mg/m2/d of TMZ and conventional fractionated radiation followed by up to six cycles of adjuvant TMZ at 150–200 mg/m2 for 5 days of every 28-day cycle. The phase 2 trial showed a median survival of 16 months, and the 1- and 2-year survival rates of 58% and 31%, respectively, and phase 3 trial showed an increase in median survival from 12.1 months to 14.6 months and an increase in 2-year survival from 10.4% to 26.5% in the TMZ + radiation group.[1,5] These clinical trials formed the basis of the current standard of care for MGs. However, this treatment regimen is often associated with significant lymphopenia, thrombocytopenia, and progressive BBB dysfunction that can result in clinical and radiological deterioration without true tumor progression.[6] TMZ-induced thrombocytopenia occurs in ~ 12 to 20% of treated patients and can substantially limit the amount of TMZ that can be administered.[1]

To overcome the natural boundaries presented by the central nervous system (CNS) and increase the delivery of chemotherapeutic agents to the tumor, several approaches have been utilized in recent years. Some of the common strategies include increasing BBB permeability, intra-arterial administration, and BBB disruption.

Increasing Blood–Brain Barrier Permeability

Existing drugs can be pharmacologically manipulated to create a more lipophilic and thus a more BBB-traversable agent. However, clinical trials utilizing systemic administration of lomustine or semustine, two lipophilic variants of a known chemotherapeutic agent, carmustine (BCNU), have shown no efficacy of these drugs over BCNU in the setting of MGs.[7] Permeability of a hydrophilic agent can be increased by linking the drug to a carrier capable of traversing the BBB; for example, redox conversion of a lipophilic dihydropyridine to an ionic, lipid-insoluble pyridinium salt can improve CNS access and retention of therapeutic agents such as antineoplastic agents.[8] Other methods of traversing the BBB include vector-mediated drug delivery that employs conjugation of a nontransportable drug to a modified protein or receptor-specific monoclonal antibody that undergoes receptor-mediated transcytosis through the BBB.[9]

Intra-arterial Administration

Direct administration of a therapeutic agent into an artery instead of a vein has a principle advantage; the tissue perfused by that artery receives a higher plasma concentration during the first passage through the circulation. Thus the greatest advantages of intra-arterial (IA) administration occur in three specific settings: (1) when there is very low tumor blood flow, (2) when there is a very high rate of systemic transformation or excretion of the drug, or (3) when the drug binds to the tissue after crossing the BBB or BTB. Once the drug passes through the tumor microvasculature, it enters the systemic circulation, and the pharmacokinetics are the same as those for an IV administration. Thus the ideal drug for IA administration is one that rapidly crosses the BBB or BTB and is either bound to tissue elements or locally metabolized in the process of exerting its anticancer effect. IA delivery is associated with several added risks, including groin hematoma, failure to cannulate the carotid or vertebral artery, and higher neuro- and systemic toxicity.[10] Developments in modern endovascular techniques and microcatheters have made the technical aspect of IA drug delivery easier and supraselective, where a drug can be injected into the artery directly supplying the tumor. However, the efficacy of combining this technique with current chemotherapeutic agents is yet to be determined.[11]

Blood–Brain Barrier Disruption

Disrupting the BBB by means of IA infusion of either hyperosmolar mannitol, which increases capillary permeability due to acute dehydration of endothelial cells and widening of the tight junctions, or vasoactive compounds, such as bradykinin or its analogue receptor mediated permeabilizer (RMP)-7, which directly disrupt the BBB,[12] or interleukin-2 (IL-2), leukotriene C4 followed by administration of chemotherapeutic agents, provides the first-pass advantage for any drug. This mode of drug delivery is most useful for drugs that, once having crossed the BBB, bind to brain or tumor tissue and do not efflux back across the BBB. There are fundamental differences between the BBB and the BTB, and mannitol has been shown to increase permeability of the normal BBB. However, its effect on the BTB is not very well defined,[13–15] and, on the other hand, RMP-7 may selectively increase permeability of the tumor.[16] In a rat glioma model intracarotid infusion of RMP-7 selectively increases transport of carboplatin into brain tumors and results in higher survival.[17] A phase 1 study of both IA and IV RMP-7 and carboplatin in patients with recurrent glioma has shown this to be safe and acceptable.[18,19] However, a randomized, controlled trial of IV carboplatin and

RMP-7 versus carboplatin and placebo in patients with recurrent MG concluded that RMP-7 had no effect on the pharmacokinetics, toxicity, or efficacy of carboplatin at the dose and schedule used in that particular trial, suggesting that higher doses of RMP-7 may be required to increase carboplatin delivery to tumor.[20] Similarly mannitol has been used with several different chemotherapeutic agents, such as bevacizumab,[21] etoposide, carboplatin,[22] and methotrexate[23]. However, there has been no randomized, controlled trial looking at the efficacy of these chemotherapeutic agents with and without mannitol.

■ Rationale for Local Drug Delivery

Evolution of local drug delivery came as a logical progression in search for better therapeutic options in a disease that is defined by local recurrence. An attractive approach that does not depend on the penetration or disruption of any physiological barrier involves the direct delivery of an antineoplastic agent to the tumor by implanting one end of a catheter within the tumor bed and leaving the opposite end easily accessible for injection, such as an Ommaya reservoir, which can be used to deliver intermittent bolus injections of chemotherapy to the tumor. Markert et al demonstrated safe administration of G207, a doubly mutated herpes simplex virus, via a stereotactically implanted catheter in the enhancing portion of recurrent MGs.[24] In a retrospective study, Boiardi et al showed that the most significant favorable prognostic factor for survival in patients with recurrent MG was the local delivery of mitoxantrone via Ommaya reservoir, which reduced the risk of death to 50%.[25] Several compounds have been delivered via this system with variable levels of success (**Table 9.1**). There are two primary limitations of this system: (1) there is a low volume of distribution given that the primary mode of drug distribution is diffusion, and (2) delivery is only as successful as the drug being delivered and is limited by neurotoxicity of the drug.

Convection-Enhanced Delivery

Fluid convection within the brain, established by maintaining the pressure gradient during interstitial infusion, can be used to overcome the distance limitation of simple diffusion and greatly enhance the distribution of small and large molecules, including high molecular weight proteins. This can be accomplished by connecting a motor-driven pumping device to a stereotactically implanted catheter in the brain to generate bulk flow, which can deliver the infusate independent of its intrinsic diffusivity in larger volumes in comparison with simple diffusive flow. Successful induction of convection in the brain is critically dependent on the infusion rate, and an infusion rate greater than a few microliters per minute causes loss of infusion pressure and leakage of infusion solution out of the cannula tract,[26] missing the target volume and draining into ventricular or subarachnoid spaces,[27,28] which leads to neurotoxicity. Tanner et al assessed the effects of drug efflux on convection and concluded that sealing the burr hole during convection-enhanced delivery (CED) prevents drug efflux while maintaining a high volume of distribution (Vd).[29] However, even with the use of a specially designed efflux-resistant catheter with a flow rate of 5 ml/min Fiandaca et al documented reflux in almost 20% of the infusion tracks.[30] Apart from the rate of infusion and rate of efflux, the geography of the targeted brain also affects the Vd, because white matter fibers offer a lower resistance pathway to convection, as compared with gray matter tissue.[31] In a retrospective analysis of 51 trajectories for CED catheters planned with neuronavigation in 21 patients with supratentorial malignant gliomas, Dörner et al defined two areas that appear most suitable as entry points in CED catheter placement: the superior parietal lobule and the superior frontal gyrus.[32]

In patients with recurrent MGs, Sampson et al retrospectively tested the ability of a software algorithm using magnetic resonance (MR) diffusion tensor imaging to predict patient-specific drug distributions by CED, where a tumor-targeted cytotoxin, cintredekin besudotox (IL-13-PE38QQR) was co-infused with iodine 123-labeled human serum albumin (^{123}I-HSA). The software algorithm was found to have a high sensitivity and specificity for identifying the proportion (7/14) of catheter trajectories that failed to deliver drug into the desired anatomical region ($p = 0.021$) when spatial distribution of ^{123}I-HSA was compared with a drug distribution simulation provided by the software algorithm. Failure in drug delivery usually occurred when catheter trajectories crossed deep sulci, resulting in leakage of the infusate into the subarachnoid CSF space. This simulation algorithm was considered clinically useful in 84.6% of catheters.[33] In a retrospective analysis of the phase 3 PRECISE trial (Phase 3 Randomized Evaluation of Convection-Enhanced Delivery of IL13-PE38QQR Compared with Gliadel Wafer with Survival Endpoint in Glioblastoma Multiforme at First Recurrence) employing the same software algorithm Sampson et al showed that the catheter positioning score (hazard ratio 0.93, $p = 0.043$) and the number of optimally positioned catheters (hazard ratio 0.72, $p = 0.038$) had a significant effect on progression-free survival, with strong correlation of estimations of drug delivery to relevant target volumes with catheter score ($p < 0.003$). Optimally positioned catheters had larger coverage volumes ($p < 0.002$).[34] To assess the effect of CED of paclitaxel in eight patients with

Table 9.1 Studies involving local drug delivery using Ommaya reservoir

Study	Compound delivered locally	Type of tumor	Type of study
Boiardi et al 2008[25]	Mitoxantrone	Recurrent GBM	Retrospective
Boiardi et al 2005[82]	Mitoxantrone + radioimmunotherapy	Recurrent GBM	Prospective
Boiardi et al 2001[83]	Mitoxantrone	Recurrent GBM	Prospective controlled
Boiardi et al 1999[84]	Mitoxantrone and bleomycin	Recurrent GBM	Prospective
Boiardi et al 1996[85]	Mitoxantrone	Recurrent GBM	Phase 1/2
Boiardi et al 2003[86]	Novantrone and pegylated liposomal doxorubicin	Recurrent GBM	Prospective
Boiardi et al 1991[87] and Silvani et al 1990[88]	Interferon (IFN)-β	Recurrent GBM	Prospective controlled
Boiardi et al 1994[89]	Autologous adherent lymphokine-activated killer (A-LAK) cells and interleukin-2 (IL-2)	Recurrent GBM	Prospective
Koch et al 2007[90]	O-6-benzylguanine (O(6)BG)	Recurrent GBM	Case report
Oshiro et al 2006[91]	Tumor necrosis factor-α (TNF-SAM2)	New and recurrent MG	Prospective
Prados et al 2003[92]	Virus-producing cells (GLI 328) containing the herpes simplex virus thymidine-kinase gene	Recurrent GBM	Phase 1/2 multi-institutional
Patchell et al 2002[93]	Bleomycin	Recurrent GBM	Phase 1
Voulgaris et al 2002[94]	Doxorubicin	Recurrent GBM	Prospective
Huang et al 2001[95]	IL-2	Recurrent GBM	Case report
Nakagawa et al 2001[96]	5-fluoro-2′-deoxyuridine (FdUrd)	Primary or recurrent GBM	Prospective
Quattrocchi et al 1999[97]	Autologous tumor-infiltrating lymphocytes and rIL-2	Recurrent GBM	Prospective
Bigner et al 1998[98]	Iodine 131 (131I)-labeled 81C6 monoclonal antibody (mAb)	Recurrent GBM	Phase 1
Naganuma et al 1997[99]	Lymphokine-activated killer (LAK) cells	Recurrent GBM	Case report
Fetell et al 1990[100]	Beta-serine-interferon (IFN-β ser17)	Recurrent GBM	Phase 1
Jereb et al 1989[101]	Human leukocyte interferon-α (HLI-α)	New and recurrent GBM	Prospective
McKeran et al 1985[102]	Bleomycin entrapped within negatively charged liposomes	GBM	Prospective

Abbreviation: GBM, glioblastoma multiforme.

recurrent GBM, Pöpperl et al evaluated the role of O-(2-[18F] fluoroethyl)-L-tyrosine (FET) positron-emission tomography (PET) in monitoring the effects of this type of direct drug delivery and concluded that FET PET is a valuable tool in monitoring the effects of CED of paclitaxel and is more reliable than magnetic resonance imaging (MRI) in differentiating stable disease from tumor regrowth. In long-term follow-up, stable or decreasing FET uptake, even in contrast-enhancing lesions, is suggestive of reactive changes, whereas increasing ratios appear to be indicative of recurrence in all cases.[35]

Because the success of this modality is very dependent on effective delivery, real-time imaging during the delivery process or monitoring with T2-weighted and diffusion-weighted (DW) MRI of the convection process could allow early identification and interruption of an ineffective delivery. Development of hyperintense signal on T2-weighted MRI scans after infusion strongly correlated with the volume and geometry of distribution of infusate in seven patients with recurrent MG receiving CB + ^{123}I-HAS, however, was of little use to estimate the Vd if delivery occurred in contrast-enhanced areas.[36] In the phase 1/2 clinical trial of CED of paclitaxel hyperintense signal that appeared on DW MRI as early as 24 hours after treatment initiation precipitated lytic responses later observed on T1-weighted images.[37] Even though MRI can monitor CED, it cannot reliably estimate the Vd without a surrogate tracer. Thus Sampson et al used ^{123}I-HAS as a surrogate tracer in seven patients treated with CB and found that single-photon emission computed tomography (SPECT) with ^{123}I-HSA can effectively estimate the Vd; however, its limited half-life requires SPECT to be performed within 2 days after initiation of CED, and it could overestimate the Vd of a drug targeted to specific receptors on brain cells because it does not bind to the receptors that the convected drug binds to.[28] Gadolinium diethylenetriamine penta-acetic acid (Gd-DTPA), a commonly used MRI contrast agent, low cost and readily available, was found to be a good surrogate tracer when co-infused with MR1–1 (a novel recombinant immunotoxin that targets the GBM tumor-specific antigen epidermal growth factor receptor variant III [EGFRvIII]) for drug distribution monitoring in a mouse model.[38] When tested in a human study, Gd-DTPA seemed to colocalize with treatment-related changes on [11C]-l-methionine (MET) PET.[39]

Level I Evidence

A randomized, open-label, active-controlled, dose-finding phase 2b study comparing current standard of care to CED of trabedersen, a synthetic antisense phosphorothioate oligodeoxynucleotide complementary to the messenger RNA (mRNA) of the human transforming growth factor (TGF)-β2 gene, indicated a threefold survival at 2 and 3 years for 10 µM trabedersen versus chemotherapy in a group with glioblastoma multiforme (GBM) and established superior efficacy and safety for 10 µM trabedersen over chemotherapy.[40] In the PRECISE study, the first randomized phase 3 evaluation comparing cintredekin besudotox (CB), a recombinant cytotoxin consisting of IL-13 and truncated *Pseudomonas* exotoxin that binds selectively to IL-13R α2 receptors, administered via CED and Gliadel Wafer (Eisai, Woodcliff Lake, NJ) in patients with GBM, Kunwar et al showed no survival difference between CB administered via CED and Gliadel Wafer (Eisai).[41] The PRECISE trial did not assess drug distribution; however, Mueller et al did a retrospective analysis of the trial data and concluded that, despite intensive onsite training, a majority of catheters were incorrectly positioned. The authors performed a detailed analysis of catheter positioning score. Overall placement score and imaging change score did not reveal any correlation of these parameters with clinical outcome.[42] In another study, patients harboring recurrent GBM were randomized to receive an intratumoral injection of the human-murine chimeric mAb Ch81C6, which had been labeled with the ^{123}I tracer, either as a bolus injection or CED via a stereotactically placed catheter. It was found that for the relatively small volumes injected, the CED did not provide a significant increase in the Vd when compared with the bolus injection.[43]

Level II Evidence

In 2006, a safety analysis study of CED of CB by Kunwar et al identified three symptomatic windows: the first one was between the surgical procedure and CED; the second was during CED and up to 1 week after its completion; and the third window was 2 to 10 weeks after treatment. Those windows generally reflected adverse events related to surgical procedures, mass effect from infusate, and drug effect on tumor-infiltrated and normal brain parenchyma, respectively.[44] Subsequently it was deemed to have a favorable risk–benefit profile in a phase 1 study of patients treated for recurrent MGs.[45] CED of CB was found to be well tolerated in the setting of newly diagnosed MGs, when tested as an adjunct to the current standard of care, TMZ, and radiation.[46] A phase 2 trial of CED of immunostimulating oligodeoxynucleotides containing CpG motifs (CpG-ODN) in patients with recurrent GBMs showed only modest activity on the 6-month progression-free survival (PFS) in this patient population.[47] In 2005 Patel et al did a safety and feasibility study of convection-enhanced delivery of Cotara (Peregrine Pharmaceuticals, Tustin, CA), a novel radioimmunotherapeutic agent, in patients with MG and showed that the majority of Cotara (Peregrine) infusions safely delivered between 90 and 110% of the prescribed administered activity to the targeted region.[48] Another similar study assessing the safety and feasibility of paclitaxel in patients with confirmed recurrent MGs determined that CED of paclitaxel is associated with a high antitumor response rate, although it is associated with a significant incidence of treatment-associated complications.[37] CED of biological agents such as the herpes simplex virus HSV-1-tk gene-bearing liposomal vector was tested in a prospective phase 1/2 clinical study and showed that the treatment was well tolerated without major side effects, with two of eight patients demonstrating greater than 50% reduction of tumor volume, and two of eight patients demonstrating focal treatment effects.[39] A dose-escalation study of CED of TP-38, a recombinant chimeric targeted toxin composed of the EGFR binding ligand TGF-α and a genetically engineered form of the *Pseudomonas* exotoxin PE-38, in 20 patients with recurrent MG showed a slight survival benefit in patients without radiographic evidence of residual

Table 9.2 Clinical trials investigating role of CED in the setting of malignant glioma

Study	Level	No. patients	Title	Conclusion
Bogdahn et al 2011[40]	I	145	Targeted therapy for high-grade glioma with the TGF-β2 inhibitor trabedersen: results of a randomized, controlled phase 2b study	10 µM is the optimal dose of trabedersen
Kunwar et al 2010[41]	I	296	Phase 3 randomized trial of CED of IL-13-PE38QQR versus Gliadel Wafers[a] for recurrent glioblastoma	No survival difference between CB administered via CED and Gliadel Wafers[a]
Vogelbaum et al 2007[46]	II	23	CED of cintredekin besudotox (IL-13-PE38QQR) followed by radiation therapy with and without temozolomide in newly diagnosed malignant gliomas: phase 1 study of final safety results	CB (0.5 mg/mL) administered via CED before standard radiochemotherapy seems to be well tolerated
Kunwar et al 2007[45]	II	51	Direct intracerebral delivery of cintredekin besudotox (IL-13-PE38QQR) in recurrent malignant glioma: a report by the Cintredekin Besudotox Intraparenchymal Study Group	CB appears to have a favorable risk–benefit profile
Carpentier et al 2010[47]	II	31	Intracerebral administration of CpG oligonucleotide for patients with recurrent glioblastoma: a phase 2 study	CpG-28 showed modest activity on the 6-month PFS
Carpentier et al 2006[103]	II	24	Phase 1 trial of a CpG oligodeoxynucleotide for patients with recurrent glioblastoma	CpG-28 was well tolerated at doses up to 20 mg per injection
Kunwar et al 2006[44]	II	51	Safety of intraparenchymal convection-enhanced delivery of cintredekin besudotox in early-phase studies	Three symptomatic windows: first one was between surgical procedure and CED; the second was during CED and up to 1 week after its completion; and the third window was 2 to 10 weeks after treatment
Patel et al 2005[48]	II	51	Safety and feasibility of convection-enhanced delivery of Cotara[b] for the treatment of malignant glioma: initial experience in 51 patients	Majority of Cotara[b] infusions delivered between 90 and 110% of the prescribed administered activity to the targeted region
Lidar et al 2004[37]	II	15	CED of paclitaxel for the treatment of recurrent malignant glioma: a phase 1/2 clinical study	Paclitaxel in patients with recurrent malignant gliomas is associated with a high antitumor response rate and a significant incidence of treatment-associated complications
Pöpperl et al 2005[35]	II	8	O-(2-[18F]fluoroethyl)-L-tyrosine PET for monitoring the effects of CED of paclitaxel in patients with recurrent glioblastoma	FET PET is a valuable tool in monitoring the effects of CED of paclitaxel
Tanner et al 2007[29]	II	8	Effects of drug efflux on CED of paclitaxel to malignant gliomas: technical note	Sealing the burr hole during CED prevented efflux
Weber et al 2003[50]	II	31	Safety, tolerability, and tumor response of IL-4-*Pseudomonas* exotoxin (NBI-3001) in patients with recurrent malignant glioma	NBI-3001 appears to have an acceptable safety and toxicity profile
Sampson et al 2007[104]	II	20	Intracerebral infusion of an EGFR-targeted toxin (TP-38) in recurrent malignant brain tumors	Intracerebral CED of TP-38 was well tolerated and produced some durable radiographic responses
Weaver, Laske 2003[105]	II	44	Transferrin receptor ligand-targeted toxin conjugate (Tf-CRM107) for therapy of malignant gliomas	Tf-CRM107 produced tumor response in patients refractory to conventional therapy without severe neurological or systemic toxicity

(Continued on page 82)

Table 9.2 *(Continued)* Clinical trials investigating role of CED in the setting of malignant glioma

Study	Level	No. patients	Title	Conclusion
Laske et al 1997[106]	II	15	Tumor regression with regional distribution of the targeted toxin TF-CRM107 in patients with malignant brain tumors	Regional perfusion with Tf-CRM107 produces tumor responses without systemic toxicity in patients
Sampson et al 2006[43]	II	10	Comparison of intratumoral bolus injection and CED of radiolabeled antitenascin monoclonal antibodies	CED did not provide a significant increase in the volume of distribution when compared with the bolus injection
Voges et al 2003[39]	II	8	Imaging-guided convection-enhanced delivery and gene therapy of glioblastoma (HSV-1-tk)	In two of eight patients, a > 50% reduction of tumor volume and in six of eight patients focal treatment effects were seen
Steven S Gill		Registered, not yet open	Phase 1 trial of carboplatin administered by CED to patients With recurrent/progressive glioblastoma multiforme	
Behnam Badie		Currently recruiting	Phase 1 study of cellular immunotherapy for recurrent/refractory malignant glioma using intratumoral infusions of GRm13Z40–2, an allogeneic CD8+ cytolytic T-cell line genetically modified to express the IL-13-Zetakine and HyTK and to be resistant to glucocorticoids, in combination with IL-2	
Jeffrey N Bruce		Currently recruiting	Phase I study of topotecan by CED (intracerebral clysis) for the treatment of recurrent primary malignant brain tumors	
Rolando Del Maestro		Terminated	Efficacy and safety of AP 12009 in adult patients with recurrent or refractory anaplastic astrocytoma or secondary glioblastoma as compared with standard chemotherapy treatment: a randomized, actively controlled, open-label clinical phase 3 study (SAPPHIRE)	Stopped due to lack of patients (no safety or efficacy issues) Reasons: Changed WHO brain tumor definitions, standard of care first-line, neurosurgical advances
Patrick M Rossi		Registered, not yet recruiting	Phase 2, multicenter, open-label, single-arm study of intratumoral infusion of PRX321 (IL-4PE) in subjects with glioblastoma multiforme at first recurrence or progression (CLARITY-1)	
James Vredenburgh		Currently recruiting	Dose-finding and safety study of PVSRIPO (poliovirus vaccine) against recurrent glioblastoma	

Abbreviations: CB, cintredekin besudotox; CED, convection-enhanced delivery; EGFR, epithelial growth factor receptor; FET PET, O-(2-[^{18}F] fluoroethyl)-L-tyrosine positron-emission tomography; PFS, progression-free survival; WHO, World Health Organization.

[a]Gliadel Wafers, Eisai, Woodcliff Lake, NJ.

[b]Cotara, Peregrine Pharmaceuticals, Tustin, CA.

disease at the time of therapy.[49] In an open-label, dose-escalation trial of intratumoral administration of IL-4 *Pseudomonas* exotoxin (NBI-3001) via CED in patients with recurrent MGs, Weber et al concluded that NBI-3001 has an acceptable safety and toxicity profile.[50] **Table 9.2** lists all the clinical trials investigating the role of CED in the setting of MG.

Polymer Based Delivery

Development of implantable nonbiodegradable ethylene vinyl acetate (EVAc) copolymer capable of sustained release of macromolecules by means of diffusion through the micropores of its matrix was first described in 1976 by Langer and Folkman.[51] The rate of diffusion of a drug from the polymer into the brain is defined by the chemical properties of the drug itself, including molecular weight, charge, and water solubility. In general, the smaller the molecule, the faster it is released from the polymer, and once released, the drug retains its biological activity. Biodegradable polymer systems such as the polyanhydride poly [bis (p-carboxyphenoxy) propane-sebacic acid] (PCPP-SA) break down to dicarboxylic acids by spontaneous reaction with water and release drugs by a combination of polymer degradation and drug diffusion at a nearly constant rate.[52] Polymer breakdown rate can be adjusted from 1 day to several years by modifying the ratio of carboxyphenoxypropane (CPP) to sebacic acid (SA), negating the need for surgical foreign body removal, and any drug can be incorporated into the polymer as long as it does not react with the matrix. Many hydrophilic agents or hydrolytically unstable compounds such as methotrexate or carboplatin are not very effectively released by PCPP-SA polymer; thus, to increase the spectrum of drugs that can be optimally released from the polyanhydride matrix a second generation of biodegradable polymers such as fatty acid dimer-sebacic acid (FAD-SA) copolymer were introduced.[53] Since then many different varieties of polymers have been introduced, such as poly (lactide-co-glycolide) polymer, that can be formed into microspheres and stereotactically injected into the brain.[54] When covalently linked to a polyethylene glycol coating, this polymer matrix has been shown to reduce opsonization and elimination by the immune system.[55] Polyethyleneglycol-coated liposomes that encapsulate anthracyclines,[56] and gelatin-chondroitin sulfate-coated microspheres have been shown to reproducibly release cytokines in vivo.[57]

Multiple chemotherapeutic agents such as 5-fluorouacil (FU), cisplatin, and bucladesine have been delivered in the form of polymer wafers. Menei et al conducted a randomized phase 2 clinical trial wherein 95 patients with a radiological diagnosis of MG were randomized to receive 130 mg of radiosensitizing 5-FU incorporated in 40 mm poly-D-lactide-co-glycolide (PLGA) microparticles stereotactically injected in the walls of the resection cavity and XRT, or XRT only, hypothesized that the implantation of 5-FU-loaded microspheres possibly did increase the overall survival; however, the study itself was not designed and sufficiently powered to demonstrate this.[58] Local chemotherapy with cisplatin incorporated into biodegradable 6-carboxylcellulose polymer (cisplatin-depot [CDDP-D]) delivering 45 mg of radiosensitizing cisplatin in 21 patients with primary GBM was well tolerated and associated with improved survival.[59] In a randomized prospective study, Dalbasti et al showed that the group treated with implantation of bucladesine-loaded biodegradable polymeric sustained release (bcl-SR) pellets with maximal doses of 20 mg bucladesine with a mean dose of 15.5 mg, and six IV infusions of fotemustine after tumor resection had a significant delay of recurrence with a survival rate of 70% at 12 months estimated by the Kaplan-Meier method.[60]

Systemic use of nitrosoureas, low-molecular-weight, lipid-soluble alkylation agents capable of crossing the BBB and well known for their activity against MGs,[61,62] is limited by its relatively short life-life (~ 15 min) and severe toxicity such as myelosuppression and pulmonary fibrosis. In an effort to improve its effectiveness and limit the dose-related side effects, BCNU was incorporated into polymers (Gliadel Wafer, Eisai) and when tested against a rat intracranial glioma clearly proved to be superior to systemic administration and led to significant prolongation of survival.[63] When tested for its toxicity in primate studies it was shown that BCNU polymers were well tolerated and that concomitant external beam radiotherapy did not increase toxicity.[64] In a phase 1/2 clinical trial of 21 patients with diagnosis of recurrent MG, treated with three different doses of BCNU loaded in PCPP-SA polymers (1.93%, 3.85%, and 6.35% BCNU by polymer weight), it was established that the treatment was well tolerated, and no patient experienced any signs of local or systemic toxicity with overall median survival of 46 weeks after implant and 87 weeks after initial diagnosis, and 86% of the patients alive more than 1 year after diagnosis.[65] On the basis of this work, the 3.85% BCNU-loaded polymers were chosen for further clinical study. In 1996, the Food and Drug Administration approved Gliadel (Eisai Inc., Woodcliff Lake, NJ) as the first new treatment against malignant brain tumors in 23 years. Overall safety of the BCNU polymer combination was also tested in a phase 1 study involving 22 patients with newly diagnosed MG, and none of the 22 patients experienced any local or systemic side effects attributable to Gliadel Wafers (Eisai).[66] A prospective, randomized, double-blind clinical trial involving 32 patients with newly diagnosed MGs, half treated with 3.85%-BCNU wafers and the other half receiving placebo wafers at the time of the initial resection showed that the median survival was 58 weeks for the BCNU treatment group and 40 weeks for the placebo group (p = 0.001). At 1 year, 63% of the patients treated with BCNU polymers were alive compared with 19% for the control group; at 2 years, the differences remained highly significant, with 31% of the Gliadel (Eisai) group surviving compared with 6% of the control group, and after 3 years, 25% of patients treated with Gliadel Wafers (Eisai) were alive compared with 6% of the control group.[67] Based on these phase 1/2 data two well-designed, randomized, controlled trials have compared Gliadel (Eisai) with placebo in recurrent and newly diagnosed MGs thus defining its role in both newly diagnosed and recurrent MGs. Both the trials concluded that Gliadel

(Eisai) was safe and effective, with the most frequent neurological adverse events being hemiplegia, brain edema, confusion, and seizures. However, serious intracranial infection, intracranial hypertension, and CSF leakage were noted to be more frequent in the Gliadel (Eisai) group than in the placebo group.[68,69]

O-6-alkylguanine DNA alkyltransferase (AGT), an important DNA-repair protein that protects cells from killing and mutagenesis by alkylation agents such as BCNU, can confer resistance to glioma cells from BCNU. Quinn et al designed a phase 2 trial to define the efficacy of Gliadel Wafers (Eisai) in combination with an infusion of O-6-benzylguanine (O-6-BG), an AGT suppressor, in patients with recurrent GBM and concluded that, although systemically administered O-6-BG can be safely coadministered with Gliadel Wafers (Eisai), it may increase the risk of hydrocephalus, CSF leakage, and CSF/brain infection.[70] A recent study by McGirt et al showed that concomitant TMZ (Stupp protocol) therapy in addition to Gliadel Wafer (Eisai) implantation was associated with a median survival of nearly 21 months without increased perioperative morbidity.[71]

Level I Evidence

To evaluate the effectiveness of biodegradable polymers impregnated with carmustine, Gliadel Wafer (Eisai), in the treatment of recurrent MGs Brem et al conducted a randomized, placebo-controlled, prospective study, wherein 222 patients with recurrent MGs requiring reoperation were randomly assigned to receive surgically implanted Gliadel Wafers (Eisai) with or without 3.85% BCNU and showed that median survival of the 110 patients who received Gliadel Wafers (Eisai) was 8 weeks longer compared with the 112 patients who received only placebo polymers (hazard ratio = 0.67, $p = 0.006$), among patients with GBM 6-month survival in the treatment group was 50% greater than in the placebo group (mortality = 32/72 [44%] versus 47/73 [64%], $p = 0.02$) with no clinically important adverse reactions related to the Gliadel Wafers (Eisai), either in the brain or systemically.[68] In a phase 3 trial in the setting of newly diagnosed GBM, 240 patients were randomized to receive either BCNU or placebo wafers at the time of primary surgical resection, and then both groups were treated with external beam radiation. Results showed a median survival of 13.9 months in the intent-to-treat group and 11.6 months for the placebo-treated group (log-rank *P*-value stratified by country = 0.03), with a 29% reduction in the risk of death in the treatment group. When adjusted for factors affecting survival, the treatment effect remained positive, with a risk reduction of 28% ($p = 0.03$), thus confirming that local chemotherapy with Gliadel Wafers (Eisai) is well tolerated and offers a survival benefit to patients with newly diagnosed MG.[69] In an attempt to address the issue whether BCNU should be recommended as part of the standard of care for patients with MG, Hart et al performed a systematic review and meta-analysis of all the available randomized, controlled trials looking at insertion of BCNU wafers in cases of newly diagnosed or recurrent MG and concluded that insertion of BCNU-impregnated wafers results in improved survival without an increased incidence of adverse events over placebo wafers when used for primary disease therapy. There is no evidence of benefit for any other outcome measures such as quality of life or progression-free survival. In the studies included in this systematic review the recurrence was treated very aggressively with re-resection, maximum XRT, and chemotherapy, and in that setting they concluded that BCNU wafers do not appear to confer any additional benefit.[72]

Level II Evidence

In a single institutional safety and feasibility study of adjunct local chemotherapy with BCNU wafers to the standard of care, Salvati et al reported that the integration of local chemotherapy with BCNU wafers and the standard adjuvant regimen with radiotherapy and concomitant chemotherapy appears to be safe and feasible without any adjunctive complication.[73] However, Noël et al's recent retrospective study of patients treated for MG, with or without Gliadel Wafers (Eisai) and according to the Stupp protocol concluded that adding Gliadel (Eisai) before performing a Stupp protocol does not improve survival.[74] Over the years Gliadel Wafers (Eisai) have been associated with many reported but not consistently replicated complications.[75–78] To shed some light on this issue Attenello et al published a retrospective study of 10 years of institutional experience with Gliadel Wafers (Eisai) and concluded that their use was not associated with an increase in perioperative morbidity after surgical treatment of MG.[79] Menei et al published a retrospective multicenter study of the French experience with Gliadel (Eisai). They compared the adverse effects and survival in patients with newly diagnosed MG receiving Gliadel (Eisai) plus radiochemotherapy with TMZ with those of previous phase 3 trials and concluded that survival rates for newly diagnosed patients were better than those reported in previous phase 3 trials. Combination of Gliadel (Eisai) and radiochemotherapy with TMZ was well tolerated and appeared to increase survival without increasing adverse effects.[80] Several studies looked at the efficacy of Gliadel Wafers (Eisai) in newly diagnosed and recurrent gliomas along with different combinations of adjuvant therapy. **Table 9.3** lists all the trials involving Gliadel Wafers (Eisai).

Table 9.3 Clinical trials involving Gliadel Wafers[a]

Study	Level	No. patients	Title	Conclusion
Hart et al 2011[72]	I	272 primary and 222 recurrent	Chemotherapy wafers for high-grade glioma	Increased survival with Gliadel Wafers[a] compared with placebo
Kunwar et al 2010[41]	I	296	Phase 3 randomized trial of convection-enhanced delivery of IL-3-PE38QQR versus Gliadel Wafers[a] for recurrent glioblastoma	No survival difference between convection-enhanced delivery of IL-13-PE38QQR and Gliadel Wafers[a]
Westphal et al 2006[107]	II	59	Gliadel Wafers[a] in initial surgery for malignant glioma: long-term follow-up of a multicenter, controlled trial	Gliadel Wafers[a] at the time of initial surgery in combination with radiation therapy demonstrated a survival advantage
Valtonen et al 1997[67]	I	32	Interstitial chemotherapy with carmustine-loaded polymers for high-grade gliomas: a randomized double-blind study	Carmustine applied locally in a biodegradable polymer at the time of primary operation seems to have a favorable effect on the life span of patients with high-grade gliomas
Noël et al 2012[74]	II	65	Retrospective comparison of chemoradiotherapy followed by adjuvant chemotherapy, with or without prior Gliadel[a] implantation (carmustine) after initial surgery in patients with newly diagnosed high-grade gliomas	Adding Gliadel[a] before performing a Stupp protocol did not improve survival
Salvati et al 2011[73]	II	32	Safety and feasibility of the adjunct of local chemotherapy with biodegradable carmustine (BCNU) wafers to the standard multimodal approach to high-grade gliomas at first diagnosis	Integration of local chemotherapy with carmustine wafers and the standard adjuvant regimen appears to be safe and feasible
Bock et al 2010[108]	II	44	First-line treatment of malignant glioma with carmustine implants followed by concomitant radiochemotherapy: a multicenter experience	Combination of local chemotherapy and concomitant radiochemotherapy carries a significant risk of toxicity that currently appears underestimated
Menei et al 2010[80]	II	163	Biodegradable carmustine wafers (Gliadel[a]) alone or in combination with chemoradiotherapy: the French experience	Combination of Gliadel[a] and radiochemotherapy with temozolomide was well tolerated and appeared to increase survival
McGirt et al 2009[71]	II	33	Gliadel (BCNU) Wafers[a] plus concomitant temozolomide therapy after primary resection of glioblastoma multiforme	Temozolomide can be safely administered to patients receiving Gliadel Wafers[a] after resection of glioblastoma multiforme
Quinn et al 2009[70]	II	52	Phase 2 trial of Gliadel[a] plus O-6-benzylguanine (O-6-BG) in adults with recurrent glioblastoma multiforme	The efficacy of implanted Gliadel Wafers[a] may be improved with the addition of O-6-BG
Smith et al 2008[109]	II	30	Prospective trial of gross total resection with Gliadel Wafers[a] followed by early postoperative Gamma Knife[b] radiosurgery and conformal fractionated radiotherapy as the initial treatment for patients with radiographically suspected, newly diagnosed glioblastoma multiforme	Aggressive local tumor control with these multimodal therapies should be approached judiciously for a select group of high-performance patients
Attenello et al 2008[79]	II	1,013	Use of Gliadel (BCNU) Wafers[a] in the surgical treatment of malignant glioma: a 10-year institutional experience	Gliadel Wafers[a] were not associated with an increase in perioperative morbidity

(Continued on page 86)

Table 9.3 *(Continued)* Clinical trials involving Gliadel Wafers[a]

Study	Level	No. patients	Title	Conclusion
Limentani et al 2005[110]	II	16	A phase 1 trial of surgery, Gliadel Wafer[a] implantation, and immediate postoperative carboplatin in combination with radiation therapy for primary anaplastic astrocytoma or glioblastoma multiforme	Administering systemic carboplatin is safe and well tolerated in the postoperative period immediately following resection and implantation of Gliadel Wafer[a]
Giese et al 2004[111]	II	24	Pattern of recurrence following local chemotherapy with biodegradable carmustine (BCNU) implants in patients with glioblastoma	Both the clinical progression and radiological progression were significantly delayed in patients treated with local chemotherapy
Kleinberg et al 2004[111]	II	46	Clinical course and pathological findings after Gliadel and radiotherapy for newly diagnosed malignant glioma: implications for patient management	Gliadel[a] followed by full-dose standard radiotherapy is well tolerated
Whittle et al 2003[112]	II	56	Gliadel[a] therapy given for first resection of malignant glioma: a single-center study of the potential use of Gliadel[a]	Only 20% of patients met the inclusion criteria
Westphal et al 2003[69]	II	240	Phase 3 trial of local chemotherapy with biodegradable carmustine (BCNU) wafers (Gliadel Wafers[a]) in patients with primary malignant glioma	Local chemotherapy with BCNU wafers is well tolerated and offers a survival benefit to patients with newly diagnosed malignant glioma
Gururangan et al 2001[78]	II	10	Phase 1 study of Gliadel Wafers[a] plus temozolomide in adults with recurrent supratentorial high-grade gliomas	Temozolomide can be given safely after placement of Gliadel (3.85%) Wafers[a]

[a]Gliadel or Gliadel Wafers, Eisai, Woodcliff Lake, NJ.
[b]Gamma Knife, Elekta, Atlanta, GA.

Level III Evidence

In a case series of four patients, three with recurrent disease and one with a newly diagnosed GBM, Balossier et al reported that treatment with Gliadel Wafers (Eisai) was well tolerated, with patient survival from diagnosis ranging from 56 to 132 weeks, which compares favorably with the survival of ~ 58 weeks seen in the European Organization for Research and Treatment of Cancer–National Cancer Institute of Canada (EORTC-NCIC) clinical trial of combined radiotherapy with concomitant and adjuvant temozolomide.[81]

Expert Recommendations

1. Local implantation of Gliadel Wafers after surgical resection increases survival in patients with primary malignant glioma compared with placebo and can be safely recommended in this group of patients (Grade 1A Recommendation, Level I Evidence).
2. Local delivery of various agents via convection-enhanced delivery has thus far failed to show any clinically significant survival advantage (Grade 2B Recommendation, Level III Evidence).

■ Summary and Conclusions

CNS anatomy and protective mechanisms pose a significant challenge in terms of drug delivery to CNS tumors. Several options have been employed to bypass these obstacles and deliver drugs in a safe and effective fashion; however, to date only Gliadel Wafers (Eisai) have shown solid evidence of effectiveness. Based on the currently available body of literature the use of Gliadel Wafers (Eisai) for primary disease is safe and effectively increases survival compared with placebo. Multiple retrospective studies also concluded that Gliadel Wafers (Eisai) could be safely combined with a Stupp protocol; however, this remains to be tested in a phase 3 randomized study. CED, even though it shows promises, has failed to show any benefit over Gliadel Wafers (Eisai). The success of local drug delivery depends on a combination of good and effective therapeutic agents in combination with an effective and efficient delivery vehicle. Future research is needed in both these aspects to formulate a perfect therapeutic option for an ever-evolving disease.

■ References

1. Stupp R, Mason WP, van den Bent MJ, et al; European Organisation for Research and Treatment of Cancer Brain Tumor and Radiotherapy Groups; National Cancer Institute of Canada Clinical Trials Group. Radiotherapy plus concomitant and adjuvant temozolomide for glioblastoma. N Engl J Med 2005;352(10):987–996
2. Hochberg FH, Pruitt A. Assumptions in the radiotherapy of glioblastoma. Neurology 1980;30(9):907–911
3. Ting CY, Fan CH, Liu HL, et al. Concurrent blood-brain barrier opening and local drug delivery using drug-carrying microbubbles and focused ultrasound for brain glioma treatment. Biomaterials 2012;33(2):704–712
4. Stewart LA. Chemotherapy in adult high-grade glioma: a systematic review and meta-analysis of individual patient data from 12 randomised trials. Lancet 2002;359(9311):1011–1018
5. Stupp R, Dietrich PY, Ostermann Kraljevic S, et al. Promising survival for patients with newly diagnosed glioblastoma multiforme treated with concomitant radiation plus temozolomide followed by adjuvant temozolomide. J Clin Oncol 2002;20(5):1375–1382
6. Holdhoff M, Grossman SA. Controversies in the adjuvant therapy of high-grade gliomas. Oncologist 2011;16(3):351–358
7. Kornblith PL, Walker M. Chemotherapy for malignant gliomas. J Neurosurg 1988;68(1):1–17
8. Prokai L, Prokai-Tatrai K, Bodor N. Targeting drugs to the brain by redox chemical delivery systems. Med Res Rev 2000;20(5):367–416
9. Pardridge WM. Vector-mediated drug delivery to the brain. Adv Drug Deliv Rev 1999;36(2-3):299–321
10. Tfayli A, Hentschel P, Madajewicz S, et al. Toxicities related to intraarterial infusion of cisplatin and etoposide in patients with brain tumors. J Neurooncol 1999;42(1):73–77
11. Shin BJ, Burkhardt JK, Riina HA, Boockvar JA. Superselective intra-arterial cerebral infusion of novel agents after blood-brain disruption for the treatment of recurrent glioblastoma multiforme: a technical case series. Neurosurg Clin N Am 2012;23(2):323–329, ix–x
12. Sanovich E, Bartus RT, Friden PM, Dean RL, Le HQ, Brightman MW. Pathway across blood-brain barrier opened by the bradykinin agonist, RMP-7. Brain Res 1995;705(1-2):125–135
13. Nakagawa H, Groothuis D, Blasberg RG. The effect of graded hypertonic intracarotid infusions on drug delivery to experimental RG-2 gliomas. Neurology 1984;34(12):1571–1581
14. Neuwelt EA, Barnett PA, Frenkel EP. Chemotherapeutic agent permeability to normal brain and delivery to avian sarcoma virus-induced brain tumors in the rodent: observations on problems of drug delivery. Neurosurgery 1984;14(2):154–160
15. Groothuis DR, Warkne PC, Molnar P, Lapin GD, Mikhael MA. Effect of hyperosmotic blood-brain barrier disruption on transcapillary transport in canine brain tumors. J Neurosurg 1990;72(3):441–449
16. Black KL, Cloughesy T, Huang SC, et al. Intracarotid infusion of RMP-7, a bradykinin analog, and transport of gallium-68 ethylenediamine tetraacetic acid into human gliomas. J Neurosurg 1997;86(4):603–609
17. Matsukado K, Inamura T, Nakano S, Fukui M, Bartus RT, Black KL. Enhanced tumor uptake of carboplatin and survival in glioma-bearing rats by intracarotid infusion of bradykinin analog, RMP-7. Neurosurgery 1996;39(1):125–133
18. Cloughesy TF, Black KL, Gobin YP, et al. Intra-arterial Cereport (RMP-7) and carboplatin: a dose escalation study for recurrent malignant gliomas. Neurosurgery 1999;44(2):270–278
19. Ford J, Osborn C, Barton T, Bleehen NM. A phase I study of intravenous RMP-7 with carboplatin in patients with progression of malignant glioma. Eur J Cancer 1998;34(11):1807–1811
20. Prados MD, Schold SC Jr, Fine HA, et al. A randomized, double-blind, placebo-controlled, phase 2 study of RMP-7 in combination with carboplatin administered intravenously for the treatment of recurrent malignant glioma. Neuro-oncol 2003;5(2):96–103
21. Boockvar JA, Tsiouris AJ, Hofstetter CP, et al. Safety and maximum tolerated dose of superselective intraarterial cerebral infusion of bevacizumab after osmotic blood-brain barrier disruption for recurrent malignant glioma. Clinical article. J Neurosurg 2011;114(3):624–632
22. Morikawa N, Mori T, Abe T, Kawashima H, Takeyama M, Hori S. Pharmacokinetics of etoposide and carboplatin in cerebrospinal fluid and plasma during hyperosmotic disruption of the blood brain barrier and intraarterial combination chemotherapy. Biol Pharm Bull 1999;22(4):428–431
23. Neuwelt EA, Diehl JT, Vu LH, Hill SA, Michael AJ, Frenkel EP. Monitoring of methotrexate delivery in patients with malignant brain tumors after osmotic blood-brain barrier disruption. Ann Intern Med 1981;94(4 pt 1):449–454
24. Markert JM, Liechty PG, Wang W, et al. Phase Ib trial of mutant herpes simplex virus G207 inoculated pre-and post-tumor resection for recurrent GBM. Mol Ther 2009;17(1):199–207
25. Boiardi A, Silvani A, Eoli M, et al. Treatment of recurrent glioblastoma: can local delivery of mitoxantrone improve survival? J Neurooncol 2008;88(1):105–113
26. Bobo RH, Laske DW, Akbasak A, Morrison PF, Dedrick RL, Oldfield EH. Convection-enhanced delivery of macromolecules in the brain. Proc Natl Acad Sci U S A 1994;91(6):2076–2080
27. Varenika V, Dickinson P, Bringas J, et al. Detection of infusate leakage in the brain using real-time imaging of convection-enhanced delivery. J Neurosurg 2008;109(5):874–880
28. Sampson JH, Brady ML, Petry NA, et al. Intracerebral infusate distribution by convection-enhanced delivery in humans with malignant gliomas: descriptive effects of target anatomy and catheter positioning. Neurosurgery 2007;60(2, Suppl 1):ONS89–ONS98
29. Tanner PG, Holtmannspötter M, Tonn JC, Goldbrunner R. Effects of drug efflux on convection-enhanced paclitaxel delivery to malignant gliomas: technical note. Neurosurgery 2007;61(4):E880–E882
30. Fiandaca MS, Forsayeth JR, Dickinson PJ, Bankiewicz KS. Image-guided convection-enhanced delivery platform in the treatment of neurological diseases. Neurotherapeutics 2008;5(1):123–127
31. Raghavan R, Brady ML, Rodríguez-Ponce MI, Hartlep A, Pedain C, Sampson JH. Convection-enhanced delivery of therapeutics for brain disease, and its optimization. Neurosurg Focus 2006;20(4):E12
32. Dörner L, Nabavi A, Mehdorn HM. Entry points for catheter placement in convection-enhanced delivery—a retrospective anatomic analysis. Minim Invasive Neurosurg 2009;52(5-6):229–232
33. Sampson JH, Raghavan R, Brady ML, et al. Clinical utility of a patient-specific algorithm for simulating intracerebral drug infusions. Neuro-oncol 2007;9(3):343–353
34. Sampson JH, Archer G, Pedain C, et al; PRECISE Trial Investigators. Poor drug distribution as a possible explanation for the results of the PRECISE trial. J Neurosurg 2010;113(2):301–309
35. Pöpperl G, Goldbrunner R, Gildehaus FJ, et al. O-(2-[18F]fluoroethyl)-L-tyrosine PET for monitoring the effects of convection-enhanced delivery of paclitaxel in patients with recurrent glioblastoma. Eur J Nucl Med Mol Imaging 2005;32(9):1018–1025
36. Sampson JH, Raghavan R, Provenzale JM, et al. Induction of hyperintense signal on T2-weighted MR images correlates with infusion distribution from intracerebral convection-enhanced delivery of a tumor-targeted cytotoxin. AJR Am J Roentgenol 2007;188(3):703–709
37. Lidar Z, Mardor Y, Jonas T, et al. Convection-enhanced delivery of paclitaxel for the treatment of recurrent malignant

glioma: a phase I/II clinical study. J Neurosurg 2004;100(3): 472–479
38. Ding D, Kanaly CW, Bigner DD, et al. Convection-enhanced delivery of free gadolinium with the recombinant immunotoxin MR1-1. J Neurooncol 2010;98(1):1–7
39. Voges J, Reszka R, Gossmann A, et al. Imaging-guided convection-enhanced delivery and gene therapy of glioblastoma. Ann Neurol 2003;54(4):479–487
40. Bogdahn U, Hau P, Stockhammer G, et al; Trabedersen Glioma Study Group. Targeted therapy for high-grade glioma with the TGF-b2 inhibitor trabedersen: results of a randomized and controlled phase IIb study. Neuro-oncol 2011;13(1): 132–142
41. Kunwar S, Chang S, Westphal M, et al; PRECISE Study Group. Phase III randomized trial of CED of IL13-PE38QQR vs Gliadel wafers for recurrent glioblastoma. Neuro-oncol 2010;12(8):871–881
42. Mueller S, Polley MY, Lee B, et al. Effect of imaging and catheter characteristics on clinical outcome for patients in the PRECISE study. J Neurooncol 2011;101(2):267–277
43. Sampson JH, Akabani G, Friedman AH, et al. Comparison of intratumoral bolus injection and convection-enhanced delivery of radiolabeled antitenascin monoclonal antibodies. Neurosurg Focus 2006;20(4):E14
44. Kunwar S, Chang SM, Prados MD, et al. Safety of intraparenchymal convection-enhanced delivery of cintredekin besudotox in early-phase studies. Neurosurg Focus 2006;20(4):E15
45. Kunwar S, Prados MD, Chang SM, et al; Cintredekin Besudotox Intraparenchymal Study Group. Direct intracerebral delivery of cintredekin besudotox (IL13-PE38QQR) in recurrent malignant glioma: a report by the Cintredekin Besudotox Intraparenchymal Study Group. J Clin Oncol 2007;25(7):837–844
46. Vogelbaum MA, Sampson JH, Kunwar S, et al. Convection-enhanced delivery of cintredekin besudotox (interleukin-13-PE38QQR) followed by radiation therapy with and without temozolomide in newly diagnosed malignant gliomas: phase 1 study of final safety results. Neurosurgery 2007;61(5):1031–1037
47. Carpentier A, Metellus P, Ursu R, et al. Intracerebral administration of CpG oligonucleotide for patients with recurrent glioblastoma: a phase II study. Neuro-oncol 2010;12(4): 401–408
48. Patel SJ, Shapiro WR, Laske DW, et al. Safety and feasibility of convection-enhanced delivery of Cotara for the treatment of malignant glioma: initial experience in 51 patients. Neurosurgery 2005;56(6):1243–1252
49. Sampson JH, Akabani G, Archer GE, et al. Progress report of a Phase I study of the intracerebral microinfusion of a recombinant chimeric protein composed of transforming growth factor (TGF)-alpha and a mutated form of the Pseudomonas exotoxin termed PE-38 (TP-38) for the treatment of malignant brain tumors. J Neurooncol 2003;65(1):27–35
50. Weber F, Asher A, Bucholz R, et al. Safety, tolerability, and tumor response of IL4-Pseudomonas exotoxin (NBI-3001) in patients with recurrent malignant glioma. J Neurooncol 2003; 64(1-2):125–137
51. Langer R, Folkman J. Polymers for the sustained release of proteins and other macromolecules. Nature 1976; 263(5580):797–800
52. Leong KW, Brott BC, Langer R. Bioerodible polyanhydrides as drug-carrier matrices, I: Characterization, degradation, and release characteristics. J Biomed Mater Res 1985;19(8): 941–955
53. Domb A, Bogdansky S, Olivi A, et al. Controlled delivery of water soluble and hydrolytically unstable anti-cancer drugs for polymeric implants. Polymer Prepr 1991;32:219–220
54. Menei P, Benoit JP, Boisdron-Celle M, Fournier D, Mercier P, Guy G. Drug targeting into the central nervous system by stereotactic implantation of biodegradable microspheres. Neurosurgery 1994;34(6):1058–1064
55. Gref R, Minamitake Y, Peracchia MT, Trubetskoy V, Torchilin V, Langer R. Biodegradable long-circulating polymeric nanospheres. Science 1994;263(5153):1600–1603
56. Gabizon AA. Liposomal anthracyclines. Hematol Oncol Clin North Am 1994;8(2):431–450
57. Golumbek PT, Azhari R, Jaffee EM, et al. Controlled release, biodegradable cytokine depots: a new approach in cancer vaccine design. Cancer Res 1993;53(24):5841–5844
58. Menei P, Capelle L, Guyotat J, et al. Local and sustained delivery of 5-fluorouracil from biodegradable microspheres for the radiosensitization of malignant glioma: a randomized phase II trial. Neurosurgery 2005;56(2):242–248
59. Sheleg SV, Korotkevich EA, Zhavrid EA, et al. Local chemotherapy with cisplatin-depot for glioblastoma multiforme. J Neurooncol 2002;60(1):53–59
60. Dalbasti T, Oktar N, Cagli S, Ozdamar N. Local interstitial chemotherapy with sustained release bucladesine in de novo glioblastoma multiforme: a preliminary study. J Neurooncol 2002;56(2):167–174
61. Green SB, Byar DP, Walker MD, et al. Comparisons of carmustine, procarbazine, and high-dose methylprednisolone as additions to surgery and radiotherapy for the treatment of malignant glioma. Cancer Treat Rep 1983;67(2):121–132
62. Walker MD, Green SB, Byar DP, et al. Randomized comparisons of radiotherapy and nitrosoureas for the treatment of malignant glioma after surgery. N Engl J Med 1980;303(23): 1323–1329
63. Tamargo RJ, Myseros JS, Epstein JI, Yang MB, Chasin M, Brem H. Interstitial chemotherapy of the 9L gliosarcoma: controlled release polymers for drug delivery in the brain. Cancer Res 1993;53(2):329–333
64. Brem H, Tamargo RJ, Olivi A, et al. Biodegradable polymers for controlled delivery of chemotherapy with and without radiation therapy in the monkey brain. J Neurosurg 1994; 80(2):283–290
65. Brem H, Mahaley MS Jr, Vick NA, et al. Interstitial chemotherapy with drug polymer implants for the treatment of recurrent gliomas. J Neurosurg 1991;74(3):441–446
66. Brem H, Ewend MG, Piantadosi S, Greenhoot J, Burger PC, Sisti M. The safety of interstitial chemotherapy with BCNU-loaded polymer followed by radiation therapy in the treatment of newly diagnosed malignant gliomas: phase I trial. J Neurooncol 1995;26(2):111–123
67. Valtonen S, Timonen U, Toivanen P, et al. Interstitial chemotherapy with carmustine-loaded polymers for high-grade gliomas: a randomized double-blind study. Neurosurgery 1997;41(1):44–48
68. Brem H, Piantadosi S, Burger PC, et al; The Polymer-brain Tumor Treatment Group. Placebo-controlled trial of safety and efficacy of intraoperative controlled delivery by biodegradable polymers of chemotherapy for recurrent gliomas. Lancet 1995;345(8956):1008–1012
69. Westphal M, Hilt DC, Bortey E, et al. A phase 3 trial of local chemotherapy with biodegradable carmustine (BCNU) wafers (Gliadel wafers) in patients with primary malignant glioma. Neuro-oncol 2003;5(2):79–88
70. Quinn JA, Jiang SX, Carter J, et al. Phase II trial of Gliadel plus O6-benzylguanine in adults with recurrent glioblastoma multiforme. Clin Cancer Res 2009;15(3):1064–1068
71. McGirt MJ, Than KD, Weingart JD, et al. Gliadel (BCNU) wafer plus concomitant temozolomide therapy after primary resection of glioblastoma multiforme. J Neurosurg 2009;110(3):583–588
72. Hart MG, Grant R, Garside R, Rogers G, Somerville M, Stein K. Chemotherapy wafers for high grade glioma. Cochrane Database Syst Rev 2011;(3):CD007294

73. Salvati M, D'elia A, Frati A, Brogna C, Santoro A, Delfini R. Safety and feasibility of the adjunct of local chemotherapy with biodegradable carmustine (BCNU) wafers to the standard multimodal approach to high grade gliomas at first diagnosis. J Neurosurg Sci 2011;55(1):1–6
74. Noël G, Schott R, Froelich S, et al. Retrospective comparison of chemoradiotherapy followed by adjuvant chemotherapy, with or without prior Gliadel implantation (carmustine) after initial surgery in patients with newly diagnosed high-grade gliomas. Int J Radiat Oncol Biol Phys 2012;82(2):749–755
75. Dörner L, Ulmer S, Rohr A, Mehdorn HM, Nabavi A. Space-occupying cyst development in the resection cavity of malignant gliomas following Gliadel® implantation incidence, therapeutic strategies, and outcome. J Clin Neurosci 2011;18(3):347–351
76. Glick JA, Graham RS, Voils SA. Candida meningitis post Gliadel wafer placement successfully treated with intrathecal and intravenous amphotericin B. Ann Pharmacother 2010;44(1):215–218
77. Weber EL, Goebel EA. Cerebral edema associated with Gliadel wafers: two case studies. Neuro-oncol 2005;7(1): 84–89
78. Gururangan S, et al. Phase I study of Gliadel wafers plus temozolomide in adults with recurrent supratentorial high-grade gliomas. Neuro Oncol 2001 Oct;3(4):246–250
79. Attenello FJ, Mukherjee D, Datoo G, et al. Use of Gliadel (BCNU) wafer in the surgical treatment of malignant glioma: a 10-year institutional experience. Ann Surg Oncol 2008;15(10): 2887–2893
80. Menei P, Metellus P, Parot-Schinkel E, et al; Neuro-oncology Club of the French Society of Neurosurgery. Biodegradable carmustine wafers (Gliadel) alone or in combination with chemoradiotherapy: the French experience. Ann Surg Oncol 2010;17(7):1740–1746
81. Balossier A, Dörner L, Emery E, et al. Incorporating BCNU wafers into malignant glioma treatment: European case studies. Clin Drug Investig 2010;30(3):195–204
82. Boiardi A, Bartolomei M, Silvani A, et al. Intratumoral delivery of mitoxantrone in association with 90-Y radioimmunotherapy (RIT) in recurrent glioblastoma. J Neurooncol 2005; 72(2):125–131
83. Boiardi A, Eoli M, Salmaggi A, et al. Efficacy of intratumoral delivery of mitoxantrone in recurrent malignant glial tumours. J Neurooncol 2001;54(1):39–47
84. Boiardi A, Eoli M, Pozzi A, Salmaggi A, Broggi G, Silvani A. Locally delivered chemotherapy and repeated surgery can improve survival in glioblastoma patients. Ital J Neurol Sci 1999;20(1):43–48
85. Boiardi A, Salmaggi A, Pozzi A, Broggi G, Silvani A. Interstitial chemotherapy with mitoxantrone in recurrent malignant glioma: preliminary data. J Neurooncol 1996;27(2):157–162
86. Boiardi A, Eoli M, Salmaggi A, et al. New approach in delivering chemotherapy: locoregional treatment for recurrent glioblastoma (rGBM). J Exp Clin Cancer Res 2003;22(4, Suppl): 123–127
87. Boiardi A, Silvani A, Milanesi I, Munari L, Broggi G, Botturi M. Local immunotherapy (beta-IFN) and systemic chemotherapy in primary glial tumors. Ital J Neurol Sci 1991;12(2):163–168
88. Silvani A, Milanesi I, Munari L, Broggi G, Botturi M, Boiardi A. Intratumoral beta interferon and systemic chemotherapy: preliminary data in GBM patients. J Neurosurg Sci 1990;34(3-4): 257–259
89. Boiardi A, Silvani A, Ruffini PA, et al. Loco-regional immunotherapy with recombinant interleukin-2 and adherent lymphokine-activated killer cells (A-LAK) in recurrent glioblastoma patients. Cancer Immunol Immunother 1994;39(3): 193–197
90. Koch D, Hundsberger T, Boor S, Kaina B. Local intracerebral administration of O(6)-benzylguanine combined with systemic chemotherapy with temozolomide of a patient suffering from a recurrent glioblastoma. J Neurooncol 2007;82(1):85–89
91. Oshiro S, Tsugu H, Komatsu F, et al. Evaluation of intratumoral administration of tumor necrosis factor-alpha in patients with malignant glioma. Anticancer Res 2006;26(6A): 4027–4032
92. Prados MD, McDermott M, Chang SM, et al. Treatment of progressive or recurrent glioblastoma multiforme in adults with herpes simplex virus thymidine kinase gene vector-producer cells followed by intravenous ganciclovir administration: a phase I/II multi-institutional trial. J Neurooncol 2003;65(3):269–278
93. Patchell RA, Regine WF, Ashton P, et al. A phase I trial of continuously infused intratumoral bleomycin for the treatment of recurrent glioblastoma multiforme. J Neurooncol 2002;60(1):37–42
94. Voulgaris S, Partheni M, Karamouzis M, Dimopoulos P, Papadakis N, Kalofonos HP. Intratumoral doxorubicin in patients with malignant brain gliomas. Am J Clin Oncol 2002;25(1): 60–64
95. Huang Y, Hayes RL, Wertheim S, Arbit E, Scheff R. Treatment of refractory recurrent malignant glioma with adoptive cellular immunotherapy: a case report. Crit Rev Oncol Hematol 2001;39(1-2):17–23
96. Nakagawa H, Maeda N, Tsuzuki T, et al. Intracavitary chemotherapy with 5-fluoro-2¢-deoxyuridine (FdUrd) in malignant brain tumors. Jpn J Clin Oncol 2001;31(6):251–258
97. Quattrocchi KB, Miller CH, Cush S, et al. Pilot study of local autologous tumor infiltrating lymphocytes for the treatment of recurrent malignant gliomas. J Neurooncol 1999;45(2): 141–157
98. Bigner DD, Brown MT, Friedman AH, et al. Iodine-131-labeled antitenascin monoclonal antibody 81C6 treatment of patients with recurrent malignant gliomas: phase I trial results. J Clin Oncol 1998;16(6):2202–2212
99. Naganuma H, Sasaki A, Satoh E, et al. Long-term survival in a young patient with anaplastic glioma. Brain Tumor Pathol 1997;14(1):71–74
100. Fetell MR, Housepian EM, Oster MW, et al. Intratumor administration of beta-interferon in recurrent malignant gliomas. A phase I clinical and laboratory study. Cancer 1990;65(1): 78–83
101. Jereb B, Petric J, Lamovec J, Skrbec M, Soss E. Intratumor application of human leukocyte interferon-alpha in patients with malignant brain tumors. Am J Clin Oncol 1989;12(1): 1–7
102. McKeran RO, Firth G, Oliver S, Uttley D, O'Laoire S. A potential application for the intracerebral injection of drugs entrapped within liposomes in the treatment of human cerebral gliomas. J Neurol Neurosurg Psychiatry 1985;48(12):1213–1219
103. Carpentier A, Laigle-Donadey F, Zohar S, et al. Phase 1 trial of a CpG oligodeoxynucleotide for patients with recurrent glioblastoma. Neuro-oncol 2006;8(1):60–66
104. Sampson JH, Akabani G, Archer GE, et al. Intracerebral infusion of an EGFR-targeted toxin in recurrent malignant brain tumors. Neuro-oncol 2008;10(3):320–329
105. Weaver M, Laske DW. Transferrin receptor ligand-targeted toxin conjugate (Tf-CRM107) for therapy of malignant gliomas. J Neurooncol 2003;65(1):3–13
106. Laske DW, Youle RJ, Oldfield EH. Tumor regression with regional distribution of the targeted toxin TF-CRM107 in patients with malignant brain tumors. Nat Med 1997;3(12):1362–1368
107. Westphal M, Ram Z, Riddle V, Hilt D, Bortey E; Executive Committee of the Gliadel Study Group. Gliadel wafer in initial surgery for malignant glioma: long-term follow-up of a mul-

ticenter controlled trial. Acta Neurochir (Wien) 2006;148(3): 269–275
108. Bock HC, Puchner MJ, Lohmann F, et al. First-line treatment of malignant glioma with carmustine implants followed by concomitant radiochemotherapy: a multicenter experience. Neurosurg Rev 2010;33(4):441–449
109. Smith KA, Ashby LS, Gonzalez LF, et al. Prospective trial of gross-total resection with Gliadel wafers followed by early postoperative Gamma Knife radiosurgery and conformal fractionated radiotherapy as the initial treatment for patients with radiographically suspected, newly diagnosed glioblastoma multiforme. J Neurosurg 2008;109(Suppl):106–117
110. Limentani SA, Asher A, Heafner M, Kim JW, Fraser R. A phase I trial of surgery, Gliadel wafer implantation, and immediate postoperative carboplatin in combination with radiation therapy for primary anaplastic astrocytoma or glioblastoma multiforme. J Neurooncol 2005;72(3):241–244
111. Kleinburg LR, et al. Clinical course and pathological findings after Gliadel and radiotherapy for newly diagnosed malignant glioma: implications for patent management. Cancer Invest 2004;22(1):1–9
112. Whittle IR, Lyles S, Walker M. Gliadel therapy given for first resection of malignant glioma: a single centre study of the potential use of Gliadel. Br J Neurosurg 2003;17(4):352–354

10

The Role of Adjuvant Therapy in Newly Diagnosed High-Grade Astrocytomas

Isabel Arrillaga-Romany, Manmeet S. Ahluwalia, and Patrick Y. Wen

Glioblastoma multiforme (GBM) and anaplastic astrocytoma (AA) are high-grade astrocytomas accounting for 54% and 8% of all gliomas in adults.[1] Their incidence is 3.2 and 0.12 per 100,000 person-years, respectively.[1] Surgical resection is the backbone of treatment for high-grade gliomas when the expected postsurgical neurological sequelae are acceptable. High-grade astrocytoma cells are highly infiltrative, and tumors almost always recur despite best efforts at resection. Adjuvant treatment with radiation and alkylating chemotherapy has been the focus of extensive research and has become the postoperative standard of care. This chapter reviews the best evidence on the role of adjuvant therapy in the treatment of high-grade astrocytomas, with a focus on high-quality, Level I evidence that guides current clinical practice.

■ Literature Review

Radiation Therapy

Level I Evidence

External beam fractionated radiation is the mainstay of postoperative adjuvant therapy for newly diagnosed high-grade astrocytomas. Early randomized studies from the 1970s and early 1980s conducted by the Brain Tumor Study Group (BTSG) demonstrated that postoperative radiotherapy provided significant survival benefit over surgery alone. One of these initial trials randomized 303 patients with newly diagnosed high-grade gliomas to receive one of the following postoperative adjuvant therapies: (1) best supportive care, (2) chemotherapy with carmustine, (3) whole-brain radiotherapy (at a cumulative dose of 50 to 60 Gy), and (4) chemotherapy with carmustine plus radiotherapy (similar dose).[2] There was a clear statistically significant survival advantage for all groups receiving radiotherapy. Median survival times were 4.3 months for the supportive care group, 6.3 for the chemotherapy alone group, 9.4 for the radiation therapy group, and 10.1 months for the group getting both radiation and chemotherapy.[2] Several follow-up randomized trials reviewed by Buatti et al[3] confirmed this benefit (**Table 10.1**). A meta-analysis further validated the utility of radiotherapy in newly diagnosed high-grade astrocytomas.[4]

Volume and Dose

Initial trials focused on whole-brain radiation therapy (WBRT), though an involved-field approach has been adopted more recently, in part based on Level II evidence demonstrating no benefit of WBRT over more-limited-field strategies.[5,6] Natural history data that demonstrate a tendency for local recurrence

Table 10.1 Randomized trials demonstrating a significant survival benefit for postoperative adjuvant radiotherapy

Study	Level	Trial
Walker et al 1980[38]	I	EBRT (60 Gy) vs nitrosourea vs combination in malignant glioma
Andersen 1978[39]	I	Supportive care vs EBRT (45 Gy) in GBM
Sandberg-Wollheim et al 1991[40]	I	PCV ± EBRT (58 Gy)
Kristiansen et al 1981[41]	II	Bleomycin ± EBRT (45 Gy)

Abbreviations: EBRT, external beam radiation therapy; PCV, procarbazine, lomustine (CCNU), and vincristine.

Source: Buatti J, Ryken TC, Smith MC, et al. Radiation therapy of pathologically confirmed newly diagnosed glioblastoma in adults. J Neurooncol 2008;89(3):313–337.

within 1 to 2 cm of the initial treatment region further support the shift away from WBRT to the use of more-limited fields.[3] Current practice frequently entails involved-field external beam radiation aimed at the gross total tumor volume + 2 cm margins.[3,4]

Various dose escalation trials have helped define the current standard dose of 60 Gy divided over fractions of 1.8 to 2.0 Gy. A randomized trial in 443 patients with newly diagnosed high-grade astrocytomas administered either 45 Gy divided over 20 fractions or 60 Gy divided over 30 fractions and revealed a significant survival advantage with the higher dose (Level I evidence).[7] One-year survival was 29% for the 45 Gy arm compared with 39% for the 60 Gy arm. Significant survival benefits were also reported at 18 months (11% and 18%, respectively).[7] Subsequent trials have found no advantage at doses higher than 60 Gy. Two trials randomized patients to receive postoperative radiation at either 60- or 70-Gy dose ± chemotherapy. Results indicated no statistically significant difference in survival between the two doses of radiation.[8,9] Further efforts to increase radiation doses to the tumor have included new techniques, such as radiosurgery and brachytherapy, that have also met with limited success. Review of the literature on radiosurgery and brachytherapy is beyond the scope of this chapter but can be found in several recent publications.[3,4,10]

Chemotherapy

Early Data

Early data from the 1970s to the 1990s failed to support a role for adjuvant chemotherapy in the treatment of high-grade gliomas. These studies focused on the effect of nitrosoureas administered alone or in combination with radiation. They were generally underpowered and provided inconsistent results.[11] Two meta-analyses (Level I evidence) were among the first published reports to support the use of adjuvant chemotherapy for high-grade gliomas.[12,13] These two systematic reviews analyzed updated patient data from available randomized trials that compared radiotherapy alone with radiotherapy plus chemotherapy. In the first review, published in 1993, Fine and colleagues evaluated 16 trials involving more than 3,000 patients.[12] Stewart and colleagues' analysis published in 2002 encompassed a total of 12 trials and 3,004 patients. Overall results favored the use of chemotherapy, with absolute improvements in 1-year survival of 10.1%[12] and 6%[13] and in 2-year survival of 8.6%[12] and 5%[13] (for the Fine and Stewart analyses, respectively). Notably, all agents led to significantly increased toxicity.

Recent Level I Evidence

Temozolomide

A landmark phase 3 trial reported in 2005 by Stupp and colleagues[14] provided some of the first Level I evidence for the use of adjuvant chemotherapy in the treatment of GBM. Temozolomide is an oral, second-generation alkylating agent with good central nervous system (CNS) penetration targeting especially the O6 position on guanine. Preclinical investigations demonstrated the agent's antitumor activity against in vitro GBM cell lines. Early clinical data further suggested an increased effect with repeated exposure to temozolomide.[15] Following successful phase 1 and 2 studies, the European Organization for Research and Treatment of Cancer (EORTC) and the National Cancer Institute of Canada (NCIC) initiated a phase 3 randomized, controlled trial evaluating the impact of temozolomide (administered concurrently and as adjuvant therapy to radiation) on survival in patients with newly diagnosed GBM.[14,16]

Patients with newly diagnosed GBM were randomized to receive either radiation therapy alone (60 Gy divided over 30 fractions administered 5 days per week for 6 weeks) or radiation in combination with temozolomide. Temozolomide was administered at a dose of 75 mg/m^2 of body surface area per day, 7 days per week, concurrently with radiation therapy for 6 weeks and following radiation therapy for 6 cycles administered 5 out of 28 days per cycle at a dose of 150 to 200 mg/m^2. A total of 573 patents were accrued and groups were well matched for prognostic factors, such as age, extent of tumor resection, and functional status. Results demonstrated significant improvements for the temozolomide arm in progression-free survival (PFS) (6.9 vs 5 months) and median survival (14.6 vs 12.1 months), and substantial improvement in survival at 2 years (27.2% vs 10.9%) and at 5 years (9.8% vs 1.9%).[14,16] Severe grade 3 or 4 hematologic toxic effects were limited to 16% of patients receiving the combined chemoradiation therapy.

Prolifeprosan 20 with Carmustine Implants

Food and Drug Administration (FDA)-approved carmustine (3-bis (2-chloroethyl1)-1-nitrosourea; BCNU) biodegradable polymer wafers (Gliadel Wafers, Eisai, Woodcliff Lake, NJ) represent a different chemotherapeutic strategy against GBM that has been validated in three phase 3 trials.[17–19] Polymer wafers are implanted into the surgical cavity at the time of resection and release carmustine over a period of 2 to 3 weeks. In the largest of the phase 3 trials, 240 patients with newly diagnosed grade III and IV gliomas were randomized to receive carmustine or placebo wafers. Both groups also received external beam radiation therapy postoperatively.[19] Results revealed statistically significant improvement in median survival time for the treatment group with grade IV gliomas (13.9 vs 11.6 months) with a risk reduction of 31%.[19] Survival advantage was maintained over 3 years,[20] and adverse effects were limited and comparable in the two groups.[19] Reported complication rates, however, have been higher in clinical practice following drug approval.[21]

Resistance to Alkylating Agents

The DNA repair enzyme O-6-methylguanine-DNA methyltransferase (MGMT) rapidly reverses alkylation at the O6 position of guanine, where agents such as temozolomide and carmustine act.[22] High levels of active MGMT in glioma cells can thereby result in resistance to alkylating agents, whereas depletion of the protein may be associated with improved outcomes.[23] Methylation of the promoter for the MGMT protein inactivates the gene, and methylation status is predictive of response to alkylating agents.[22,23,24] Among patients whose tumors contained a methylated MGMT protein, treatment with both radiotherapy and temozolomide resulted in a prolonged median survival at both 2 and 5 years compared with treatment with radiotherapy alone. In the absence of methylation of the MGMT promoter, there was a much smaller, although statistically significant, difference in survival between the treatment groups. Notably, an overall survival (OS) benefit irrespective of treatment was also evident in patients with methylated MGMT promoters, suggesting that it is also a favorable prognostic factor (**Table 10.2**).[16,24]

In an effort to overcome resistance to alkylating agents, mechanisms aimed at manipulating MGMT activity have been the subject of various research studies. O-6-benzylguanine is an agent that inactivates and depletes MGMT. This agent has been effective at promoting alkylating agents' antitumor activity in preclinical trials,[25,26] though phase 2 trials in both adults and children with GBM were disappointing in both outcome and discovery of significant related marrow toxicities.[27,28]

A more recent strategy has been to use a dose-intensified regimen of adjuvant temozolomide. MGMT activity can be significantly decreased following prolonged exposure to alkylating agents, even at relatively low doses.[29] An international phase 3 clinical trial (RTOG 0525) led by the Radiotherapy Oncology Group (RTOG) and the EORTC investigated whether an alternative "dose-dense" temozolomide regimen improved outcomes in patients with GBM (Level I evidence). A total of 823 patients were enrolled at the time of diagnosis and received standard 60 Gy of fractionated radiation therapy plus 42 days

Table 10.2 Survival benefit of radiotherapy alone or with temozolomide (TMZ) stratified by MGMT methylation status

	Median survival (months)	2-year survival (%)	5-year survival (%)
Unmethylated			
EBRT alone	11.8	1.8	0
EBRT + TMZ	12.6	14.8	8.3
Methylated			
EBRT alone	15.3	23.9	5.2
EBRT + TMZ	23.4	48.9	13.8

Abbreviations: EBRT, external beam radiation therapy; MGMT, O6-methylguanine-DNA methyltransferase.

Source: Stupp R, Hegi ME, Mason WP, et al; European Organisation for Research and Treatment of Cancer Brain Tumour and Radiation Oncology Groups; National Cancer Institute of Canada Clinical Trials Group. Effects of radiotherapy with concomitant and adjuvant temozolomide versus radiotherapy alone on survival in glioblastoma in a randomized phase III study: 5-year analysis of the EORTC-NCIC trial. Lancet Oncol 2009;10(5):459–466.

of temozolomide as initial treatment. Patients were then randomized to receive standard treatment (150 to 200 mg/m^2/d temozolomide on days 1 through 5 of each 28-day cycle for up to 12 cycles) or a "dose-dense" regimen (85 to 100 mg/m^2/d temozolomide on days 1 through 21 of each 28-day cycle for up to 12 cycles).[30] Results were unfortunately disappointing and did not demonstrate a significant difference between the two arms in OS (18.9 months for the standard regimen; 16.8 months for the dose-dense regimen) or PFS (7.5 months for the standard regimen; 8.8 months for the dose-dense regimen). Subgroup analysis based on methylation status did not alter these results, though it did confirm the overall prognostic utility of MGMT gene methylation on improved outcome.[30] Given these results, standard adjuvant therapy remains that outlined in the EORTC/NCIC trial,[14] where temozolomide is administered in 5 out of 28 days following a period of concomitant chemoradiation. Further research is needed to identify mechanisms that limit resistance and enhance the effectiveness of alkylating agents.

■ Adjuvant Therapy in Elderly Patients

The incidence of GBM is highest in patients aged 75 to 84 (incidence rate of 14.49 per 100,000 person-years).[1] Higher age and poor functional status have been associated with decreased survival. Treatment of elderly patients remains a significant challenge, complicated by poor tolerance of therapy and poor performance status at disease onset. There is not yet consensus on the appropriate treatment protocol for elderly patients and little data to guide decision making, in part because this patient population has been excluded from many of the large, randomized trials in the field.[31]

Radiation Therapy

Radiotherapy remains the mainstay of adjuvant treatment of high-grade gliomas in elderly patients, and various studies endorse its utility in this population despite concerns for increased neurotoxicity. A randomized, prospective, controlled trial of 85 patients of ages 70 and over demonstrated the effectiveness and relative safety of radiotherapy in elderly patients (Level I evidence).[32] Patients were randomized to receive radiation therapy (1.8 Gy administered 5 days per week for a total dose of 50 Gy) plus supportive treatment or supportive treatment alone. Results indicated a significant survival benefit in the treatment group (19.1 vs 16.9 weeks), and importantly no further deterioration in performance status or quality of life.[32] Notably, the dose of radiation therapy at 50 Gy, slightly lower than the standard 60 Gy used in younger patients, was selected given concerns for neurotoxicity at higher doses.

Subsequent trials have investigated the equivalence of shorter versus standard protracted courses of radiotherapy in the management of high-grade gliomas. A prospective, randomized trial of 100 patients over age 60 (Level I evidence) revealed no difference in mean survival time (5.1 vs 5.6 months) between the standard radiotherapy arm (60 Gy over 6 weeks) and a short-course treatment arm (40 Gy in 15 fractions over 3 weeks).[33] The shortened course was better tolerated, with fewer patients requiring corticosteroid increases (23% vs 49%).[33] A single-arm trial (Level IV evidence) composed of elderly patients with poor performance status (Karnofsky performance scale [KPS] score < 70) and compared with historical controls also suggests that shorter courses of radiotherapy (30 Gy in 10 fractions over 2 weeks) may be equivalent to and better tolerated in this population than more aggressive courses of radiotherapy.[34] Importantly, higher doses of radiation therapy did provide a survival benefit in elderly patients with good performance status.[34]

Although no consensus exists, the current data support the use of radiotherapy for the treatment of GBM in elderly patients, and a shorter course may be most appropriate for patients with poor performance status. Standard-dose radiotherapy may have its utility in this population but should be reserved for patients with a higher performance status.

Chemotherapy

Given concerns about radiation-induced toxicity, chemotherapy as a solo adjunctive treatment strategy has been evaluated in small phase 2 trials. In the most recent of these investigations (Level IV evidence), elderly patients over the age of 70 with a KPS < 70 were treated with temozolomide (dose of 150 to 200 mg/m^2/d for 5 days every 4 weeks). Median PFS was 16 weeks and median OS was 25 weeks, a modest improvement over the 12- to 16-week OS expected from a purely supportive approach.[35]

The utility of adjuvant chemotherapy over radiation therapy in this population remains controversial in light of recent inconsistent preliminary results from randomized trials presented at the 2010 American Society of Clinical Oncology (ASCO) meeting. The Methusalem trial enrolled 373 patients over the age of 65 (mean age 72) and KPS > 60 with AA or GBM. Patients were randomized to receive either a truncated course of radiotherapy (30 fractions of 1.8 to 2.0 Gy administered over 6 weeks) or chemotherapy (temozolomide administered at a dose of 100 mg/m^2/d for 7 days, repeated every 14 days). Results revealed prolonged OS in the radiation therapy group (median survival 293 vs 245 days, 1-year survival rate 38 vs 31%) and increased toxicity in the temozolomide group.[36]

The Nordic Clinical Brain Tumor Study Group trial enrolled 342 patients over age 60 (mean age 70) with GBM. Patients were randomized to one of the following three treatment arms: (1) radiation therapy at 60 Gy administered in 30 fractions, (2) radiation therapy at 34 Gy administered in 10 fractions, or (3) chemotherapy with temozolomide at a dose of 200 mg/m^2 for 5 days with cycles repeated every 28 days. OS was significantly increased in the temozolomide group compared with the 60-Gy radiation therapy group (6.0 vs 8.3 months). There was no difference in OS between the 30-Gy radiation and other treatment arms.[37]

Expert Recommendations

1. Postsurgical adjuvant radiation therapy provides significant survival benefit to patients with high-grade gliomas over surgery alone (Grade 1A Recommendation, Level I Evidence).
2. WBRT offers no benefit over more limited field strategies (Grade 1B Recommendation, Level I Evidence).
3. Fractionated involved-field external beam radiation at 60 Gy is the current standard of practice. The total dose of 60 Gy provides significant survival advantage over the dose of 45 Gy and is equivalent to the higher 70-Gy dose (Grade 1A Recommendatin, Level I Evidence).
4. The addition of concomitant and adjuvant chemotherapy with temozolomide to radiation therapy provides a significant survival benefit to patients with newly diagnosed GBM (Grade 1A Recommendation, Level I Evidence).
5. In elderly GBM patients with a poor performance status, shorter courses of radiation at lower doses may be equivalent to and better tolerated than standard treatments (Grade 2C Recommendation, Level IV Evidence).
6. The utility of adjuvant chemotherapy alone over radiation in the elderly population remains controversial in light of recent inconsistent preliminary results from randomized trials (Grade 2B Recommendation).

■ Summary and Conclusions

The treatment of high-grade astrocytomas, including GBM and AA, has been the focus of extensive neuro-oncological research. Level I evidence supports the utility of postsurgical adjuvant radiation in the treatment of GBM and AA. Additional Level I evidence demonstrates that adjuvant chemotherapy with temozolomide plus radiation therapy provides a significant survival benefit in patients with newly diagnosed GBM. These data underpin the current standard of care for GBM with adjuvant postoperative chemoradiation (including involved-field radiation at a total dose of 60 Gy and temozolomide). The role of adjuvant chemotherapy in patients with AA remains less clear. The phase 3 trials that established the survival benefits with temozolomide were limited to patients with GBM, and no randomized trials exist that evaluate the role of adjuvant chemotherapy in addition to radiotherapy in patients with AA. Treatment usually models the standard of care used in GBM, though this approach is not evidence based. The ongoing Concurrent and Adjuvant Temozolomide Chemotherapy in Non-1P/19Q Deleted Anaplastic Glioma (CATNON) trial will address this issue.

Demonstration of the utility of postoperative chemoradiation in the treatment of GBM was a landmark advance, though observed survival benefits remain poor. The vast majority of high-grade astrocytomas will recur following initial treatment. Further research is urgently needed and is ongoing to improve upon our current standards of care and to delineate new strategies for the treatment of recurrent high-grade malignant gliomas.

■ References

1. CBTRUS. CBTRUS Statistical Report: Primary Brain and Central Nervous System Tumors Diagnosed in the United States in 2004–2008. In: Hinsdale, IL: Central Brain Tumor Registry of the United States; 2012. www.cbtrus,org
2. Walker MD, Alexander E Jr, Hunt WE, et al. Evaluation of BCNU and/or radiotherapy in the treatment of anaplastic gliomas: a cooperative clinical trial. J Neurosurg 1978;49(3):333–343
3. Buatti J, Ryken TC, Smith MC, et al. Radiation therapy of pathologically confirmed newly diagnosed glioblastoma in adults. J Neurooncol 2008;89(3):313–337
4. Laperriere N, Zuraw L, Cairncross G; Cancer Care Ontario Practice Guidelines Initiative Neuro-Oncology Disease Site Group. Radiotherapy for newly diagnosed malignant glioma in adults: a systematic review. Radiother Oncol 2002;64(3):259–273
5. Kita M, Okawa T, Tanaka M, Ikeda M. Radiotherapy of malignant glioma—prospective randomized clinical study of whole brain vs local irradiation [in Japanese]. Gan No Rinsho 1989;35(11):1289–1294
6. Shapiro WR, Green SB, Burger PC, et al. Randomized trial of three chemotherapy regimens and two radiotherapy regimens in postoperative treatment of malignant glioma. Brain Tumor Cooperative Group Trial 8001. J Neurosurg 1989;71(1):1–9
7. Bleehen NM, Stenning SP; The Medical Research Council Brain Tumour Working Party. A Medical Research Council trial of two radiotherapy doses in the treatment of grades 3 and 4 astrocytoma. Br J Cancer 1991;64(4):769–774
8. Nelson DF, Diener-West M, Horton J, Chang CH, Schoenfeld D, Nelson JS. Combined modality approach to treatment of

malignant gliomas—re-evaluation of RTOG 7401/ECOG 1374 with long-term follow-up: a joint study of the Radiation Therapy Oncology Group and the Eastern Cooperative Oncology Group. NCI Monogr 1988;6(6):279–284
9. Chang CH, Horton J, Schoenfeld D, et al. Comparison of postoperative radiotherapy and combined postoperative radiotherapy and chemotherapy in the multidisciplinary management of malignant gliomas. A joint Radiation Therapy Oncology Group and Eastern Cooperative Oncology Group study. Cancer 1983;52(6):997–1007
10. Tsao MN, Mehta MP, Whelan TJ, et al. The American Society for Therapeutic Radiology and Oncology (ASTRO) evidence-based review of the role of radiosurgery for malignant glioma. Int J Radiat Oncol Biol Phys 2005;63(1):47–55
11. Khan MK, Hunter GK, Vogelbaum M, Suh JH, Chao ST. Evidence-based adjuvant therapy for gliomas: current concepts and newer developments. Indian J Cancer 2009;46(2):96–107
12. Fine HA, Dear KB, Loeffler JS, Black PM, Canellos GP. Meta-analysis of radiation therapy with and without adjuvant chemotherapy for malignant gliomas in adults. Cancer 1993;71(8): 2585–2597
13. Stewart LA; Group GM-aTG. Chemotherapy in adult high-grade glioma: a systematic review and meta-analysis of individual patient data from 12 randomised trials. Lancet 2002; 359(9311):1011–1018
14. Stupp R, Mason WP, van den Bent MJ, et al; European Organisation for Research and Treatment of Cancer Brain Tumor and Radiotherapy Groups; National Cancer Institute of Canada Clinical Trials Group. Radiotherapy plus concomitant and adjuvant temozolomide for glioblastoma. N Engl J Med 2005;352(10):987–996
15. Stupp R, Gander M, Leyvraz S, Newlands E. Current and future developments in the use of temozolomide for the treatment of brain tumours. Lancet Oncol 2001;2(9):552–560
16. Stupp R, Hegi ME, Mason WP, et al; European Organisation for Research and Treatment of Cancer Brain Tumour and Radiation Oncology Groups; National Cancer Institute of Canada Clinical Trials Group. Effects of radiotherapy with concomitant and adjuvant temozolomide versus radiotherapy alone on survival in glioblastoma in a randomised phase III study: 5-year analysis of the EORTC-NCIC trial. Lancet Oncol 2009; 10(5):459–466
17. Brem HH, Piantadosi SS, Burger PCP, et al; The Polymer-brain Tumor Treatment Group. Placebo-controlled trial of safety and efficacy of intraoperative controlled delivery by biodegradable polymers of chemotherapy for recurrent gliomas. Lancet 1995;345(8956):1008–1012
18. Valtonen S, Timonen U, Toivanen P, et al. Interstitial chemotherapy with carmustine-loaded polymers for high-grade gliomas: a randomized double-blind study. Neurosurgery 1997;41(1):44–48
19. Westphal M, Hilt DC, Bortey E, et al. A phase 3 trial of local chemotherapy with biodegradable carmustine (BCNU) wafers (Gliadel wafers) in patients with primary malignant glioma. Neuro-oncol 2003;5(2):79–88
20. Westphal M, Ram Z, Riddle V, Hilt D, Bortey E; Executive Committee of the Gliadel Study Group. Gliadel wafer in initial surgery for malignant glioma: long-term follow-up of a multicenter controlled trial. Acta Neurochir (Wien) 2006;148(3): 269–275
21. Bota DA, Desjardins A, Quinn JA, Affronti ML, Friedman HS. Interstitial chemotherapy with biodegradable BCNU (Gliadel) wafers in the treatment of malignant gliomas. Ther Clin Risk Manag 2007;3(5):707–715
22. Esteller M, Garcia-Foncillas J, Andion E, et al. Inactivation of the DNA-repair gene MGMT and the clinical response of gliomas to alkylating agents. N Engl J Med 2000;343(19): 1350–1354
23. Hegi ME, Diserens AC, Godard S, et al. Clinical trial substantiates the predictive value of O-6-methylguanine-DNA methyltransferase promoter methylation in glioblastoma patients treated with temozolomide. Clin Cancer Res 2004;10(6): 1871–1874
24. Hegi ME, Diserens A-C, Gorlia T, et al. MGMT gene silencing and benefit from temozolomide in glioblastoma. N Engl J Med 2005;352(10):997–1003
25. Wedge SR, Newlands ES. O6-benzylguanine enhances the sensitivity of a glioma xenograft with low O6-alkylguanine-DNA alkyltransferase activity to temozolomide and BCNU. Br J Cancer 1996;73(9):1049–1052
26. Rhines LD, Sampath P, Dolan ME, Tyler BM, Brem H, Weingart J. O6-benzylguanine potentiates the antitumor effect of locally delivered carmustine against an intracranial rat glioma. Cancer Res 2000;60(22):6307–6310
27. Quinn JA, Jiang SX, Reardon DA, et al. Phase II trial of temozolomide plus O-6-benzylguanine in adults with recurrent, temozolomide-resistant malignant glioma. J Clin Oncol 2009; 27(8):1262–1267
28. Warren KE, Gururangan S, Geyer JR, et al. A phase II study of O6-benzylguanine and temozolomide in pediatric patients with recurrent or progressive high-grade gliomas and brainstem gliomas: a Pediatric Brain Tumor Consortium study. J Neurooncol 2012;106(3):643–649
29. Tolcher AWA, Gerson SLS, Denis LL, et al. Marked inactivation of O6-alkylguanine-DNA alkyltransferase activity with protracted temozolomide schedules. Br J Cancer 2003; 88(7):1004–1011
30. Gilbert MR, Wang M, Aldape KD, et al. A randomized phase III trial comparing standard adjuvant temozolomide (TMZ) with a dose-dense (dd) schedule in newly diagnosed glioblastoma (GBM). J Clin Oncol 2011;29:2006
31. Nayak L, Iwamoto FM. Primary brain tumors in the elderly. Curr Neurol Neurosci Rep 2010;10(4):252–258
32. Keime-Guibert F, Chinot O, Taillandier L, et al; Association of French-Speaking Neuro-Oncologists. Radiotherapy for glioblastoma in the elderly. N Engl J Med 2007;356(15): 1527–1535
33. Roa W, Brasher PM, Bauman G, et al. Abbreviated course of radiation therapy in older patients with glioblastoma multiforme: a prospective randomized clinical trial. J Clin Oncol 2004;22(9):1583–1588
34. Bauman GS, Gaspar LE, Fisher BJ, Halperin EC, Macdonald DR, Cairncross JG. A prospective study of short-course radiotherapy in poor prognosis glioblastoma multiforme. Int J Radiat Oncol Biol Phys 1994;29(4):835–839
35. Gállego Pérez-Larraya J, Ducray F, Chinot O, et al. Temozolomide in elderly patients with newly diagnosed glioblastoma and poor performance status: an ANOCEF phase II trial. J Clin Oncol 2011;29(22):3050–3055
36. Wick W, Platten M, Meisner C, et al. NOA-08 study group of Neuro-oncology Working Group (NOA) of German Cancer Society. Lancet Oncol 2012 July;13(7):707–715
37. Malmstrom A, Gronberg BH, Marosi C, Stupp R, Frappaz D, Schultz H, et al. Nordic Clinical Brain Study Group (NCBTSG). Lancet Oncol 2012 Sep;13(9):916–926
38. Walker MD, Green SB, Byar DP, et al. Randomized comparisons of radiotherapy and nitrosoureas for the treatment of malignant glioma after surgery. N Engl J Med 1980;303(23): 1323–1329
39. Andersen AP. Postoperative irradiation of glioblastomas. Results in a randomized series. Acta Radiol Oncol Radiat Phys Biol 1978;17(6):475–484
40. Sandberg-Wollheim M, Malmström P, Strömblad LG, et al; al S-WMe. A randomized study of chemotherapy with procarbazine, vincristine, and lomustine with and without radiation therapy for astrocytoma grades 3 and/or 4. Cancer 1991; 68(1):22–29
41. Kristiansen K, Hagen S, Kollevold T, et al. Combined modality therapy of operated astrocytomas grade III and IV: confirmation of the value of postoperative irradiation and lack of potentiation of bleomycin on survival time: a prospective multicenter trial of the Scandinavian Glioblastoma Study Group. Cancer 1981;47(4):649–652

11

Salvage Therapy for High-Grade Gliomas

David S. Wolf and John Laterra

High-grade astrocytomas, including anaplastic astrocytomas (World Health Organization [WHO] grade III) and glioblastoma multiforme (GBM, WHO grade IV), are the most prevalent primary brain tumors in adults. GBM represents the majority of these tumors, accounting for nearly 60% of primary brain tumors. Both tumors carry a poor prognosis, with 2-year survival rates up to 50% for anaplastic astrocytoma[1] and 20 to 37% in GBM.[2]

The current standard of care for high-grade gliomas is based on the pivotal 2005 European Organization for Research and Treatment of Cancer/National Cancer Institute of Canada Clinical Trials Group (EORTC/NCIC) phase 3 trial and involves radiation therapy with concurrent daily temozolomide (Temodar, Merck, Whitehouse Station, NJ) 75 mg/m^2 daily for 6 weeks followed by six cycles of temozolomide 200 mg/m^2 for 5 out of 28 days.[3] Temozolomide is a cytotoxic alkylating chemotherapy. This regimen offered a significant survival benefit compared with radiation alone. Although median survival increased modestly from 12.1 months with radiation therapy alone to 14.6 months with combination therapy, combination therapy increased 2-year survival from 10.9 to 27.2%, increased 3-year survival from 3.0 to 10.1%, and increased 5-year survival from 1.9 to 9.8%.

In the last decade, it was demonstrated that the DNA repair enzyme O-6-methylguanine-DNA methyltransferase (MGMT) repairs the damage to DNA caused by temozolomide, thereby allowing tumor cell resistance to chemotherapy. MGMT gene silencing through promoter methylation predicts better response to temozolomide with improved survival. Hegi and others showed that 34.7% of MGMT-methylated patients who received temozolomide and radiation therapy survived at 24 months, as compared with 11.7% of patients who were unmethylated.[4] Currently, MGMT status has helped with prognosis but has not altered initial treatment decisions. The absence of MGMT methylation provides a molecular rationale for not treating with alkylating agents at time of recurrence.

Despite chemoradiation, and regardless of MGMT methylation status, disease progression is nearly universal. The EORTC recently reviewed prognostic factors for outcome in patients with recurrent GBM previously enrolled in phase 1 or 2 trials.[5] Poor performance status and more than one lesion had a significant negative prognostic impact for both progression-free survival (PFS) and overall survival. Tumors localized to the frontal lobe had better survival. Age and sex did not show independent prognostic values. Survival from time of progression is 25 to 30 weeks. Thus, salvage therapy is needed in most patients, but currently there is no consensus for the treatment of recurrent high-grade gliomas. This chapter addresses the wide range of options available.

■ Pseudoprogression

One of the challenges in the management of recurrent high-grade astrocytomas is distinguishing true tumor progression from treatment-induced pseudoprogression. Pseudoprogression is a well-recognized phenomenon that typically occurs in the initial months following the completion of chemoradiation treatment. The severest form of pseudoprogression represents radionecrosis, consisting of frank tissue necrosis, gliosis, vessel hyalinization, and occlusions. Magnetic resonance imaging (MRI) of radiation necrosis typically shows increased enhancement within the radiation field, most often within regions of preexisting elevated T2 signal (**Fig. 11.1**), with increased surrounding edema. Often the patient is asymptomatic,[6] but signs and symptoms from increased localized mass effect or increased intracranial pressure or focal neurological deficits can be seen.

Pseudoprogression typically occurs within 3 months of completing radiation therapy. MGMT methylation has been shown to correlate with pseudoprogression, and increased survival is seen in patients who develop pseudoprogression.[7] Determination of pseudoprogression based on standard MRI alone can be challenging. New areas of gadolinium enhancement are insufficient to diagnose tumor recurrence. Diffusion-weighted imaging (DWI), MR spectroscopy, fluorodeoxyglucose positron-emission tomography (FDG-PET), and perfusion-weighted imaging all have been able to differentiate between

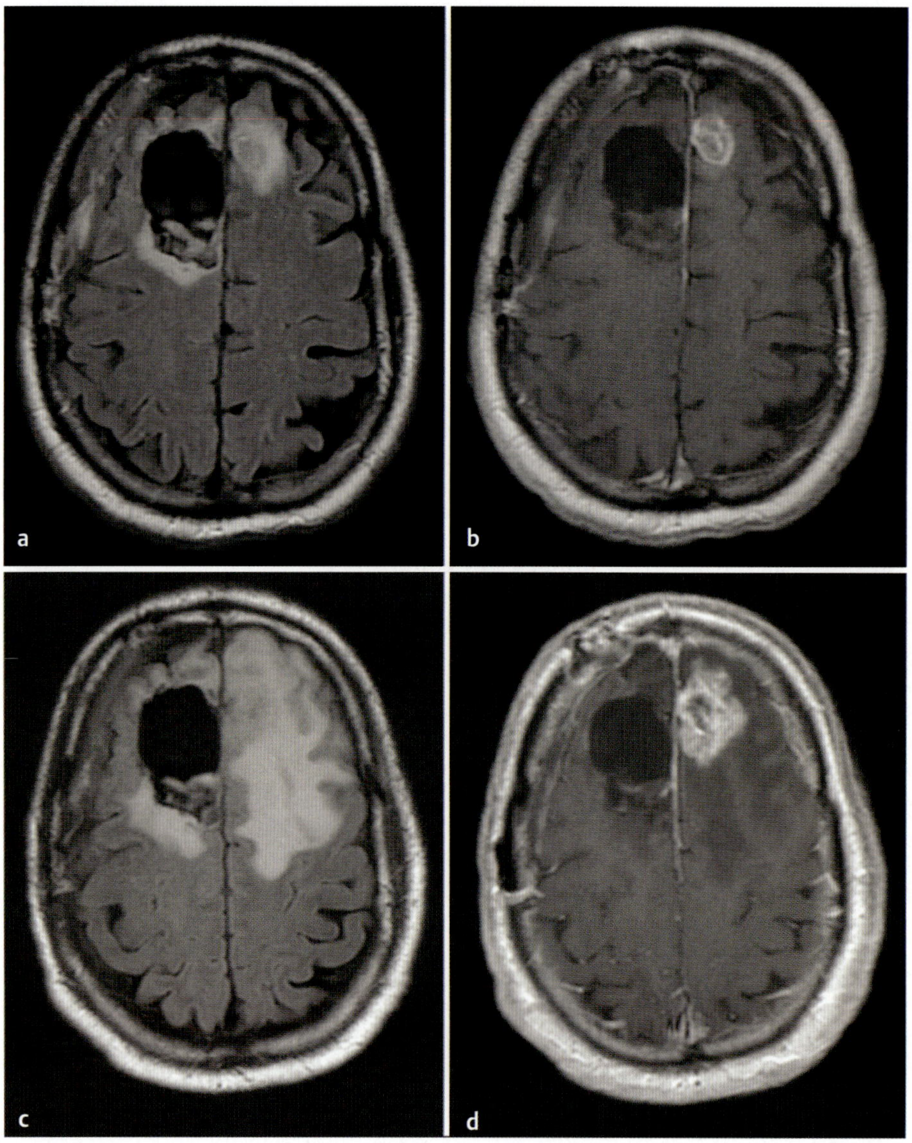

Fig. 11.1 Characteristic magnetic resonance imaging findings in pseudoprogression. **(a)** Immediate post-X-ray therapy fluid-attenuated inversion recovery (XRT FLAIR). **(b)** Immediate post-XRT postcontrast. **(c)** Three months post-XRT FLAIR. **(d)** Three months post-XRT postcontrast.

true progression and radiation necrosis in retrospective studies, although the sensitivity and specificity of each modality are suboptimal.[8]

The gold standard for determining whether there is pseudoprogression or tumor recurrence is stereotactic or excisional biopsy. There is no clear consensus for when to proceed to surgery to obtain confirmation of tumor progression. The Canadian Glioblastoma Recommendations Committee recommended not classifying progressive disease by gadolinium enhancement alone within the first 12 weeks after the end of radiotherapy unless new enhancement is observed outside the radiation field or active tumor is confirmed by pathology.[9] Temozolomide should not be halted until true tumor progression is confirmed. If there is a concern for progression in the initial months following radiation therapy, follow-up imaging should be obtained on a monthly basis. Should the MRI changes progressively enlarge, then proceeding to surgery to confirm progression is recommended. Once the decision is made to obtain a tissue diagnosis, it is not always possible to distinguish radiation-induced injury from active tumor. A mixture of both residual/recurrent tumor and radiation necrosis is often seen, and sampling errors from stereotactic surgery may lead to nondiagnostic results.[10]

Treatment of Pseudoprogression

For symptomatic pseudoprogression, steroids are the mainstay of initial therapy. If steroids are not sufficient to relieve symptoms, and surgery is not being considered, few options are available.

Level I to Level II Evidence

Bevacizumab (Avastin, Genentech, South San Francisco, CA) has been shown in a randomized, double-blind, placebo-controlled study to reduce both the radiographic signs of pseudoprogression and the neurological deficits.[11] There were only 14 patients in this study, and two had anaplastic astrocytoma. In a report of six patients with histologically proven radiation necrosis treated with either bevacizumab or bevacizumab with irinotecan, all had a radiographic response to therapy, the duration of which ranged from 6 weeks to 18 months.[12]

Level III to Level IV Evidence

Antioxidant therapy with a combination of pentoxifylline and vitamin E has been shown to reduce radiation-induced fibrosis, primarily in women with breast cancer.[13] In a pilot study involving 11 patients (none with primary brain tumors) with radiation-associated injury after intracranial stereotactic radiosurgery, 10 showed evidence of reduced edema on MRI after receiving pentoxifylline and vitamin E.[14] Hyperbaric oxygen has also been used to treat radiation-induced injury from stereotactic radiosurgery for arteriovenous malformations[15] and radiation therapy in central nervous system (CNS) lymphoma,[15,16] although these are only case reports.

■ Treatment Options for Recurrent High-Grade Gliomas

Chemotherapy

Level I Evidence

A randomized, double-blind, placebo-controlled study investigating placement of carmustine wafers (Gliadel Wafers, Eisai, Woodcliff Lake, NJ) at the time of surgery for recurrent malignant glioma demonstrated extended median survival by 8 weeks.[17] In patients with glioblastoma, 6-month survival was 50% greater than that of recipients of placebo. This therapy is a viable option in patients with a unilateral, single focus of disease who require open resection. It is approved by the Food and Drug Administration (FDA) for therapy in both newly diagnosed and recurrent malignant glioma.

Level II Evidence

Temozolomide remains the backbone of chemotherapies used at the time of relapse. Multiple dosing strategies have been investigated to assess whether they offer any benefit above the traditional 5 out of 28 days dosing regimen used in the adjuvant phase of up-front therapy. These regimens are more dose intense, the rationale being that they will help overcome MGMT-dependent DNA repair. They include 150 mg/m^2/d on days 1 through 7 and 15 through 21 (7 days on/7 days off), 75 mg/m^2/d for 21 out of 28 days, and metronomic at 50 mg/d. A temozolomide dosing schedule of 21 out of 28 days offered 6-month progression-free survival in 30% of patients.[18] This treatment regimen led to a greater incidence of side effects, including thrombocytopenia. A 7 days on/7 days off regimen was better tolerated, with 6-month progression-free survival of 48%.[19] Metronomic temozolomide, at 50 mg/m^2/d, led to 57% progression-free survival at 6 months.[20] This dosing strategy appears to work better in patients who fail traditional temozolomide treatment early, or those who are restarted after a break in therapy. Wick and others showed that these temozolomide rechallenge regimens have possible benefit in recurrent GBM, even if there was progression while a patient was on initial temozolomide treatment.[21]

Multiple other cytotoxic chemotherapy agents have been used in the treatment of recurrent disease. When compared with temozolomide, procarbazine offered decreased PFS6 (21% vs 8%) and was less tolerated.[22] The combination of procarbazine, lomustine N-(2-chloroethyl)-N′-cycloexyl-N-nitrosourea (CCNU) and vincristine was shown to be as effective as temozolomide, although the degree of improvement in quality-of-life measures relative to baseline was higher in the temozolomide group.[23] In a retrospective analysis of patients treated with carmustine (3-bis (2-chloroethyl)-1-nitrosourea; BCNU) at recurrence, median progression-free survival was 11 weeks and median overall survival 22 weeks.[24] The rate of adverse events, especially hematological toxicity, was relatively high.

Repeat Radiation Therapy

Given the short time between initial radiation therapy and tumor progression, repeat radiation therapy is often not considered a viable option due to the risk to healthy brain tissue. However, modern techniques in radiotherapy have opened new opportunities to revisit this option.[25] The primary focus of reirradiation strategies has been on stereotactic modalities using either single or fractionated treatments.

Level I to Level II Evidence

None.

Level II to Level IV Evidence

Stereotactic radiosurgery has been shown in retrospective analyses to result in median survival times ranging from 7.5 to 30 months.[26] Combs and others' overall survival from the point of stereotactic radiotherapy was extended by 8 months.[27] Hypofractionated radiotherapy (35 Gy in 3.5-Gy fractions) has also been tried, with a mean survival time of 10 months for patients with anaplastic astrocytoma and 11 months in patients with GBM.[28] Most patients were able to reduce their steroid dependence and had improvement in symptoms.

Antiangiogenesis Therapy

As the tumorigenesis pathways in malignant gliomas have been elucidated, the development and use of selective therapeutic agents have exploded. A hallmark of GBM is that it is highly vascular; this angiogenesis is driven by tumor-derived vascular endothelial growth factor (VEGF). Bevacizumab (Avastin, Genentech), a humanized monoclonal antibody that selectively binds VEGF-A, is FDA approved in the treatment of recurrent GBM.

Although the majority of patients tolerate bevacizumab very well, it can cause serious or fatal adverse events, including spontaneous gastrointestinal perforation, hypertension, and increased risk of both hemorrhagic and thromboembolic events. Wound healing is also delayed, and most surgeons require a 4-week period off therapy before allowing any major surgical procedure.

The ideal time to start bevacizumab is not clear. If surgery is a consideration, then bevacizumab is best deferred due to the problems with wound healing. Patients who receive bevacizumab are often excluded from clinical trials; thus other experimental therapies or more established second-line agents are tried first.

Level I Evidence

None.

Level II Evidence

FDA approval was based on two trials. One was a single-arm phase 2 study of patients with recurrent GBM given bevacizumab with or without irinotecan.[29] Objective response in the trial was 28% in the bevacizumab-alone arm, although an independent review by the FDA determined it to be only 26%.[30] Progression-free survival of 6 months was 36%, and median overall survival was 9.2 months. The second trial looked at bevacizumab monotherapy in 48 patients.[31] This phase 2 trial showed an FDA-determined response rate of 19.6% (35% in the original trial).[30] In both trials, steroid doses were able to be reduced in a majority of cases. It also must be noted that in all prior studies, bevacizumab failed to offer any survival benefit, although they were not properly powered to demonstrate patient survival.

Bevacizumab has been less successful in treating recurrent anaplastic gliomas. In 31 patients, the median overall survival was 12 months and progression-free survival of 6 months was 20.9%; both were similar to historical controls.[32] Radiographic response was seen in up to 20 of the subjects, depending on response criteria used.

Level III to Level IV Evidence

A review of a European registry of 225 patients with recurrent high-grade gliomas (176 glioblastoma, 49 anaplastic glioma) treated off-study with bevacizumab showed median survival of 8.5 months; 75.1%

of patients died.[33] Clinical improvement or stability was seen in 78% of patients. Steroids were able to be discontinued in 37.6%.

Patients on bevacizumab show radiographic improvement in their disease (**Fig. 11.2**) but can also have functional improvement. Nagpal and others showed bevacizumab increased independent living after GBM recurrence when compared with patients who did not receive bevacizumab.[34] Reduction in steroid dose may have contributed to prolonged independence. In patients who responded to bevacizumab, neurocognitive function was improved or stable, whereas those with progressive disease had neurocognitive decline at the time of progression.[35]

Tumor progression is often very rapid followed by very short survival in patients who develop bevacizumab resistance (**Fig. 11.2**). Tumors that progress during bevacizumab therapy are refractory to most treatment regimens. Median overall survival was 4.5 months in one series of 37 patients treated with standard chemotherapy regimens following bevacizumab failure.[36] The addition of cytotoxic chemotherapy to bevacizumab at the time of progression similarly failed to show any benefit. Median PFS was merely 6 weeks, with no patients surviving at 6 months.[37] Once bevacizumab is stopped, there can be rapid decompensation, both clinically and radiographically.

Emerging Molecular Targeting Agents

Numerous other targeted therapies are being investigated. A partial list of these agents is presented in **Table 11.1**. Unfortunately, the use of these newer-generation therapies has resulted in poor response rates and minimal, if any, effect on progression-free survival. These include erlotinib (epidermal growth factor receptor [EGFR] inhibitor),[38] cilengitide (integrin inhibitor),[39] imatinib (platelet-derived growth factor receptor [PDGFR] inhibitor),[40] and vorinostat (histone deacetylase inhibitor).[41] This has been attributed to the coactivation of multiple tyrosine kinases and redundant signaling pathways, thus limiting the success of single agents. In addition, compensatory pathways can be upregulated in response to molecular blockade.[42]

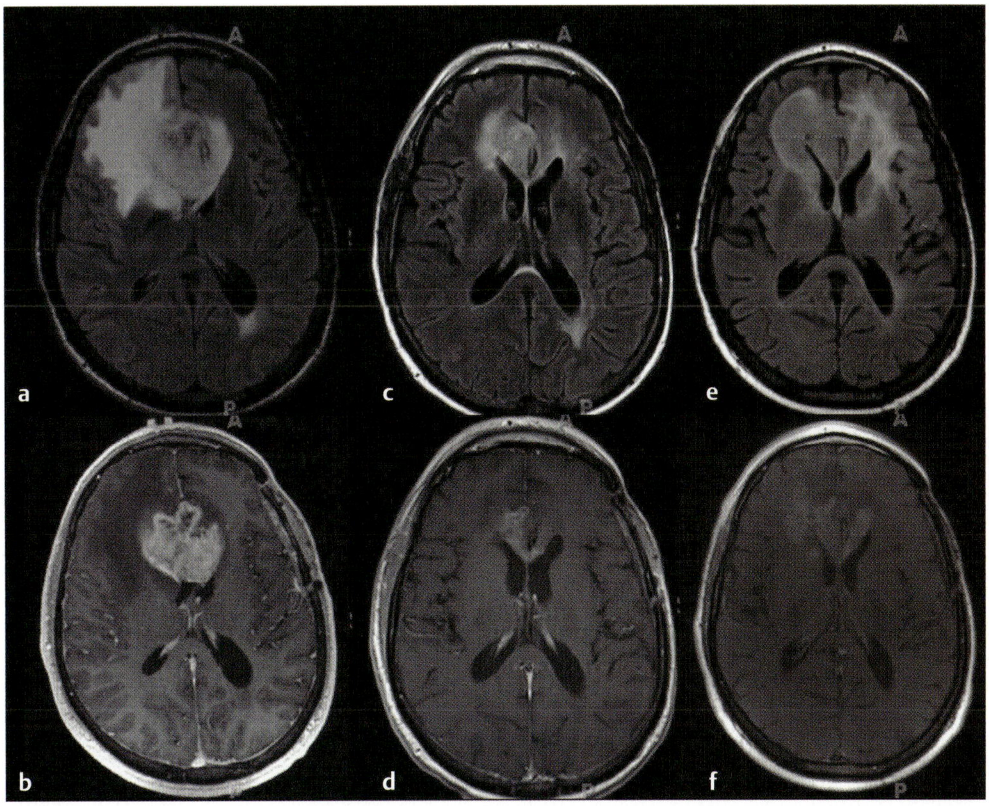

Fig. 11.2 Evolution of magnetic resonance imaging response of glioblastoma multiforme to bevacizumab therapy. **(a)** Pretreatment fluid-attenuated inversion recovery (FLAIR). **(b)** Pretreatment postcontrast. **(c)** On bevacizumab for 3 months, FLAIR. **(d)** On bevacizumab for 3 months postcontrast. **(e)** Treatment failure on bevacizumab for 5 months, FLAIR. **(f)** Treatment failure on bevacizumab for 5 months postcontrast.

Table 11.1 Selected molecular targets in glioblastoma multiforme

Primary target	Drug name	Mechanism of action
EGFR	Erlotinib Gefitinib Lapatinib Cetuximab	TKI TKI TKI Monoclonal antibody
HDAC	Vorinostat Valproic acid	HDAC inhibitor HDAC inhibitor
Integrins	Cilengitide	Synthetic peptide
mTOR	Everolimus Sirolimus	mTOR inhibitor mTOR inhibitor
PDGFR	Imatinib Dasatinib	TKI TKI
VEGF	Afibercept Bevacizumab	Soluble decoy receptor Monoclonal antibody
VEGFR	Cediranib Sorafenib Sunitinib	TKI TKI TKI
PARP	ABT-888 BSI-201	PARP inhibitor PARP inhibitor

Abbreviations: EGFR, epidermal growth factor receptor; HDAC, histone deacetylase; mTOR, mammalian target of rapamycin; PARP, poly (ADP ribose) polymerase; PDGFR, platelet-derived growth factor receptor; TKI, tyrosine kinase inhibitor; VEGFR, vascular endothelial growth factor receptor.

Source: Walbert T, Mikkelsen T. Recurrent high-grade glioma: a diagnostic and therapeutic challenge. Expert Rev Neurother 2011; 11(4):509–518. Adapted with permission.

Expert Recommendations

1. Current imaging modalities do not reliably differentiate pseudoprogression from recurrent active tumor; the gold standard for this determination is pathological confirmation by excisional (preferred) or stereotaxic biopsy.
2. For symptomatic pseudoprogression, steroids are the mainstay of initial therapy (Grade 1C Recommendation, Level II Evidence).
3. Bevacizumab (Avastin) has been shown to improve neurologic deficits and radiographic signs in patients with pseudoprogression (Grade 1B Recommendation, Level I Evidence).
4. Carmustine wafers (Gliadel) have been shown to extend median survival by 8 weeks (Grade 1B Recommendation, Level I Evidence).
5. Temozolomide remains the backbone of chemotherapeutic strategies used at the time of relapse. Different dosing strategies may be employed during recurrence in patients who fail traditional temozolomide early or those patients restarting after a break in therapy (Grade 1C Recommendation, Level II Evidence).
6. Repeat radiation therapy has not traditionally been considered a viable option during the management of recurrent disease; new data is emerging regarding potential uses of repeat radiation including stereotactic radiotherapy (Grade 2C Recommendation, Level II–IV Evidence).
7. For recurrent disease, the role of bevacizumab is unclear. Studies have demonstrated improvement in symptoms, radiographic findings, and time to radiographic progression, bevacizumab has yet to be found to offer any survival benefit (Grade 2C Recommendation, Level II–IV Evidence).

■ Summary and Conclusions

The diagnosis and treatment of recurrent gliomas remain challenging despite advances in imaging techniques and development of molecularly targeted therapies. The first, critical step is confirming that tumor progression, and not pseudoprogression, has occurred. Once tumor progression is confirmed (either radiographically or through tissue diagnosis), multiple treatment options are available. Repeat temozolomide treatment should be considered as a first option, particularly in patients with MGMT methylation. Gliadel is an FDA-approved option for resectable solitary lesions. Bevacizumab is also approved for use in recurrent glioblastoma. Other molecularly targeted therapies have yet to demonstrate efficacy in the treatment of recurrent malignant gliomas, but several exciting new treatments are currently under investigation.

■ References

1. Central Brain Tumor Registry of the United States. CBTRUS statistical report: primary brain and central nervous system tumors diagnosed in the United States in 2004–2008. 2012. Central Brain Tumor Registry of the United States, Hinsdale, IL. www.cbtrus.org
2. Grossman SA, Ye X, Piantadosi S, et al; NABTT CNS Consortium. Survival of patients with newly diagnosed glioblastoma treated with radiation and temozolomide in research studies in the United States. Clin Cancer Res 2010;16(8):2443–2449
3. Stupp R, Mason WP, van den Bent MJ, et al; European Organisation for Research and Treatment of Cancer Brain Tumor and Radiotherapy Groups; National Cancer Institute of Canada Clinical Trials Group. Radiotherapy plus concomitant and adjuvant temozolomide for glioblastoma. N Engl J Med 2005; 352(10):987–996
4. Hegi ME, Diserens AC, Gorlia T, et al. MGMT gene silencing and benefit from temozolomide in glioblastoma. N Engl J Med 2005;352(10):997–1003

5. Gorlia T, Stupp R, Brandes AA, et al. New prognostic factors and calculators for outcome prediction in patients with recurrent glioblastoma: a pooled analysis of EORTC Brain Tumour Group phase I and II clinical trials. Eur J Cancer 2012; 48(8):1176–1184
6. Brandes AA, Franceschi E, Tosoni A, et al. MGMT promoter methylation status can predict the incidence and outcome of pseudoprogression after concomitant radiochemotherapy in newly diagnosed glioblastoma patients. J Clin Oncol 2008; 26(13):2192–2197
7. Brandsma D, van den Bent MJ. Pseudoprogression and pseudoresponse in the treatment of gliomas. Curr Opin Neurol 2009;22(6):633–638
8. Yang I, Aghi MK. New advances that enable identification of glioblastoma recurrence. Nat Rev Clin Oncol 2009;6(11): 648–657
9. Easaw JC, Mason WP, Perry J, et al; Canadian Glioblastoma Recommendations Committee. Canadian recommendations for the treatment of recurrent or progressive glioblastoma multiforme. Curr Oncol 2011;18(3):e126–e136
10. Perry A, Schmidt RE. Cancer therapy-associated CNS neuropathology: an update and review of the literature. Acta Neuropathol 2006;111(3):197–212
11. Levin VA, Bidaut L, Hou P, et al. Randomized double-blind placebo-controlled trial of bevacizumab therapy for radiation necrosis of the central nervous system. Int J Radiat Oncol Biol Phys 2011;79(5):1487–1495
12. Torcuator R, Zuniga R, Mohan YS, et al. Initial experience with bevacizumab treatment for biopsy confirmed cerebral radiation necrosis. J Neurooncol 2009;94(1):63–68
13. Delanian S, Balla-Mekias S, Lefaix JL. Striking regression of chronic radiotherapy damage in a clinical trial of combined pentoxifylline and tocopherol. J Clin Oncol 1999;17(10): 3283–3290
14. Williamson R, Kondziolka D, Kanaan H, Lunsford LD, Flickinger JC. Adverse radiation effects after radiosurgery may benefit from oral vitamin E and pentoxifylline therapy: a pilot study. Stereotact Funct Neurosurg 2008;86(6):359–366
15. Wanebo JE, Kidd GA, King MC, Chung TS. Hyperbaric oxygen therapy for treatment of adverse radiation effects after stereotactic radiosurgery of arteriovenous malformations: case report and review of literature. Surg Neurol 2009;72(2): 162–167
16. Cihan YB, Uzun G, Yildiz S, Dönmez H. Hyperbaric oxygen therapy for radiation-induced brain necrosis in a patient with primary central nervous system lymphoma. J Surg Oncol 2009;100(8):732–735
17. Brem H, Piantadosi S, Burger PC, et al; The Polymer-brain Tumor Treatment Group. Placebo-controlled trial of safety and efficacy of intraoperative controlled delivery by biodegradable polymers of chemotherapy for recurrent gliomas. Lancet 1995;345(8956):1008–1012
18. Brandes AA, Tosoni A, Cavallo G, et al; GICNO. Temozolomide 3 weeks on and 1 week off as first-line therapy for recurrent glioblastoma: phase II study from Gruppo Italiano Cooperativo di Neuro-oncologia (GICNO). Br J Cancer 2006;95(9): 1155–1160
19. Wick W, Steinbach JP, Küker WM, Dichgans J, Bamberg M, Weller M. One week on/one week off: a novel active regimen of temozolomide for recurrent glioblastoma. Neurology 2004;62(11):2113–2115
20. Perry JR, Bélanger K, Mason WP, et al. Phase II trial of continuous dose-intense temozolomide in recurrent malignant glioma: RESCUE study. J Clin Oncol 2010;28(12):2051–2057
21. Wick A, Pascher C, Wick W, et al. Rechallenge with temozolomide in patients with recurrent gliomas. J Neurol 2009; 256(5):734–741
22. Yung WK, Albright RE, Olson J, et al. A phase II study of temozolomide vs. procarbazine in patients with glioblastoma multiforme at first relapse. Br J Cancer 2000;83(5):588–593
23. Brada M, Stenning S, Gabe R, et al. Temozolomide versus procarbazine, lomustine, and vincristine in recurrent high-grade glioma. J Clin Oncol 2010;28(30):4601–4608
24. Reithmeier T, Graf E, Piroth T, Trippel M, Pinsker MO, Nikkhah G. BCNU for recurrent glioblastoma multiforme: efficacy, toxicity and prognostic factors. BMC Cancer 2010;10:30
25. Combs SE, Debus J, Schulz-Ertner D. Radiotherapeutic alternatives for previously irradiated recurrent gliomas. BMC Cancer 2007;7:167
26. Romanelli P, Conti A, Pontoriero A, et al. Role of stereotactic radiosurgery and fractionated stereotactic radiotherapy for the treatment of recurrent glioblastoma multiforme. Neurosurg Focus 2009;27(6):E8
27. Combs SE, Gutwein S, Thilmann Ch, Huber P, Debus J, Schulz-Ertner D. Stereotactically guided fractionated re-irradiation in recurrent glioblastoma multiforme. J Neurooncol 2005;74(2):167–171
28. Fogh SE, Andrews DW, Glass J, et al. Hypofractionated stereotactic radiation therapy: an effective therapy for recurrent high-grade gliomas. J Clin Oncol 2010;28(18):3048–3053
29. Friedman HS, Prados MD, Wen PY, et al. Bevacizumab alone and in combination with irinotecan in recurrent glioblastoma. J Clin Oncol 2009;27(28):4733–4740
30. Cohen MH, Shen YL, Keegan P, Pazdur R. FDA drug approval summary: bevacizumab (Avastin) as treatment of recurrent glioblastoma multiforme. Oncologist 2009;14(11):1131–1138
31. Kreisl TN, Kim L, Moore K, et al. Phase II trial of single-agent bevacizumab followed by bevacizumab plus irinotecan at tumor progression in recurrent glioblastoma. J Clin Oncol 2009; 27(5):740–745
32. Kreisl TN, Zhang W, Odia Y, et al. A phase II trial of single-agent bevacizumab in patients with recurrent anaplastic glioma. Neuro-oncol 2011;13(10):1143–1150
33. Hofer S, Elandt K, Greil R, et al. Clinical outcome with bevacizumab in patients with recurrent high-grade glioma treated outside clinical trials. Acta Oncol 2011;50(5):630–635
34. Nagpal S, Harsh G, Recht L. Bevacizumab improves quality of life in patients with recurrent glioblastoma. Chemother Res Pract 2011;2011:602812. doi: 10.1155/2011/602812. Epub 2011 Oct 2
35. Wefel JS, Cloughesy T, Zazzali JL, et al. Neurocognitive function in patients with recurrent glioblastoma treated with bevacizumab. Neuro-oncol 2011;13(6):660–668
36. Quant EC, Norden AD, Drappatz J, et al. Role of a second chemotherapy in recurrent malignant glioma patients who progress on bevacizumab. Neuro-oncol 2009;11(5):550–555
37. Iwamoto FM, Abrey LE, Beal K, et al. Patterns of relapse and prognosis after bevacizumab failure in recurrent glioblastoma. Neurology 2009;73(15):1200–1206
38. Yung WK, Vredenburgh JJ, Cloughesy TF, et al. Safety and efficacy of erlotinib in first-relapse glioblastoma: a phase II open-label study. Neuro-oncol 2010;12(10):1061–1070
39. Gilbert MR, Kuhn J, Lamborn KR, et al. Cilengitide in patients with recurrent glioblastoma: the results of NABTC 03-02, a phase II trial with measures of treatment delivery. J Neurooncol 2012;106(1):147–153
40. Wen PY, Yung WK, Lamborn KR, et al. Phase I/II study of imatinib mesylate for recurrent malignant gliomas: North American Brain Tumor Consortium Study 99-08. Clin Cancer Res 2006;12(16):4899–4907
41. Galanis E, Jaeckle KA, Maurer MJ, et al. Phase II trial of vorinostat in recurrent glioblastoma multiforme: a North Central Cancer Treatment Group study. J Clin Oncol 2009;27(12): 2052–2058
42. Walbert T, Mikkelsen T. Recurrent high-grade glioma: a diagnostic and therapeutic challenge. Expert Rev Neurother 2011; 11(4):509–518

▪ SECTION II ▪

Pineal Region Tumors

12

Intracranial Germ Cell Tumors—Treatment Paradigms

Soriaya Motivala, Mustafa Nadi, and James T. Rutka

Intracranial germ cell tumors (GCTs) are a rare group of tumors most often found in children and adolescents.[1] The World Health Organization (WHO) classifies central nervous system (CNS) GCTs in two distinct groups based on their histological profile and the presence or absence of the tumor markers β-human chorionic gonadotropin (β-HCG) or α-fetoprotein (AFP) on immunohistochemistry of tumor specimens, in serum, or in cerebrospinal fluid (CSF). Germinomas account for approximately half to two thirds of cases and consist of those with a syncytiotrophoblastic component, which secrete β-HCG, and pure germinomas, which are nonsecretors.[2–6] Pure germinomas are the most common GCT, representing 60% of all CNS GCTs.[2,4,7] A nongerminomatous GCT is the second subtype of intracranial GCTs. These can be divided into embryonal carcinoma, endodermal sinus tumors (yolk sac), choriocarcinoma, and teratomas. Teratomas can further be subdivided into benign (mature) or malignant (immature) tumors. GCTs can also present as mixed tumors consisting of any number of different germ cell components.

■ Terminology

The majorities of GCTs present extracranially and are most frequently found in the gonads. They are termed dysgerminomas when present in the ovaries, and seminomas when they originate in the testes. Interestingly, extragonadal GCTs typically occur in a midline location, and, accordingly, intracranial GCTs are often found in the pineal or suprasellar regions.

■ Incidence

The incidence of GCTs is low and has been reported as being anywhere from 1 to 5% of pediatric brain tumors in North America.[8,9] Ninety percent of patients with intracranial GCTs will present with symptoms prior to the age of 20, with a median age of diagnosis of 16 years (Central Brain Tumor Registry of USA data 1998–2002). Goodwin et al, in a review of 638 cases of CNS GCT, described most patients in the age category below age 30. They found that throughout childhood, adolescence, and early adulthood males had significantly higher rates of CNS GCTs than females. They also noted that, although both sexes showed a spike in incidence of these tumors at the 10- to 12-year age mark, male risk remained elevated into the third decade of life, whereas female risk decreased substantially by the second decade. In both sexes, the incidence of these tumors declined after the age of 30. Furthermore, tumor location appears to be related to gender, because pineal region tumors have a statistically significant male predominance ($p < 0.0001$). Race was also determined to be a factor, in that Asians have a significantly higher rate of CNS GCTs than do other races. This finding mirrors previous literature in which Asian populations outside of North America have been found to have an overall increase in CNS GCTs.[9] In 5 to 10% of cases, lesions will occur in a synchronous fashion in both the pineal and the suprasellar regions. This type of bifocal disease occurs with increasing frequency in males as well.

The frequency of adult primary GCTs of the CNS has been quoted as less than 1%, though the true incidence is somewhat difficult to establish because the majority of studies include young adults up to the age of 30 in descriptions of the pediatric population. In an extensive review, the majority of nonpineal CNS GCTs were found in those aged 0 to 14 years (45.3%), followed by those aged 15 to 29 years (38.9%), with those adults over 30 having a frequency of only 15.8%.[10] The authors also noted that for children and young adults, the majority of the tumors were malignant (86.8 and 89%, respectively), whereas in adults (those > 30 years of age), more than half were benign tumors (56.8%).[10]

■ Clinical Presentation

The presentation of children with intracranial GCTs is highly dependent on tumor location. In the case of pineal region tumors, the aqueduct of Sylvius often becomes obstructed, leading to hydrocephalus. Patients will consequently develop signs and symptoms of increased intracranial pressure (ICP), such as headache, vomiting, and somnolence. Furthermore, mass effect of the lesion on the tectal region can result in Parinaud syndrome, or upward gaze palsy, which is often considered pathognomonic for pineal region masses. Tumors of the suprasellar region often present with visual disturbances caused by compression of the optic apparatus as well as endocrine dysfunction due to mass effect on the hypothalamic–pituitary axis. Diabetes insipidus (DI), growth retardation, precocious or delayed puberty, and menstrual irregularities in women are often common manifestations of endocrinopathy. In many cases, DI can precede all other disturbances. Thus any patient with unexplained central DI with or without other associated endocrinopathies requires a mandatory magnetic resonance imaging (MRI) scan to exclude suprasellar mass lesions. Endocrine disturbance is exceedingly rare in patients with pineal region lesions only; however, in those with bifocal disease the tendency is toward presenting symptoms being consistent with a suprasellar lesion.

■ Diagnosis

Once the suspicion of an intracranial GCT has been raised, the algorithm for diagnosis remains the same in children as well as adults. Neuroimaging should be used to confirm the presence of an intracranial mass lesion. MRI remains the most sensitive modality for detecting intracranial GCT and demonstrates the relationship to surrounding normal brain and blood vessels. Computed tomography (CT) has some advantages over MRI in detection of calcification, fat, and acute hemorrhage. Calcification and fat signals suggest teratoma, whereas hemorrhage is a sign of choriocarcinoma.

Germinoma is usually solid, with iso- or high density on CT and iso- or low intensity on T1-weighted MRI, with homogeneous enhancement and no surrounding edema. Calcification is minimal in extrapineal regions. Synchronous lesions involving pineal and suprasellar regions are pathognomonic of germinoma (**Fig. 12.1**). Nongerminomatous GCTs (NGGCTs) are more heterogeneous and surrounding edema is more prominent than in germinomas. The degree of enhancement is variable in teratomas (**Fig. 12.2a,b**). Additionally, in children with pineal tumors, pineal parenchymal tumors, dermoid or epidermoid cysts, gliomas, and cavernous malformation should be differentiated from the GCTs. When

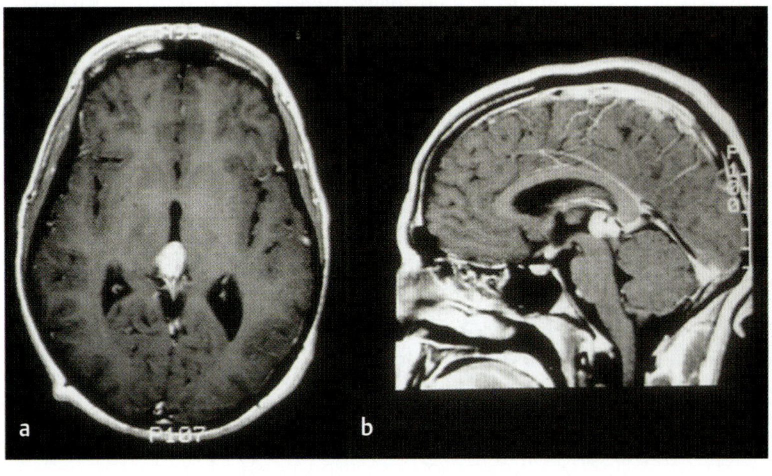

Fig. 12.1 Axial **(a)** and sagittal **(b)** gadolinium-enhanced T1-weighted magnetic resonance imaging of an 8-year-old male with Parinaud syndrome showing synchronous lesions in the pineal region **(a)** and suprasellar region **(b)**. The diagnosis is germinoma.

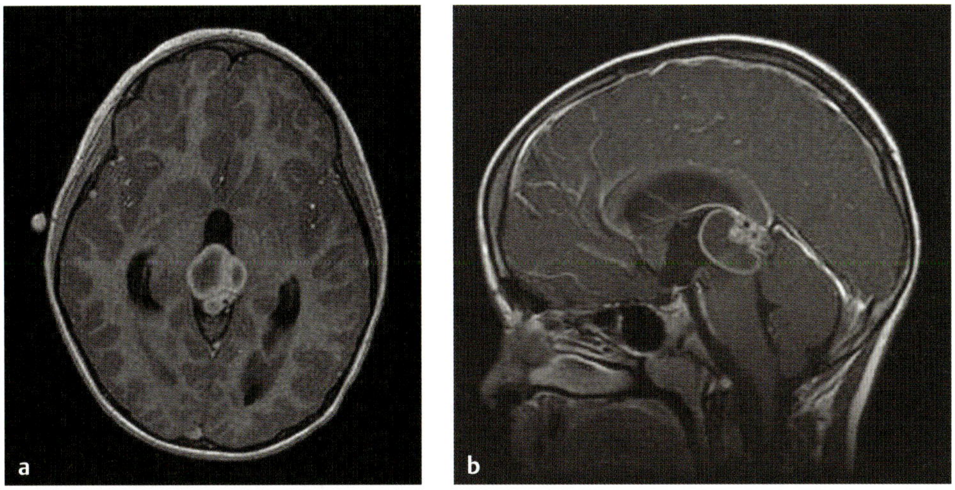

Fig. 12.2 **(a)** Axial gadolinium-enhanced T1-weighted magnetic resonance imaging (MRI) showing a pineal region lesion with central cystic change. **(b)** Sagittal gadolinium-enhanced T1-weighted MRI showing the same lesion, which proved to be a mature teratoma.

a suprasellar tumor is detected by neuroimaging, craniopharyngioma, optic glioma, Langerhans cell histiocytosis, and lymphocytic infundibuloneurohypophysitis are the main differentials for germinoma.

It should be noted that there can occasionally be a lag time between onset of symptoms relating to endocrinopathy (Level III evidence), especially DI, and detection of the GCT on MRI. In many instances, the first clue to the presence of an intracranial GCT is thickening of the pituitary stalk. A thorough clinical exam, with particular attention being paid to symptoms suggestive of endocrine dysfunction or visual disturbance, should be initiated.

Tumor markers in the serum and the CSF, β-HCG, and AFP should be assessed. Pure germinomas and teratomas usually present with negative markers, whereas NGGCTs often present with tumor marker elevation. Interestingly, however, very low levels of β-HCG can be detected in pure germinomas with leptomeningeal spread or among those that contain syncytiotrophoblastic giant cells. Elevated levels of AFP can also be seen in teratomas on occasion. The laboratory tests used to detect tumor markers have become more reliable during the last decade, but the exact interpretation and meaning of specific values often vary within study groups. Many of the European and U.S. groups have traditionally classified tumors as "secreting" if the serum CSF AFP is ≥ 10 or ≥ 25 ng/dL (or higher than the laboratory normal values) and when the β-HCG is > 50 IU/L (or higher than the laboratory normal values). Some Asian groups, however, use higher levels of β-HCG to categorize a patient into differing risk groups. Also, different study groups place more or less significance upon the importance of an isolated elevation in β-HCG (Level II to III evidence).[8,11–13]

Given the similarity in appearance of the various GCTs in the brain on MRI, it is not possible to categorize them into their histological subgroups based on imaging appearance alone. In general, whenever possible, a tumor biopsy is necessary to confirm the diagnosis and direct treatment. In some cases where CSF tumor markers are elevated and highly suggestive of a malignant GCT, treatment may be initiated without biopsy and tissue diagnosis. Unlike the situation decades ago when a "test dose" of radiation therapy was considered good initial treatment, this approach is no longer recommended.

Intracranial GCTs exhibit a wide variety of behaviors and responses to treatment paradigms. Their response is predicted by their histopathological subtype (**Fig. 12.3**); therefore, this delineation is exceedingly important prior to initiation of a treatment algorithm. Even germinomas may have a tendency

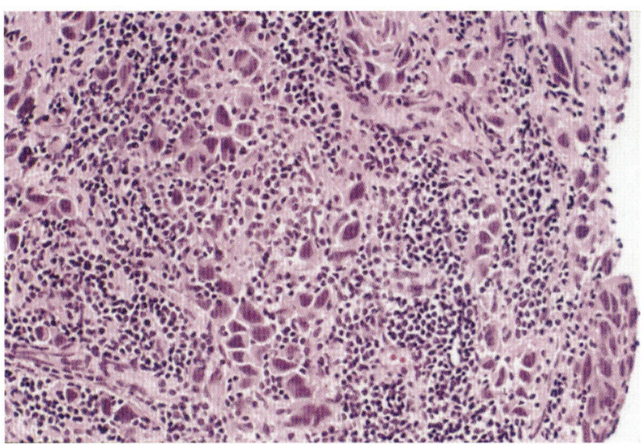

Fig. 12.3 Histopathology of pineal region germinoma shows malignant tumor cells with heavy lymphoplasma cell infiltration. The neoplastic cells show large vesicular nuclei and prominent cytoplasm. The cytoplasm is clear because of cytoplasmic glycogen and lipid.

to seed the ependyma through CSF dissemination (**Fig. 12.4**). Prognostication is also highly dependent on this information, because the 5-year survival rates vary considerably based on tumor classification. Sawamura et al divided intracranial GCTs into three groups based on available treatment paradigms (Level III evidence)[14] (**Table 12.1**).

■ Surgical Treatment

The indications for surgical intervention for patients with intracranial GCTs have changed remarkably over the years (see Expert Recommendations). For those patients presenting with obstructive hydrocephalus, endoscopic third ventriculostomy (ETV) with simultaneous biopsy is becoming the procedure of choice[11,15] (Level III evidence) except for some suprasellar GCTs where it is difficult to approach the floor of the third ventricle. ETV allows for CSF diversion and obviates the need for ventriculoperitoneal (VP) shunting in patients with intracranial GCTs. ETV diminishes the complications associated with VP shunting, including shunt infection and blockages, and prevents the risk of peritoneal seeding of tumor cells.

Given the potential for extraneural metastasis with shunting and given that the success rate of ETV for tumor-induced hydrocephalus can be as high as 70%, as well as the fact that endoscopic biopsy can be performed at the time of ETV, most centers prefer to perform an ETV with simultaneous biopsy whenever possible (Level III evidence).[15] Recent studies have also suggested that there is no increased rate of tumor dissemination with performance of an ETV with concomitant biopsy (Level III evidence).[16]

Improvements of stereotactic and endoscopic technique have dramatically increased the safety profile

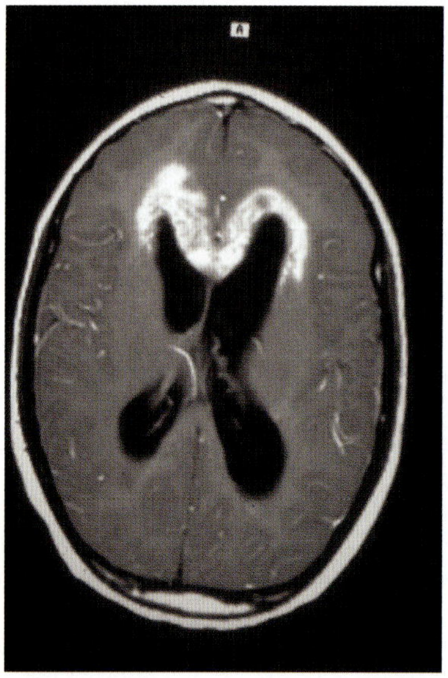

Fig. 12.4 Axial gadolinium-enhanced T1-weighted magnetic resonance imaging through the level of the lateral ventricles showing dissemination of intracranial germinoma within the frontal horns.

of biopsy in these tumors. Furthermore, accuracy in diagnosis with endoscopic biopsy has been found to be 90 to 98% in recent reviews.[7,17–19]

In the case of germinoma, partial or gross total resection has been shown to offer no further survival benefit as compared with biopsy with radiotherapy (Level III evidence).[20] For NGGCTs, which have been notoriously resistant to chemoradiation, a subsequent secondary surgery may be required to achieve a gross total resection where possible, subsequently prolonging survival.

Table 12.1 Classification of intracranial germ cell tumors

Prognosis	Tumor	5-Year survival
Good	Germinoma Mature teratoma	> 90%
Intermediate	Immature teratoma Mixed: germinoma with mature or immature teratoma	~ 70%
Poor	Malignant teratoma Embryonal carcinoma Choriocarcinoma Endodermal sinus (yolk sac) Mixed: including embryonal carcinoma, endodermal sinus (yolk sac), choriocarcinoma or any other malignant tumor	< 50%

■ Adjuvant Therapy

Germinoma

For pure germinomas, complete neurosurgical resection is not required or recommended; the literature has shown that chemotherapy and radiation therapy are highly effective treatments. Radiation therapy for intracranial GCTs has resulted in a 5-year survival rate of greater than 90%.[21,22] Radiation dose and field have remained somewhat controversial subjects. Current treatment paradigms suggest that local radiation along with whole ventricular radiation provides control rates similar to those of whole neuraxis radiation (Level III evidence).[23] Given the concerns for cognitive impairment after craniospinal irradiation, this treatment option is now reserved for those patients with radiological or cytological evidence of metastatic disease.

The use of platinum-based chemotherapy in conjunction with radiation has made it possible to significantly reduce the dosage of radiation needed without affecting outcomes. Chemotherapy as a stand-alone treatment, although showing initial efficacy, resulted in a significantly greater recurrence rate and thus is not recommended as a single-agent modality (Level II evidence).[24]

The current treatment recommendation for germinomas is for whole ventricular radiation 24 Gy with local boost 45 Gy where there is no evidence of metastatic spread.[8,23,25] If metastatic disease is present, craniospinal irradiation should be employed. The use of adjuvant chemotherapy remains controversial, and, although it has the potential to decrease radiation dosage, it has its own significant side effects, both short and long term, which must be taken into consideration,[25] though new evidence shows some promising results (Level III evidence) (**Table 12.2**).[23]

Table 12.2 Recommendations for adjuvant and neoadjuvant therapy

Germinoma
1. For germinoma, after tissue biopsy confirmation, radiation therapy is the main treatment (Grade 1C+, Level III Evidence).
2. The field of radiation is local, along with whole ventricular or whole brain radiation if there is no metastasis. In cases of metastatic germinoma, whole neuraxis radiation is recommended (Grade 1C+, Level III Evidence).
3. Dose of radiation is whole ventricular radiation 24 Gy with local boost 45 Gy + no metastasis (Grade 1C+, Level III Evidence).
4. The dose of radiation should be more than 40 Gy (Grade 1C, Level III Evidence).
5. Chemotherapy is not recommended as a single-agent modality (Grade 1C+, Level II Evidence).
6. Chemotherapy is being used in conjunction with radiation therapy to minimize radiation's long-term side effects (Grade 2C, Level III Evidence).
Nongerminomatous germ cell tumor (NGGCT)
1. Combined radiation therapy, chemotherapy, and radical resection as an initial or salvage treatment achieved excellent tumor control in the intermediate-prognosis NGGCT group (Grade 1C, Level III Evidence).
2. For the poor-prognosis NGGCT group, initial therapy is gross total resection where possible (Grade 2C, Level III Evidence).
3. Neoadjuvant chemotherapy and second-look surgery are an acceptable combination (Grade 2C, Level III Evidence).

Nongerminomatous Germ Cell Tumors

Standard treatment for this mixed group of tumors has not been completely elucidated. Certainly, some mixed tumors containing germinoma and immature teratoma have shown a 70% recurrence-free survival at 5 years when treated with radiation therapy and chemotherapy. However, choriocarcinoma, embryonal carcinoma, yolk sac tumors, and malignant teratomas have shown extremely low survival rates (**Table 12.1**). They have been shown to have an extremely poor response to chemoradiation. Patients with this group of tumors may benefit most from gross total resection where possible (class 1C+, Level II evidence).

To facilitate this, a combination of craniospinal irradiation and multidrug chemotherapy is often initiated after diagnostic biopsy prior to radical surgical resection. Preoperative chemoradiation has been shown in some instances to decrease tumor bulk and vascularity and may limit tumor spread during surgery.[26] Kochi et al treated 11 consecutive patients with NGGCTs with neoadjuvant therapy consisting of chemotherapy and radiation followed by radical resection. Ten of 11 of these patients were disease free at a mean of 96 months, and only one patient suffered a recurrence ultimately resulting in mortality.[26]

Salvage or second-look surgery may incur an interesting paradigm shift in treating these intracranial tumors. Its role is seemingly increasingly important in NGGCTs after induction chemotherapy, which despite reversal of serum/CSF markers may have radiographic evidence of residual disease. After postchemotherapy resection, many tumors were found to have a predominantly teratomatous component—the so-called growing teratoma syndrome.[7] In this context, surgery is often the optimum potentially curative treatment. The International Symposium on Central Nervous System GCTs suggested that second-look surgery may be most beneficial in those NGGCTs with reversion of serum/CSF markers and radiographic residual showing growth (Level III evidence).[7]

The role of surgery in those patients with NGGCTs with continued elevation of serum/CSF markers after adjuvant treatment is controversial because it is unclear if it offers any survival benefit. Furthermore, in this setting, the exact timing of surgical intervention also remains ill defined.

Long-Term Effects of Treatment

Radiation is one of the mainstays of treatment of intracranial germinoma, offering excellent long-term survival. Due to the fact that germinoma mainly affects the pediatric population, increasing concerns over the long-term effects of radiation are important to consider and resolve if possible. Late neuropsychological decline, endocrine dysfunction, development of moyamoya disease or cavernous malformations, and the possibility of a radiation-induced tumor are of significant concern. The literature relating to the effects of cranial irradiation on the brain is burgeoning.[27–32] Because there is typically a delay before cognitive decline is recognized in children, it is imperative that all children with GCTs who undergo cranial irradiation undergo early and long-term neuropsychological testing.

A recent study by O'Neil et al evaluated 20 patients with germinoma treated first with chemotherapy followed by whole ventricular radiation with a boost to the tumor field, thus allowing for a lower radiation dosage. After extensive neuropsychological testing, they were not able to find any significant difference pre- and posttreatment with no reduction in efficacy of treatment.[33]

The subject of radiation-induced tumors is one that all treating physicians should be aware of, especially for children with GCTs. Kamoshima et al report on a 20-year-old survivor of a childhood CNS germinoma who developed a progressively enlarging intraparenchymal meningioma occurring in an area that had received radiation 6 years prior.[34] Of concern is that previously reported radiation-induced meningiomas have shown themselves to have an aggressive biological behavior despite a benign gross appearance.[35,36]

Expert Recommendations

1. The clinical presentation, biochemical data, and neuroimaging must be considered in combination before any surgical intervention.
2. Tissue biopsy is crucial and mandatory.
3. Neuroendoscopy is the first step that we recommend wherever possible for biopsy and CSF diversion.
4. Neuronavigation is a helpful neurosurgical tool to aid with tumor biopsy in difficult situations such as a small ventricular system.
5. For germinomas, biopsy is a sufficient first step, followed by radiation therapy and chemotherapy.
6. 24-Gy whole ventricular radiation and 45-Gy local boost are the current recommendations.
7. A test dose of radiation therapy without biopsy is not recommended.
8. For NGGCT, chemoradiation and maximum safe resection are recommended whenever they are possible.
9. Neuropsychological tests before and after radiation therapy are preferred for all patients.
10. Attempts to reduce radiation dose may improve long-term morbidity.

■ Summary and Conclusions

CNS GCTs are a significant subgroup of pediatric brain tumors that decline in incidence after the second decade of life. Approximately 60% of these tumors are of the germinoma subgroup in which the survival rate with best treatment practice paradigms is greater than 90%. NGGCTs are much more difficult to treat effectively and continue to show a fairly dismal survival rate. Although current treatment regimens offer increasing survival advantages, they also cause concern for late complications, which are being more fully documented at this point.

Given the advances in microneurosurgical techniques, there is decreasing morbidity and mortality when these techniques are used within the deep structures of the brain. Neurosurgical procedures, whether ETV, tumor biopsy, or aggressive resection using neuronavigation, neuromonitoring, and other strategies, are increasingly being used for children with these tumors.

■ References

1. Villano JL, Propp JM, Porter KR, et al. Malignant pineal germ-cell tumors: an analysis of cases from three tumor registries. Neuro-oncol 2008;10(2):121–130
2. Matsutani M, Sano K, Takakura K, et al. Primary intracranial germ cell tumors: a clinical analysis of 153 histologically verified cases. J Neurosurg 1997;86(3):446–455
3. Crawford JR, Santi MR, Vezina G, et al. CNS germ cell tumor (CNSGCT) of childhood: presentation and delayed diagnosis. Neurology 2007;68(20):1668–1673
4. Jennings MT, Gelman R, Hochberg F. Intracranial germ-cell tumors: natural history and pathogenesis. J Neurosurg 1985;63(2):155–167
5. Sano K. Pathogenesis of intracranial germ cell tumors reconsidered. J Neurosurg 1999;90(2):258–264
6. Jooma R, Kendall BE. Diagnosis and management of pineal tumors. J Neurosurg 1983;58(5):654–665
7. Souweidane MM, Krieger MD, Weiner HL, Finlay JL. Surgical management of primary central nervous system germ cell tumors: proceedings from the Second International Symposium on Central Nervous System Germ Cell Tumors. J Neurosurg Pediatr 2010;6(2):125–130
8. Balmaceda C, Finlay J. Current advances in the diagnosis and management of intracranial germ cell tumors. Curr Neurol Neurosci Rep 2004;4(3):253–262

9. Goodwin TL, Sainani K, Fisher PG. Incidence patterns of central nervous system germ cell tumors: a SEER Study. J Pediatr Hematol Oncol 2009;31(8):541–544
10. Villano JL, Virk IY, Ramirez V, Propp JM, Engelhard HH, McCarthy BJ. Descriptive epidemiology of central nervous system germ cell tumors: nonpineal analysis. Neuro-oncol 2010; 12(3):257–264
11. Echevarría ME, Fangusaro J, Goldman S. Pediatric central nervous system germ cell tumors: a review. Oncologist 2008; 13(6):690–699
12. Calaminus G, Bamberg M, Baranzelli MC, et al. Intracranial germ cell tumors: a comprehensive update of the European data. Neuropediatrics 1994;25(1):26–32
13. Calaminus G, Andreussi L, Garré ML, Kortmann RD, Schober R, Göbel U. Secreting germ cell tumors of the central nervous system (CNS): first results of the cooperative German/Italian pilot study (CNS sGCT). Klin Padiatr 1997;209(4):222–227
14. Sawamura Y. Current diagnosis and treatment of central nervous system germ cell tumours. Curr Opin Neurol 1996;9(6):419–423
15. Ray P, Jallo GI, Kim RY, et al. Endoscopic third ventriculostomy for tumor-related hydrocephalus in a pediatric population. Neurosurg Focus 2005;19(6):E8
16. Shono T, Natori Y, Morioka T, et al. Results of a long-term follow-up after neuroendoscopic biopsy procedure and third ventriculostomy in patients with intracranial germinomas. J Neurosurg 2007;107(3, Suppl):193–198
17. Souweidane MM. Endoscopic management of pediatric brain tumors. Neurosurg Focus 2005;18(6A):E1
18. Souweidane MM, Sandberg DI, Bilsky MH, Gutin PH. Endoscopic biopsy for tumors of the third ventricle. Pediatr Neurosurg 2000;33(3):132–137
19. Badie B, Brooks N, Souweidane MM. Endoscopic and minimally invasive microsurgical approaches for treating brain tumor patients. J Neurooncol 2004;69(1-3):209–219
20. Sawamura Y, de Tribolet N, Ishii N, Abe H. Management of primary intracranial germinomas: diagnostic surgery or radical resection? J Neurosurg 1997;87(2):262–266
21. Kersh CR, Constable WC, Eisert DR, et al. Primary central nervous system germ cell tumors. Effect of histologic confirmation on radiotherapy. Cancer 1988;61(11):2148–2152
22. Shirato H, Nishio M, Sawamura Y, et al. Analysis of long-term treatment of intracranial germinoma. Int J Radiat Oncol Biol Phys 1997;37(3):511–515
23. Kanamori M, Kumabe T, Saito R, et al. Optimal treatment strategy for intracranial germ cell tumors: a single institution analysis. J Neurosurg Pediatr 2009;4(6):506–514
24. Kellie SJ, Boyce H, Dunkel IJ, et al. Intensive cisplatin and cyclophosphamide-based chemotherapy without radiotherapy for intracranial germinomas: failure of a primary chemotherapy approach. Pediatr Blood Cancer 2004;43(2):126–133
25. Rogers SJ, Mosleh-Shirazi MA, Saran FH. Radiotherapy of localised intracranial germinoma: time to sever historical ties? Lancet Oncol 2005;6(7):509–519
26. Kochi M, Itoyama Y, Shiraishi S, Kitamura I, Marubayashi T, Ushio Y. Successful treatment of intracranial nongerminomatous malignant germ cell tumors by administering neoadjuvant chemotherapy and radiotherapy before excision of residual tumors. J Neurosurg 2003;99(1):106–114
27. Grill J, Renaux VK, Bulteau C, et al. Long-term intellectual outcome in children with posterior fossa tumors according to radiation doses and volumes. Int J Radiat Oncol Biol Phys 1999; 45(1):137–145
28. Edelstein K, D'agostino N, Bernstein LJ, et al. Long-term neurocognitive outcomes in young adult survivors of childhood acute lymphoblastic leukemia. J Pediatr Hematol Oncol 2011;33(6):450–458
29. Edelstein K, Spiegler BJ, Fung S, et al. Early aging in adult survivors of childhood medulloblastoma: long-term neurocognitive, functional, and physical outcomes. Neuro-oncol 2011;13(5):536–545
30. Mabbott DJ, Monsalves E, Spiegler BJ, et al. Longitudinal evaluation of neurocognitive function after treatment for central nervous system germ cell tumors in childhood. Cancer 2011;117(23):5402–5411
31. Mabbott DJ, Spiegler BJ, Greenberg ML, Rutka JT, Hyder DJ, Bouffet E. Serial evaluation of academic and behavioral outcome after treatment with cranial radiation in childhood. J Clin Oncol 2005;23(10):2256–2263
32. Spiegler BJ, Bouffet E, Greenberg ML, Rutka JT, Mabbott DJ. Change in neurocognitive functioning after treatment with cranial radiation in childhood. J Clin Oncol 2004;22(4):706–713
33. O'Neil S, Ji L, Buranahirun C, et al. Neurocognitive outcomes in pediatric and adolescent patients with central nervous system germinoma treated with a strategy of chemotherapy followed by reduced-dose and volume irradiation. Pediatr Blood Cancer 2011;57(4):669–673
34. Kamoshima Y, Terasaka S, Kobayashi H, et al. Radiation induced intraparenchymal meningioma occurring 6 years after CNS germinoma: case report. Clin Neurol Neurosurg 2012; 114(7):1077–1080
35. Sadetzki S, Flint-Richter P, Ben-Tal T, Nass D. Radiation-induced meningioma: a descriptive study of 253 cases. J Neurosurg 2002;97(5):1078–1082
36. Umansky F, Shoshan Y, Rosenthal G, Fraifeld S, Spektor S. Radiation-induced meningioma. Neurosurg Focus 2008;24(5): E7

13

Surgery versus Initial Trial of Radiation in the Management of Pineal Region Tumors

Ramiro Del Valle, Javier Avendaño, and Juan Barges Coll

Primary pineal tumors (PTs) represent only 0.4 to 1.0% of all cranial lesions. The individual surgeon's experience with these tumors is thus limited, and their location in relation to vascular and neural structures constitutes a surgical challenge.[1] Germ cell tumors (GCTs) are the most common PTs (35%), followed by pineal parenchymal tumors (PPTs, 30%). Other less common pineal region tumors include astrocytomas and ependymomas. In 2007, the World Health Organization (WHO) introduced a new class of PTs called papillary pineal tumors. Among the PPTs, there are three major subgroups: pineocytoma (WHO grade I), PPTs of intermediate differentiation (WHO grade II/III), and pineoblastoma (PB) (WHO grade IV).[2,3] Malignant tumors of the pineal region account for 75%, and their proximity to vital venous structures makes them unsuitable for gross total resection. However, their response to radiation after biopsy has had a positive impact on the outcome.[4,5] Indications for surgical management of PTs depend on tumor markers, pathology findings on biopsy, and associated hydrocephalus.[6–8] Although it is impossible to differentiate among the different histological subtypes based on magnetic resonance imaging (MRI), its role in decision making is currently significant.[9–11] Contrasted MRI is indicated prior to any nonurgent management; it is thus used for planning the operative approach, identifying the relationships between the tumor and other anatomical structures, and determining whether total resection can be safely attempted.

■ Clinical Presentation and Initial Management

Patients with PT commonly present with elevated intracranial pressure (ICP) (headache, nausea/vomiting, and decreased level of consciousness) as a result of obstructive hydrocephalus due to compression of the cerebral aqueduct by the tumor mass. Patients may also exhibit Parinaud syndrome (upgaze paralysis, convergence nystagmus, and near-light dissociation) as a result of compression of the dorsal midbrain structures. Focal neurological deficits are present in ~ 25% of patients and are found incidentally in 5%.[7]

Initial workup includes a careful neurological history and physical examination, including funduscopic examination. If a significant level of suspicion is present, the next step should be an intracranial imaging protocol.[10]

Tumor Markers

Considering the attendant morbidity of pineal region surgery (resection or biopsy), noninvasive means should be employed to detect a radiosensitive tumor promptly. Detection of β-human chorionic gonadotropin (β-HCG), α-fetoprotein, or both, in blood or cerebrospinal fluid (CSF) suggests a malignant GCT and is an indication for radiotherapy and chemotherapy without resection or biopsy, though management of hydrocephalus is still usually warranted.[12] CSF can be obtained during external ventricular drain placement, endoscopic third ventriculostomy, or shunting, or via low-volume lumbar puncture. It must be noted that pineal masses cause obstructive hydrocephalus, and lumbar puncture in this setting could precipitate herniation.

Hydrocephalus Treatment and Cerebrospinal Fluid Sampling

Given that most patients with PTs present with symptoms related to hydrocephalus, a common first procedure is an endoscopic third ventriculostomy (ETV) or ventriculoperitoneal shunt. Either procedure allows for both CSF sampling (important for ruling out GCTs as already discussed) and alleviation of obstructive hydrocephalus, which is the most pressing concern during acute management of patients with PB. Patients with CSF positive for GCT markers should then receive adjuvant therapy without the need of further surgical intervention.[12]

Among the CSF diversion options, most neurosurgeons prefer ETV due to its permanent relief of hydrocephalus without indwelling hardware and the possibility of performing an endoscopic biopsy during the same surgical procedure.[13–15]

■ Literature Review

Role of Surgery

Since its first description in the early 20th century, surgery of the pineal region has matured, reflecting an understanding of the region's varied pathologies as well as evolution of surgical technologies and techniques, creating a modern, nuanced, multidisciplinary approach to these tumors.[16–18] The interhemispheric transcallosal approach was among the earliest descriptions of operative approaches to PTs. This approach was published in 1913 and modified by Dandy in the 1920s. PT surgery from the 1910s through the early 1930s was dangerous for a multitude of reasons beyond the anatomical challenges, including the lack of experience, operative microscope, and adequate lighting.[19]

Four possible surgical corridors or approaches to the pineal region are generally used: transcallosal, transventricular, occipital transtentorial, and infratentorial supracerebellar.[20] The transcallosal interforniceal approach has been used extensively in adults with PTs and less frequently in pediatric patients. Poppen used the supratentorial approach for a parietoccipital craniotomy followed by transection of the tentorium to access the posterior third ventricle.[21] This approach typically places the veins at the top of the tumor, adding the risk of injury.[17,22] Krause described the supracerebellar infratentorial approach, which provides excellent visualization of the posterior third ventricular wall and pineal region.[23] The precentral vein is usually sacrificed, with no clinical significance to the blood flow drainage of the cerebellum. This approach has the limitation of not being suitable for lesions extending beyond the tentorial notch.[17]

With the development of microneurosurgery in 1970, the anterior transcallosal interforniceal approach became widely used.[24] It allows further posterior enlargement of the foramen of Monro without scarifying any other neural structure on the way to the pineal region. There are a few advantages of this approach: it protects normal anatomy, it provides great visualization of the total region, it facilitates the separation of the internal veins, and it reduces the risk of injury to the cerebral cortex and thus lowers the risk of epilepsy.[21]

Surgery versus Biopsy

Level I to Level II Evidence

No randomized clinical trials are published comparing surgery and biopsy.

Level III to Level IV Evidence

The decision between biopsy alone or resection should take into account the treatment objectives as well as the risks of each of the possible procedures. The primary objective in the surgical management of pineal region tumors is to establish accurate pathological diagnosis, which dictates further surgical strategy, adjuvant therapy, metastatic workup, prognosis, and follow-up plans. The secondary objective is resection, whether partial or complete. Considering the diversity of histological findings in pineal masses, in the absence of positive tumor markers, accurate tissue diagnosis is essential. The most reliable strategy for accurate diagnosis is adequate tissue sampling, which is limited in stereotactic and endoscopic biopsy and much more feasible in open procedures.[13,25–27] A major advantage of open microsurgical techniques is resection. Approximately one third of PTs are benign, and resection affords the best opportunity for long-term recurrence-free survival. For malignant tumors, the clinical impact of maximal tumor resection is less well documented, though several reports have correlated extent of tumor resection with improved response to adjuvant therapy and increased survival. Other advantages of more aggressive resection include the potential control of hydrocephalus without a second procedure and a reduced risk of postoperative hemorrhage into the residual tumor bed.[14]

These advantages are contingent on avoidance of complications. Favorable results are achievable but are considerably dependent on the experience and judgment of the surgeon, beyond what is typically necessary for an intracranial tumor operation. Indeed, the risk–benefit balance may shift depending on the surgeon as much as on the anatomy

Role of Radiosurgery

Level I to Level II Evidence

Only retrospective analyses have been conducted regarding the role of radiosurgery.

Level III to Level IV Evidence

The role of radiosurgery (RS) remains controversial. Traditionally, pineal region tumors have been approached surgically with or without conventional radiation depending on the histopathological features. Due to the heterogeneity of the PTs, MRI does not always provide an adequate diagnostic conclusion. Biopsy is necessary in most cases before definite treatment is decided. Conversely, some groups argue that empirical treatment of pineal region tumors should be avoided. Radiosurgery is most effective when used as a secondary treatment for high-grade lesions rather than when used as a primary treatment, whereas low-grade lesions respond adequately to gamma knife surgery as a stand-alone therapy.

Conventional radiation therapy is highly effective in the treatment of GCTs and therefore for most pineal region tumors. Nonetheless, concerns about radiation toxicity, especially regarding to the intellect and to the function of the hypothalamic–pituitary axis in children, have prompted efforts to reduce or avoid conventional radiation therapy. For the treatment of GCTs, these efforts have led to the adoption of chemotherapy regimens shown to be efficacious in the treatment of gonadal GCTs. Intracranial GCTs, however, are not amenable to treatment with chemotherapy alone; they can be treated successfully with a combination of chemotherapy and reduced-dose radiation. The rationale for radiosurgery for radiation-sensitive tumors, either as a boost to reduce the dose of conventional radiation or to replace it, is similar to that for chemotherapy.[28–29]

Level V Evidence

The Gamma Knife Unit in Mexico City has treated over 24 patients with pineal region tumors since 2000 (**Table 13.1**). All patients were treated using Leksell Gamma Plan treatment planning software (Version 5.34, Elekta, Atlanta, GA). All doses were prescribed to the 50% isodose line (IDL). The database was obtained from all patients treated at our facility from 2000 to December 2011. Volumetric analysis was performed in the entire follow-up protocol as described previously by the senior author.[30] Fifteen patients had histological diagnosis made with endoscopic biopsy (EB), SB, or open surgery. All other patients underwent MRI, CSF markers, and an initial trial of radiation with GKS. Out of 15 patients with confirmed histological diagnosis, 3 were germinomas, 6 astrocytomas, 1 gangliocytoma, 1 pineoblastoma, 2 pineocytomas, 1 mixed tumor, and 1 metastasis. Follow-up ranged from 3 months to 12 years, with a mean follow-up of 3.6 years. There were no neurological deficits or complications that could be attributable to GKS. The advantages of GKS over conventional wide-field radiation therapy include single-fraction radiation, less radiation to normal tissues, rapid patient recovery, and no bone marrow toxicity. Also, the patient can begin systemic chemotherapy management immediately after tissue diagnosis.[31]

Discussion

Treatment of pineal region tumors remains challenging and controversial. No topic can better fit the aim of this book. Classically, pineal region tumors have been treated either surgically or with radiotherapy. Although the role of stereotactic radiosurgery has been increasing, few radiosurgery studies for pineal region tumors have been reported. Whereas some authors suggest radiosurgery as the initial treatment without biopsy,[33] other groups believe that empirical treatment of pineal region tumors with radiosurgery should never be performed, and tissue must be obtained before definitive treatment is indicated.[32,34] Concerning the cohort of patients treated empirically in our center, two showed total response and complete tumor involution (**Figs. 13.1** and **13.2**), and three presented partial but significant response measured by volumetric analysis. Four patients were lost to follow-up, and we could not conduct a strong statistical analysis as a result. Seemingly, a trial of radiation without biopsy is justified due to the biological radiosensitivity of these tumors; this statement is supported by our series. However, prospective analysis with a larger sample size and longer follow-up is needed to delineate factors associated with outcome. Meanwhile, we have confirmed the importance of obtaining tissue for histopathological analysis and present our recommendations for the management of the most common pineal region tumors.

Table 13.1 Treatment considerations for 24 cases of pineal region tumors

Case No.	Age-Sex	Diagnosis	Method of diagnosis	Vol (cm³)	Doses (Gy) IDL 50%	Max dose	Duration of FU	Response and current vol (cm³)	Multimodality treatment
1	29, F	Pineoblastoma	EB	11.33	14.45	28.89	7 mo	PR, NA	VPS, QT, RT
2	22, M	PPT	SB	6.02	14	28	12 y	Total	VPS, QT, boost, RT
3	12, M	PRT	MRI	14.2	13.6	27.3	1 y	PR, 1.9	VPS
4	3, M	LGA	SB	22.4	11	22	12 y	PR, 1.2	Boost (2)
5	10, M	MNGGCT	EB	5.7	14	28	2 y	PR, 3.0	None
6	9 mo, M	Germinoma	SB, PM	3.6	14	35	7 y	NA	NA
7	37, M	Pineocytoma	EB	4.7	12	27.91	12 y	PR, 1.9	RT
8	61, F	LGA	EB	0.489	14	28	7 y	Total	None
9	33, F	PRT	MRI	4.1	16.25	32.5	8 y	Total	None
10	13, M	PRT	MRI	8	12	24	5 y	Total	RT, QT
11	18, M	LGA	SB	7.2	18	36	9 y	PR, 0.919	Boost
12	22, M	PRT	MRI	5.95	13.95	27.91	NFU	PR, NA	VPS
13	9, M	Pineocytoma	EB	3.19	14	28	NFU	NA	NA
14	11, M	LGA	EB	4.8	10	25	7 y	PR, 0.48	None
15	16, M	Gangliocytoma	SB	6.1	14	28	NFU	NA	VPS, QT
16	36, F	PRT	MRI	7.9	10.8	21.67	NFU	NA	NA
17	60, F	PRT	MRI	1.6	14	28	6 y	PR, 0.046	None
18	7, M	HGA	SB	13.9	14	28	1 y	NR, 24	VPS, RT, QT
19	19, M	Germinoma	QX	8.87	13	26	NFU	NA	VPS, SR
20	12, F	PRT	MRI	1.1	16.25	32.5	NFU	NA	VPS
21	11, M	PRT	MRI, PM	12.6	13	26	1 y	PR, 13MM	VPS, QT
22	10, F	Mixed	SB	9.92	14	28	5 mo	PR, 661	QT, RT
23	12, M	PRT	MRI	2.1	15	30	3 mo	PR, NA	VPS
24	39, F	Metastasis	MRI	4.5	14	28	3 mo	PR, 2.1	None

Abbreviations: EB, endoscopic biopsy; FU, follow-up; HGA, high-grade astrocytoma; IDL, isodose line; LGA, low-grade astrocytoma; MNGGCT, malignant nongerminomatous germ cell tumor; MRI, magnetic resonance imaging; NA, not available; NFU, no follow-up; NR, no response; PM, positive markers; PPT, pineal parenchymal tumor; PR, partial response; PRT, pineal region tumor; QT, chemotherapy; RT, radiotherapy; SB, stereotactic biopsy; SR, surgical resection; VPS, ventricular peritoneal shunt.

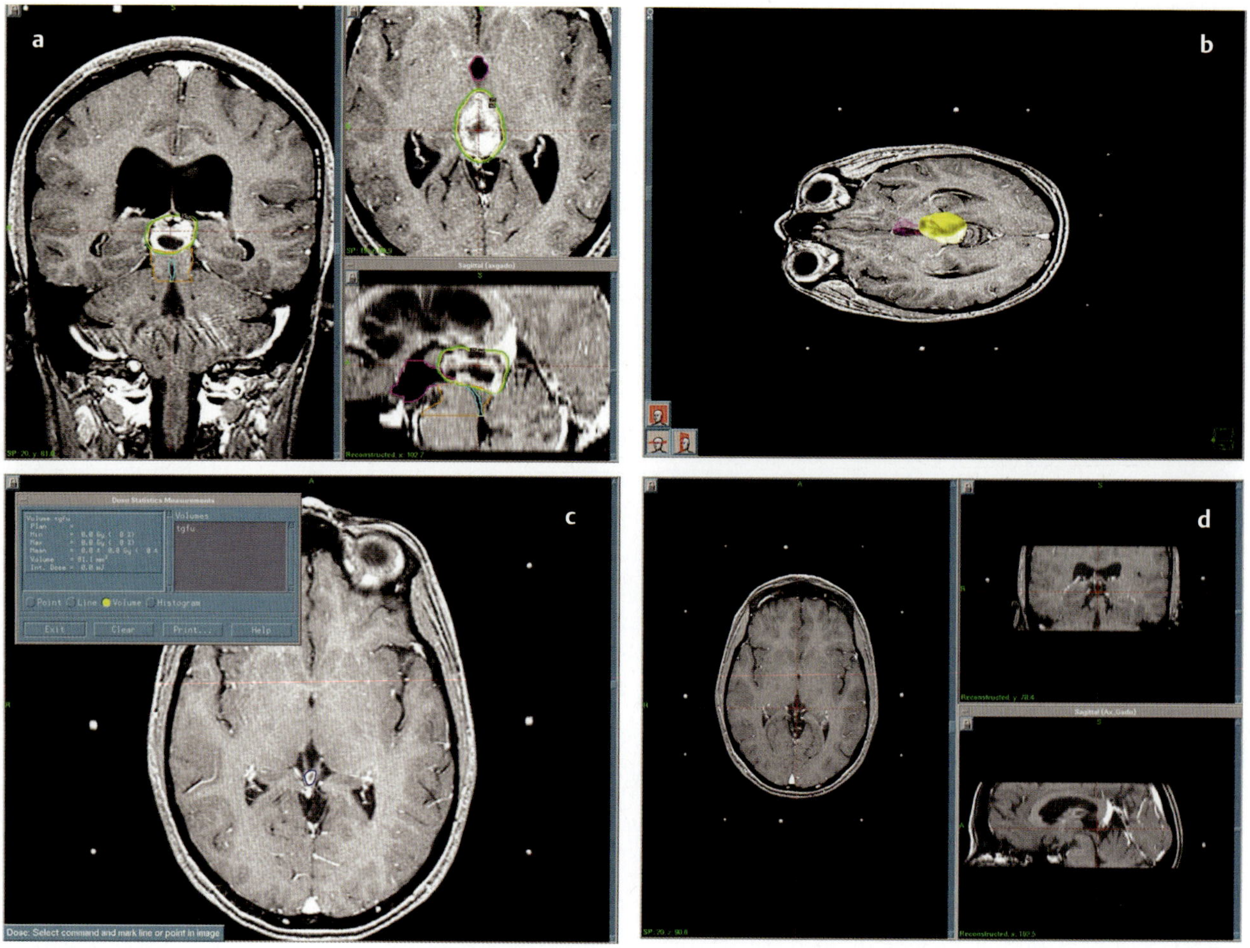

Fig. 13.1 Thirty-three-year-old female (case 9, **Table 13.1**) referred from a fertility physician who found a pineal region mass during standard protocol. Gamma knife radiosurgery (GKRS) without biopsy was performed and close follow-up was planned. **(a)** Planning 2003. **(b)** Three-dimensional GKRS treatment plan, 13 Gy/40% IDL. **(c)** Four-year follow-up with remarkable tumor involution. **(d)** Last follow-up in 2011 shows total response. Patient's fertility problem was solved.

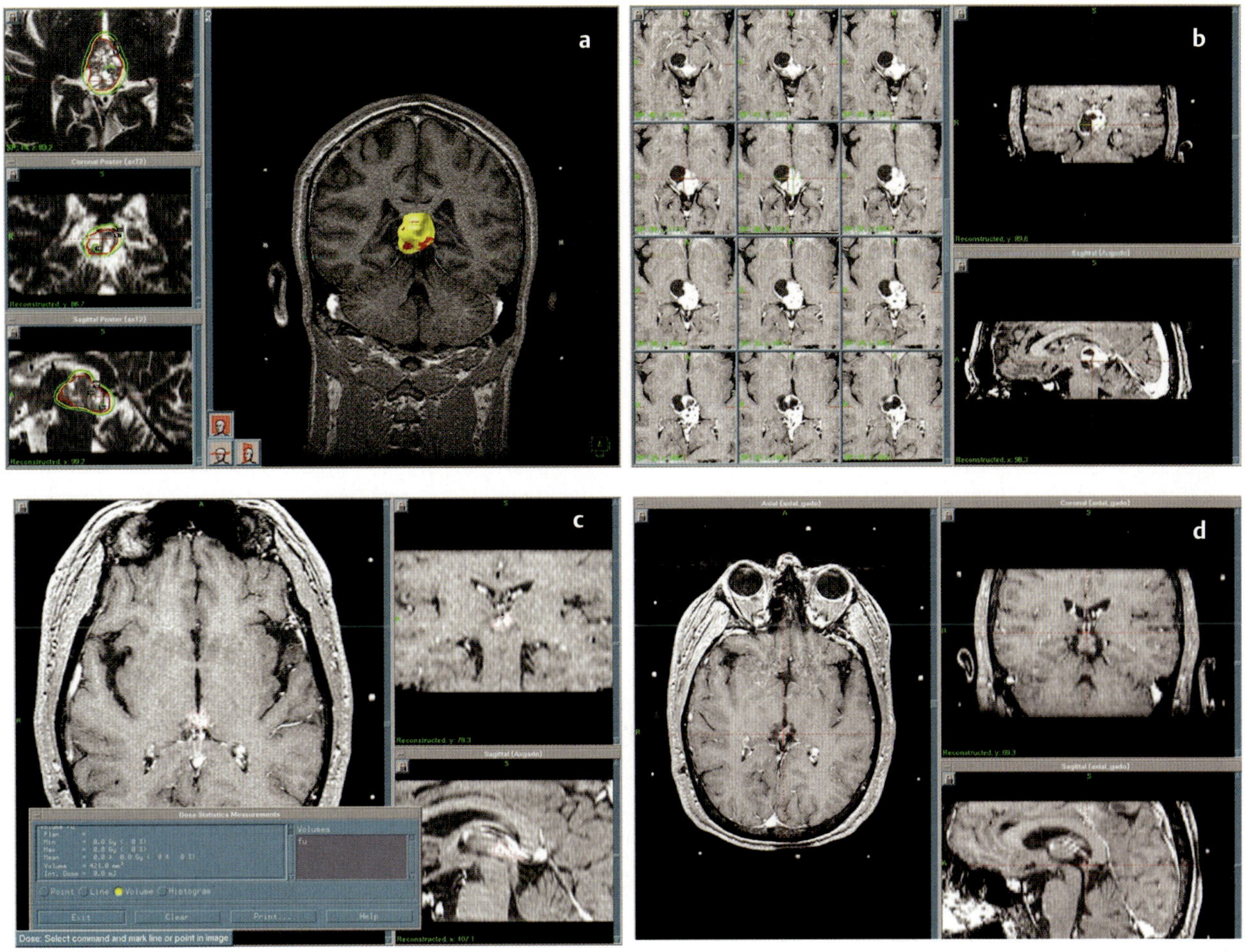

Fig. 13.2 Male student (case 2, **Table 13.1**) presented with increased intracranial pressure due to hydrocephalus and was treated with ventriculoperitoneal shunt (VPS). Initial treatment with gamma knife radiosurgery (GKRS) was performed with close follow-up. First follow-up showed significant tumor involution. Six-year follow-up magnetic resonance imaging showed a significant tumor regrowth with an important cyst component. Stereotactic biopsy was performed to decompress the cyst and obtain tissue for diagnosis. Pineal parenchymal tumor and radiation-induced changes were reported by pathology and a GKRS boost was indicated. **(a)** Initial planning; **(b)** recurrence with cyst component; **(c)** follow-up, significant involution is highlighted; and **(d)** twelve-year follow-up, total response is achieved.

Expert Recommendations

1. Stereotactic or endoscopic biopsy may be pursued in tumors smaller than 3 cm. All other lesions should be referred for open biopsy with microsurgical techniques. This approach provides adequate tissue for diagnosis, may be curative in low-grade tumors, and may substantially improve survival in patients with malignant tumors (Grade 1C Recommendation, Level II and IV Evidence).
2. Radiation therapy is the first-line therapy for germinomas. It has been reported that biopsy-confirmed germinomas had superior survival rates compared with nonbiopsied patients with a presumptive diagnosis of germinomas. Treatment recommendation should be based on assessment of histological type and extent of disease. Intracranial germinomas are highly radiocurable tumors, and major surgery should be avoided to prevent serious damage to the region, which could result in undesirable neurological deficits. For pure germinomas with no evidence of dissemination, local radiotherapy plays a curative role. Based on the rarity of pineocytoma and the long follow-up required to adequately document recurrence and overall survival, a prospective trial to address management concerns is unlikely. In the absence of information, current evidence indicates that surgical resection is the appropriate treatment for these tumors. When anatomically possible, gross total resection should be attempted because it has been associated with improved tumor control and longer progression-free and overall survivals. Adjuvant fractionated radiotherapy does not improve the rate of tumor control or survival when used to treat a subtotally resected tumor[31] (Grade 1C Recommendation, Level II and IV Evidence).
3. Any of the malignant tumors (non-GCTs, pineoblastomas, and parenchymal tumors of intermediate determination) also require craniospinal radiation (with local tumor doses of at least 50 Gy) and adjuvant chemotherapy (generally platinum based). Patients with tectal gliomas may undergo excision with or without postoperative radiation; however, they also may be observed with vigilant follow-up alone. Pineoblastomas represent the most aggressive of the PPTs. Routine treatment consists of operative management of obstructive hydrocephalus and CSF studies followed by maximal resection and adjuvant chemotherapy/radiotherapy, resulting in a median survival of 20 months. Important prognostic factors for survival of patients with PB include the extent of resection, age at presentation, disseminated disease, and craniospinal radiotherapy. Novel strategies are being evaluated for the treatment of PB and include high-dose chemotherapy with autologous stem cell therapy, stereotactic radiosurgery, and histone deacetylase inhibitors.

■ Summary and Conclusions

There are few studies that explore the efficacy of radiosurgery in treating pineal region tumors. In those analyses, authors have mainly used gamma knife radiosurgery (GKRS) as an adjuvant therapy rather than as a primary treatment modality. There is controversy about using GKS as a stand-alone procedure without histological confirmation. According to our records, GKS can be an option as a stand-alone procedure when pineocytoma or low-grade glioma has been confirmed and the lesion is less than 3 cm in diameter because few complications and a high rate of adequate response have been observed.

■ References

1. Mamelak AN, Drazin D, Shirzadi A, Black KL, Berci G. Infratentorial supracerebellar resection of a pineal tumor using a high definition video exoscope (VITOM®). J Clin Neurosci 2012;19(2):306–309
2. Hanft SJ, Isaacson SR, Bruce JN. Stereotactic radiosurgery for pineal region tumors. Neurosurg Clin N Am 2011;22(3):413–420, ix
3. Dumrongpisutikul N, Intrapiromkul J, Yousem DM. Distinguishing between germinomas and pineal cell tumors on MR imaging. AJNR Am J Neuroradiol 2012;33(3):550–555
4. Márquez J, Rivero M. Pineal cysts. J Neurosurg Pediatr 2011;8(4):422, author reply 422
5. Idris Z, Ghani AR, Idris B, et al. Neuronavigation-guided endoscopic management of a pineal region tumour with obscured floor of the third ventricle: case report. Minim Invasive Neurosurg 2011;54(3):125–127
6. Harris LM, Davies NP, Wilson S, et al. Short echo time single voxel ^{1}H magnetic resonance spectroscopy in the diagnosis and characterisation of pineal tumours in children. Pediatr Blood Cancer 2011;57(6):972–977
7. Al-Holou WN, Terman SW, Kilburg C, et al. Prevalence and natural history of pineal cysts in adults. J Neurosurg 2011;115(6):1106–1114
8. Fèvre-Montange M, Vasiljevic A, Champier J, Jouvet A. Histopathology of tumors of the pineal region. Future Oncol 2010;6(5):791–809
9. Ellenbogen RG, Moores LE. Endoscopic management of a pineal and suprasellar germinoma with associated hydrocephalus: technical case report. Minim Invasive Neurosurg 1997;40(1):13–15
10. Evans RW, Peres MF. Headaches and pineal cysts. Headache 2010;50(4):666–668

11. Fujimaki T. Pineal tumors. Ryoikibetsu Shokogun Shirizu 2000;28(28 Pt 3):316–321
12. Allen J, Chacko J, Donahue B, et al. Diagnostic sensitivity of serum and lumbar CSF bHCG in newly diagnosed CNS germinoma. Pediatr Blood Cancer 2012;59(7):1180–1182
13. Parker JJ, Waziri A. Preoperative evaluation of pineal tumors. Neurosurg Clin N Am 2011;22(3):353–358, vii–viii
14. Novák Z, Chrastina J, Ríha I, Jancálek R. Neuroendoscopic biopsy of a brain tumor [in Czech]. Klin Onkol 2011;24(5): 348–355
15. Navas-Garcia M, Goig-Revert F, Villarejo-Ortega FJ, et al. Tumours in the pineal region in the paediatric age. Reports of 23 cases and a review of the literature [in Spanish]. Rev Neurol 2011;52(11):641–652
16. Hanada T, Oyoshi T, Hirano H, Arita K. Metastatic pineal tumors treated by neuroendoscopic surgery—two case reports. Neurol Med Chir (Tokyo) 2010;50(3):232–236
17. Pollack IF. Surgical options for pineal region tumors. World Neurosurg 2012;77(2):302–303
18. Morgenstern PF, Souweidane MM. Pineal region tumors: simultaneous endoscopic third ventriculostomy and tumor biopsy. World Neurosurg 2012 Feb 10. doi:pii: S1878-8750(12) 00153-2. 10.1016/j.wneu.2012.02.020. [Epub ahead of print]
19. Kaye AH, Leslie K. The sitting position for neurosurgery: yet another case series confirming safety. World Neurosurg 2012;77(1):42–43
20. Raza SM, Recinos PF, Avendano J, Adams H, Jallo GI, Quinones-Hinojosa A. Minimally invasive trans-portal resection of deep intracranial lesions. Minim Invasive Neurosurg 2011;54(1): 5–11
21. Poppen JL, Marino R Jr. Pinealomas and tumors of the posterior portion of the third ventricle. J Neurosurg 1968;28:357–364
22. Zhang HW, Zhang MS, Xia L, et al. Experiences of transcallosal-interforniceal approach for resection of the third ventrical and the pineal region tumors: report of 24 cases [in Chinese]. Zhonghua Wai Ke Za Zhi 2012;50(2):139–143
23. Stein BM. The infratentorial supracerebellar approach to pineal lesions. J Neurosurg 1971;35:197–202
24. Ture U. The transcallosal-tranforaminal approach to the third ventricle with regard to the venous variations in this region. Neurosurg 1997;87:706–715
25. Linstadt D, Wara WM, Edwards MS, Hudgins RJ, Sheline GE. Radiotherapy of primary intracranial germinomas: the case against routine craniospinal irradiation. Int J Radiat Oncol Biol Phys 1988;15(2):291–297
26. Edwards MS, Hudgins RJ, Wilson CB, Levin VA, Wara WM. Pineal region tumors in children. J Neurosurg 1988;68(5): 689–697
27. Han SJ, Clark AJ, Ivan ME, Parsa AT, Perry A. Pathology of pineal parenchymal tumors. Neurosurg Clin N Am 2011;22(3): 335–340, vii
28. Yianni J, Rowe J, Khandanpour N, et al. Stereotactic radiosurgery for pineal tumours. Br J Neurosurg 2012;26(3):361–366
29. Tate MC, Rutkowski MJ, Parsa AT. Contemporary management of pineoblastoma. Neurosurg Clin N Am 2011;22(3): 409–412, ix
30. del Valle R, Pérez M, Ortiz J, et al. Stereotactic noninvasive volume measurement compared with geometric measurement for indications and evaluation of gamma knife treatment. J Neurosurg 2005;102(Suppl):140–142
31. Kano H, Niranjan A, Kondziolka D, Flickinger JC, Lunsford D. Role of stereotactic radiosurgery in the management of pineal parenchymal tumors. Prog Neurol Surg 2009;23:44–58
32. Anisimov VN. Pineal gland, biorhythms and aging of an organism [in Russian]. Usp Fiziol Nauk 2008;39(4):40–65
33. Cardenas RJ, Javalkar V, Ezer H, Burnham J, Nanda A. Occipital interhemispheric transtentorial approach to the superior cerebellum. J Clin Neurosci 2011;18(1):128–130
34. Lekovic GP, Gonzalez LF, Shetter AG, et al. Role of gamma knife surgery in the management of pineal region tumors. Neurosurg Focus 2007;23(6):E12

14

The Role of Gross Total Resection in the Management of Pineal Region Tumors

Hani R. Malone, Victoria Ebiana, and Jeffrey N. Bruce

Tumors of the pineal region account for 0.4 to 1.0% of intracranial tumors in adults and 3.0 to 8.0% of brain tumors in children. Neoplastic lesions in this region are histologically diverse and can generally be divided into germ cell and non–germ cell derivatives. Most tumors are the result of displaced embryonic tissue, malignant transformation of pineal parenchymal cells, or transformation of surrounding astroglia. Initial management of patients with pineal region tumors should be directed at treating hydrocephalus and establishing a diagnosis. Preoperative evaluation should include high-resolution magnetic resonance imaging (MRI) with gadolinium, measurement of serum and cerebrospinal fluid (CSF) markers, cytologic examination of CSF, and evaluation of pituitary function if endocrine abnormalities are suspected.

The role of surgery in the management of pineal region tumors is influenced by the histological heterogeneity of these tumors and the favorable response of many lesions to evolving multimodality adjuvant therapies. In most cases, optimal management requires surgically secured tissue diagnosis. Maximal tumor resection is often pursued as a primary treatment modality or as a means of improving the efficacy of adjuvant therapy. Surgical outcome analyses for pineal tumors have largely been hindered by small sample size, retrospective study design, and controversial results regarding the importance of achieving gross total resection (GTR) for different tumor subtypes. Recent meta-analysis and population-based studies have furthered this debate without providing conclusive evidence regarding the role of GTR for all pineal tumor subtypes.

This chapter reviews current evidence and controversies associated with surgery for pineal region tumors and provides evidence-based recommendations for treatment, with special attention to the importance of gross total resection for different tumor subtypes.

■ Surgical History

Early attempts at radical resection of pineal region tumors, prior to the use of the operating microscope and sophisticated critical care, were mostly tragic. Although surgery to excise pineal region tumors was the original mainstay of treatment, these surgeries were as often as not fatal. Even the adept Cushing stated that he "never succeeded in exposing a pineal tumor sufficiently well to justify an attempt to remove it."[1] Dandy reported the first complete excision of a pineal tumor in 1921,[2] employing an interhemispheric, transcallosal (IHTC) approach, but later recanted in 1936, stating that it was not until "a decade [after his original paper] that the first pineal tumor was successfully extirpated [again by Dandy]." In the interim, Van Wagenen reported a subtotal resection of a pineal region tumor with a transcortical, transventricular approach in 1931.[3] Attempts to emulate the approaches described by Dandy and Van

Wagenen in the 1940s and 1950s resulted in unacceptable rates of morbidity and mortality described in several small clinical series.

These poor surgical outcomes coincided with reports of successful radiation therapy, particularly in Japan, where radiosensitive germinomas account for 60 to 70% of all pineal tumors. Prior to the 1970s, a treatment paradigm consisting of empirical radiation with shunting for hydrocephalus became routine treatment for pineal region tumors, with surgery reserved for nonresponders.[4,5] However, this approach resulted in ineffective and unnecessary whole-brain radiation to many patients with benign and low-grade lesions resistant to radiotherapy.

In 1971, two seminal papers from Stein, detailing the infratentorial supracerebellar approach[6] and Jamieson, detailing the occipital transtentorial approach,[7] established the safety and efficacy of pineal region surgery with the use of the operating microscope. Advances in microsurgical technique, coupled with the varying sensitivity of pineal lesions to radiotherapy, demanded that the role of radical surgery be reexamined. The renaissance of pineal region surgery that followed increased awareness of the heterogeneity of pineal pathology and emphasized the need for individualized therapy based on accurate histological diagnosis.

Extent of Resection

Numerous studies have shown a correlation between extent of resection and improved response to adjuvant therapy and survival for various pineal region tumor subtypes.[8–11] However, the potential morbidity associated with aggressive attempts at total resection has led some neurosurgeons to advocate a minimally invasive approach, consisting of stereotactic biopsy followed by appropriate multimodality adjuvant therapy.[12] The pathological diversity of pineal region tumors complicates the importance of extent of resection for neoplastic lesions in this region. In general, the literature supports aggressive tumor resection for benign/low-grade tumors because this can be curative. However, in high-grade and malignant lesions, the added benefit of aggressive resection is less clear and dependent on the variable efficacy of adjuvant chemotherapy and radiation for different tumor subtypes.

Unfortunately, the bulk of clinical data in the current literature related to surgical intervention is derived from retrospective analyses that often include cases performed over a decade ago. Furthermore, attempts to analyze the role of surgical resection are limited by small numbers of patients within each histological grouping, favorable long-term survival for many pineal region tumors resulting in insufficient follow-up, and evolving indications and treatment strategies for different tumor types. Accordingly, evidence for the role of gross total resection of pineal tumors must be examined according to tumor pathology.

■ Clinical Considerations

Pathology

Neoplastic transformation in the pineal region can lead to ependymomas, astrocytomas, choroid plexus papillomas, pineal parenchymal tumors, and meningiomas.[13–15] This diversity is a reflection of the normal cell types that reside in the pineal gland and adjacent structures. The pineal gland is composed of pineal parenchymal cells, astrocytes, and sympathetic neurons. Adjacent to the gland are ependymal cells lining the third ventricle, cells forming the choroid plexus, arachnoid cells forming the velum interpositum, and glial cells from the brainstem and thalamus. Additionally, primitive germ cell rests are frequently retained in midline structures like the pineal gland, resulting in the full complement of germ cell tumor subtypes, of which germinomas are the most common. The pineal region may also be the site of miscellaneous histological subtypes, including metastases, neuronal tumors, endothelial tumors, and lymphomas.

The diagnostic difficulties associated with pineal region lesions are complicated by the potential for mixed cell types as well as the full spectrum of anaplasia, ranging from benign to highly malignant.[16] Pineal region pathology is further complicated by the range of nonneoplastic lesions that can occur, including pineal cysts, vascular abnormalities, and infectious lesions.

Preoperative Evaluation

Standard preoperative evaluation for patients with pineal tumors includes high-resolution MRI with gadolinium enhancement and analysis of germ cell markers.[16] MRI provides critical anatomical information about the tumor's relationship to surrounding structures as well as the presence and severity of hydrocephalus. Although predictive of tumor histology, radiographic data are not sufficient to distinguish histological subtypes.

The germ cell markers α-fetoprotein and β-human chorionic gonadotropin (β-HCG) should be measured in the CSF and serum in all patients. The presence of one or both markers is pathognomonic for a malignant germ cell tumor.[8] When markers are elevated, a tissue diagnosis is not necessary, and patients should be treated with radiation and chemotherapy.[17] The value of surgical resection to improve the prognosis or outcome for this group of patients is suggestive but inconclusive (see Germ Cell Tumors later in the chapter).

Treating Hydrocephalus

Patients with pineal region tumors often present with obstructive hydrocephalus from compression of the cerebral aqueduct. The optimal surgical strategy for treating hydrocephalus in these patients involves endoscopic third ventriculostomy.[16,18] This procedure is safe, highly effective, and preferred over ventriculoperitoneal shunting, which is associated with higher rates of infection and metastasis, as well as malfunction, symptomatic overshunting, and subdural hematoma. Occasionally, patients with mild hydrocephalus from a well-encapsulated tumor can be managed with a simple ventricular drain placed prior to tumor resection.

■ Surgical Considerations

Advances in surgical technique and neuroanesthesia have significantly lowered the morbidity and mortality associated with pineal region surgery. In patients for whom primary surgical resection is the best therapeutic and diagnostic option, several well-described approaches are currently in use. In general, surgical approaches to the pineal region can be categorized as supratentorial or infratentorial. Supratentorial approaches include the parietal-interhemispheric approach described by Dandy[19] and the occipital-transtentorial approach originally described by Horrax and later modified by Poppen.[20] The infratentorial approach is through a supracerebellar corridor.[6]

Surgical Objectives

The primary objective of surgical management of pineal region tumors is the establishment of an accurate histological diagnosis.[13,15,16,21–27] Given the variety of histological subtypes and the nuances of mixed tumor pathologies, diagnostic accuracy is essential for making optimal management decisions regarding adjuvant therapy, for establishing prognosis, and for planning long-term follow-up. A secondary surgical objective is tumor debulking, with the relative benefits of maximal tumor removal.[8,9,11,15,16,23,28–32] Gross total resection has been clearly established as the optimal therapy for benign tumors that are treated surgically. However, the benefit of aggressive attempts for complete surgical removal of malignant lesions remains controversial.

Biopsy versus Open Resection

The first surgical decision involves choosing between stereotactic biopsy or an "open" microsurgical procedure. Strong advocates can be found for either strategy; however, each technique is most effective when used for specific indications rather than exclusively for all tumors in the pineal region. Open resection facilitates the maximal removal of tumor volume, offering diagnostic accuracy and, in many cases, improved prognosis. Stereotactic biopsy is less invasive and is generally considered to have a lower risk of complications. Advocates of "minimally invasive" management favor stereotactic biopsy followed by radiosurgery as the primary strategy for pineal tumors.[12] Outcomes from this strategy are provocative yet inconclusive because they have not withstood sufficient tests of time and patient numbers.

The pineal region is considered by many to be among the most hazardous areas of the brain to biopsy because of potential bleeding from multiple sources, including the deep venous system, the choroidal vessels, and the multiple pial surfaces that must be traversed during biopsy. The increased vascularity of many malignant pineal region tumors is an added risk.[33,34] The consequences of bleeding in the pineal region are magnified by the lack of tissue turgor provided by adjacent ventricular and cisternal surfaces, limiting the brain's innate ability to tamponade even minor bleeding. Stereotactic biopsy also provides limited tissue sampling, which can be problematic for even experienced neuropathologists.[23,35] A recent review of all major series reporting stereotactic biopsy for pineal region lesions revealed a mean diagnostic yield of 94%.[36]

In addition to improved diagnostic accuracy, microsurgical tumor resection has important clinical implications. In benign pineal lesions, surgical resection clearly provides the best opportunity for long-term recurrence-free survival.[15,26,31,37] Although the clinical impact of maximal tumor resection in malignant tumors remains controversial, numerous reports have correlated extent of tumor resection with improved response to adjuvant therapy and increased survival.[8,10,11,29,30,38,39] Additional benefits of aggressive tumor resection include the potential to control hydrocephalus without a second procedure and reduced risk of postoperative hemorrhage into the residual tumor bed.

Stereotactic Radiosurgery

Stereotactic radiosurgery (SRS) serves as an alternative to whole-brain radiation for radiosensitive malignant pineal region tumors and for local control of benign lesions.[12,40–42] Clinical outcomes following SRS for pineal region tumors are summarized in **Table 14.1**. For

Table 14.1 Series reporting stereotactic radiosurgery for pineal region tumors

Study	Cases	Adjuvant cases	Modality	Tumor histology	Mean follow-up	CR (%)	PR (%)	NC (%)	PG (%)	Death during follow-up (%)
Manera et al 1996[43]	11	NA	GKRS	All	12.3 (mo)	NA	NA	NA	0	0
Raco et al 2000[81]	11	NA	LINAC	All	NA	36	9	0	5	45
Kobayashi et al 2001[40]	33	11	GKRS	All	23.3	24	42	0	24	21
Hasegawa et al 2002[12]	16	13	GKRS	PPT	61	29	50	6	0	5
Hasegawa et al 2003[42]	4	NA	GKRS	NGGCT	25	0	25	25	25	25
Reyns et al 2006[82]	13	NA	GKRS	PPT	34	42	50	17	8	17
Lekovic et al 2007[83]	17	NA	GKRS	All	31	13	44	31	13	31
Kano et al 2009[84]	20	NA	GKRS	PPT	54.1	26	47	11	11	30

Abbreviations: CR, complete response; GKRS, gamma knife radiosurgery; NA, not available; NC, no change; NGGCT, nongerminomatous germ cell tumors; PG, progression; PPT, pineal parenchymal tumors; PR, partial response.

malignant pineal parenchymal tumors, SRS alone does not appear to provide adequate regional control or increase overall survival. With the exception of Manera et al,[43] all authors report treatment failures. For pineocytomas, patients receiving SRS have fared well, reflecting the benign nature of these lesions; however, the reporting of several pineocytoma treatment failures is cause for concern.[12]

Over all, SRS results parallel the outcomes of fractionated radiation, and some authors have advocated using radiosurgery in place of conventional radiotherapy to limit the morbidity associated with whole-brain radiation, particularly in children.[28,43] Existing studies have shown that SRS is safe in the pineal region and effective for some tumors; however, the evidence is limited by small sample size, the wide range of pathologies treated, and insufficient follow-up.

■ Surgical Procedures

Stereotactic Biopsy

Advances in stereotactic technology and navigation systems have improved the precision and safety of stereotactic biopsy acquisition. Frame-based image guidance is generally preferred given its widespread availability, ease of use, and accuracy. Associated planning software that facilitates viewing of the entire trajectory helps minimize the number of ventricular or cisternal surfaces that must be traversed (**Fig. 14.1**). The most common trajectory is via an anterolateral–superior approach, originating anterior to the coronal suture and lateral to the midpupillary line.[36] This trajectory traverses the frontal lobe such that optimal entry points and targets should be chosen to minimize pathways through ependymal surfaces and adjacent vasculature. Alternatively, a posterolateral-superior approach through a parieto-occipital junction entry point can be utilized, preferably for tumors with lateral extension.

Local anesthesia with mild sedation is usually sufficient and minimizes morbidity. Multiple serial biopsy specimens are desirable, but the decision to obtain additional specimens depends on the clinical situation and must take into account the reliability of the frozen specimen diagnosis, the risk of bleeding, and the likelihood of tumor heterogeneity. Although stereotactic biopsy in the pineal region is often associated with higher complication rates than those in other areas of the brain, results by experienced neurosurgeons have validated its use on a routine basis. Large consecutive series examining complication rates from intracranial stereotactic biopsies conducted by experienced neurosurgeons report no difference in complication rate between pineal

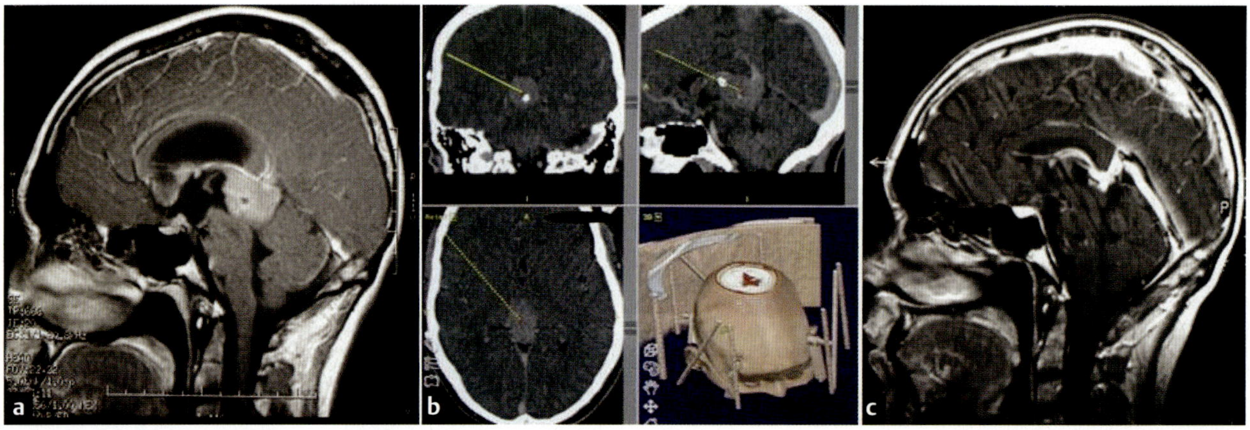

Fig. 14.1 **(a)** A disseminated tumor involving the third ventricle at the foramen of Monro, infundibulum, and pineal region in a young male patient. Despite negative serum markers, suspicion remained high that the lesion was a radiosensitive germinoma. **(b)** This diagnosis was histologically confirmed following frame-based stereotactic needle biopsy. **(c)** The germinoma was subsequently treated successfully with radiation therapy.

region biopsies and biopsies of other regions of the brain.[44,45] Perioperative mortality following stereotactic pineal region biopsies ranges from 0 to 2%, with a permanent major morbidity of 0 to 1.2% and transient minor morbidity of 7.0 to 8.4%.[22,34,46,47]

Microsurgery

Open microsurgical resection has three roles in the management of pineal region tumors: optimal management of benign lesions, cytoreduction prior to adjuvant chemotherapy/radiation for malignant lesions, and "second-look" surgery to remove residual tumor following chemotherapy.[16,28] Additional advantages of surgery include accurate diagnosis and correction of obstructive hydrocephalus without the need for CSF diversion. The importance of gross total resection is still being defined for many types of pineal region tumors, but it is generally accepted to be the treatment of choice for benign and low-grade pineal lesions, including meningiomas, pineocytomas, epidermoids, and mature teratomas.[14] With the exception of germinomas, malignant pineal region tumors respond poorly to radiation, and maximum surgical resection, while not curative, reduces tumor burden and may improve response to adjuvant therapy.[48,49]

Given the accepted benefit of maximal tumor removal with open surgery, current controversy centers on the degree of morbidity tolerable to achieve this goal. Microsurgical approaches to the pineal region have evolved to the extent that favorable results can be expected by experienced microsurgeons. Nevertheless, the approaches are not trivial, and optimal results require a degree of planning, judgment, and experience beyond what is necessary for most intracranial tumor operations. Results of pineal surgery vary significantly with surgical expertise, and debates about optimal procedures must be framed in this context.[15]

■ Surgical Approach

Several commonly used operative approaches to the pineal region are available, consisting of variations of either the supracerebellar–infratentorial (SCIT) approach or the occipital–transtentorial (OTT) approach.[6,16] The optimal approach for a specific patient depends on the anatomical features of the tumor. The SCIT approach is the most widely used and has the benefit of providing a direct midline approach through a natural corridor between the dorsal cerebellum and the tentorium. This approach facilitates the dissection of the tumor from its attachment along the velum interpositum and deep venous system, which often represents the most difficult aspect of surgical removal (**Fig. 14.2**). Supratentorial approaches, including the OTT and the transcallosal–interhemispheric approaches, provide wider exposure than the SCIT approach and are often preferable for tumors extending superiorly or laterally (**Fig. 14.3**). However, supratentorial approaches have the disadvantage of exposing the deep venous system overlying the tumor, forcing the surgeon to work around these vessels to avoid injury.

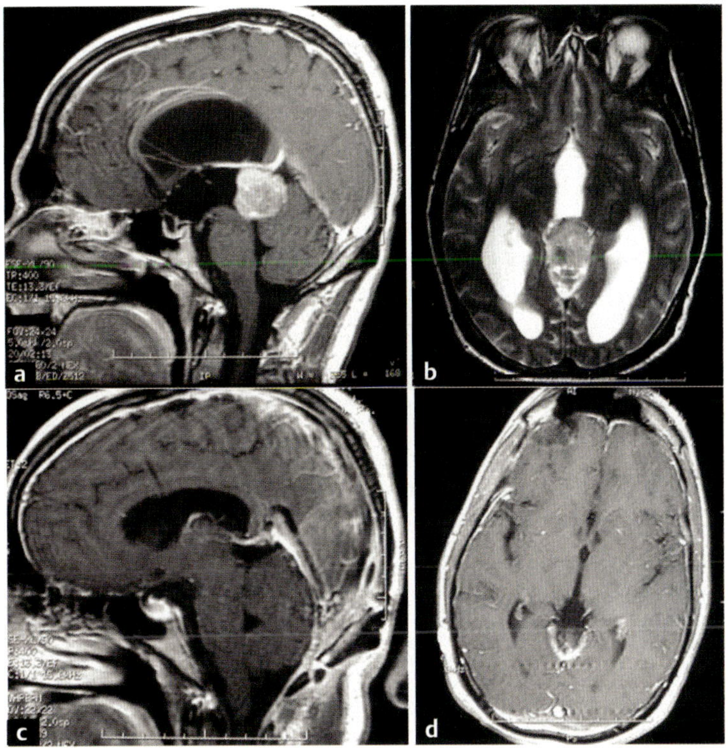

Fig. 14.2 Preoperative imaging **(a,b)** of a benign enhancing pineal tumor. Gross total resection was achieved **(c,d)** via the supracerebellar infratentorial approach.

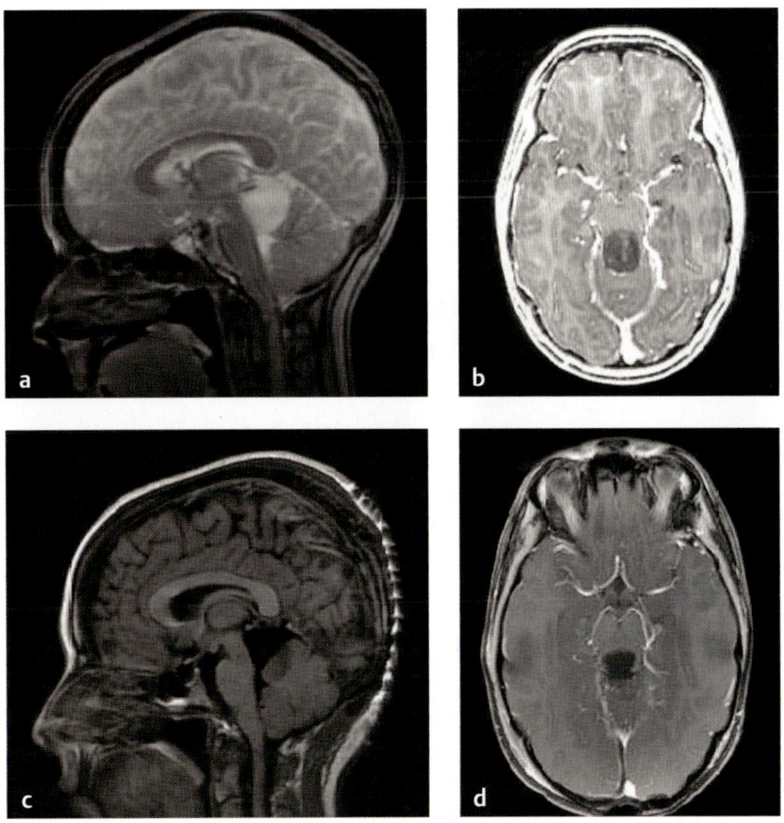

Fig. 14.3 Preoperative magnetic resonance imaging **(a,b)** of a nonenhancing low-grade glioma involving the dorsal midbrain. The inferior extension of this tumor makes complete resection via the supracerebellar infratentorial approach challenging. In this case, the surgical trajectory achieved via the occipital transtentorial approach allowed for safe gross total resection **(c,d)**.

Surgical Outcomes

Relatively low morbidity and mortality from patients operated on in the microsurgical era suggest that surgical resection is the preferred strategy for most pineal region tumors (**Table 14.2**).[13,27,28,50] Large microsurgical series report major surgical morbidity rates of 3 to 6.8% following radical resection, and minor morbidity rates of 3 to 28%.[14] Of note, series with higher rates of morbidity include many cases from over a quarter century ago. Perioperative deaths are rare in the modern era, with a mortality rate of ~ 1.8% in cases reported since 1990.[13,27,28,50]

The most serious complications from pineal surgery involve postoperative hemorrhage, which may occur in a delayed fashion and is more common with malignant and vascular tumors that have been incompletely resected.[14,16,28] Brainstem manipulation and cerebellar retraction intraoperatively can lead to extraocular movement dysfunction, pupillary abnormalities, and ataxia. Fortunately, these deficits tend to be transient. Increased severity and incidence of complications are correlated with prior radiation, invasive/malignant tumors, and the presence of preoperative symptoms.[16,28]

Endoscopy

The morbidity and mortality associated with endoscopic surgery in the pineal region have not been well established in large studies. By virtue of their vascularity, many pineal tumors present hemostatic difficulties that limit endoscopic resection to carefully selected patients. Nevertheless, small case series have shown that both endoscopic biopsy and

Table 14.2 Modern series reporting results of microsurgery for pineal region tumors utilizing different surgical approaches

Study	Cases	Approach	Population	Pathology	GTR (%)	Mortality (%)	Major morbidity (%)	Minor morbidity (%)
Hoffman et al 1983[86]	61	TC/SCIT	Peds	All	NA	20[a]	NA	NA
Neuwelt 1985[25]	13	OTT	Adult/Peds	All	60	0	0	20
Lapras et al 1987[26]	86	TC/OTT	Adult/Peds	All	65	5.8[b]	5.80	28
Edwards et al 1988[23]	36	TT/OTT/SCIT	Peds	All	NA	0	3.30	3.30
Pluchino et al 1989[87]	40	SCIT	Adult/Peds	All	25	5	NA	NA
Luo et al 1989[88]	64	OTT	Adult/Peds	All	21	10	NA	NA
Vaquero et al 1992[50]	29	TC/SCIT/OTT	Adult/Peds	All	NA	11	NA	NA
Herrmann et al 1990[89]	49	IHTC/SCIT	Adult/Peds	All	NA	8	NA	NA
Bruce, Stein 1995[15]	160	SCIT/TC/OTT	Adult/Peds	All	45	4	3	19
Chandy, Damaraju 1998[90]	48	SCIT/OTT	Adult/Peds	"Benign lesions"	55	0	NA	NA
Kang et al 1998[91]	16	OTT/SCIT/TC	Adult/Peds	All	37.50	0	0	19
Shin et al 1998[92]	21	OTT	Adult/Peds	All	54.50	0	0	5
Konovalov, Pitskhelauri 2003[27]	201	OTT (54%) SCIT (34%)	Adult/Peds	All	58	10[c]	NA	> 20
Bruce 2004[16]	81	SCIT/TC/OTT	Adult/Peds	All	47	1	2	NA
Jan 2011[93]	150	TCIF	Peds	All	86	0	NA	NA

Abbreviations: GTR, % of patients with gross total resection; IHTC, interhemispheric transcallosal; NA, not available; OTT, occipital–transtentorial; SCIT, supracerebellar–infratentorial; TC, transcallosal; TCIF, transcallosal interforniceal.

[a] All except one mortality prior to 1975.

[b] Combined major morbidity/mortality reduced to 2.8% in last 40 patients.

[c] Mortality rate of 1.8% in the 168 resections after 1990.

endoscopic resection of pineal tumors can be safe and effective (**Table 14.3**).[51–54] In regard to pineal region biopsy, Pople and colleagues[54] reported the largest consecutive series of patients consistently managed endoscopically. Diagnostic yield of biopsy was 94% in 34 patients, but 74% required a second operation for CSF diversion. More recent retrospective studies by Uschold et al[55] and Broggi et al[56] have reported promising results related to the safety and efficacy of endoscopically assisted microsurgical resection of pineal tumors.[55,56] Although limited by small sample size (9 and 15 patients), both studies indicate that use of the endoscope, combined with an open craniotomy approach, increases the ability of neurosurgeons to achieve gross total resection of pineal region tumors without increased morbidity.

■ The Importance of Gross Total Resection by Tumor Subtype

An analysis of the importance of gross total resection for pineal tumors is most instructive in the context of specific histopathology. In general, complete resection confers clear benefit for tumors that are benign or low grade. However, the importance of extent of resection on pineal tumors of intermediate and malignant grades remains controversial. Attempts to more clearly delineate the importance of maximal surgical resection in the treatment of these lesions are hindered by (1) the continued evolution of indications and treatment strategies for various pineal tumor types, (2) favorable long-term survival for most pineal tumors and insufficient follow-up in most studies, (3) inaccuracies in assessing degree of resection, (4) small numbers of patients within specific histologic subtypes, (5) historical inaccuracies in establishing definitive diagnoses, and (6) retrospective study design.

Benign Pineal Region Tumors: Meningiomas, Epidermoids, Teratomas, and Pineal Cysts

Approximately one third of pineal region tumors are benign, including meningiomas, epidermoids, teratomas, and pineal cysts.[22,28,31] Gross total resection of these lesions invariably results in long-term remission and is potentially curative. In addition, patients with benign pathology have fewer operative complications.[57,58] Pineal cysts are anatomical variants of the pineal gland and can be managed expectantly when stable and asymptomatic. Pineal cysts that demonstrate progression on serial imaging or cause obstructive hydrocephalus should be removed surgically.[57]

Germinomas

Germinomas are the most common tumor in the pineal region. Fortunately, these tumors are highly radiosensitive with long-term survival rates as high as 80 to 90% when adequate doses of radiation (> 5,500 cGy) are given to the tumor and surrounding ventricles.[59,60] Given the cognitive and endocrine morbidity associated with whole-brain radiation, especially in pediatric patients, radiosurgery and chemotherapy have been investigated as promising alternatives. Platinum-based chemotherapy regimens have been shown to be particularly effective, achieving results

Table 14.3 Series reporting endoscopic biopsy and endoscopic resection of pineal region tumors

Study	Cases	Diagnostic (%)	Mortality (%)	MM (%)	TMM (%)	VP shunt (%)
Endoscopic biopsy						
Ferrer et al 1997[51]	4	75	0	25	50	25
Oi et al 2001[52]	6	100	0	0	0	17
Gangemi et al 2001[53]	5	100	0	0	20	NA
Pople et al 2001[54]	34	94	0	2.9	2.9	74
Endoscopic resection						
Broggi et al 2010[56]	15	100	0	7	60	100
Uschold et al 2011[55]	9	100	0	0	11.1	88.9
Sood et al 2011[85]	2	100	0	0	NA	100

Abbreviations: GTR, gross total resection; MM, major morbidity; NA, not available; TMM, transient minor morbidity; VP, ventriculoperitoneal.

comparable to those of whole-brain radiation.[61,62] Ongoing trials are evaluating SRS and chemotherapy as a first-line therapy, reserving whole-brain radiation for nonresponders. However, because an accurate diagnosis of germinoma cannot be made from radiographic or serological data, surgical biopsy remains a vital role in diagnosis and treatment. Multimodality therapy for germinoma without surgical biopsy and histological diagnosis is considerably less effective because many presumed germinomas are actually radioresistant teratomas or mixed tumors with nongerminomatous components.

The proven success of adjuvant therapy for germinomas has rendered questions related to the importance of gross total resection less clinically salient for these lesions. Studies that have examined the effect of surgical debulking for germinomas have shown conflicting results. Advocates of limited resection with adjuvant therapy cite a clinical series reported by Sawamura and colleagues,[63] in which 29 patients with intracranial germinomas had a 100% survival rate, regardless of degree of resection. However, the relatively short mean follow-up of 42 months in this study may have concealed any survival advantage offered by greater extent of resection. Indeed, the International CNS Germ Cell Tumor Study observed a non–statistically significant trend toward improved survival in patients who underwent radical resection and chemotherapy versus those who underwent chemotherapy alone.[8] Importantly, patients were not randomized to treatment arms in this study, and thus the survival benefit seen in the radical resection group may be secondary to favorable biological tumor characteristics associated with resectability.

Nongerminomatous Germ Cell Tumors

Nongerminomatous germ cell tumors (NGGCTs), including embryonal cell carcinomas, endodermal sinus tumors, and choriocarcinomas, exhibit highly aggressive behavior. When embryonal cell carcinomas differentiate, they follow either the yolk sac pathway to become endodermal sinus tumors or the trophoblast differentiation pathway to form choriocarcinomas. These malignant lesions are generally diagnosed on the basis of elevated markers in the serum and CSF (α-fetoprotein for endodermal sinus tumors and β-HCG for choriocarcinomas), making biopsy unnecessary in most cases, although each can occur without elevated markers.

Accurate assessments of the natural history of NGGCTs are limited by the rarity of these lesions and their propensity toward mixed pathology. Accordingly, consensus regarding the optimal treatment algorithm for these tumors remains elusive. Nongerminomatous germ cell tumors are radiosensitive, and the best results appear to be achieved when patients receive both radiation and chemotherapy. Clinical trials have investigated radical surgery as a primary intervention followed by adjuvant chemotherapy and radiation,[64–66] or in a second-look capacity for persistent lesions on MRI following radiation and chemotherapy and the normalization of CSF markers.[61,62,67]

Several studies have indicated the beneficial effects of primary radical resection, including one report with statistical significance.[29] However, in most reports the benefits of maximal resection as a primary treatment have either been anecdotal or not statistically significant.[8,11] Second-look trials appear to have identified the most effective use of surgical resection for NGGCTs.[68,69] In the surgical arms of these studies, radical resection is pursued when a residual mass is present following radiation and chemotherapy. Using this strategy, 5-year survival rates of 90% have been achieved, a remarkable improvement from the less than 2-year median survival reported in the early 1990s.[15,28,67]

Pineal Region Astrocytomas

These exceedingly rare tumors arise from astrocytes within the pineal gland, brainstem, or thalamus. The histology of these tumors is identical to that of astrocytomas in other CNS locations, ranging from the relatively benign grade I lesions (pilocytic astrocytoma) to highly malignant glioblastoma. Astrocytomas in the pineal region are usually cystic, and gross total resection is often achievable, as well as potentially curative.[28,70] The role of surgery is less clearly defined in the management of astrocytomas stemming from the quadrigeminal plate because there is some evidence that these tumors often follow an indolent natural history.[71]

Pineal Parenchymal Tumors

Pineal parenchymal tumors exist along a spectrum of malignancy ranging from benign pineocytomas to aggressive pineoblastomas. Treatment paradigms vary according to tumor grade, as does the importance of maximal surgical resection. Patient age also has an important impact on tumor behavior, even in histologically similar pineal parenchymal tumors. As with other tumors in the pineal region, accurate tissue diagnosis is essential before initiating therapy.

Pineocytoma

Pineocytomas are slow-growing, benign tumors that are best treated with gross total resection. In a recent meta-analysis, Clark and colleagues demonstrated that gross total resection was superior to subtotal resection, as well as subtotal resection with adjuvant radiation, in the treatment of pineocytomas.[72,73] Exceptions to this rule may be pediatric cases of pineocytoma, which may behave more aggressively. However, in adults, surgical resection with or without radiation therapy is associated with complete long-term remission.[30,50]

Pineoblastoma

Pineoblastomas are aggressive tumors that are prone to metastasis and are histologically identical to primitive neuroectodermal tumors (PNETs). Similar to other PNETs, pineoblastomas carry a much worse prognosis in the pediatric population, leading many to evaluate pediatric and adult pineoblastomas as separate entities. Although some authors have advocated treatment of pediatric pineoblastoma with radiation alone, most neurosurgeons pursue a course of treatment similar to that for more common PNETs, whose prognosis is closely tied to extent of resection.[74] Clinical trials with both pineal and nonpineal PNETs have advocated gross total resection in pediatric patients and have emphasized the development of chemotherapy regimens to reduce effective doses of radiation in children.[38,75–78]

The benefit of gross total resection in the treatment of adult patients with pineoblastoma remains controversial (**Table 14.4**). Despite the aggressive nature of these lesions, long-term remission is not unusual, and aggressive surgical resection has been shown to be beneficial in many studies. In a multicenter, retrospective review of 101 cases by Lutterbach and colleagues, 56 patients received surgery followed by radiation and/or chemotherapy and 44 were treated primarily with radiotherapy after diagnostic biopsy.[10] Although tumor control was achieved in numerous cases using both strategies, patients undergoing surgery were twice as likely to be tumor free as patients who received radiation alone. Although the study did not analyze extent of resection directly, the absence of residual tumor following treatment resulted in 100% 10-year survival.

Lee and colleagues similarly found gross total resection to be an important predictor of survival in their review of 39 adult patients with pineoblastoma from the Brain Tumor Registry of Japan (BTRJ).[47] In this study, extent of resection was stratified into six groups—0% (biopsy), 1 to 49%, 50 to 74%, 75 to 94%, 95 to 99%, and 100% (gross total resection)—with a median surgical resection of 75 to 94% and median survival from diagnosis of 25.7 months. In the final

Table 14.4 Retrospective cohort studies, case series, and a recent meta-analysis have produced conflicting reports regarding the potential survival benefit conferred by aggressive resection

Level of evidence	Study	Conclusion
Level I	None	
Level II	None	
Level III	[a]Fauchon et al 2000[24]	No value in increased extent of resection in pineal parenchymal tumors
	[a]Lutterbach et al 2002[10]	Residual disease carries negative prognostic value in pineal parenchymal tumors
	[a]Al-Hussaini et al 2009[94]	No effect of extent of resection on survival in pineal parenchymal tumors
	[a]Tate et al 2012[80]	Improved survival with increased extent of resection in pineoblastoma
Level IV	Vaquero et al 1990[50]	Surgical resection associated with long-term remission in pineocytomas
	[a]Lee et al 2005[47]	Craniospinal irradiation greater than 40 Gy and gross total resection are associated with increased survival in pineoblastoma
	[b]Gilheeney et al 2008[95]	Correlation between gross total resection, craniospinal irradiation, multiagent chemotherapy, and increased survival in pediatric pineoblastoma
	[a]Clark et al 2010[72]	Gross total resection improves tumor control more than subtotal resection with radiation for pineocytomas
	Broggi et al 2010[56]	Use of endoscope increases rate of gross total resection, which may extend survival and obviate need for adjuvant radiotherapy

[a]Pineal parenchymal tumors.
[b]Pediatric population.

Note: None of these studies offers class I or II evidence.

multivariate model, radiotherapy and gross total resection were the only factors associated with improved survival. No patient who received gross total resection ($n = 5$) died during follow-up, a period ranging from 21.7 to 107.5 months in this cohort.[47]

These findings do not support earlier work done by Fauchon and colleagues,[24] who collected clinical data from 12 different centers across Europe. In this study, 76 consecutive adult patients treated for histologically confirmed pineoblastoma were retrospectively identified. Final multivariate analysis confirmed histology and tumor volume to be significant independent prognostic factors, but extent of surgery had no clear influence on survival.[24] Recent analysis of the Surveillance, Epidemiology, and End Results (SEER) cancer registry by Selvanathan and colleagues supports this position.[79] Following multivariate analysis, only age at diagnosis and localized disease emerged as important prognostic factors, and extent of resection was not found to be a significant predictor of outcome. Of note, the SEER database has limited information on tumor size, extent of resection, dose and type of radiotherapy, and use of chemotherapy. Furthermore, there were no data available on time to tumor recurrences, performance status, complications, or comorbidity, and an independent pathologist could not confirm the diagnosis of pineoblastoma.

The most extensive dataset regarding the importance of gross total resection in the treatment of adult pineoblastoma comes from a recent meta-analysis by Tate and colleagues.[80] The authors performed an exhaustive review of 109 studies in the literature. Two hundred ninety-nine patients met inclusion criteria, making this study more than three times larger than any preexisting analysis of pineoblastoma surgical outcomes. Multivariate analysis indicated that not achieving gross total resection markedly worsened patient survival, with hazard ratios of 6.47 and 9.27 for subtotal resection and debulking, respectively. Importantly, a graded increase in survival was observed with increasing degrees of resection (5-year survival rate: 84% for patients who underwent gross total resection, 53% for patients who underwent subtotal resection, 29% for patients who underwent debulking), leading the authors to emphasize the importance of aggressive surgical resection in the treatment of pineoblastoma.

The disparate conclusions detailed in this chapter highlight the need for higher-level evidence addressing the benefit of gross total resection in pineoblastoma. Although aggressive resection appears to result in improved tumor control and survival, the existing evidence is not strong enough to make a Level 1A recommendation.

■ Summary and Conclusions

The pineal region harbors a histologically diverse set of tumor subtypes. Optimal therapeutic strategies vary with tumor type, making accurate diagnosis the

Expert Recommendations

1. In general, gross total resection confers clear benefit for benign or low-grade tumors; the importance of extent of resection of intermediate and malignant grade tumors remains controversial.
2. Gross total resection of benign pineal region tumors (meningiomas, epidermoids, teratomas and pineal cyts) is associated with long-term remission and is potentially curative (Grade 1C Recommendation, Level II–IV Evidence).
3. Due to the radiosensitive nature, the role of surgery in germinomas is limited to biopsy for histological diagnosis. Therapy without tissue diagnosis is considerably less effective because a presumed germinoma might be a radiosensitive tumor of another histology (Grade 1C, Level II/III Evidence).
4. The role of surgery in the management of nongerminomatous germ cell tumors (NGGCTs) is limited by the paucity of accurate information of their natural history. The potential benefit of radical resection is confounded by anecdotal data or studies demonstrating benefit without statistical significant. Several studies indicate a benefit for radical resection (Grade 1C Recommendation, Level II–IV Evidence).
5. Gross total resection is superior to subtotal resection in the management of pineocytomas (Grade 1C Recommendation, Level II/III Evidence).
6. There is conflicting data regarding the role of resection with pineoblastomas; this is a result of the relative rarity of these tumors and the limitations of the studies published to date. There is data to suggest that resection is associated with improved survival (Grade 2C Recommendation, Level II/III Evidence).

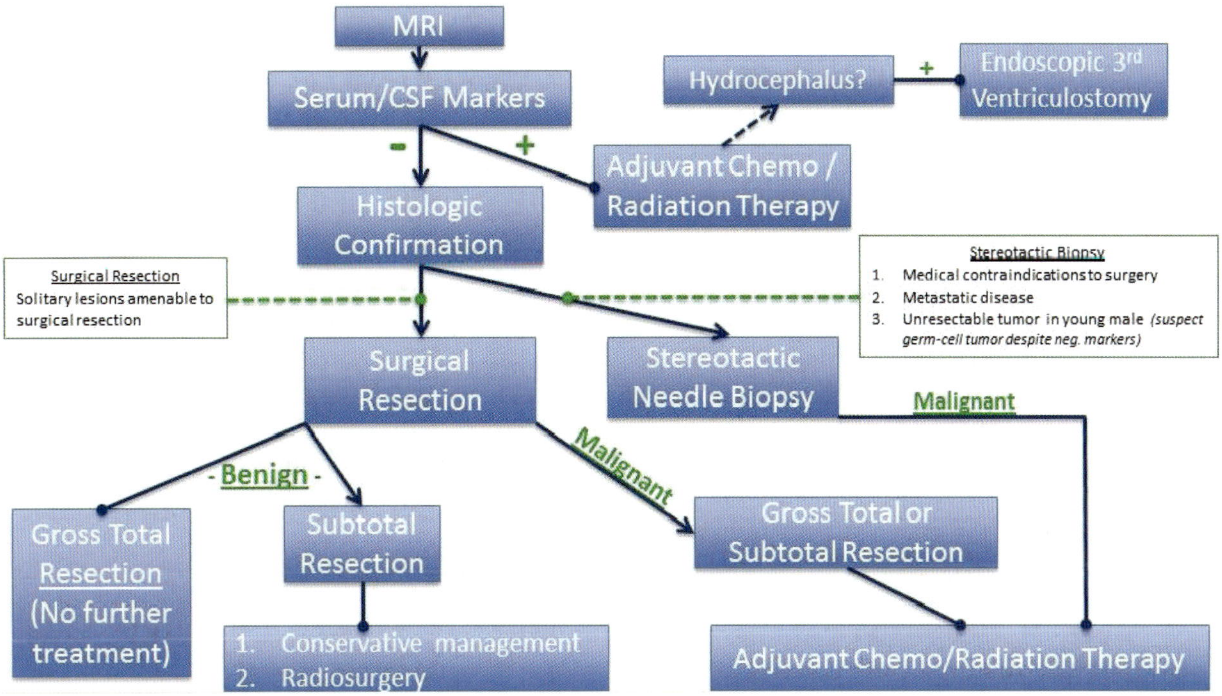

Fig. 14.4 The pineal region is host to a pathologically diverse set of neoplastic lesions along a spectrum of malignancy with varying sensitivity to adjuvant therapies. Accordingly, surgical strategy and the importance of gross total resection (GTR) differ considerably according to tumor subtype. The authors support obtaining tissue for accurate diagnosis in all pineal region tumors. In rare instances, when the anatomy of a tumor or the medical condition of the patient increases the morbidity associated with open surgery, a stereotactic needle biopsy may be performed to obtain tissue. In all other cases, an attempt at maximal surgical resection should be made. For benign lesions, GTR is generally curative. For malignant lesions, no Level I or II evidence exists supporting the clinical importance of GTR. However, recent meta-analysis of smaller clinical series suggests that maximal surgical resection confers a survival benefit for both benign and malignant lesions, including pineoblastoma.

foundation of appropriate management decisions. As an initial step, surgical intervention by either stereotactic biopsy or open surgery is necessary to obtain tissue for pathological examination. The further benefit of aggressive surgical resection is clearly defined for some tumors but is less evident for others. For pineal tumors that are benign or low grade, complete surgical resection is generally achievable and should be considered the standard of care, with excellent long-term recurrence-free survival. The benefit of maximal surgical resection for malignant pineal region tumors is less clearly defined and must be weighed against the potential morbidity of more aggressive surgical goals (**Fig. 14.4**). Retrospective cohort studies, case series, and meta-analyses have correlated degree of tumor removal with improved outcome for high-grade pineal lesions. However, these findings are not consistent across the literature, and no class I or II evidence exists. The rarity and vast histological diversity of tumors in the pineal region have prevented the proper conduction of randomized, controlled trials to date.

The authors are of the opinion that aggressive surgical resection is beneficial in all pineal region tumors (benign and malignant) that are not exquisitely sensitive to adjuvant therapy, provided that the neurosurgeon can achieve such a resection with minimal morbidity. The proper application of emerging endoscopic techniques may enhance the ability of neurosurgeons trained in this discipline to more fully excise pineal region tumors without increasing surgical morbidity, but the endoscopic approach is probably limited to carefully selected patients. Advances in neuroanesthesia and postoperative intensive care unit care have also reduced surgical morbidity and justify increasingly aggressive approaches. Nevertheless, surgery in the pineal region can be technically challenging, and advanced judgment and expertise are necessary to achieve rates of success sufficient to justify aggressive management.

■ References

1. Cushing H. Intracranial Tumors: Notes Upon a Series of Two Thousand Verified Cases with Surgical Mortality Pertaining Thereto. Charles C Thomas; 1932
2. Dandy W. An operation for the removal of pineal tumors. Surg Gynecol Obstet 1921;33:113–119
3. Van Wagenen W. A surgical approach for removal of certain pineal tumors: report of a case. Surg Gynecol Obstet 1931;53:216–220
4. Jenkin RD, Simpson WJ, Keen CW. Pineal and suprasellar germinomas: results of radiation treatment. J Neurosurg 1978;48(1):99–107
5. Marsh WR, Laws ER Jr. Shunting and irradiation of pineal tumors. Clin Neurosurg 1985;32:384–396
6. Stein BM. The infratentorial supracerebellar approach to pineal lesions. J Neurosurg 1971;35(2):197–202
7. Jamieson KG. Excision of pineal tumors. J Neurosurg 1971;35(5):550–553
8. Weiner HL, Finlay JL. Surgery in the management of primary intracranial germ cell tumors. Childs Nerv Syst 1999;15(11-12):770–773
9. Matsutani M. Pineal germ cell tumors. Prog Neurol Surg 2009;23:76–85
10. Lutterbach J, Fauchon F, Schild SE, et al. Malignant pineal parenchymal tumors in adult patients: patterns of care and prognostic factors. Neurosurgery 2002;51(1):44–55
11. Matsutani M, Sano K, Takakura K, et al. Primary intracranial germ cell tumors: a clinical analysis of 153 histologically verified cases. J Neurosurg 1997;86(3):446–455
12. Hasegawa T, Kondziolka D, Hadjipanayis CG, Flickinger JC, Lunsford LD. The role of radiosurgery for the treatment of pineal parenchymal tumors. Neurosurgery 2002;51(4):880–889
13. Bruce JN, Stein BM. Pineal tumors. Neurosurg Clin N Am 1990;1(1):123–138
14. Kennedy BC, Bruce JN. Surgical approaches to the pineal region. Neurosurg Clin N Am 2011;22(3):367–380, viii
15. Bruce JN, Stein BM. Surgical management of pineal region tumors. Acta Neurochir (Wien) 1995;134(3-4):130–135
16. Bruce JN. Pineal tumors. In: Winn HR, ed. Youman's Neurological Surgery. Philadelphia, PA: WB Saunders; 2004:1011–1029
17. Choi JU, Kim DS, Chung SS, Kim TS. Treatment of germ cell tumors in the pineal region. Childs Nerv Syst 1998;14(1-2): 41–48
18. Goodman RR. Magnetic resonance imaging-directed stereotactic endoscopic third ventriculostomy. Neurosurgery 1993;32(6):1043–1047
19. Dandy W. Operative experience in cases of pineal tumor. Arch Surg 1936;(33):19–46
20. Poppen JL. The right occipital approach to a pinealoma. J Neurosurg 1966;25(6):706–710
21. Stein BM. Supracerebellar-infratentorial approach to pineal tumors. Surg Neurol 1979;11(5):331–337
22. Dempsey PK, Kondziolka D, Lunsford LD. Stereotactic diagnosis and treatment of pineal region tumours and vascular malformations. Acta Neurochir (Wien) 1992;116(1):14–22
23. Edwards MS, Hudgins RJ, Wilson CB, Levin VA, Wara WM. Pineal region tumors in children. J Neurosurg 1988;68(5): 689–697
24. Fauchon F, Jouvet A, Paquis P, et al. Parenchymal pineal tumors: a clinicopathological study of 76 cases. Int J Radiat Oncol Biol Phys 2000;46(4):959–968
25. Neuwelt EA. An update on the surgical treatment of malignant pineal region tumors. Clin Neurosurg 1985;32: 397–428
26. Lapras C, Patet JD, Mottolese C, Lapras C Jr. Direct surgery for pineal tumors: occipital-transtentorial approach. Prog Exp Tumor Res 1987;30:268–280
27. Konovalov AN, Pitskhelauri DI. Principles of treatment of the pineal region tumors. Surg Neurol 2003;59(4):250–268
28. Bruce JN, Ogden AT. Surgical strategies for treating patients with pineal region tumors. J Neurooncol 2004;69(1-3): 221–236
29. Schild SE, Scheithauer BW, Haddock MG, et al. Histologically confirmed pineal tumors and other germ cell tumors of the brain. Cancer 1996;78(12):2564–2571
30. Schild SE, Scheithauer BW, Schomberg PJ, et al. Pineal parenchymal tumors. Clinical, pathologic, and therapeutic aspects. Cancer 1993;72(3):870–880
31. MacKay CI, Baeesa SS, Ventureyra EC. Epidermoid cysts of the pineal region. Childs Nerv Syst 1999;15(4):170–178
32. Chandy MJ, Damaraju SC. Benign tumours of the pineal region: a prospective study from 1983 to 1997. Br J Neurosurg 1998;12(3):228–233
33. Field M, Witham TF, Flickinger JC, Kondziolka D, Lunsford LD. Comprehensive assessment of hemorrhage risks and outcomes after stereotactic brain biopsy. J Neurosurg 2001;94(4):545–551
34. Pecker J, Scarabin JM, Vallee B, Brucher JM. Treatment in tumours of the pineal region: value of stereotaxic biopsy. Surg Neurol 1979;12(4):341–348
35. Kraichoke S, Cosgrove M, Chandrasoma PT. Granulomatous inflammation in pineal germinoma: a cause of diagnostic failure at stereotaxic brain biopsy. Am J Surg Pathol 1988;12(9):655–660
36. Zacharia BE, Bruce JN. Stereotactic biopsy considerations for pineal tumors. Neurosurg Clin N Am 2011;22(3):359–366, viii
37. Barker FG II, Carter BS, Ojemann RG, Jyung RW, Poe DS, McKenna MJ. Surgical excision of acoustic neuroma: patient outcome and provider caseload. Laryngoscope 2003;113(8): 1332–1343
38. Reddy AT, Janss AJ, Phillips PC, Weiss HL, Packer RJ. Outcome for children with supratentorial primitive neuroectodermal tumors treated with surgery, radiation, and chemotherapy. Cancer 2000;88(9):2189–2193
39. Mena H, Rushing EJ, Ribas JL, Delahunt B, McCarthy WF. Tumors of pineal parenchymal cells: a correlation of histological features, including nucleolar organizer regions, with survival in 35 cases. Hum Pathol 1995;26(1):20–30
40. Kobayashi T, Kida Y, Mori Y. Stereotactic gamma radiosurgery for pineal and related tumors. J Neurooncol 2001;54(3): 301–309
41. Mori Y, Kobayashi T, Hasegawa T, Yoshida K, Kida Y. Stereotactic radiosurgery for pineal and related tumors. Prog Neurol Surg 2009;23:106–118
42. Hasegawa T, Kondziolka D, Hadjipanayis CG, Flickinger JC, Lunsford LD. Stereotactic radiosurgery for CNS nongerminomatous germ cell tumors: report of four cases. Pediatr Neurosurg 2003;38(6):329–333
43. Manera L, Régis J, Chinot O, et al. Pineal region tumors: the role of stereotactic radiosurgery. Stereotact Funct Neurosurg 1996;66(Suppl 1):164–173
44. Apuzzo ML, Chandrasoma PT, Cohen D, Zee CS, Zelman V. Computed imaging stereotaxy: experience and perspective related to 500 procedures applied to brain masses. Neurosurgery 1987;20(6):930–937
45. Sawin PD, Hitchon PW, Follett KA, Torner JC. Computed imaging-assisted stereotactic brain biopsy: a risk analysis of 225 consecutive cases. Surg Neurol 1998;49(6):640–649
46. Kreth FW, Schätz CR, Pagenstecher A, Faist M, Volk B, Ostertag CB. Stereotactic management of lesions of the pineal region. Neurosurgery 1996;39(2):280–289
47. Lee JYK, Wakabayashi T, Yoshida J. Management and survival of pineoblastoma: an analysis of 34 adults from the brain tumor registry of Japan. Neurol Med Chir (Tokyo) 2005;45(3):132–141

48. Ogawa K, Toita T, Nakamura K, et al. Treatment and prognosis of patients with intracranial nongerminomatous malignant germ cell tumors: a multiinstitutional retrospective analysis of 41 patients. Cancer 2003;98(2):369–376
49. Kanamori M, Kumabe T, Saito R, et al. Optimal treatment strategy for intracranial germ cell tumors: a single institution analysis. J Neurosurg Pediatr 2009;4(6):506–514
50. Vaquero J, Ramiro J, Martínez R, Coca S, Bravo G. Clinicopathological experience with pineocytomas: report of five surgically treated cases. Neurosurgery 1990;27(4):612–618
51. Ferrer E, Santamarta D, Garcia-Fructuoso G, Caral L, Rumià J. Neuroendoscopic management of pineal region tumours. Acta Neurochir (Wien) 1997;139(1):12–20
52. Oi S, Kamio M, Joki T, Abe T. Neuroendoscopic anatomy and surgery in pineal region tumors: role of neuroendoscopic procedure in the 'minimally-invasive preferential' management. J Neurooncol 2001;54(3):277–286
53. Gangemi M, Maiuri F, Colella G, Buonamassa S. Endoscopic surgery for pineal region tumors. Minim Invasive Neurosurg 2001;44(2):70–73
54. Pople IK, Athanasiou TC, Sandeman DR, Coakham HB. The role of endoscopic biopsy and third ventriculostomy in the management of pineal region tumours. Br J Neurosurg 2001;15(4):305–311
55. Uschold T, Abla AA, Fusco D, Bristol RE, Nakaji P. Supracerebellar infratentorial endoscopically controlled resection of pineal lesions: case series and operative technique. J Neurosurg Pediatr 2011;8(6):554–564
56. Broggi M, Darbar A, Teo C. The value of endoscopy in the total resection of pineocytomas. Neurosurgery 2010;67(3, Suppl Operative):ons159–ons165
57. Fetell MR, Bruce JN, Burke AM, et al. Non-neoplastic pineal cysts. Neurology 1991;41(7):1034–1040
58. Radovanovic I, Dizdarevic K, de Tribolet N, Masic T, Muminagic S. Pineal region tumors—neurosurgical review. Med Arh 2009;63(3):171–173
59. Sawamura Y. Strategy of combined treatment of germ cell tumors. Prog Neurol Surg 2009;23:86–95
60. Rich TA, Cassady JR, Strand RD, Winston KR. Radiation therapy for pineal and suprasellar germ cell tumors. Cancer 1985; 55(5):932–940
61. Balmaceda C, Heller G, Rosenblum M, et al. Chemotherapy without irradiation—a novel approach for newly diagnosed CNS germ cell tumors: results of an international cooperative trial. The First International Central Nervous System Germ Cell Tumor Study. J Clin Oncol 1996;14(11):2908–2915
62. Buckner JC, Peethambaram PP, Smithson WA, et al. Phase II trial of primary chemotherapy followed by reduced-dose radiation for CNS germ cell tumors. J Clin Oncol 1999;17(3): 933–940
63. Sawamura Y, de Tribolet N, Ishii N, Abe H. Management of primary intracranial germinomas: diagnostic surgery or radical resection? J Neurosurg 1997;87(2):262–266
64. Robertson PL, DaRosso RC, Allen JC. Improved prognosis of intracranial non-germinoma germ cell tumors with multimodality therapy. J Neurooncol 1997;32(1):71–80
65. Camins MB, Schlesinger EB. Treatment of tumours of the posterior part of the third ventricle and the pineal region: a long term follow-up. Acta Neurochir (Wien) 1978;40(1-2): 131–143
66. Matsutani M, Sano K, Takakura K, Fujimaki T, Nakamura O. Combined treatment with chemotherapy and radiation therapy for intracranial germ cell tumors. Childs Nerv Syst 1998; 14(1-2):59–62
67. Kochi M, Itoyama Y, Shiraishi S, Kitamura I, Marubayashi T, Ushio Y. Successful treatment of intracranial nongerminomatous malignant germ cell tumors by administering neoadjuvant chemotherapy and radiotherapy before excision of residual tumors. J Neurosurg 2003;99(1):106–114
68. Friedman JA, Lynch JJ, Buckner JC, Scheithauer BW, Raffel C. Management of malignant pineal germ cell tumors with residual mature teratoma. Neurosurgery 2001;48(3): 518–522
69. Weiner HL, Lichtenbaum RA, Wisoff JH, et al. Delayed surgical resection of central nervous system germ cell tumors. Neurosurgery 2002;50(4):727–733
70. Barnett DW, Olson JJ, Thomas WG, Hunter SB. Low-grade astrocytomas arising from the pineal gland. Surg Neurol 1995;43(1):70–75
71. Yeh DD, Warnick RE, Ernst RJ. Management strategy for adult patients with dorsal midbrain gliomas. Neurosurgery 2002;50(4):735–738
72. Clark AJ, Sughrue ME, Ivan ME, et al. Factors influencing overall survival rates for patients with pineocytoma. J Neurooncol 2010;100(2):255–260
73. Clark AJ, Ivan ME, Sughrue ME, et al. Tumor control after surgery and radiotherapy for pineocytoma. J Neurosurg 2010;113(2):319–324
74. Packer RJ, Sutton LN, Rorke LB, et al. Prognostic importance of cellular differentiation in medulloblastoma of childhood. J Neurosurg 1984;61(2):296–301
75. Gururangan S, McLaughlin C, Quinn J, et al. High-dose chemotherapy with autologous stem-cell rescue in children and adults with newly diagnosed pineoblastomas. J Clin Oncol 2003;21(11):2187–2191
76. Kurisaka M, Arisawa M, Mori T, et al. Combination chemotherapy (cisplatin, vinblastin) and low-dose irradiation in the treatment of pineal parenchymal cell tumors. Childs Nerv Syst 1998;14(10):564–569
77. Jakacki RI, Zeltzer PM, Boyett JM, et al. Survival and prognostic factors following radiation and/or chemotherapy for primitive neuroectodermal tumors of the pineal region in infants and children: a report of the Childrens Cancer Group. J Clin Oncol 1995;13(6):1377–1383
78. Graham ML, Herndon JE II, Casey JR, et al. High-dose chemotherapy with autologous stem-cell rescue in patients with recurrent and high-risk pediatric brain tumors. J Clin Oncol 1997;15(5):1814–1823
79. Selvanathan SK, Hammouche S, Smethurst W, Salminen HJ, Jenkinson MD. Outcome and prognostic features in adult pineoblastomas: analysis of cases from the SEER database. Acta Neurochir (Wien) 2012;154(5):863–869
80. Tate M, Sughrue ME, Rutkowski MJ, et al. The long-term postsurgical prognosis of patients with pineoblastoma. Cancer 2012;118(1):173–179
81. Raco A, Raimondi AJ, D'Alonzo A, Esposito V, Valentino V. Radiosurgery in the management of pediatric brain tumors. Childs Nerv Syst 2000;16(5):287–295
82. Reyns N, Hayashi M, Chinot O, et al. The role of gamma knife radiosurgery in the treatment of pineal parenchymal tumours. Acta Neurochir (Wien) 2006;148(1):5–11
83. Lekovic GP, Gonzalez LF, Shetter AG, et al. Role of gamma knife surgery in the management of pineal region tumors. Neurosurg Focus 2007;23(6):E12
84. Kano H, Niranjan A, Kondziolka D, Flickinger JC, Lunsford D. Role of stereotactic radiosurgery in the management of pineal parenchymal tumors. Prog Neurol Surg 2009;23: 44–58
85. Sood S, Hoeprich M, Ham SD. Pure endoscopic removal of pineal region tumors. Childs Nerv Syst 2011;27(9):1489–1492
86. Hoffman HJ, Yoshida M, Becker LE, Hendrick EB, Humphreys RP. Pineal region tumors in childhood. Experience at the Hospital for Sick Children. 1983. Pediatr Neurosurg 1994; 21(1):91–103
87. Pluchino F, Broggi G, Fornari M, Franzini A, Solero CL, Allegranza A. Surgical approach to pineal tumours. Acta Neurochir (Wien) 1989;96(1-2):26–31

88. Luo SQ, Li DZ, Zhang MZ, Wang ZC. Occipital transtentorial approach for removal of pineal region tumors: report of 64 consecutive cases. Surg Neurol 1989;32(1):36–39
89. Herrmann HD, Winkler D, Westphal M. Treatment of tumours of the pineal region and posterior part of the third ventricle. Acta Neurochir (Wien) 1992;116(2-4):137–146
90. Chandy MJ, Damaraju SC. Benign tumours of the pineal region: a prospective study from 1983 to 1997. Br J Neurosurg 1998;12(3):228–233
91. Kang JK, Jeun SS, Hong YK, et al. Experience with pineal region tumors. Childs Nerv Syst 1998;14(1-2):63–68
92. Shin HJ, Cho BK, Jung HW, Wang KC. Pediatric pineal tumors: need for a direct surgical approach and complications of the occipital transtentorial approach. Childs Nerv Syst 1998; 14(4-5):174–178
93. Jia W, Ma Z, Liu IY, Zhang Y, Jia G, Wan W. Transcallosal interforniceal approach to pineal region tumors in 150 children. J Neurosurg Pediatr 2011;7(1):98–103
94. Al-Hussaini M, Sultan I, Abuirmileh N, Jaradat I, Qaddoumi I. Pineal gland tumors: experience from the SEER database. J Neurooncol 2009;94(3):351–358
95. Gilheeney SW, Saad A, Chi S, et al. Outcome of pediatric pineoblastoma after surgery, radiation and chemotherapy. J Neurooncol 2008;89(1):89–95

▪ SECTION III ▪

Intraventricular Tumors

15

The Role of Adjuvant Therapy in Subtotal Resection and High-Grade Ependymomas

Carmen Kut and Kristin Janson Redmond

Ependymoma is a rare tumor seen predominantly in the pediatric population. Approximately two thirds of ependymomas arise adjacent to the ventricles and are infratentorial, whereas the remaining third of cases occur supratentorially, often in the periventricular region. Rare cases of ependymoma develop within the filum terminale or spinal cord but are often viewed as an entity distinct from intracranial ependymomas.[1] Metastases from supratentorial ependymomas are rare but are reported in one third of infratentorial cases; however, this number could be overestimated given that primitive neuroectodermal tumors (PNETs) are also included within the data, which could account for part of the metastasis cases.[2]

The role of adjuvant therapy in ependymoma patients is a commonly disputed issue. This chapter summarizes the current surgical standard of care and reviews the literature related to the practice of surgical, radiation, and chemotherapeutic care in patients with ependymoma.

■ Best Evidence Medicine for Treatment in Ependymoma Patients

Surgery

Level I to Level II Evidence

A 2009 prospective study reports that overall survival was affected by the extent of resection (hazard ratio of 0.16; $p < 0.0001$), event-free survival (hazard ratio of 0.20; $p < 0.0001$), as well as local failure (hazard ratio of 0.16; $p < 0.001$) for gross total resection (GTR) versus near-total or subtotal resection (STR).[3]

Level III to Level IV Evidence

The current standard of care for most ependymoma patients includes maximal safe resection, followed by consideration of postoperative radiation therapy to the primary site.[4] A study at the Children's Hospital of Los Angeles followed 28 children in 1993 to 2003 and reported 33 versus 6.5 months of progression-free survival (PFS) and 44 versus 15 months of overall survival (OS) for GTR versus STR patients.[1] Other studies have placed 3-year event-free survival at 77.6% versus 42.9% for GTR versus STR patients ($p = 0.0031$), and 5-year OS of GTR and STR at ~ 67 to 80% versus 22 to 47%, and 5-year PFS at 51 to 75% versus 0 to 26%.[4–10]

Despite the significance of complete resection in long-term PFS and OS, complete resection is only achieved in 42 to 62% of patients.[8,9,11] The extent of surgical resection depends on the location of the ependymoma. Myxopapillary spinal ependymomas tend to be most amenable to GTR, followed by supratentorial and infratentorial tumors[5]. According to some studies, complete resection is more easily accomplished, and radical surgery alone may be sufficient for patients with supratentorial low-grade ependymomas.[1,4] Infratentorial ependymomas, especially those closely adjacent to lower cranial nerves, are associated with increased morbidity when aggressive resection is attempted.[4]

Recommendations for Surgical Treatment in Ependymoma Patients

1. Aggressive gross total resection should be attempted if it does not significantly compromise a patient's neurofunctional outcome.
2. GTR is associated with improved overall survival, event-free survival, and local control (Grade 1C Recommendation, Level II/III Evidence).

Radiation

Controversy

Adjuvant radiation is frequently administered following surgical resection of ependymoma. The role of radiation therapy remains controversial. This section explores the arguments in favor of and against radiation therapy.

Level I to Level II Evidence

A 2009 prospective study reports no significant difference in OS and event-free survival for patients receiving 54 versus 59.4 Gy (p = 0.67 and 0.82). The same study also describes no significant difference in OS and event-free survival for patients receiving conformal radiation therapy either before or after the age of 3 years (p = 0.37 and 0.46).[3]

Level III to Level IV Evidence

Numerous studies suggest improved OS, event-free survival, and PFS for patients receiving radiation.[11-14] For example, 5-year local control and OS are both improved in patients receiving postoperative radiation therapy. A retrospective review of 40 patients with posterior fossa ependymoma reports a 10-year actuarial local control rate at 50% versus 100%, and a 10-year OS rate at 67% versus 83% for GTR/observation versus GTR/irradiation.[13]

The rationale for the postoperative radiation therapy lies in the observation that GTR is difficult for infratentorial or posterior fossa lesions, which are often proximal to the fourth ventricle. As a result, postoperative radiation therapy is important in controlling the rates of local recurrences. If the ependymoma is located close to any critical structures or large vessels, this will increase the rates of local recurrences if the patient does not receive postoperative radiation therapy, perhaps because of increased likelihood of microscopic residual disease.[5]

Level V Evidence

Nevertheless, there are contradicting expert opinions on the use of radiation therapy following resection of ependymoma. Some authors argue that the existing literature is limited and does not provide strong evidence for the use of adjuvant therapies.[1,15] More specifically, these authors argue that the survival advantages of adjuvant therapies are not statistically significant, and that both chemotherapy and radiation only fare "slightly better" compared with surgery alone.[1] According to these authors, the existing literature is inconclusive for two major reasons: (1) too few patients have been recruited in published multivariate analyses, and (2) the universal use of radiotherapy (except in younger children known to have a higher recurrence risk) makes it difficult to establish an independent benefit for postoperative irradiation.[15]

Treatment Guidelines (Level V Evidence)

The radiation field for ependymoma typically includes the tumor/tumor bed plus a 1- to 2-cm margin to account for microscopic spread and setup error. The prescription dose is generally 54 to 59 Gy. Craniospinal irradiation (36 Gy with supplemental chemotherapy vincristine ± carboplatin) is reserved for cases with positive cerebrospinal fluid, positive magnetic resonance imaging neuroaxis, or ependymoblastoma.[5] Craniospinal radiation is typically followed by a boost to the cavity or gross disease to a total of 54 to 59 Gy.

One manner of stratifying the need for adjuvant radiation therapy is by tumor location. For example, at Johns Hopkins, patients with supratentorial ependymoma are often observed, whereas patients with infratentorial ependymoma generally receive postoperative radiation treatment.

In spinal ependymoma, radiation is indicated if the resection is incomplete or if the patient has anaplastic histology. Radiation fields often include two vertebral bodies or sacral nerve roots above and below the ependymoma, at a dose of 45.0 to 50.4 Gy; if the ependymoma is below the spinal cord, a boost to 54.0 to 59.4 Gy is implemented.

Spinal Myxopapillary Ependymoma (Level III to Level IV Evidence)

Spinal myxopapillary ependymoma (MPE) is a grade I spinal ependymoma that presents commonly in adults and very occasionally in children[2]. Despite conventional opinions that complete resection is sufficient, an evolving literature has pointed out the benefits of adjuvant radiation therapy in improving patient outcomes. Multiple studies, including a large study series with 85 MPE patients, have demonstrated that radiation provides improved PFS in both adult and pediatric patients with STR,[10,16,17] as well as improved long-term disease control rates in both recurrent and metastatic patients.[16,18] One study even reports significant improvement in PFS and decreased rates of local failure with adjuvant radiation therapy, *regardless* of the extent of surgery (GTR or STR) in adult patients.[10]

Radiation Side Effects

Despite the efficacy of radiation therapy, patients undergoing irradiation may be at risk of severe side effects, including cognitive, endocrine, and neurological dysfunction.[1]

Level I to Level II Evidence

Preliminary results from a phase 2 prospective study report stable IQ testing and minimal neurocognitive side effects in children 2 years after receiving small and local radiation fields.[19]

Level III to Level IV Evidence

There is considerable concern that radiation therapy in young children can lead to neurodevelopmental problems. A 1995 study shows that the intellectual outcome in children with malignant ependymoma in the posterior fossa is dependent on the radiation field and the surgical outcome.[20] In this study, 70 to 80% of pediatric patients maintained an IQ of over 90 if there were no postoperative complications versus 20 to 40% in children with postoperative complications. As for radiation fields, 90% of children maintained an IQ > 90 at 5 to 10 years after radiation to the posterior fossa. In a separate meta-analysis, children who receive cranial irradiation (including the neuroaxis) had significantly lower IQ values than children without radiation therapy. For children receiving focal irradiation, there was no difference in IQ values versus those without radiation therapy.[21]

Recommendations for Radiation Treatment in Ependymoma Patients

1. Role of adjuvant radiation therapy remains controversial, especially for patients under 3 years old who may be at increased risk of neurocognitive side effects (Grade 1C Recommendation, Level III/IV Evidence).
2. Studies overall suggest improved OS, event-free survival, and PFS for patients receiving adjuvant radiation therapy (Grade 1C Recommendatin, Level III Evidence).
3. The radiation field typically includes the tumor plus a 1- to 2-cm margin at a cumulative dose of 54 to 59 Gy.

Chemotherapy

Controversy

The role of chemotherapy in ependymoma patients is uncertain and demonstrated little to no independent benefit.[4,8,22]

Level I Evidence

There is no Level I evidence about the use of chemotherapy in ependymoma patients.

Level II to Level III Evidence

Single-agent studies have been disappointing, with cisplatin having the highest response rate at 30% in a literature review of Level 3 studies.[22] A phase 2 prospective study quotes literature that supports the use of carboplatin and reports a 40% response rate for patients who have been previously treated with cisplatin.[23]

Prospective studies evaluating combination chemotherapy have been more optimistic, with a 16 to 86% response rate to various combination regimens that involve cisplatin, vincristine, etoposide, and cyclophosphamide.[24] Previous POG infant studies (8633 and 9233) demonstrated significant improvement in event-free survival for infants with brain tumors, including ependymoma, but no difference in OS.

By contrast, preliminary results from a phase 2 prospective study describe worse 3-year PFS for chemotherapy (60% with chemotherapy vs 78.1% without chemotherapy).[19] However, it is possible that this could be a result of selection bias, where patients with a worse prognosis may have been more likely to receive adjuvant chemotherapy.

In summary, studies suggest that ependymomas are potentially responsive to combination chemotherapy, but results so far have not demonstrated a clear overall survival advantage.

Level V Evidence

Because the efficacy of chemotherapy is uncertain, many experts advocate that it should be reserved for patients who have failed surgery and radiation therapy.[1,25]

Use of Chemotherapy to Delay Radiation in Children < 3 Years Old

Level I Evidence

There is no Level I evidence associated with the use of chemotherapy in children under 3 years old.

Level II to Level III Evidence

One application of chemotherapy is in pediatric ependymoma patients below the age of 3, who may be especially vulnerable to neurocognitive effects and other complications of radiation. In these patients, chemotherapy may be used to delay radiation treatment up to a few years after diagnosis.[3,5] This approach is controversial because patients younger than 3 years old often demonstrate worse outcomes. It remains uncertain whether the poor outcome is due to the young age or the avoidance of radiation therapy during treatment. Some authors suggest that 42% of patients receive chemotherapy and avoid irradiation for up to 5 years after diagnoses without compromising OS.[26] Others argue that fewer than 22% of patients may benefit from such an approach and that the efficacy of chemotherapy remains unproven.[22]

■ Treatment Guidelines

There is no conventional chemotherapy regimen nor are there established chemotherapy treatment guidelines because the efficacy of chemotherapy remains in dispute for ependymoma patients.

Recommendations for Chemotherapy Treatment in Ependymoma Patients

1. The role of adjuvant chemotherapy is uncertain and should be reserved for patients who have failed surgery or radiation therapy (Grade 2C Recommendation, Level V Evidence).
2. Chemotherapy may be used to delay radiation treatment for children under 3 years old (Grade 1C Recommendation, Level II/III Evidence).
3. There is no conventional chemotherapy regimen available, and the efficacy of chemotherapy remains disputable.

Treatment Guidelines for Recurrent Tumor

The management of recurrent ependymoma is controversial. Management options include repeat resection, observation, radiation therapy, and/or chemotherapy.

At least 10 years of follow-up are required for ependymoma patients because late recurrences as many as 12 years postsurgery have been reported.[5] During the follow-up, craniospinal magnetic resonance imaging is required every 6 months for the first 2 years, followed by annual scans.

Level I to Level II Evidence

Although some groups give empirical recommendations for observation, a randomized trial at St. Jude's Children's Research Hospital (SJCRH) performed systematic evaluation of second resections prior to radiation therapy. From April 1997 to April 2000, 40 children were referred to SJCRH for ependymoma treatment; following initial surgery, 24 patients (60%) were considered to have a complete resection, whereas the remaining 16 (40%) had residual tumor. Twelve of these 16 patients were candidates for additional resection, and complete resection was achieved in 10 of 12 patients undergoing a second surgery. If we combine patients with complete resection after initial surgery with those having complete resection after a second surgery, the percentage of complete resection for the whole group increased from 60 to 85%.[27]

Level III Evidence

There is no Level III evidence concerning the treatment of recurrent ependymomas.

Level IV to Level V Evidence

The efficacy of single chemotherapeutic agents in recurrent ependymoma has been disappointing.[4] However, chemotherapy may play a role between initial and salvage surgery for residual tumor. One study used chemotherapy between the initial and second surgery and reports that tumors appear better defined and easier to resect following chemotherapy regimens.[28] The rationale is that chemotherapy may exert a series of cytotoxic and antiangiogenesis effects, which in turn make tumors more amenable to resection. However, these were mostly subjective impressions from the neurosurgeons, and to our knowledge, there is no study that quantitatively correlates the intensity of, or the response to, chemotherapy with the ease of resection at second surgery.[4]

Expert Recommendations

1. At least 10-year follow-up is required for postoperative patients.
2. There may be a benefit in second surgery for patients with recurrent ependymoma (Grade 2B Recommendation, Level I/II Evidence).
3. Adjuvant radiation may benefit recurrent ependymoma patients (Grade 2C Recommendation, Level IV Evidence).
4. Chemotherapy may have some minimal benefit prior to a second surgery (Grade 2C Recommendation, Level V Evidence).

■ Summary and Conclusions

The most important prognostic factor in management of ependymoma is the extent of surgical resection. Extent of resection correlates closely with local control, and surgeons should aim for a GTR when it is safely achievable.[1,3,5] A study at the University of Pittsburgh following 40 children with ependymomas identifies a dramatic increase in PFS at 68% (5-year) and 54% (10-year), versus a 3-year PFS of 8.9% in subtotal resection.[9] The rate of local recurrence following subtotal resection remains elevated even in patients receiving adjuvant radiation therapy.[4]

Patients younger than age 4 at the time of diagnosis have a worse prognosis than older patients.[1,5,9,29] Patients 3 years old or older at the time of diagnosis have a PFS at 60% (5-year) and 45% (10-year), compared to patients younger than 3 years old, who have PFS at 12% (5-year and 10-year).[9] Nevertheless, few patients younger than 3 years old receive radiation treatment due to the possibility of negative cognitive defects, and some receive adjuvant chemotherapy in place of radiation treatment. Consequently, the true factor limiting survival for younger patients could be adjuvant therapy, rather than age.

Factors such as tumor location, grade, and histology show little significance in predicting the treatment outcome. Some studies report a worse prognosis in infratentorial ependymomas, whereas others show no statistical significance and a lack of clear prognostic indicators.[29,30] There is considerable variation in grading and it is unclear whether tumor grade has any prognostic significance.[1]

Currently, there are no reliable molecular prognostic markers for ependymoma, and the prognostic role of histological subtype or grading remains controversial.[4] Pilot data suggest that different cytogenetic aberrations are responsible for intracranial tumors in younger (loss of 9p in patients < 3 years old) and older patients (loss of 9q in patients > 7 years old).[31] Other common chromosomal aberrations in intracranial tumors include a gain of 1q; losses of 61, 9, and 13; and spinal cord tumors, which are sometimes associated with a gain on chromosome 7.[4]

Additionally, overexpression of erbB-2/erbB-4 is often associated with poorer outcomes in ependymoma patients.[5] Better understanding of genetic and expression profiles could potentially help to subclassify ependymomas and identify better chemotherapeutic targets in the future.

New methods in radiation delivery (e.g., conformal radiation therapy, proton beam radiotherapy) and neurosurgery (more complete resections) may also lead to increased local control, reduced toxicity, and improved OS in these young patients.

■ References

1. Krieger MD, Bowen IE. Effects of surgical resection and adjuvant therapy on pediatric intracranial ependymomas. Expert Rev Neurother 2005;5(4):465–471
2. Pierre-Kahn A, Hirsch JF, Roux FX, Renier D, Sainte-Rose C. Intracranial ependymomas in childhood. Survival and functional results of 47 cases. Childs Brain 1983;10(3):145–156
3. Merchant TE, Li C, Xiong X, Kun LE, Boop FA, Sanford RA. Conformal radiotherapy after surgery for paediatric ependymoma: a prospective study. Lancet Oncol 2009;10(3):258–266
4. Merchant TE, Kiehna EN, Kun LE, et al. Phase II trial of conformal radiation therapy for pediatric patients with craniopharyngioma and correlation of surgical factors and radiation dosimetry with change in cognitive function. J Neurosurg 2006;104(2, Suppl):94–102

5. Hristov B, Lin SH, Christodouleas JP. Radiation Oncology: A Question-Based Review. Philadelphia, PA: Lippincott Williams & Wilkins; 2011:581
6. Foreman NK, Love S, Thorne R. Intracranial ependymomas: analysis of prognostic factors in a population-based series. Pediatr Neurosurg 1996;24(3):119–125
7. Goldwein JW, Glauser TA, Packer RJ, et al. Recurrent intracranial ependymomas in children. Survival, patterns of failure, and prognostic factors. Cancer 1990;66(3):557–563
8. Sutton LN, Goldwein J, Perilongo G, et al. Prognostic factors in childhood ependymomas. Pediatr Neurosurg 1990-1991;16(2):57–65
9. Pollack IF, Gerszten PC, Martinez AJ, et al. Intracranial ependymomas of childhood: long-term outcome and prognostic factors. Neurosurgery 1995;37(4):655–666
10. Nazar GB, Hoffman HJ, Becker LE, Jenkin D, Humphreys RP, Hendrick EB. Infratentorial ependymomas in childhood: prognostic factors and treatment. J Neurosurg 1990;72(3):408–417
11. Rousseau P, Habrand JL, Sarrazin D, et al. Treatment of intracranial ependymomas of children: review of a 15-year experience. Int J Radiat Oncol Biol Phys 1994;28(2):381–386
12. Mørk SJ, Løken AC. Ependymoma: a follow-up study of 101 cases. Cancer 1977;40(2):907–915
13. Rogers L, Pueschel J, Spetzler R, et al. Is gross-total resection sufficient treatment for posterior fossa ependymomas? J Neurosurg 2005;102(4):629–636
14. Perilongo G, Massimino M, Sotti G, et al. Analyses of prognostic factors in a retrospective review of 92 children with ependymoma: Italian Pediatric Neuro-oncology Group. Med Pediatr Oncol 1997;29(2):79–85
15. Little A, Teo C. Response to the letter by Dr. Massimino et al. "Do we really need class 1 evidence to give adjuvant radiation therapy to childhood ependymoma?" Childs Nerv Syst 2009;25(6):643–644
16. Grill J, Renaux VK, Bulteau C, et al. Long-term intellectual outcome in children with posterior fossa tumors according to radiation doses and volumes. Int J Radiat Oncol Biol Phys 1999;45(1):137–145
17. Donahue B, Steinfeld A. Intracranial ependymoma in the adult patient: successful treatment with surgery and radiotherapy. J Neurooncol 1998;37(2):131–133
18. Tomita T, McLone DG, Das L, Brand WN. Benign ependymomas of the posterior fossa in childhood. Pediatr Neurosci 1988;14(6):277–285
19. Merchant TE, Mulhern RK, Krasin MJ, et al. Preliminary results from a phase II trial of conformal radiation therapy and evaluation of radiation-related CNS effects for pediatric patients with localized ependymoma. J Clin Oncol 2004;22(15):3156–3162
20. Hoppe-Hirsch E, Brunet L, Laroussinie F, et al. Intellectual outcome in children with malignant tumors of the posterior fossa: influence of the field of irradiation and quality of surgery. Childs Nerv Syst 1995;11(6):340–345
21. Mulhern RK, Hancock J, Fairclough D, Kun L. Neuropsychological status of children treated for brain tumors: a critical review and integrative analysis. Med Pediatr Oncol 1992;20(3):181–191
22. Bouffet E, Perilongo G, Canete A, Massimino M. Intracranial ependymomas in children: a critical review of prognostic factors and a plea for cooperation. Med Pediatr Oncol 1998;30(6):319–329
23. Gaynon PS, Ettinger LJ, Baum ES, Siegel SE, Krailo MD, Hammond GD. Carboplatin in childhood brain tumors: a children's cancer study group phase II trial. Cancer 1990;66(12):2465–2469
24. White L, Kellie S, Gray E, et al. Postoperative chemotherapy in children less than 4 years of age with malignant brain tumors: promising initial response to a VETOPEC-based regimen. A Study of the Australian and New Zealand Children's Cancer Study Group (ANZCCSG). J Pediatr Hematol Oncol 1998;20(2):125–130
25. Gornet MK, Buckner JC, Marks RS, Scheithauer BW, Erickson BJ. Chemotherapy for advanced CNS ependymoma. J Neurooncol 1999;45(1):61–67
26. Grundy RG, Wilne SA, Weston CL, et al; Children's Cancer and Leukaemia Group (formerly UKCCSG) Brain Tumour Committee. Primary postoperative chemotherapy without radiotherapy for intracranial ependymoma in children: the UKCCSG/SIOP prospective study. Lancet Oncol 2007;8(8):696–705
27. Osterdock RJ, Sanford RA, Merchant TE. Pediatric ependymoma (40 in 36 months). Paper presented at AANS/CNS Section on Pediatric Neurological Surgery Annual Meeting, California, 2000:6–9
28. Foreman NK, Love S, Gill SS, Coakham HB. Second-look surgery for incompletely resected fourth ventricle ependymomas: technical case report. Neurosurgery 1997;40(4):856–860
29. Tamburrini G, D'Ercole M, Pettorini BL, Caldarelli M, Massimi L, Di Rocco C. Survival following treatment for intracranial ependymoma: a review. Childs Nerv Syst 2009;25(10):1303–1312
30. Mansur DB, Perry A, Rajaram V, et al. Postoperative radiation therapy for grade II and III intracranial ependymoma. Int J Radiat Oncol Biol Phys 2005;61(2):387–391
31. Hirose Y, Aldape K, Bollen A, et al. Chromosomal abnormalities subdivide ependymal tumors into clinically relevant groups. Am J Pathol 2001;158(3):1137–1143

16

The Role of Surgery in the Management of Asymptomatic Colloid Cysts without Hydrocephalus

David A. Wilson and Peter Nakaji

Colloid cysts of the third ventricle are histologically benign lesions found in ~ 1 in 10,000 individuals at autopsy.[1–3] Although most colloid cysts are believed to be asymptomatic, sudden death is a rare but well-documented complication of previously undetected colloid cysts.[4–14] This feared complication is believed to occur by cyst expansion and blockage of cerebrospinal fluid (CSF) pathways at the foramen of Monro, leading to acute hydrocephalus and cerebral herniation.[4,15] Alternative explanations for sudden death associated with colloid cysts include more distal blockage of the cerebral aqueduct by cystic contents and pressure-related hypothalamic dysfunction.[16,17]

Prior to the era of modern neuroimaging, virtually all colloid cysts encountered in the clinical setting were symptomatic. Given the potential for progressive hydrocephalus and sudden death, the management of symptomatic colloid cysts is well accepted and largely uncontroversial; most would agree that, in the setting of headache and hydrocephalus, prompt neurosurgical treatment via either an open microsurgical approach or an endoscopic approach is indicated.[18,19]

However, with the increased use of neuroimaging, today more colloid cysts are discovered incidentally (**Figs. 16.1** and **16.2**). Because most colloid cysts remain asymptomatic throughout life and, as autopsy studies suggest, most are never detected, the management of incidentally discovered colloid cysts is controversial.[20–23] Decisions to operate may be based on the perceived fear of sudden death posed by an untreated colloid cyst, whereas conservative wait-and-see approaches are supported by the rarity of this complication and the small, but real, risks of surgical intervention. This chapter explores the controversies surrounding the management of asymptomatic colloid cysts, in terms of both the decision to treat versus observe and the available surgical options.

■ Epidemiology

Colloid cysts are believed to arise from ectopic endodermal elements within the velum interpositum at the roof of the third ventricle.[10,24] These lesions are rare, accounting for, at most, 1 to 2% of all primary intracranial brain tumors.[11,25] Because most colloid cysts are asymptomatic and undetected, there are no solid data regarding the true prevalence of colloid cysts in the general population and their natural history.

Because the complications of colloid cysts, specifically sudden death, are rare but devastating, an estimate of the prevalence of colloid cysts in the general population is necessary to approximate the risk of harboring an asymptomatic lesion. Autopsy studies suggest that the prevalence of colloid cysts in the general population ranges from 1 in 5,800 to 1 in 10,995.[1–3] Population-wide magnetic resonance imaging (MRI) studies have found rates of 0 in 1,000 individuals and 1 in 3,672 individuals.[26,27]

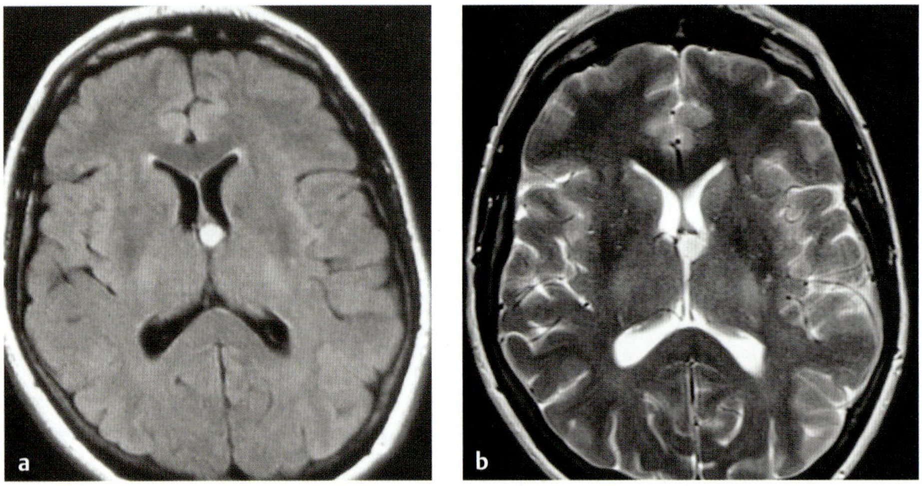

Fig. 16.1 **(a)** Axial T1- and **(b)** T2-weighted magnetic resonance imaging (MRI) of an asymptomatic colloid cyst discovered incidentally. Given the lack of symptoms, the small size of the cyst, and the absence of ventriculomegaly, this cyst has been observed without surgical intervention and without complications thus far. (Used with permission from Barrow Neurological Institute.)

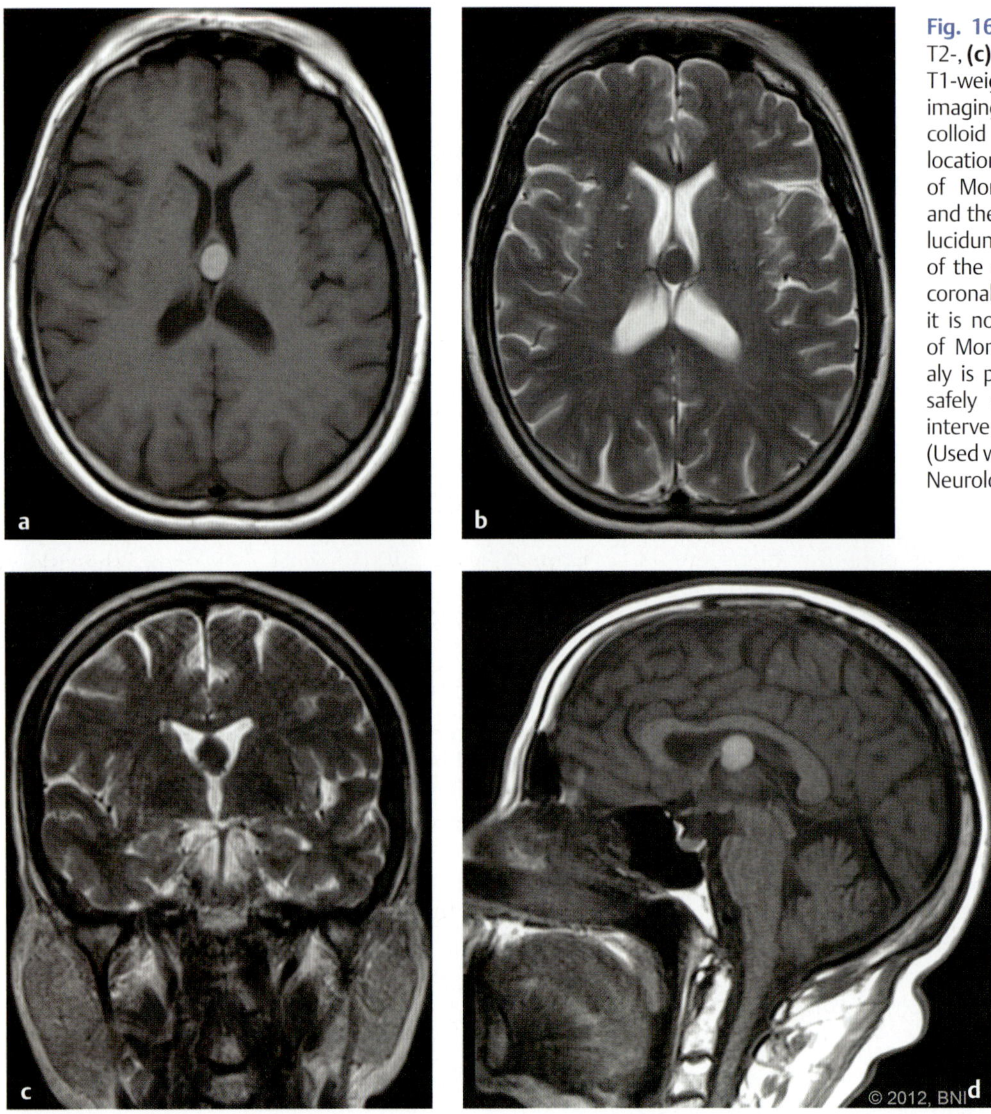

Fig. 16.2 **(a)** Axial T1-, **(b)** axial T2-, **(c)** coronal T2-, and **(d)** sagittal T1-weighted magnetic resonance imaging (MRI) of an asymptomatic colloid cyst located in a nonclassic location, posterior to the foramen of Monro between the fornices and the leaflets of the septum pellucidum. Although the diameter of the cyst exceeds 1 cm, **(c)** the coronal image demonstrates that it is not obstructing the foramen of Monro and no ventriculomegaly is present. This cyst has been safely observed without surgical intervention for more than 4 years. (Used with permission from Barrow Neurological Institute.)

After weighing the data, some authors believe that the most accurate rate is near 1:8,500.[19] Estimates of the incidence of symptomatic colloid cysts range between 1:1,000,000 per person per year to 3:1,000,000 per person per year depending on the population under investigation.[19,20] These data suggest that most colloid cysts remain asymptomatic and undetected. One Dutch study estimated that, of 1,800 individuals likely harboring a colloid cyst in the general population, only 78 were diagnosed.[19] Although the data are scarce, most clinicians agree that most colloid cysts are asymptomatic and are never detected.

■ Clinical Symptoms

Colloid cysts are slow-growing lesions, and symptoms, when they do develop, usually appear between the ages of 20 and 50 years.[15,28,29] Most symptoms are related to gradually progressive hydrocephalus as cyst expansion causes blockage of cerebrospinal fluid (CSF) pathways.[30] Headache is the most common symptom. Classically, colloid cyst headaches are frontal, paroxysmal, improve in the recumbent position, and are associated with nausea and vomiting in as many as 50% of cases.[15] However, headaches are very common in the general population and often occur in patients with small cysts (< 5 mm) that are neither obstructing the foramen of Monro nor associated with ventricular enlargement. Whether these should be classified as symptomatic is controversial. Furthermore, even in the setting of biventricular hydrocephalus, the clinical presentation of symptomatic colloid cysts can be quite variable and nonspecific. Patients may have vague complaints of dizziness, gait disturbance, cognitive slowing, memory dysfunction, and urinary incontinence.[15,31] In most cases, symptoms progress gradually, reflecting the slow-growing nature of these lesions and the possibility that CSF obstruction is intermittent and associated with some degree of cerebral compensation.

Acute Hydrocephalus and Sudden Death

Sudden death is a rare but well-documented complication of previously undetected colloid cysts.[4–14] Several case reports describe sudden neurological deterioration in previously healthy patients found to harbor a colloid cyst causing acute hydrocephalus on presentation. Over 60 such reports exist in the literature, although, because most cases of sudden death are not published, the true number of instances is higher. In most cases, sudden death is believed to be due to obstruction at the foramen of Monro.[4,15] Some reports, however, offer alternative explanations, such as more distal obstruction of the cerebral aqueduct by cyst contents, pressure-related hypothalamic dysfunction, and sudden sympathetic discharge causing cardiac dysrhythmias.[16,17]

Sudden death associated with colloid cysts is thought to affect younger patients disproportionately.[32] One study determined that the mean age of patients suffering sudden death was 27 years, compared with a mean age of 41 years among 372 symptomatic colloid cyst patients reported over a 25-year period.[6,11] Proposed explanations for this predilection include a lower cerebral tolerance to CSF obstruction in younger patients and the possibility that colloid cysts have greater potential to grow more rapidly earlier in life.[23,32] A disproportionate number of cases of sudden death also appear to affect airline travelers.[6,15] Some postulate that this is due to the effect of changes in atmospheric pressure on intracranial pressure.[33]

The true risk of sudden death in patients harboring a colloid cyst is difficult to ascertain and likely depends on the patient's age, symptoms, and the presence of hydrocephalus. In some early reports the rates of sudden death were as high as 11 to 20% among colloid cyst patients seeking medical attention.[22,25] In a more recent retrospective study of 78 Dutch colloid cyst patients, the authors estimated a 34% lifetime risk of sudden neurological decline among symptomatic patients.[19] Other studies suggest that rates of acute life-threatening neurological decline between 21 and 37%.[20]

Although these rates are high, a significant limitation of all of these studies is their retrospective nature and substantial selection bias. In most studies, the only patients studied were those who presented with symptoms, often acutely to an emergency room. Consequently, these studies do not address the question of risk for patients harboring incidental lesions. As a result, the appropriate management of asymptomatic colloid cysts is controversial. Some clinicians cite the high rates of sudden death as evidence that incidental lesions should be treated, and others question the applicability of these results to the asymptomatic population. Even among those who agree that the risk of sudden death associated with asymptomatic colloid cysts is low, the desire to avoid a low-probability but catastrophic event may continue to influence treatment decisions. Although no firm conclusions can be drawn, sudden death without preceding symptoms is believed to be a rare occurrence.

■ Management Options

The management options of asymptomatic colloid cysts include surgical treatment or observation. Surgical treatment may consist of open microsurgical cyst resection, endoscopic cyst resection, or stereotactic cyst aspiration. Ventriculoperitoneal shunting provides treatment of cyst-associated hydrocephalus but does not directly treat the cyst itself. No known lifestyle modifications, additional medical risk factors, drug, chemotherapy, or radiation options have been shown to affect colloid cyst progression.

Observation

Observation with periodic surveillance imaging is an option sometimes advocated for asymptomatic colloid cysts. A caveat to this approach is that conscientious routine clinical and radiographic follow-up is required for early detection of cyst-related symptoms, cystic enlargement, or ventriculomegaly. Patients and families are instructed to pay strict attention to symptoms of headache, dizziness, gait instability, memory problems, and urinary incontinence in particular. The literature does not provide an objective indication of how often patients should undergo imaging. Anecdotal evidence and expert opinion (class IV) favor annual imaging, preferably with MRI.

Microsurgical Cyst Resection

Open microsurgical resection is the gold standard for the treatment of symptomatic colloid cysts.[18,34] Open surgery offers direct visualization of the cyst and an opportunity for gross total removal with standard microsurgical techniques. In most instances, complete cyst removal (including removal of the cyst wall) will represent a cure. The deep location of colloid cysts and the preponderance of important surrounding neurovascular structures, particularly the fornices, can create surgical challenges.

Endoscopic Cyst Resection

In more recent years, endoscopic approaches have gained popularity for the treatment of colloid cysts. As experience with endoscopic techniques and instrumentation has grown, endoscopic case series have demonstrated excellent results in treating these lesions.[35–41] The underlying philosophy of endoscopic approaches to colloid cysts is to achieve cure rates comparable to those associated with open approaches but with less approach-related morbidity.

Stereotactic Cyst Aspiration

Prior to the development and refinement of microsurgical and endoscopic approaches to colloid cysts, cyst decompression was frequently achieved through stereotactic aspiration of the cystic contents. This approach was thought to be associated with minimal risk. However, because the cyst wall is not resected, recurrence rates with an aspiration-only technique remain higher, with two studies reporting cyst recurrence rates of 39% and 69%.[42,43] Subsequently, stereotactic aspiration has fallen from favor as a treatment of colloid cysts. In patients with significant comorbid conditions and an unacceptable microsurgical risk, stereotactic aspiration may have a role in achieving cyst decompression despite high recurrence rates.

Ventriculoperitoneal Shunting

The goal of placing a ventriculoperitoneal shunt in the setting of a colloid cyst is to treat the hydrocephalus caused by cyst obstruction of CSF pathways. Shunt placement does not directly address the cyst itself. As such, shunting is not considered a first-line treatment of colloid cysts and is reserved for patients with hydrocephalus in whom microsurgery or endoscopic resection are deemed too high risk or in patients with intractable hydrocephalus despite cyst resection. This approach is definitely not recommended for asymptomatic patients with no objective signs of hydrocephalus. In fact, it may not be adequate treatment if hydrocephalus does develop, because a unilateral shunt may not prevent herniation caused by a cyst that obstructs both ventricles.

In cases of acute neurological decline due to hydrocephalus, emergent external ventricular drain placement effectively treats hydrocephalus and may be life-saving. In such cases, placement of an external ventricular drain should not be delayed. Endoscopic third ventriculostomy is seldom an effective treatment for colloid cyst–associated hydrocephalus because the main point of CSF blockage is at the foramen of Monro, proximal to the ventriculostomy site on the floor of the third ventricle.

Surgical Indications

The surgical indications for colloid cysts include any colloid cyst causing clear symptoms of CSF obstruction, including headaches, nausea, vomiting, dizziness, and acute neurological deterioration. As noted, in cases of acute neurological decline, an emergent external ventricular drain should be placed without delay before surgical intervention.

In cases of asymptomatic colloid cysts, the indications for surgery remain controversial and no absolute indications for surgery exist. As is discussed here, relative indications for treatment of an asymptomatic colloid cyst include the following: (1) age < 50 years, (2) maximum cyst diameter > 10 mm, (3) ventriculomegaly, and (4) hyperintense cyst contents on T2-weighted MRI sequences. Decisions to observe asymptomatic colloid cysts require close long-term clinical and radiographic follow-up. Therefore, an inability to closely follow patients (for social, economic, or other reasons) may be considered a relative indication for surgical intervention.

The psychological burden of harboring a colloid cyst may weigh heavily on some patients and this should be addressed through counseling. A particularly difficult problem is posed by patients with ongoing vague or protean symptoms or headaches from another cause (for example, migraine) with small cysts and normal-sized ventricles. Such patients or their neurosurgeons may think the patient should seek a surgical reevaluation each time they have symptoms because they fear that the cyst is the actual cause and neurological deterioration is imminent. In this setting, patients may request cyst removal although they do not meet the other criteria. Whether removal is offered or not and by what means must be addressed on a case-by-case basis.

Level I Evidence

No studies provide Level I evidence comparing surgical treatment to observation for asymptomatic colloid cysts.

Level II Evidence

No studies provide Level II evidence comparing surgical treatment to observation for asymptomatic colloid cysts. However, Level II studies that investigate the natural history of asymptomatic colloid cysts and the risk factors for symptom development have been conducted.

Pollock and Huston performed an observational retrospective study of 68 patients with incidentally discovered colloid cysts treated conservatively to delineate the long-term prognosis of patients harboring asymptomatic lesions.[23] Fifty-eight (85%) patients were followed clinically for a mean of 79 months. One (2%) patient eventually developed symptoms 101 months after initial diagnosis. No other patient developed symptoms or required surgical treatment. An additional patient experienced asymptomatic cyst growth at 81 months with no ventriculomegaly and did not require treatment. Of the 34 patients followed radiographically, only these two (6%) patients demonstrated cyst growth or change in ventricular size during the follow-up period. This study was an update of a prior study demonstrating that no symptoms developed over a mean follow-up period of 19 months in 24 patients with incidental colloid cysts managed conservatively.[44]

Pollock and colleagues also retrospectively compared clinical and radiographic features of 87 symptomatic and 68 asymptomatic colloid cyst patients to delineate factors associated with symptom development.[32] Using multivariate logistic regression, the authors identified younger patient age, larger cyst size, ventriculomegaly, and increased T2-weighted signal as independent risk factors for symptom development. Recursive partitioning analysis was used to stratify patients based on these risk factors. This analysis yielded three groups with significantly different risk levels of symptom development. Group 1 included patients with normal ventricular size and cysts less than 10 mm in maximum diameter. Symptoms were present in 12% of these patients. Group 2 included patients with ventriculomegaly who were older than 50 years and had a cyst less than 10 mm in diameter; 50% of group 2 had symptoms. Group 3, the highest-risk group, included all patients with cysts greater than 10 mm in maximum diameter as well as all young patients (age < 50 years) with ventriculomegaly. Eighty-five percent of group 3 had symptoms. These findings suggest that patients with small cysts and normal-sized ventricles have a low risk of developing symptoms, whereas those with cysts larger than 10 mm or young patients with ventriculomegaly have a high risk of becoming symptomatic. Notably, many patients fell in the intermediate category for which symptom development was difficult to predict.

Level III Evidence

No studies provide Level III evidence comparing surgical treatment to observation for asymptomatic colloid cysts.

Level IV Evidence

Sporadic case reports and case series provide mixed evidence regarding the safety of observing asymptomatic colloid cysts. In a retrospective series of 40 patients with a colloid cyst, Hernesniemi and Leivo encountered two patients with small (3 mm and 7 mm) asymptomatic cysts that were observed.[20] During a follow-up period of 1 and 3 years, respectively, both patients remained well with no symptoms. Kondziolka and Lunsford elected to observe six patients with small (< 7 mm) asymptomatic cysts.[21] During a follow-up period ranging from 3 to 7 years, all six patients remained well with no need for surgical intervention. Mathiesen and colleagues retrospectively reviewed 37 colloid cysts patients.[22] Of these, seven patients were initially observed because they were either asymptomatic or had minimal symptoms. During a follow-up period of 6 to 37 months, four (57%) of these patients developed new or worsening symptoms and required treatment. The authors concluded that most young patients will eventually develop symptoms and require treatment.

In addition to these retrospective series of asymptomatic colloid cyst patients, more than 60 cases of colloid cyst–related sudden death or acute neurological decline have been reported.[4–14] In most of these cases, the colloid cyst was a new diagnosis, although a definitive lack of symptoms prior to presentation cannot be established.

Autopsy and epidemiological studies suggest that most colloid cysts are asymptomatic and remain undetected throughout life. Most autopsy studies report a prevalence of colloid cysts in the general population of ~ 1 in 10,000.[1–3] Other authors report that the prevalence of colloid cysts is ~ 1 in 8,500.[19] The incidence of symptomatic colloid cysts diagnosed each year ranges from 1 in 1,000,000 to 3 in 1,000,000.[19,20] These data may be extrapolated and compared with the frequency of reported sudden death events. Such an analysis indirectly suggests that the vast majority of colloid cysts never become symptomatic or cause sudden death.

Conclusion

Asymptomatic colloid cysts present a dilemma to clinicians. Sudden death related to CSF obstruction is a rare but feared complication. The perceived risk of this catastrophic event is often cited as a reason to treat even incidental colloid cysts.

The literature provides no data directly comparing surgery to observation for asymptomatic colloid cysts. However, epidemiological and autopsy studies suggest that most incidental colloid cysts never cause symptoms and are never detected.

Level II data suggest that 98% of asymptomatic cysts will remain asymptomatic and not require treatment over long-term follow-up.[23] Additional Level II natural history data suggest that among cases of asymptomatic colloid cysts, a cyst size < 10 mm, lack of ventriculomegaly, and patient age > 50 years are associated with continued lack of symptoms over long-term follow-up.[32] Small case series suggest that observation for asymptomatic colloid cysts is safe, although in one study four of seven patients eventually developed symptoms.[20–22]

In conclusion, although definite data are lacking, the literature supports observation as a safe treatment for most asymptomatic colloid cysts. The risk of observation may be higher among young patients and those with large colloid cysts. Asymptomatic ventriculomegaly alone does not clearly affect risk in older patients.

■ Surgical Approach

If a decision to treat an asymptomatic colloid cyst is reached, definitive treatment options include open microsurgical resection and endoscopic resection. The goals of treatment are to decompress the cyst to restore normal CSF dynamics and to remove the cyst completely to achieve cure. Stereotactic cyst aspiration and ventriculoperitoneal shunt placement are not accepted definitive colloid cyst treatments and therefore are not discussed.

Microsurgical resection emerged before the advent of neuroendoscopy. For this reason, it remains the gold standard to which endoscopic results are measured. The goal of endoscopic colloid cyst resection is to achieve results comparable (or superior) to those of microsurgical approaches, with shorter hospital stays and less perioperative morbidity.

Microsurgical Treatment

Historically, microsurgical colloid cyst resection was achieved via a transcortical route. This approach takes advantage of noneloquent frontal cortex to create a transcortical corridor to the lateral ventricle. Once the ventricle is accessed, the foramen of Monro is identified, and the colloid cyst may be visualized near the foramen, attached to the roof of the third ventricle.

One disadvantage of the transcortical approach is the amount of normal brain tissue that must be traversed to reach the cyst. As microsurgical techniques have advanced, the interhemispheric transcallosal approach has largely replaced the transcortical approach and obviates the need to place normal cortex at risk.[18,34,45] When the transcallosal approach is performed, a craniotomy is turned two thirds in front of and one third behind the coronal suture, just over and lateral to the superior sagittal sinus. The interhemispheric fissure is opened, and the pericallosal arteries over the corpus callosum are identified and preserved. A small (1 cm) corpus callosotomy is made to gain entrance into the lateral ventricle. Once inside the ventricle, the foramen of Monro is identified. The colloid cyst is usually in the vicinity of the foramen with an attachment point connected to the velum interpositum at the roof of the third ventricle. If necessary, the choroidal fissure may be split from the foramen of Monro posteriorly to increase posterior access into the third ventricle. The position of the fornices must be noted, and these structures demand surgical respect. The proximity or adherence of colloid cysts to the body of the fornices may limit the ability to resect the cyst wall completely. Colloid cysts rarely adhere to the columns of the fornix within the foramen of Monro itself.

Endoscopic Treatment

Although several variations of the endoscopic approach to colloid cysts have been described, they all share the common goal of safe resection of a cyst with minimal disruption of normal tissue and without the need for a formal craniotomy.[35–41] An optimal endoscopic trajectory to colloid cysts utilizes an anterolateral entry point, anterior to the coronal suture and up to 7 cm lateral to midline. This trajectory, just above the head of the caudate nucleus, offers a more direct view of the attachment point of the cyst at the roof of the third ventricle. Endoscopic colloid cyst resection is one of the few purely endoscopic procedures in neurosurgery—all instruments are passed through the working channels of the endoscope itself. Once the shaft of the endoscope has reached the lateral ventricle, the cyst is removed with a combination of aspiration and sharp dissection with gentle countertraction.

Level I Evidence

No studies offer Level I evidence comparing microsurgical to endoscopic approaches to colloid cysts.

Level II Evidence

No studies offer Level II evidence comparing microsurgical to endoscopic treatment of colloid cysts.

Level III Evidence

Five studies provide Level III evidence comparing open microsurgical resection to endoscopic treatment of colloid cysts (**Table 16.1**). In the largest study comparing these two approaches, Horn and colleagues retrospectively compared completeness of cyst resection, length of hospital stay, perioperative morbidity, and need for re-treatment in 55 patients with a colloid cyst who underwent an open transcallosal approach (27 patients) or endoscopic resection (28 patients).[18] Compared with the patients who underwent open surgery, endoscopic treatment was associated with shorter operative times and shorter lengths of hospital stay but with higher rates of residual cyst. No patients in either cohort demonstrated cyst recurrence, although the follow-up period (10.1 and 10.9 months) was brief. The authors conclude that endoscopic resection is a viable first-line treatment, with the understanding that some patients may require re-treatment for incomplete cyst resection.

Stachura and colleagues retrospectively compared 23 patients with a colloid cyst of whom 10 patients underwent endoscopic treatment and 13 underwent an open transcortical-transventricular approach.[46] There were no significant differences in the rates of perioperative morbidity. Although the rate of complete resection was higher in the open microsurgical group, only one endoscopic patient required re-treatment. The authors concluded that endoscopic treatment was a safe and effective treatment option.

Grondin and colleagues retrospectively compared the outcomes of 25 patients with endoscopically treated colloid cysts with nine patients who underwent microsurgical treatment.[47] Endoscopic treatment was associated with a shorter length of procedure, shorter hospital stay, and lower complication rate. The rates of complete cyst resection were high in both groups. The authors concluded that endoscopic treatment was associated with lower risk than open microsurgery, with equivalent efficacy.

Two early retrospective cohort studies also compared open to endoscopic approaches for the treatment of colloid cysts but are limited by small sample sizes. In 2001 Kehler and colleagues compared the outcomes of 10 patients with a colloid cyst treated endoscopically with 10 patients who underwent open microsurgery.[35] Endoscopic treatment was associated with fewer complications but higher rates of incomplete resection. In 1994 Lewis and colleagues published results of the first study comparing open and endoscopic approaches for colloid cysts.[48] Seven patients underwent endoscopic treatment and eight underwent microsurgery. Endoscopic treatment was

Table 16.1 Retrospective studies comparing open microsurgical to endoscopic treatment of colloid cysts

Study	No. patients		Rate of complete cyst resection (%)		Residual cyst requiring re-treatment (%)		Recurrence rate (%)		Length of stay (days)		Operative or neurological complications (%)	
	Open	Endo	Open	Endo	Open	Endo	Open	Endo	Open	Endo	Open	Endo
Horn et al 2007[18]	27	28	94	53	0	7	0	0	6.3	5.4	33	13
Stachura et al 2009[46]	13	10	100	60	0	10	NA	NA	NA	NA	38	30
Grondin et al 2007[47]	9	25	100	96	0	0	11	4	8.4	3.8	33	4
Kehler et al 2001[35]	10	10	80	30	NA	NA	0	10	18.9	5.1	50	30
Lewis et al 1994[48]	8	7	NA	NA	NA	NA	NA	NA	9.5	4	63	14

Abbreviations: Open, open microsurgical approach; Endo, endoscopic approach; NA, data not assessed by the study.

associated with shorter hospital stays, fewer complications, and a faster return to work than microsurgery. Completeness of cyst resection and recurrence rates were not evaluated.

Level IV Evidence

Several endoscopic and microsurgical case series have delineated the success and complication rates of these respective approaches (**Table 16.2**). Symss and colleagues published a series of 78 patients treated with a transcallosal microsurgical approach.[49] The rate of complete cyst resection was 99%, and the recurrence rate was 3%. There were no instances of neurocognitive disconnection syndromes. A recent series of ten patients undergoing transcallosal microsurgical resection demonstrated short operative times (mean 124 minutes), a 100% rate of complete cyst excision, 0 recurrences, and 20% rate of new memory deficits.[45] In 2009 Shapiro and colleagues published the results of 57 patients with a colloid cyst who underwent transcallosal-subchoroidal resection and who were followed for a mean of 12 years.[34] Their rate of complete excision was 100%, and the recurrence rate was 0%, as was the rate of permanent neurological morbidity. Hernesniemi and Leivo reported outcomes for 134 patients with colloid cysts treated from an open transcallosal approach and found high rates of complete removal, no surgical mortality, and low surgical morbidity that was primarily transient.[20] Desai and colleagues reported an 86% rate of complete excision and 2% rate of permanent memory deficits in 105 patients with a colloid cyst treated via open microsurgery.[50]

Several case series have investigated the safety and efficacy of endoscopic approaches to colloid cysts (**Table 16.3**). Boogaarts and colleagues retrospectively reviewed 90 patients undergoing endoscopic colloid cyst resection.[40] Eighty-five of the 90 patients had follow-up for 51 months. There was one case of permanent neurological morbidity. Of 80 patients with follow-up imaging, residual cyst was noted in 42.5%. Six of these cases (7%) eventually required re-treatment. Engh and colleagues reported results using an endoscopic port system.[51] Among 32 cases, complete excision was achieved in 97% and there were no cases of permanent neurological morbidity. Among 59 patients undergoing endoscopic resection, Mishra and colleagues reported a 78% rate of complete excision, no recurrences over a 99-month follow-up period, and one death due to meningitis.[52] Hellwig and colleagues reported a 90% rate of excellent clinic outcomes and a 5% recurrence rate among 20 colloid cyst patients treated with an endoscopic approach over a 10-year period.[39] Greenlee and colleagues reported 35 consecutive patients with a colloid cyst treated with an endoscopic approach.[41] Although six cases required conversion to open craniotomy, the cyst was resected completely in all patients. Over a mean follow-up of 88 months, one patient had an asymptomatic recurrence. In other endoscopic case series, recurrence rates have ranged between 0 and 11.5%, depending on the length of follow-up.[18,53]

Expert Recommendations

1. Observation with close long-term clinical and radiographic follow-up is a safe management strategy for most asymptomatic colloid cysts without hydrocephalus (Grade 1C Recommendation, Level II/IV Evidence).
2. The risk with observation may be higher in patients younger than 50 years and colloid cysts greater than 1 cm in diameter (Grade 1C Recommendation, Level II Evidence).
3. The development of symptoms attributable to the cyst, new ventriculomegaly, or increases in cyst size should prompt treatment in previously asymptomatic colloid cysts (Grade 1 C Recommendation, Level II/IV Evidence).
4. Both endoscopic resection and open microsurgical resection are appropriate treatment options for colloid cysts. Endoscopic approaches may be associated with shorter hospital stays and less morbidity, whereas open microsurgery may be associated with lower recurrence rates. In either treatment, complete cyst removal is the operative goal (Grade 1C Recommendation, Level III/IV Evidence).

Table 16.2 Recent retrospective series of colloid cysts resected via an open microsurgical approach

Study	No. patients	Rate of complete cyst resection (%)	Recurrence rate (%)	Permanent morbidity (%)
Symss et al 2011[49]	78	99	3	NA
Sampath et al 2010[45]	10	100	0	20
Shapiro et al 2009[34]	57	100	0	0

Abbreviation: NA, not assessed by the study.

Table 16.3 Recent retrospective series of colloid cysts resected via an endoscopic approach

Study	No. patients	Rate of complete cyst resection (%)	Recurrence rate (%)	Permanent morbidity (%)
Boogaarts et al 2011[40]	85	57.5	7	1
Engh et al 2010[51]	47	97	NA	0
Mishra et al 2010[52]	59	78	0	2
Greenlee et al 2008[41]	35	83[a]	3	0
Hellwig et al 2003[39]	29	0	5	10

Abbreviation: NA, not assessed by the study.
[a]Six patients required conversion to open approach.

Summary and Conclusions

No Level I, II, or III evidence supports whether one should operate on asymptomatic colloid cysts of the third ventricle. Cysts larger than 1 cm associated with hydrocephalus or with nonspecific symptoms may be considered for elective treatment.

Once a decision is made to pursue surgery, the literature supports either open microsurgical or endoscopic approaches as a first-line treatment for colloid cysts. Both approaches provide excellent rates of cyst removal associated with low rates of morbidity. No Level I or II data are available to compare the safety and efficacy of the open microsurgical and endoscopic approaches. Level III evidence suggests that operative time, length of hospital stay, and time to return to work are shorter when an endoscopic approach is used, although rates of complete cyst excision may be lower with endoscopic techniques. Level IV studies demonstrate excellent clinical and radiographic outcomes in patients undergoing either microsurgical or endoscopic resection, although rates of incomplete resection may be higher among endoscopically treated patients.

■ References

1. Di Maio TM, Di Maio DJ. Sudden death due to colloid cysts of third cerebral ventricle. N Y State J Med 1974;74(10):1832–1834
2. DiMaio SM, DiMaio VJ, Kirkpatrick JB. Sudden, unexpected deaths due to primary intracranial neoplasms. Am J Forensic Med Pathol 1980;1(1):29–45
3. Gezelius C, Eriksson A. Neoplastic disease in a medicolegal autopsy material: a retrospective study in northern Sweden. Z Rechtsmed 1988;101(2):115–130
4. Opeskin K, Anderson RM, Lee KA. Colloid cyst of the 3rd ventricle as a cause of acute neurological deterioration and sudden death. J Paediatr Child Health 1993;29(6):476–477
5. Aronica PA, Ahdab-Barmada M, Rozin L, Wecht CH. Sudden death in an adolescent boy due to a colloid cyst of the third ventricle. Am J Forensic Med Pathol 1998;19(2):119–122
6. Büttner A, Winkler PA, Eisenmenger W, Weis S. Colloid cysts of the third ventricle with fatal outcome: a report of two cases and review of the literature. Int J Legal Med 1997;110(5):260–266
7. Byard RW, Moore L. Sudden and unexpected death in childhood due to a colloid cyst of the third ventricle. J Forensic Sci 1993;38(1):210–213
8. Chan RC, Thompson GB. Third ventricular colloid cysts presenting with acute neurological deterioration. Surg Neurol 1983;19(4):358–362
9. Filkins JA, Cohle S, Levy BK, Graham M. Unexpected deaths due to colloid cysts of the third ventricle. J Forensic Sci 1996;41(3):521–523
10. Macaulay RJ, Felix I, Jay V, Becker LE. Histological and ultrastructural analysis of six colloid cysts in children. Acta Neuropathol 1997;93(3):271–276
11. Ryder JW, Kleinschmidt-DeMasters BK, Keller TS. Sudden deterioration and death in patients with benign tumors of the third ventricle area. J Neurosurg 1986;64(2):216–223
12. Shemie S, Jay V, Rutka J, Armstrong D. Acute obstructive hydrocephalus and sudden death in children. Ann Emerg Med 1997;29(4):524–528
13. Stoodley MA, Nguyen TP, Robbins P. Familial fatal and near-fatal third ventricle colloid cysts. Aust N Z J Surg 1999;69(10):733–736
14. Williams DJ, Tannenberg AE. Unusual presentation of colloid cyst of the third ventricle. Med Sci Law 1997;37(3):254–256
15. Humphries RL, Stone CK, Bowers RC. Colloid cyst: a case report and literature review of a rare but deadly condition. J Emerg Med 2011;40(1):e5–e9
16. Jarquin-Valdivia AA, Rich AT, Yarbrough JL, Thompson RC. Intraventricular colloid cyst, hydrocephalus and neurogenic stunned myocardium. Clin Neurol Neurosurg 2005;107(5):361–365
17. Brun A, Egund N. The pathogenesis of cerebral symptoms in colloid cysts of the third ventricle: a clinical and pathoanatomical study. Acta Neurol Scand 1973;49(4):525–535
18. Horn EM, Feiz-Erfan I, Bristol RE, et al. Treatment options for third ventricular colloid cysts: comparison of open microsurgical versus endoscopic resection. Neurosurgery 2007;60(4):613–618
19. de Witt Hamer PC, Verstegen MJ, De Haan RJ, et al. High risk of acute deterioration in patients harboring symptomatic colloid cysts of the third ventricle. J Neurosurg 2002;96(6):1041–1045
20. Hernesniemi J, Leivo S. Management outcome in third ventricular colloid cysts in a defined population: a series of 40 patients treated mainly by transcallosal microsurgery. Surg Neurol 1996;45(1):2–14

21. Kondziolka D, Lunsford LD. Microsurgical resection of colloid cysts using a stereotactic transventricular approach. Surg Neurol 1996;46(5):485–490
22. Mathiesen T, Grane P, Lindgren L, Lindquist C. Third ventricle colloid cysts: a consecutive 12-year series. J Neurosurg 1997;86(1):5–12
23. Pollock BE, Huston J III. Natural history of asymptomatic colloid cysts of the third ventricle. J Neurosurg 1999;91(3):364–369
24. Ho KL, Garcia JH. Colloid cysts of the third ventricle: ultrastructural features are compatible with endodermal derivation. Acta Neuropathol 1992;83(6):605–612
25. Little JR, MacCarty CS. Colloid cysts of the third ventricle. J Neurosurg 1974;40(2):230–235
26. Katzman GL, Dagher AP, Patronas NJ. Incidental findings on brain magnetic resonance imaging from 1000 asymptomatic volunteers. JAMA 1999;282(1):36–39
27. Yue NC, Longstreth WT Jr, Elster AD, Jungreis CA, O'Leary DH, Poirier VC. Clinically serious abnormalities found incidentally at MR imaging of the brain: data from the Cardiovascular Health Study. Radiology 1997;202(1):41–46
28. Nitta M, Symon L. Colloid cysts of the third ventricle: a review of 36 cases. Acta Neurochir (Wien) 1985;76(3-4):99–104
29. Hwang DH, Townsend JC, Ilsen PF, Bright DC. Colloid cyst of the third ventricle. J Am Optom Assoc 1996;67(4):227–234
30. Spears RC. Colloid cyst headache. Curr Pain Headache Rep 2004;8(4):297–300
31. Upadhyaya AK, Sud PD. Psychiatric presentation of third ventricular colloid cyst. A case report. Br J Psychiatry 1988; 152:567–569
32. Pollock BE, Schreiner SA, Huston J III. A theory on the natural history of colloid cysts of the third ventricle. Neurosurgery 2000;46(5):1077–1081
33. ter Meulen BC, Kros JM, Jacobs BC. Sudden death after air travel in a patient with colloid cyst. Neurology 2006;67(6): 1005
34. Shapiro S, Rodgers R, Shah M, Fulkerson D, Campbell RL. Interhemispheric transcallosal subchoroidal fornix-sparing craniotomy for total resection of colloid cysts of the third ventricle. J Neurosurg 2009;110(1):112–115
35. Kehler U, Brunori A, Gliemroth J, et al. Twenty colloid cysts—comparison of endoscopic and microsurgical management. Minim Invasive Neurosurg 2001;44(3):121–127
36. Souweidane MM, Luther N. Endoscopic resection of solid intraventricular brain tumors. J Neurosurg 2006;105(2): 271–278
37. Abdou MS, Cohen AR. Endoscopic treatment of colloid cysts of the third ventricle: technical note and review of the literature. J Neurosurg 1998;89(6):1062–1068
38. Decq P, Le Guerinel C, Brugières P, et al. Endoscopic management of colloid cysts. Neurosurgery 1998;42(6): 1288–1294
39. Hellwig D, Bauer BL, Schulte M, Gatscher S, Riegel T, Bertalanffy H. Neuroendoscopic treatment for colloid cysts of the third ventricle: the experience of a decade. Neurosurgery 2003;52(3):525–533
40. Boogaarts HD, Decq P, Grotenhuis JA, et al. Long-term results of the neuroendoscopic management of colloid cysts of the third ventricle: a series of 90 cases. Neurosurgery 2011; 68(1):179–187
41. Greenlee JD, Teo C, Ghahreman A, Kwok B. Purely endoscopic resection of colloid cysts. Neurosurgery 2008;62(3, Suppl 1): 51–55
42. Rajshekhar V. Rate of recurrence following stereotactic aspiration of colloid cysts of the third ventricle. Stereotact Funct Neurosurg 2012;90(1):37–44
43. Mathiesen T, Grane P, Lindquist C, von Holst H. High recurrence rate following aspiration of colloid cysts in the third ventricle. J Neurosurg 1993;78(5):748–752
44. Camacho A, Abernathey CD, Kelly PJ, Laws ER Jr. Colloid cysts: experience with the management of 84 cases since the introduction of computed tomography. Neurosurgery 1989;24(5):693–700
45. Sampath R, Vannemreddy P, Nanda A. Microsurgical excision of colloid cyst with favorable cognitive outcomes and short operative time and hospital stay: operative techniques and analyses of outcomes with review of previous studies. Neurosurgery 2010;66(2):368–374
46. Stachura K, Libionka W, Moskała M, Krupa M, Polak J. Colloid cysts of the third ventricle: endoscopic and open microsurgical management. Neurol Neurochir Pol 2009;43(3): 251–257
47. Grondin RT, Hader W, MacRae ME, Hamilton MG. Endoscopic versus microsurgical resection of third ventricle colloid cysts. Can J Neurol Sci 2007;34(2):197–207
48. Lewis AI, Crone KR, Taha J, van Loveren HR, Yeh HS, Tew JM Jr. Surgical resection of third ventricle colloid cysts. Preliminary results comparing transcallosal microsurgery with endoscopy. J Neurosurg 1994;81(2):174–178
49. Symss NP, Ramamurthi R, Rao SM, Vasudevan MC, Jain PK, Pande A. Management outcome of the transcallosal, transforaminal approach to colloid cysts of the anterior third ventricle: an analysis of 78 cases. Neurol India 2011;59(4):542–547
50. Desai KI, Nadkarni TD, Muzumdar DP, Goel AH. Surgical management of colloid cyst of the third ventricle—a study of 105 cases. Surg Neurol 2002;57(5):295–302
51. Engh JA, Lunsford LD, Amin DV, et al. Stereotactically guided endoscopic port surgery for intraventricular tumor and colloid cyst resection. Neurosurgery 2010;67(3, Suppl Operative):ons198–ons204
52. Mishra S, Chandra PS, Suri A, Rajender K, Sharma BS, Mahapatra AK. Endoscopic management of third ventricular colloid cysts: eight years' institutional experience and description of a new technique. Neurol India 2010;58(3):412–417
53. Acerbi F, Rampini P, Egidi M, Locatelli M, Borsa S, Gaini SM. Endoscopic treatment of colloid cysts of the third ventricle: long-term results in a series of 6 consecutive cases. J Neurosurg Sci 2007;51(2):53–60

17

Evidence-Based Management of Central Neurocytoma (Gross Total Resection versus Subtotal Resection and the Role of Adjunctive Therapies)

J. Dawn Waters, David Gonda, Clark C. Chen, and Bob S. Carter

The archetypal central neurocytoma is a benign tumor of phenotypically neuronal cells arising within the cerebral ventricles.[1] Initial case reports appeared in the literature in the 1980s.[2,3] Central neurocytoma is extremely rare and estimated to account for only 0.1 to 0.5% of brain tumors.[1,4] With such a short history and rarity, data about these tumors are less robust than for more common entities. Most of what is known comes from retrospective studies. This chapter first reviews pertinent characteristics of these tumors before delving into the best available evidence guiding current management recommendations.

■ Presentation

Central neurocytomas typically present in the second or third decade, although cases have been reported in children as young as 1 year old[4–6] and in adults into the sixth decade.[7] In general, presentation results from nonfocal and nonspecific signs and symptoms of increased intracranial pressure from obstructive hydrocephalus or tumor mass-effect. Symptoms such as headache, nausea-vomiting, visual loss, gait imbalance, bladder incontinence, seizure, and memory disturbances prompt neuroimaging with computed tomography (CT) and magnetic resonance imaging (MRI) to reveal the brain mass (**Fig. 17.1a–d**).[8] Classically, these symptoms evolve subtly with characteristic benign tumor behavior and growth within the ventricles. However, acute intratumoral hemorrhage or acute obstructive hydrocephalus may lead to sudden symptom onset, impaired consciousness, and coma.[7,9,10] Less commonly, neurocytomas appear within the brain parenchyma or spinal cord, either primarily or from cerebrospinal fluid (CSF) seeding, leading to focal neurological deficits related to the location of the lesion.[11–13]

■ Pathology

Macroscopically and intraoperatively, central neurocytomas have been described as soft, grayish tumors with gritty calcifications.[14] Under light microscopy (**Fig. 17.2a**), cells are often arranged in a honeycomb pattern, in perivascular or irregular rosettes, and on a fibrillary background of neuropil. Hematoxylin and eosin (H&E)-stained cells display finely stippled "salt and pepper" chromatin and artifactual cytoplasmic vacuolations, giving cells a "fried egg" appearance.[14] This histological architecture is often mistaken for oligodendrogliomas or ependymomas. Reliable diagnosis of central neurocytoma is achieved by demonstrating positive immunostaining with synaptophysin (**Fig. 17.2b**).[1,14]

Consistent with a benign tumor, central neurocytomas typically lack aggressive histological features, such as mitotic activity.[1] Historically, clinicians expected a benign clinical course consistent with the

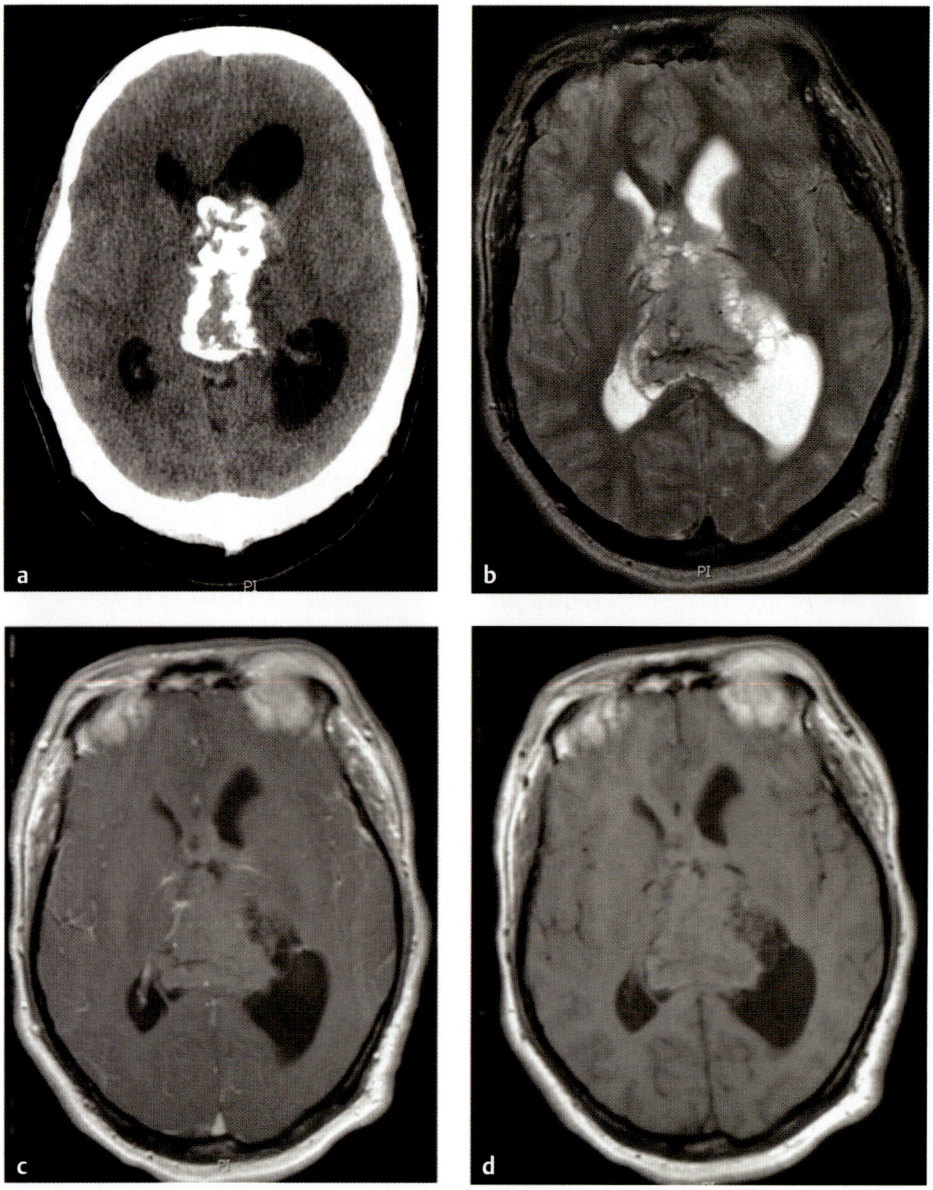

Fig. 17.1 Imaging of central neurocytoma. **(a)** Noncontrast computed tomography of the head demonstrating calcified intraventricular mass and hydrocephalus. **(b)** T2 magnetic resonance imaging (MRI) demonstrating the iso- to hyperintense mass within the enlarged ventricles. **(c)** Contrast-enhanced T1 MRI demonstrating a nonenhancing intraventricular mass with some vasculature delineated. **(d)** T1 MRI demonstrating an isointense mass within the ventricles.

tumor's benign histology. However, as additional experiences with central neurocytoma were reported, clinicians were vexed by the occasional more malignant clinical course in some patients.[1,15] Eventually, MIB-1 labeling of proliferating tumor cells at a rate greater than 2 to 3% emerged as a useful predictor of poor clinical outcome, even in the absence of histological atypia.[16–18] Subsequent studies found that 20% of central neurocytomas have a MIB-1 index greater than 3%.[19] Atypical central neurocytomas are variably defined as having either atypical histological features or a MIB-1 labeling index of greater than 2 or 3% with or without atypical histological features.[19,20] Management of "atypical" or "proliferating" central neurocytomas requires special consideration due to its more aggressive natural history.[16,18]

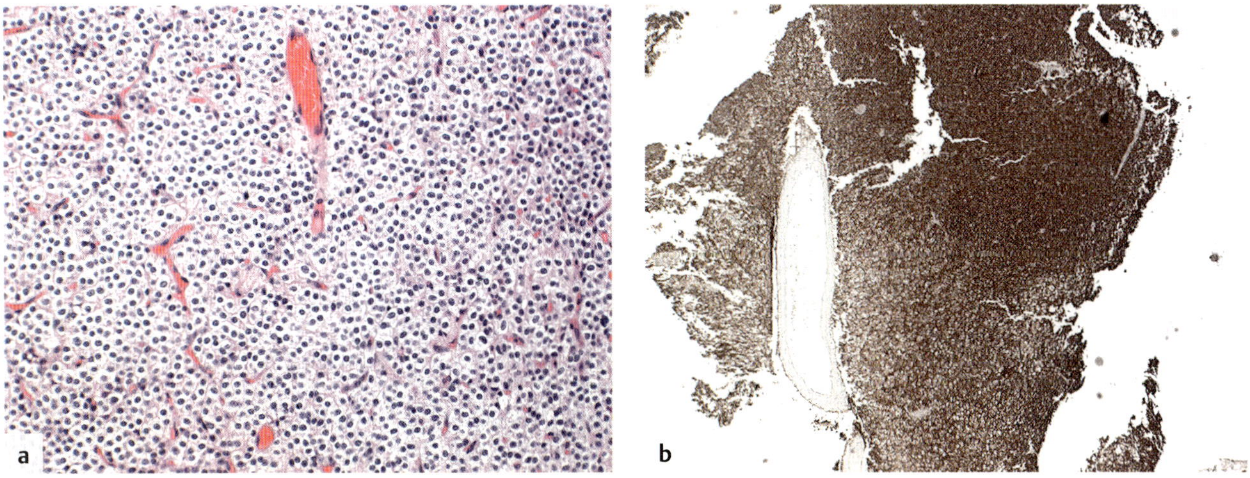

Fig. 17.2 Histology. **(a)** Appearance of a central neurocytoma on hematoxylin and eosin staining under light microscopy. **(b)** Synaptophysin positive immunostaining of a central neurocytoma.

■ Management of Central Neurocytoma

To summarize the principal management concerns, central neurocytoma is a rare intraventricular tumor presenting with ominous neurological symptoms in young patients. Youth and symptomatology favor aggressive yet safe intervention to effect a cure. Surgery is an important mainstay because CSF diversion is often necessary, and safely performed gross total resection of this benign tumor is considered curative.[19] In further support of gross total resection, transformation of tissue-confirmed residual central neurocytoma (MIB-1 of 0.5%) into a tumor with anaplastic oligodendroglioma and anaplastic astrocytoma features has been reported, with subsequent transformation into a glioblastoma.[21] Although gross total resection is favorable for many reasons, the following subsections review the best available evidence guiding current management recommendations for surgical management, management after subtotal resection, stereotactic radiosurgery, chemotherapy, and management of "atypical" central neurocytoma.

Gross Total Resection Is Superior to Subtotal Resection

Level I to Level II Evidence

There are no Level I or Level II evidence studies comparing gross total resection to subtotal resection.

Level III to Level IV Evidence

Surgical resection for central neurocytoma has been widely recognized as an important mainstay of treatment.[1,19] At the conservative management extreme, in 2002, Kulkarni et al published a case series of eight patients treated with stereotactic biopsy and radiation therapy. Three of the patients received ventricular shunts. Follow-up ranged from 15 to 114 months. One patient in the series died after 5 years from a shunt malfunction, and another suffered subependymal spread and increased tumor growth before being lost to follow-up. Somewhat surprisingly, the remaining six patients remained asymptomatic, with stable to reduced tumor size.[22] This strategy of management without attempted surgical resection has not been widely adopted but serves as an important reminder as to the often benign nature of this tumor and its radiosensitivity.

There are clear data supporting the superiority of safely performed gross total resection. In the largest reported series, Rades and Schild[19] performed a meta-analysis drawing from 520 patients. For this study, patients were identified from previously published reports, which were found by searches of Medline, Current Contents, and PubMed using the keywords "neurocytoma" and "neurocytomas." Rades and Schild then contacted ~ 75% of the authors of the previous reports for additional information to complete the dataset. After excluding patients with incomplete data, outcomes for 438 patients were analyzed in terms of survival, local control, and treatments received. Their results are summarized in **Table 17.1**.

Table 17.1 Neurocytoma outcomes at 5 years by histology and ranked by survival

Histology	Treatment	Survival (%)	Local control (%)
Typical	GTR (*n* = 137)	100	87
	GTR + RT (*n* = 29)	100	100
	STR + RT ≤ 54 Gy (*n* = 38)	97	85
	STR + RT > 54 Gy (*n* = 34)	96	93
	STR (*n* = 90)	90	52
Atypical	GTR + RT (*n* = 14)	93	63
	GTR (*n* = 15)	91	59
	STR + RT > 54 Gy (*n* = 20)	79	79
	STR + RT ≤ 54 Gy (*n* = 17)	58	48
	STR (*n* = 19)	46	5

Abbreviations: GTR, gross total resection; RT, radiation therapy; STR, subtotal resection.

Source: Rades D, Schild SE. Treatment recommendations for the various subgroups of neurocytomas. J Neurooncol 2006;77(3): 305–309. Adapted with permission.

After gross total resection of a benign (typical) central neurocytoma in an adult, 5-year survival was 100% with an 87% local control rate. With gross total resection and radiation therapy, 5-year survival remained 100% and the local control rate was boosted to 100%. Because radiation therapy fails to improve survival after gross total resection of a benign central neurocytoma, most discourage routine postoperative radiation and encourage careful consideration of the risks of radiation versus the benefits of improved local control.[23] In contrast, after subtotal resection of a benign (typical) central neurocytoma in an adult, 5-year survival was only 90% with a 52% local control rate. Administration of radiation therapy after subtotal resection increased 5-year survival and local control to 97% and 90%, respectively. For subtotal resection of benign (typical) central neurocytoma, > 54 Gy resulted in a 93% 5-year local control rate, versus 85% at 54 Gy or less, but the difference was not statistically significant ($p = 0.24$), suggesting a dose of 50 to 54 Gy may be sufficient for typical neurocytomas.[19,24] Beyond survival and tumor control, a principal advantage of gross total resection is the possible avoidance of subsequent adjuvant therapies, such as chemotherapy, radiation therapy, and radiosurgery.

It is intuitive that gross total resection would be superior to subtotal resection. However, it is important to recognize that outcomes with subtotal resection with radiation therapy are quite excellent for benign (typical) central neurocytomas. Although gross total resection is a worthy goal, uncomplicated surgery remains the primary goal. In particularly risky or difficult surgical cases, the surgeon may acknowledge that subtotal resection with radiation therapy yields excellent results and avoid an overzealous pursuit of a gross total resection. Historically, gross total resection is achieved in 45 to 70% of cases.[14,19,25] Perioperative deaths have been reported in a few series at a rate of 5 to 7% and attributed to hemorrhage, infection, and cerebral edema.[8,26,27] Hallock et al additionally reported permanent motor or cognitive deficits in three out of a series of 19 (15.7%) patients treated with surgery with and without radiation and chemotherapy between 1984 and 2009.[27] Beyond survival and tumor control, cognitive outcomes are not commonly reported in the central neurocytoma literature; thus it is unclear if subtotal or gross total resection is superior in this dimension. This is particularly important due to the proximity of the fornix to most intraventricular tumors. In addition, improvements in surgical safety are yet to be demonstrated with the adoption of neuronavigation and advanced surgical techniques, such as endoscopy.[28,29]

For atypical (proliferating) central neurocytomas, the superiority of gross total resection is echoed.[19] However, the ability of adjuvant therapies to compensate for a subtotal resection in atypical tumors deserves special consideration. Adjuvant therapies in these special cases are addressed in the following subsections.

Recommendations for Management of Typical Neurocytoma

1. In all cases, attempt gross total resection over a subtotal resection if it can be performed safely without permanent or significant complication (Grade 1C Recommendation, Level III/IV Evidence).
2. In cases where gross total resection is particularly high risk, keep in mind radiation therapy added after subtotal resection yields similar outcomes and consider a more conservative resection (Grade 1C Recommendation, Level III/IV Evidence).
3. Use of radiation therapy after subtotal resection of typical (MIB < 2%) central neurocytoma is recommended at a dose of 50 to 54 Gy (Grade 1C Recommendation, Level III/IV Evidence).[19,24]
4. Routine use of radiation therapy after gross total resection of typical (MIB < 2%) central neurocytoma is not recommended because it does not improve survival. Consider risk of radiation (e.g., higher risk in pediatric patients) against the benefit of improved local control (e.g., tumor arises near critical structures) before recommending adjunctive radiation (Grade 2C Recommendation, Level III/IV Evidence).
5. Stereotactic biopsy with CSF diversion and radiation therapy but without resection is sometimes effective, but apparently inferior to resection (Grade 2C Recommendation, Level IV Evidence).

Evidence-Based Management of Atypical Central Neurocytoma

Level I to Level II Evidence

There are no Level I or Level II evidence studies addressing the management of atypical central neurocytoma.

Level III to Level IV Evidence

Previously considered benign, the first atypical central neurocytoma was reported in 1989.[20,30] In 2004, Rades et al conducted a meta-analysis of atypical central neurocytoma case reports and series in the literature. For their analysis, atypical central neurocytomas were defined as having a MIB-1 index of > 2% or atypical histological features, such as necrosis or increased mitotic activity. The authors collected complete data on 85 patients and compared survival and local control between the subsets of patients who received gross total resection, gross total resection with radiation therapy, subtotal resection, or subtotal resection with radiation therapy.[20]

After gross total resection of an atypical central neurocytoma, the survival rate at 5 years was 93%, and local control at 5 years was 57%.[20] For comparison, gross total resection of typical neurocytoma leads to 100% survival and 87% local control at 5 years. In fact, 5-year rates for atypical neurocytoma are lower than even 10-year rates for typical neurocytomas reported by Rades, further emphasizing the distinctly aggressive nature of atypical neurocytomas.[19] Despite its aggression, completely resected atypical neurocytomas did not respond to radiation therapy with significantly improved survival or local control rates (only 90% survival and 53% local control at 5 years), leading the authors to recommend against radiation therapy after complete resection of atypical neurocytoma.[19,20]

After subtotal resection of an atypical neurocytoma, the survival rate is 43% and the rate of local control is 7% without radiation therapy.[20] These rates improve dramatically with the addition of radiation therapy, with a 5-year survival rate of 78% and local control rate of 70%.[20] In a subsequent review, Rades and Schild recommend a radiation dose of 56 to 60 Gy after subtotal resection of atypical neurocytomas because this appeared to improve 5-year local control rates from 48% with ≤ 54 Gy versus 79% with > 54 Gy ($p = 0.05$).[19] Importantly, survival rates after subtotal resection of atypical neurocytomas do not approach the survival rates after gross total resection (again, 93% at 5 years), even with adjunctive radiation therapy (78% at 5 years). Thus gross total resection, if possible, is especially crucial to the management of atypical neurocytoma. Results from Rades and Schild's 2006 review[19] are summarized in **Table 17.1**.

Recommendations for Management of Atypical Neurocytoma

1. In all cases, attempt gross total resection over a subtotal resection if it can be performed safely without permanent or significant complication (Grade 1C Recommendation, Level III/IV Evidence).
2. Use of radiation therapy after gross total resection of atypical central neurocytoma has not been shown to significantly improve survival or local control and is thus not recommended (Grade 1C Recommendation, Level III/IV Evidence).
3. Use of radiation therapy after subtotal total resection of atypical central neurocytoma is recommended at a dose of 56 to 60 Gy (Grade 1C Recommendation, Level III/IV Evidence).

Stereotactic Radiosurgery and Other Adjuncts

Level I to Level II Evidence

There are no Level I or Level II evidence studies addressing stereotactic radiosurgery or chemotherapy.

Level III to Level IV Evidence

Stereotactic radiosurgery (SRS) has emerged as an appealing alternative to conventional radiation therapy due to expected benefits from focused radiation delivery to a target with minimized off-target radiation exposure. For central neurocytoma patients specifically, Paek et al reported on the long-term outcomes, including Karnofsky performance scale (KPS) scores, from six patients treated with surgical resection (three were gross total resections) and conventional radiation therapy. In Paek et al's series, two patients suffered a decline in KPS score related to demyelination after radiation therapy, and one patient developed a posterior fossa meningioma.[31] In contrast, Kim et al found no incidence of diminished KPS score related to SRS in their case series of 13 patients treated with Gamma Knife (Elekta, Atlanta, GA) for central neurocytoma. The expectation with SRS is that equivalent treatment outcomes from focused radiation would reduce late radiation toxicities well known to occur with conventional radiation therapy, such as cognitive dysfunction and secondary malignancies.[31–33]

Schild reported the first use of SRS in 1997 in which Gamma Knife (Elekta) was used in one patient upon recurrence after subtotal resection.[34] Stereotactic radiosurgery has potential utility in many phases of central neurocytoma management: up front without resection, after subtotal resection, or upon recurrence.[35] In 2012, Park and Chang published a quantitative systematic review of SRS for central neurocytoma, including previously published case series of at least five patients. Five studies qualified for Park and Chang's review, which accounted for 64 cases of central neurocytoma treated with either Gamma Knife (Elekta) or a linear accelerator SRS system. Although some studies in the review did not distinguish subtotal resection from recurrence, eight cases were identified as using SRS without surgical resection.[35–38] Park and Chang concluded that the overall rate of local control was 91.1% at a mean follow-up of ~ 5 years, which the authors note is comparable to conventional radiation therapy.[35] Of the four cases that did recur after SRS, one received a low marginal dose (12 Gy) and two recurred outside of the SRS target area.[35,38–40] This led authors to recommend using a marginal dose of more than 13 Gy and trying to include all portions of the tumor, even nonenhancing portions, in the SRS planning.[35,38,39]

Although Park and Chang did not directly compare SRS to conventional radiation therapy, one of the publications included in their review attempted this comparison.[35,40] Rades and Schild compared outcomes from the use of SRS ($n = 21$) to radiation therapy ($n = 41$) after subtotal resection of typical neurocytomas. Local control rates at 5 years were 100% with SRS, versus 87% with radiation therapy; however, this difference was not statistically significant ($p = 0.45$).[40] Similarly, 5-year survival was 100% for both SRS and radiation therapy groups. The authors conclude that SRS is comparable to conventional radiation therapy in terms of survival and local tumor control for the management of residual typical neurocytomas. Additionally, the authors note that data are insufficient to support or reject SRS for the treatment of residual atypical central neurocytoma.[40]

Experience treating neurocytomas with chemotherapy, either alone or as an adjunct to surgery or radiation, is limited. In 2008 Amini et al published a case report and review of the literature for cases of neurocytoma treated with chemotherapy. They note that theirs was the only case out of ~ 20 that demonstrated complete remission after any chemotherapy regimen. With such limited evidence and overall poor rates of remission, there is no demonstrated benefit of chemotherapy in neurocytoma. Thus, chemotherapy is generally reserved as a salvage therapy for recurrent tumor or failed response to radiation-based adjuncts. Likewise, the ideal chemotherapy regimen in these cases is yet to be identified.[4]

Expert Recommendations

1. Use of radiosurgery after subtotal resection of typical central neurocytoma is comparable to conventional radiation therapy (Grade 1C Recommendation, Level III/IV Evidence).
2. It is unclear if radiosurgery after subtotal total resection of atypical central neurocytoma is comparable to conventional radiation therapy.
3. There is no demonstrated benefit of chemotherapy in neurocytoma, and it is generally reserved as a salvage therapy for recurrent tumor or failed response to radiation-based adjuncts (Grade 2C Recommendation, Level III/IV Evidence).[4]

■ Summary and Conclusions

Central neurocytoma is a rare tumor with a benign typical phenotype and a malignant atypical phenotype. Evidence-based management of this tumor is largely founded upon case reports, case series, and meta-analyses. Prospective studies of central neurocytoma are difficult given the rarity of the disease. In terms of survival, the best available data suggest gross total resection is superior to subtotal resection by a margin defined by the effectiveness of adjunctive therapies, such as radiation therapy and SRS. Efforts to improve and define optimal surgical technique to increase the chances for a gross total resection are warranted. Future studies of gross neurological and cognitive outcomes, in addition to survival and local control rates, will inform surgical decision making. Furthermore, developing and defining optimal adjunctive treatments may help close the outcome gap between subtotal and gross total resection.

■ References

1. Choudhari KA, Kaliaperumal C, Jain A, et al. Central neurocytoma: a multi-disciplinary review. Br J Neurosurg 2009; 23(6):585–595
2. Hassoun J, Gambarelli D, Grisoli F, et al. Central neurocytoma: an electron-microscopic study of two cases. Acta Neuropathol 1982;56(2):151–156
3. Townsend JJ, Seaman JP. Central neurocytoma—a rare benign intraventricular tumor. Acta Neuropathol 1986;71(1-2): 167–170

4. Amini E, Roffidal T, Lee A, et al. Central neurocytoma responsive to topotecan, ifosfamide, carboplatin. Pediatr Blood Cancer 2008;51(1):137–140
5. Tacconi L, Rossi M, Foy P. Central neurocytoma: long-term follow-up of a paediatric case. J Clin Neurosci 2000;7(6): 548–552
6. Rades D, Schild SE, Fehlauer F. Defining the best available treatment for neurocytomas in children. Cancer 2004; 101(11):2629–2632
7. Gallina P, Mouchaty H, Buccoliero AM, Di Lorenzo N. Haemorrhagic central neurocytoma of the fourth ventricle. Acta Neuro chir (Wien) 2005;147(11):1193–1194
8. Leenstra JL, Rodriguez FJ, Frechette CM, et al. Central neurocytoma: management recommendations based on a 35-year experience. Int J Radiat Oncol Biol Phys 2007;67(4): 1145–1154
9. Terakawa Y, Tsuruno T, Ishibashi K, Okada Y, Shimotake K, Murata T. Central neurocytoma presenting with massive hemorrhage leading to coma—case report. Neurol Med Chir (Tokyo) 2010;50(2):139–143
10. Jamshidi J, Izumoto S, Yoshimine T, Maruno M. Central neurocytoma presenting with intratumoral hemorrhage. Neurosurg Rev 2001;24(1):48–52
11. Takao H, Nakagawa K, Ohtomo K. Central neurocytoma with craniospinal dissemination. J Neurooncol 2003;61(3): 255–259
12. Sgouros S, Jackowski A, Carey MP. Central neurocytoma without intraventricular extension. Surg Neurol 1994;42(4): 335–339
13. Eng DY, DeMonte F, Ginsberg L, Fuller GN, Jaeckle K. Craniospinal dissemination of central neurocytoma: report of two cases. J Neurosurg 1997;86(3):547–552
14. Sharma MC, Deb P, Sharma S, Sarkar C. Neurocytoma: a comprehensive review. Neurosurg Rev 2006;29(4):270–285
15. Elek G, Slowik F, Eross L, Tóth S, Szabó Z, Bálint K. Central neurocytoma with malignant course: neuronal and glial differentiation and craniospinal dissemination. Pathol Oncol Res 1999;5(2):155–159
16. Mackenzie IRA. Central neurocytoma: histologic atypia, proliferation potential, and clinical outcome. Cancer 1999;85(7):1606–1610
17. Söylemezoglu F, Scheithauer BW, Esteve J, Kleihues P. Atypical central neurocytoma. J Neuropathol Exp Neurol 1997;56(5):551–556
18. Rades D, Schild SE, Fehlauer F. Prognostic value of the MIB-1 labeling index for central neurocytomas. Neurology 2004;62(6):987–989
19. Rades D, Schild SE. Treatment recommendations for the various subgroups of neurocytomas. J Neurooncol 2006; 77(3):305–309
20. Rades D, Fehlauer F, Schild SE. Treatment of atypical neurocytomas. Cancer 2004;100(4):814–817
21. Kanamori M, Kumabe T, Watanabe M, Tominaga T. Anaplastic astrocytoma and anaplastic oligodendroglioma occurring 6 years after subtotal resection of a central neurocytoma. Case report. J Neurosurg 2007;107(1):185–189
22. Kulkarni V, Rajshekhar V, Haran RP, Chandi SM. Long-term outcome in patients with central neurocytoma following stereotactic biopsy and radiation therapy. Br J Neurosurg 2002;16(2):126–132
23. Rades D, Fehlauer F, Lamszus K, et al. Well-differentiated neurocytoma: what is the best available treatment? Neuro-oncol 2005;7(1):77–83
24. Rades D, Schild SE. Is 50 Gy sufficient to achieve long-term local control after incomplete resection of typical neurocytomas? Strahlenther Onkol 2006;182(7):415–418
25. Sharma MC, Rathore A, Karak AK, Sarkar C. A study of proliferative markers in central neurocytoma. Pathology 1998; 30(4):355 359
26. Vasiljevic A, François P, Loundou A, et al. Prognostic factors in central neurocytomas: a multicenter study of 71 cases. Am J Surg Pathol 2012;36(2):220–227
27. Hallock AHB, Hamilton B, Ang LC, et al. Neurocytomas: long-term experience of a single institution. Neuro-oncol 2011;13(9):943–949
28. Romano A, Chibbaro S, Makiese O, Marsella M, Mainini P, Benericetti E. Endoscopic removal of a central neurocytoma from the posterior third ventricle. J Clin Neurosci 2009; 16(2):312–316
29. Cheng C-H, Liu C-L, Chen C-C, Lin S-Z, Cho D-Y. Single-port endoscopic removal of intraventricular central neurocytoma. J Clin Neurosci 2010;17(11):1417–1420
30. Ferreol E Sr, Sawaya R, de Courten-Myers GM. Primary cerebral neuroblastoma (neurocytoma) in adults. J Neurooncol 1989;7(2):121–128
31. Paek SH, Han J-H, Kim JW, et al. Long-term outcome of conventional radiation therapy for central neurocytoma. J Neurooncol 2008;90(1):25–30
32. Anderson RC, Elder JB, Parsa AT, Issacson SR, Sisti MB. Radiosurgery for the treatment of recurrent central neurocytomas. Neurosurgery 2001;48(6):1231–1237
33. Chen M-C, Pan DH-C, Chung W-Y, et al. Gamma knife radiosurgery for central neurocytoma: retrospective analysis of fourteen cases with a median follow-up period of sixty-five months. Stereotact Funct Neurosurg 2011;89(3):185–193
34. Schild SE, Scheithauer BW, Haddock MG, et al. Central neurocytomas. Cancer 1997;79(4):790–795
35. Park HK, Steven D C. Stereotactic radiosurgery for central neurocytoma: a quantitative systematic review. J Neurooncol 2012;108(1):115–121
36. Chen S-Y, Chen C-H, Sun M-H, Lee H-T, Shen C-C. Stereotactic biopsy for brainstem lesion: comparison of approaches and reports of 10 cases. J Chin Med Assoc 2011;74(3):110–114
37. Yen CP, Sheehan J, Patterson G, Steiner L. Gamma knife surgery for neurocytoma. J Neurosurg 2007;107(1):7–12
38. Kim C-Y, Paek SH, Jeong SS, et al. Gamma knife radiosurgery for central neurocytoma: primary and secondary treatment. Cancer 2007;110(10):2276–2284
39. Matsunaga S, Shuto T, Suenaga J, Inomori S, Fujino H. Gamma knife radiosurgery for central neurocytomas. Neurol Med Chir (Tokyo) 2010;50(2):107–112, 112–113
40. Rades D, Schild SE. Value of postoperative stereotactic radiosurgery and conventional radiotherapy for incompletely resected typical neurocytomas. Cancer 2006;106(5):1140–1143

18

The Role of Surgery in Intraventricular High-Grade Astrocytomas

Edjah K. Nduom and Costas G. Hadjipanayis

Intraventricular glioblastoma multiformes (GBMs) and anaplastic astrocytomas (AAs) represent a small subset of these most common malignant primary brain tumors. These lesions are particularly interesting to the neuro-oncological community due to the relatively recent discovery of the subventricular zone (SVZ) as a stem-cell niche. Neural stem cells (NSCs) are self-renewing multipotent cells with astrocytic features[1] that can generate most differentiated tissue components of the brain.[2] These cells were first discovered in the SVZ in mice.[3] When cultured in serum-free media supplemented with defined growth factors, NSCs grow in suspended cell aggregates (called neurospheres) and self-renew. Upon exposure to differentiation signals such as serum, they can generate all of the different cell types within the adult brain. Estimates number these cells as 0.77% of those within the SVZ, using Ki67 staining to identify mitotically active cells.[4] Given the mitotic activity in this area, it is not surprising that a significant subset of GBMs arise in periventricular areas.

The management of high-grade astrocytomas can vary based on their location within the ventricular system. The lesions tend to grow into the ventricles from various periventricular structures, such as the thalamus, into the lateral/third ventricles. They may also extend from the brainstem into the fourth ventricle or arise primarily within the ventricles from the fornix or septum. This chapter examines the experience with treating these lesions that is described in the literature. Although there has been a significant effort of the neuro-oncology community to provide evidence in support of extent of resection in the treatment of high-grade astrocytomas, the resection of intraventricular high-grade astrocytomas has not been widely reported specifically, limiting our ability to extrapolate these studies to this patient population. The deep location of these lesions can increase the risk of postoperative neurological decline because eloquent areas are often traversed in the approach. However, recent advances in operative techniques may make increase the feasibility and safety of surgery on these lesions, and this could bring the indications for resection of intraventricular lesions closer in line with those for all high-grade astrocytomas. The chapter discusses the available open and neuro-endoscopic surgical approaches to these tumors within the ventricular system.

Diagnosis

In the literature reviewed for this chapter, the most common presenting complaint with an intraventricular AA or GBM was headache (**Table 18.1**), followed by nausea and vomiting, similar to the presentation of most high-grade astrocytomas.[5-10] In most case series and case reports, radiological diagnosis was made using contrast-enhanced magnetic resonance imaging (MRI) (**Fig. 18.1**), though earlier radiographic evaluation was performed with contrast-enhanced computed tomography (CT).

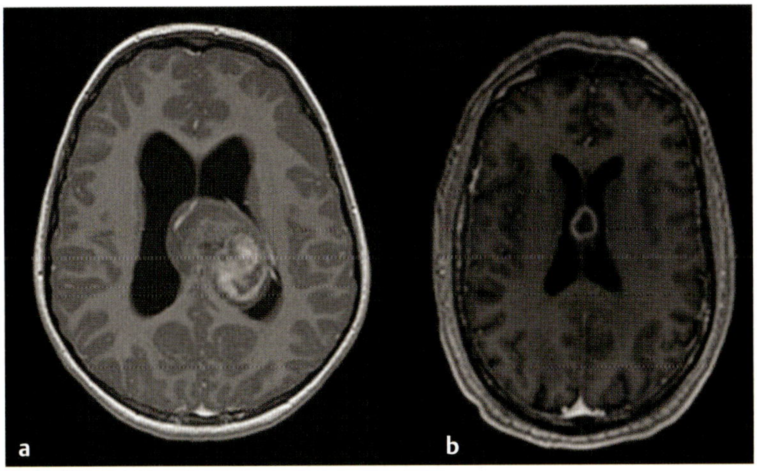

Fig. 18.1 **(a)** T1-weighted, contrast-enhanced magnetic resonance imaging (MRI) scan depicting a lateral ventricular glioblastoma in an 11-year-old male. **(b)** T1-weighted, contrast-enhanced MRI of a septum pellucidum glioblastoma in a 60-year-old male.

■ Literature Review

Indications for Surgical Resection of Intraventricular High-Grade Astrocytomas

Level I and Level II Evidence

There is no Level I or Level II evidence regarding the surgical indications for the treatment of intraventricular high-grade astrocytomas.

Level III Evidence

There is a preponderance of Level III evidence that describes the indications for resection for high-grade astrocytomas, but there is no Level III evidence that specifically references the indications for resection of intraventricular lesions. The evidence supporting extent of resection of high-grade gliomas is addressed in Chapter 3.

Level IV Evidence

Table 18.1 summarizes the case reports and case series reporting the treatment of intraventricular high-grade astrocytomas.[11,12] Studies were identified by searching PubMed for all human studies using the keywords “ventricular” and “astrocytoma” together or “ventricular” and “glioma.” Studies were excluded that included only subependymal giant cell astrocytomas, pilocytic astrocytomas, or fibrillary astrocytomas. Studies were also excluded if they described the resection of intraventricular astrocytomas but did not report the pathological grading of the lesion or lesions in question. Most studies discovered were individual case reports.

In one of the earliest reports, Wakamatsu et al described the metastasis of an intraventricular GBM to the pleura through a ventriculopleural shunt.[13] The patient presented with headache and lethargy. Angiography and pneumoencephalography revealed obstructive hydrocephalus along with a space-occupying lesion in the left thalamic region. A ventriculopleural shunt was placed, and the patient subsequently underwent telecobalt therapy (6000R). He underwent a ventriculoatrial shunt 5 months later after developing a pleural effusion at the site of his pleural catheter and eventually succumbed to the disease 9 months after his presentation. At autopsy, it was discovered he had widespread GBM involvement of his lateral ventricles in addition to his pleural cavity where the distal catheter of his shunt resided prior to placement in the atrium.

Secer et al[5] reported a case series of intraventricular GBMs that presented to their institution over a 10-year period. GBM tumors represented nine of the 46 cases (19.5%) of lateral ventricle tumors that were treated during that period. They achieved one gross total resection in their nine cases, and eight out of nine resections had greater than 78% resection (mean 85.8% ± 7.3, range 77 to 100), though they do not report how these volumes were calculated. One patient developed hepatic encephalopathy 3 days postoperatively, then subsequently developed an intraventricular hemorrhage, leading to death at 1 month postsurgery. Two patients developed neurological deficits that were not further specified in this study, and one patient required a postoperative ventriculoperitoneal shunt. Although only three of the patients received temozolomide, all patients other than the perioperative mortality received at least 54 Gy of radiation in the postoperative period. The three patients who received temozolomide were

Table 18.1 Reported cases of intraventricular high-grade astrocytomas

Study	Path	Age	Sex	Presenting symptom	Size of tumor (mm³)	Location	Surgical approach	Survival (months)	Resection %
Andoh et al[4]	GBM	44	F	HA, N/V	60 × 54 mm	lateral (trigone)	R middle temporal gyrus	–	Partial removal
Chernov et al 2004[15]	AA	17	M	HA, diplopia, N/V	–	3rd	Endoscopic biopsy	9	Biopsy
Chernov et al 2004[15]	AA	15	F	–	–	3rd	Endoscopic biopsy	–	Biopsy
El-Bahy 2005[16]	AA	–	–	–	–	4th	–	–	95
Gaab et al[6]	AA	13	M	HA	–	Lateral + 3rd	Microsurgical resection	8	–
Gaab et al[6]	AA	16	M	HA, N/V	–	3rd	Biopsy, radiation	21	Biopsy
Jelinek et al 1990[12]	2 GBM	> 30	M	–	–	Body lateral	–	–	–
Klein, Marchal 2007[19]	GBM	9	M	–	–	Lateral	R anterior transcallosal	12	100
Lee et al[2]	GBM	59	M	Memory	–	3rd	R anterior transcallosal	–	–
Mendhekar et al 2005[17]	GBM	35	F	Depression	–	Lateral	–	–	–
Nishio et al 2002[14]	AA	56	M	AMS	–	Lateral/3rd	Transcallosal	9	Partial
Osztie et al 2009[20]	8 GBM, 3 AA	mean 49	–	–	–	–	–	5 pt < 30 days, 6 pt < 1 year	–
Park et al[3]	GBM	32	F	HA, N/V	–	Lateral (trigone)	R parieto-occipital	–	Near total
Pendl et al 1992[11]	5 GBM	–	–	–	–	3 body, 2 lateral (trigone)	–	–	–

alive at the time of submission of the case series, with follow-up at 21, 27, and 33 months, and thus were excluded from the survival analysis. The remaining six patients had a mean survival of 15.8 ± 9.2 months (range 1 to 28). For the five patients with tumors located within the body of the lateral ventricle and extending into the corpus callosum, an interhemispheric transcallosal approach was used (*N* = 5). Tumors with thalamic extension were resected via a transfrontal transcortical approach (*N* = 4).

In a case series of lateral ventricular lesions, Nishio et al reported a lateral and third ventricular "malignant astrocytoma" partially resected by a transcallosal approach and subsequent radiation, leading to death 9 months after treatment.[14] Chernov et al reported on a single third ventricular AA in a 17-year-old male treated by endoscopic biopsy and radiation with complete radiological resolution at 9 months follow-up.[15] El-Bahy reported the removal of a fourth ventricular AA via a posterior fossa telovelar approach, but he did not describe the clinical features of this specific patient beyond the approach and radiographic results.[16] In a published letter to the editor, one group reported a lateral ventricular GBM resected through a frontal interhemispheric transcallosal approach with near total resection and resolution of her presenting symptom of depression.[17]

There were two other case reports of gross total resection of intraventricular high-grade astrocytomas,[18,19] but only one of these reported survival, with

Table 18.1 *(Continued)* Reported cases of intraventricular high-grade astrocytomas

Study	Path	Age	Sex	Presenting symptom	Size of tumor (mm³)	Location	Surgical approach	Survival (months)	Resection %
Secer et al[1]	GBM	19	M	–	7,500	Lateral	R frontal transcortical	12	87
Secer et al[1]	GBM	21	M	–	51,450	Lateral	R anterior transcallosal	–	89
Secer et al[1]	GBM	28	F	–	6,804	Septum	R frontal transcortical	19	82
Secer et al[1]	GBM	43	M	–	10,500	Lateral	R anterior transcallosal	–	79
Secer et al[1]	GBM	45	M	–	25,500	Lateral	L anterior transcallosal	14	82
Secer et al[1]	GBM	45	F	–	31,620	Lateral	L anterior transcallosal	21	77
Secer et al[1]	GBM	54	M	–	4,500	Septum	L frontal transcortical	1	100
Secer et al[1]	GBM	63	M	–	112,996	Lateral	R frontal transcortical	–	93
Secer et al[1]	GBM	67	M	–	125,000	Lateral	R anterior transcallosal	28	83
Tamura et al[5]	AA	56	F	HA, diplopia	–	–	–	Biopsy	–
Wakamatsu et al 1971[13]	GBM	22	M	HA, lethargy	–	Lateral	VPS placement, dx on autopsy	9	Not biopsied
Yurtseven et al 2003[21]	3 GBM, 1 AA	–	–	–	–	–	Transfrontal/ transcortical endoscopic	–	Biopsy
Zuccaro et al 1999[18]	AA	11	M	–	–	Septum	–	–	100

Abbreviations: AA, anaplastic astrocytoma; AMS, altered mental status; dx, diagnosis; GBM, glioblastoma; HA, headache; N/V, nausea/vomiting; VPS, ventriculoperitoneal shunt.

the pediatric patient dying of recurrence of his GBM at 1 year postsurgery.[19]

Osztie et al reported on the resection of eight GBMs and three AAs, but they did not present disaggregated data for these patients, so we were not able to evaluate the individual outcomes of each patient's resection.[20] Five of their patients died in the perioperative period, and all of the remaining cases died within 1 year of presentation. Yurtseven et al reported on neuroendoscopic biopsies in three GBMs and one AA, but no survival data were presented in this case series.[21] There have been no comparative studies between attempted gross total resection and biopsy of intraventricular malignant astrocytomas in the literature.

Consensus Statements

The recommendations applicable to intraventricular high-grade astrocytomas are pulled from the literature regarding the treatment of high-grade astrocytomas throughout the brain, which is covered in detail in Chapter 3. In summary, attempting a gross total resection without causing further neurological deficits is felt to impact the overall survival in these patients.

Surgical Approach to Intraventricular High-Grade Astrocytomas

In cases where resection is pursued, there are many different ways to approach tumors of the ventricular system (**Fig. 18.2**). The approach to intraventricular lesions has been studied a great deal due to the difficulty in approaching these deep-seated lesions while attempting to protect normal brain from injury.

Level IV Evidence

Open Microsurgical Approaches to Intraventricular Lesions

There have been numerous case reports and case series detailing the resection of intraventricular high-grade astrocytomas. In all reported cases in the literature, microsurgical resections were performed. Most authors have reported approaching these lesions through a transcortical frontal or interhemispheric transcallosal approach depending on the location of the lesion. Transcortical frontal approaches are predominantly used for resection of tumors located within the frontal horn, some within the body of the lateral ventricle, and some with thalamic extension, whereas transcallosal approaches are used for third ventricular lesions and some medial or midline tumors of the lateral ventricle. These approaches allow the surgeon to perform bimanual dissection with the microscope to resect the tumor using a wide range of microscopic instruments. While the interhemispheric transcallosal approach may minimize the amount of normal tissue traversed during the approach,[22] retraction injury during the interhemispheric approach is known to cause neurological deficits.[23] A recent study has shown that the interhemispheric transcallosal approach to the ventricular system may also be associated with a higher risk of seizures than with the transcortical approach,[24] though transcortical approaches are associated with seizures in 8% of patients. Another group has advocated the use of tubular retractors in pediatric[25] and adult patient populations for deep-seated lesions[26] during microsurgical approaches. However, their experience with intraventricular lesions is limited in both case series, and neither series included the resection of intraventricular high-grade astrocytomas.

Endoscopic Approaches to Intraventricular Lesions

Neuroendoscopic approaches for intraventricular tumors through a burr hole and transcortical approach have traditionally been performed for biopsy purposes and simultaneous restoration of cerebrospinal fluid (CSF) pathways due to obstruction by the tumor (i.e., endoscopic third ventriculostomy or septum pellucidum fenestration). Fukushima described his initial experience with neuroendoscopic intraventricular biopsy of lesions using a "ventriculofiberscope" in 1978.[27] Currently, rigid rod-lens endoscopes are used with working channel sheaths (< 1 cm in diameter) for high-definition intraventricular visualization while also providing working channels for instruments, irrigation, and suction.

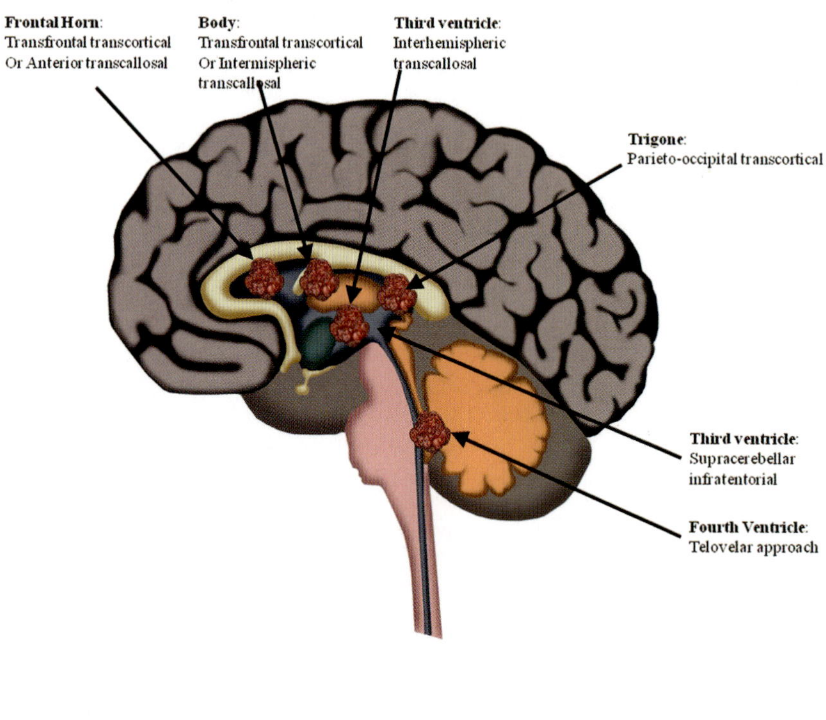

Fig. 18.2 Various microsurgical approaches to high-grade astrocytomas of the ventricular system. Not pictured is the transcortical middle temporal gyrus approach to tumors of the temporal horn or atrium of the lateral ventricle.

Conventional working channel instruments include grasping forceps, cutting instruments, and cautery for tumor biopsy and resection purposes (**Fig. 18.3**).[28] Souweidane and Luther reported the resection of seven solid intraventricular brain tumors and outlined the difficulties associated with resecting these lesions in a piecemeal fashion due to the limited instrumentation available to them at that time.[29] Their experience was also similar to that of Gaab and Schroeder, who reported on the purely endoscopic resection of intraventricular lesions.[30] In both series, the attempted resection of solid lesions with diameters greater than 20 mm was extremely difficult due to the small working channels of the endoscopes used and the length of surgery required in these cases.

Some groups have tried to use bimanual techniques while utilizing the endoscope to visualize tumors in the ventricular system. Interhemispheric endoscopically assisted approaches have been reported, but they require a large craniotomy and access near the superior sagittal sinus that may pose greater risk to the patient.[31] Kassam et al recently evaluated the use of a port-assisted endoscopic technique for the resection of intraventricular lesions, allowing the use of a bimanual technique.[32] This approach requires a small craniotomy and placement of a 1.2-cm port through the brain to the tumor or cyst.

Controlled-aspiration tissue-resection devices that are inserted through the working-channel endoscope may become a key tool for endoscopic approaches for resection of intraventricular lesions. Dlouhy et al have reported their use of the NICO Myriad device (NICO Corp., Indianapolis, IN) through a working-channel endoscope for resection of colloid cysts and a pineoblastoma.[33] The precise side-cutting aperture and pedal-controlled variable aspiration permitted intraventricular tumor resections in a safe manner due to the ability to rotate and direct the side-cutting aperture away from normal structures.

High-grade astrocytomas may not be currently amenable to minimally invasive endoscopic approaches for several reasons. They tend to be very vascular lesions, and instrumentation for tumor resection of these lesions includes only rudimentary bipolar cautery for tumor resection. Ineffective control of bleeding from the tumor resection makes visualization difficult during the neuroendosopic approach and can compromise the tumor resection and also result in significant intraventricular hemorrhage. In addition, because the lesions tend to be aggressive and rapidly growing, they may present at sizes larger than 2 cm in diameter. Tumors of this size are more challenging to resect by a neuroendoscopic route due to the small amount of tumor tissue that can be resected piecemeal through the working channel.

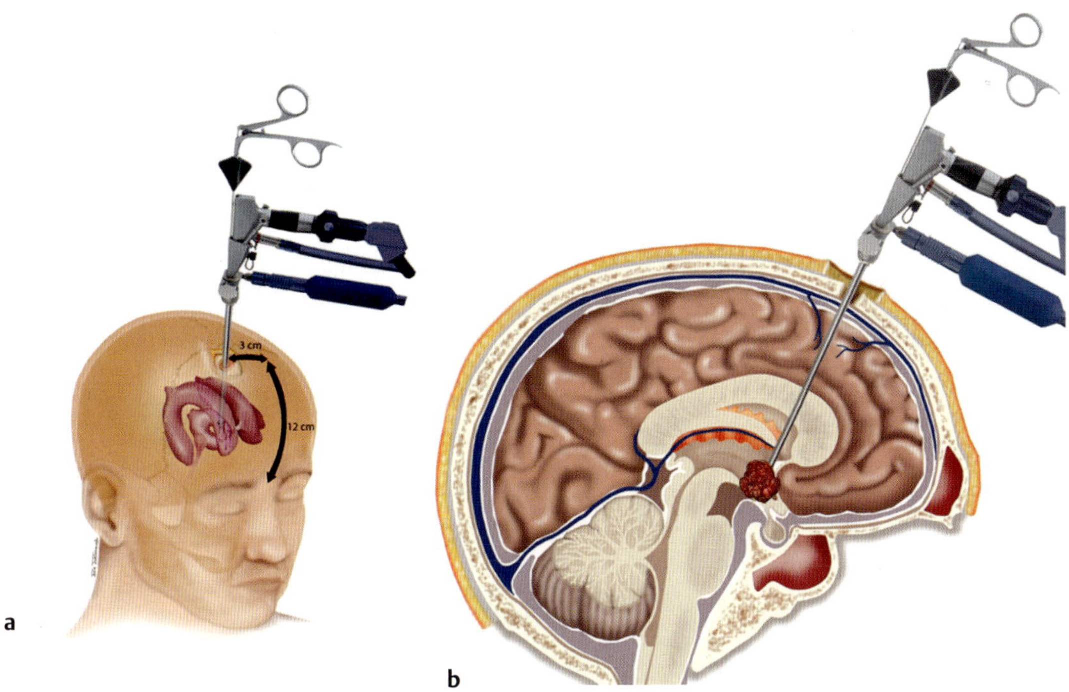

Fig. 18.3 The working channel neuroendoscope is **(a)** placed through a coronal burr hole and positioned within the ventricular system for an endoscopic approach to a lateral or third ventricular tumor and **(b)** placed within the third ventricle (in a sagittal illustration) for access to a tumor.

Currently, neuroendoscopic intraventricular approaches for high-grade astrocytomas are limited to small tumor resections for biopsy purposes and treatment of the associated obstructive hydrocephalus in patients. Newer cautery and other instrumentation may make it more feasible for resection of these tumors by a neuroendoscopic approach. Both frontal transcortical and interhemispheric transcallosal microsurgical approaches remain the most popular treatment options for intraventricular high-grade astrocytomas depending on the location of the lesion and the preference of the neurosurgeon.

Expert Recommendations

1. Recommendations regarding the management of intraventricular astrocytomas are extrapolated from literature dealing with this pathology elsewhere in the brain. No comparative studies specifically addressing this tumor have yet been published. In general, gross total resection without sacrificing neurologic function is thought to be the goal of surgical intervention (Grade 2C Recommendation, Level III/IV Evidence).
2. Current Grade 1C Recommendation, Level IV Evidence supports the use of open microscopic approaches for the resection of intraventricular high-grade astrocytomas.
3. The approach is dictated by the experience and judgment of the treating neurosurgeon together with the location of the lesion within the ventricular system.
4. There is currently no evidence to support the use of endoscopic approaches for resection of these lesions, though this may change with advances in working-channel endoscopes and ports. Such approaches have been shown to be useful for biopsy and cerebrospinal fluid diversion.
5. Further study specifically on the surgical resection of intraventricular high-grade gliomas may be needed to determine firm indications for surgical resection versus medical management.

■ Summary and Conclusions

Intraventricular high-grade astrocytomas remain a treatment dilemma because their deep-seated location often makes them difficult to resect. An interhemispheric transcallosal or transcortical approach with the microscope provides the best access to the ventricle for treating these lesions. Given the current recommendations regarding the resection of all high-grade astrocytomas, there is enough evidence to support an attempted gross total resection when possible. Preservation of neurological function remains an important consideration in any approach. Currently, neuroendoscopic approaches to intraventricular high-grade astrocytomas are limited to tumor biopsy and restoration of CSF pathways due to the vascularity and larger size of these tumors. Development of new instrumentation, including better cautery and resection devices that can be inserted through the working channel, may permit more effective resection of these tumors in a safe manner by a neuroendoscopic approach.

■ References

1. Doetsch F, Caillé I, Lim DA, García-Verdugo JM, Alvarez-Buylla A. Subventricular zone astrocytes are neural stem cells in the adult mammalian brain. Cell 1999;97(6):703–716
2. Alvarez-Buylla A, García-Verdugo JM, Tramontin AD. A unified hypothesis on the lineage of neural stem cells. Nat Rev Neurosci 2001;2(4):287–293
3. Reynolds BA, Tetzlaff W, Weiss S. A multipotent EGF-responsive striatal embryonic progenitor cell produces neurons and astrocytes. J Neurosci 1992;12(11):4565–4574
4. Sanai N, Tramontin AD, Quiñones-Hinojosa A, et al. Unique astrocyte ribbon in adult human brain contains neural stem cells but lacks chain migration. Nature 2004;427(6976):740–744
5. Secer HI, Dinc C, Anik I, Duz B, Gonul E. Glioblastoma multiforme of the lateral ventricle: report of nine cases. Br J Neurosurg 2008;22(3):398–401
6. Lee TT, Manzano GR. Third ventricular glioblastoma multiforme: case report. Neurosurg Rev 1997;20(4):291–294
7. Park P, Choksi VR, Gala VC, Kaza AR, Murphy HS, Ramnath S. Well-circumscribed, minimally enhancing glioblastoma mul-

tiforme of the trigone: a case report and review of the literature. AJNR Am J Neuroradiol 2005;26(6):1475–1478
8. Andoh T, Shinoda J, Miwa Y, et al. Tumors at the trigone of the lateral ventricle—clinical analysis of eight cases. Neurol Med Chir (Tokyo) 1990;30(9):676–684
9. Tamura Y, Kuroiwa T, Kajimoto Y, Miki Y, Miyatake S, Tsuji M. Endoscopic identification and biopsy sampling of an intraventricular malignant glioma using a 5-aminolevulinic acid-induced protoporphyrin IX fluorescence imaging system. Technical note. J Neurosurg 2007;106(3):507–510
10. Gaab MR, Schroeder HW. Neuroendoscopic approach to intraventricular lesions. Neurosurg Focus 1999;6(4):e5
11. Pendl G, Oztürk E, Haselsberger K. Surgery of tumours of the lateral ventricle. Acta Neurochir (Wien) 1992;116(2-4): 128–136
12. Jelinek J, Smirniotopoulos JG, Parisi JE, Kanzer M. Lateral ventricular neoplasms of the brain: differential diagnosis based on clinical, CT, and MR findings. AJR Am J Roentgenol 1990; 155(2):365–372
13. Wakamatsu T, Matsuo T, Kawano S, Teramoto S, Matsumura H. Glioblastoma with extracranial metastasis through ventriculopleural shunt. Case report. J Neurosurg 1971;34(5): 697–701
14. Nishio S, Morioka T, Suzuki S, Fukui M. Tumours around the foramen of Monro: clinical and neuroimaging features and their differential diagnosis. J Clin Neurosci 2002;9(2): 137–141
15. Chernov M, Kamikawa S, Toledo R, et al. Minimally invasive management of the third ventricle glioma in a patient without hydrocephalus: neurofiberscopic biopsy followed by gamma knife radiosurgery. Minim Invasive Neurosurg 2004;47(4):238–241
16. El-Bahy K. Telovelar approach to the fourth ventricle: operative findings and results in 16 cases. Acta Neurochir (Wien) 2005;147(2):137–142
17. Mendhekar DN, Inamdar A, Singh AK. Disappearance of specific phobia after removal of ventricular glioblastoma. Psychiatry Clin Neurosci 2005;59(3):362
18. Zuccaro G, Sosa F, Cuccia V, Lubieniecky F, Monges J. Lateral ventricle tumors in children: a series of 54 cases. Childs Nerv Syst 1999;15(11-12):774–785
19. Klein O, Marchal JC. Intraventricular glioblastoma: a paediatric case report. Br J Neurosurg 2007;21(4):411–413
20. Osztie E, Hanzély Z, Afra D. Lateral ventricle gliomas and central neurocytomas in adults diagnosis and perspectives. Eur J Radiol 2009;69(1):67–73
21. Yurtseven T, Erşahin Y, Demirtaş E, Mutluer S. Neuroendoscopic biopsy for intraventricular tumors. Minim Invasive Neurosurg 2003;46(5):293–299
22. Apuzzo ML, Chikovani OK, Gott PS, et al. Transcallosal, interfornicial approaches for lesions affecting the third ventricle: surgical considerations and consequences. Neurosurgery 1982;10(5):547–554
23. Shucart WA, Stein BM. Transcallosal approach to the anterior ventricular system. Neurosurgery 1978;3(3):339–343
24. Milligan BD, Meyer FB. Morbidity of transcallosal and transcortical approaches to lesions in and around the lateral and third ventricles: a single-institution experience. Neurosurgery 2010;67(6):1483–1496
25. Recinos PF, Raza SM, Jallo GI, Recinos VR. Use of a minimally invasive tubular retraction system for deep-seated tumors in pediatric patients. J Neurosurg Pediatr 2011;7(5):516–521
26. Raza SM, Recinos PF, Avendano J, Adams H, Jallo GI, Quinones-Hinojosa A. Minimally invasive trans-portal resection of deep intracranial lesions. Minim Invasive Neurosurg 2011;54(1): 5–11
27. Fukushima T. Endoscopic biopsy of intraventricular tumors with the use of a ventriculofiberscope. Neurosurgery 1978;2(2):110–113
28. Cappabianca P, Cinalli G, Gangemi M, et al. Application of neuroendoscopy to intraventricular lesions. Neurosurgery 2008;62(Suppl 2):575–597
29. Souweidane MM, Luther N. Endoscopic resection of solid intraventricular brain tumors. J Neurosurg 2006;105(2): 271–278
30. Gaab MR, Schroeder HW. Neuroendoscopic approach to intraventricular lesions. J Neurosurg 1998;88(3):496–505
31. Sood S, Nundkumar N, Ham SD. Interhemispheric endoscopic resection of large intraventricular and thalamic tumors. J Neurosurg Pediatr 2011;7(6):596–599
32. McLaughlin N, Prevedello DM, Engh J, Kelly DF, Kassam AB. Endoneurosurgical resection of intraventricular and intraparenchymal lesions using the port technique. World Neurosurg 2012;1:S1878
33. Dlouhy BJ, Dahdaleh NS, Greenlee JD. Emerging technology in intracranial neuroendoscopy: application of the NICO Myriad. Neurosurg Focus 2011;30(4):E6

■ SECTION IV ■

Hemangioblastomas

19

The Role of Surgery in von Hippel-Lindau Disease with Craniospinal Hemangioblastomas

David B. Weintraub and Russell R. Lonser

Von Hippel-Lindau disease (VHL) is a familial multiple neoplasia syndrome that occurs in ~ 0.003% of live births. VHL is autosomal dominantly inherited and has over 95% lifetime penetrance.[1] VHL is caused by a germline mutation of the *VHL* gene. This gene has a tumor suppressor function and is found on chromosome 3p.[2] VHL central nervous system (CNS) manifestations include retinal and craniospinal axis hemangioblastomas, as well as endolymphatic sac tumors. Patients with VHL also develop visceral cysts and tumors, including pheochromocytomas, renal cell carcinomas, adnexal organ cystadenomas, pancreatic cysts, and pancreatic islet cell tumors.[3]

CNS hemangioblastomas are benign vascular neoplasms often associated with peritumoral cysts (cyst forming at the edge of the tumor capsule). These tumors may occur in the retina and along the craniospinal axis (most often arising in the cerebellum or spinal cord).[4] Although surgical resection of sporadic hemangioblastomas is curative, patients with VHL often have multiple CNS tumors that develop over their lifetime in an unpredictable manner. Often, tumors will remain asymptomatic for long periods of time or indefinitely. Consequently, careful selection and timing of tumor resection are critical to maintain neurological function and quality of life, while avoiding unnecessary surgery.

This chapter summarizes the salient features of imaging, laboratory, clinical, and histopathological findings. The natural history and management of VHL-associated hemangioblastomas are reviewed in the context of their biological features, as well as the outcomes associated with resection of these tumors in the various anatomical regions of the CNS. Adjuvant treatment modalities, including radiosurgery and chemotherapy, are addressed in other chapters of this book.

There is no Level I or II evidence regarding any surgical treatment of hemangioblastomas in VHL. Data regarding surgery for hemangioblastomas in VHL are derived from retrospective series. Therefore, only Level III and IV evidence is currently available.

■ Imaging and Pathological Features

Imaging Features

Contrast-enhanced magnetic resonance imaging (MRI) provides the most accurate and useful imaging information for identifying and characterizing CNS hemangioblastomas (**Fig. 19.1**). Hemangioblastomas are usually isointense or mildly hyperintense on precontrast T1 sequences and hyperintense on T2 sequences. Postcontrast T1 sequences demonstrate avid enhancement of the solid tumor. The solid tumor often demonstrates serpentine flow voids due to the rich vascular supply. Peritumoral cysts are frequently associated with hemangioblastomas. Peritumoral cysts are hyperintense on T2-weighted MRI and are hypointense on T1-weighted MRI.[5,6]

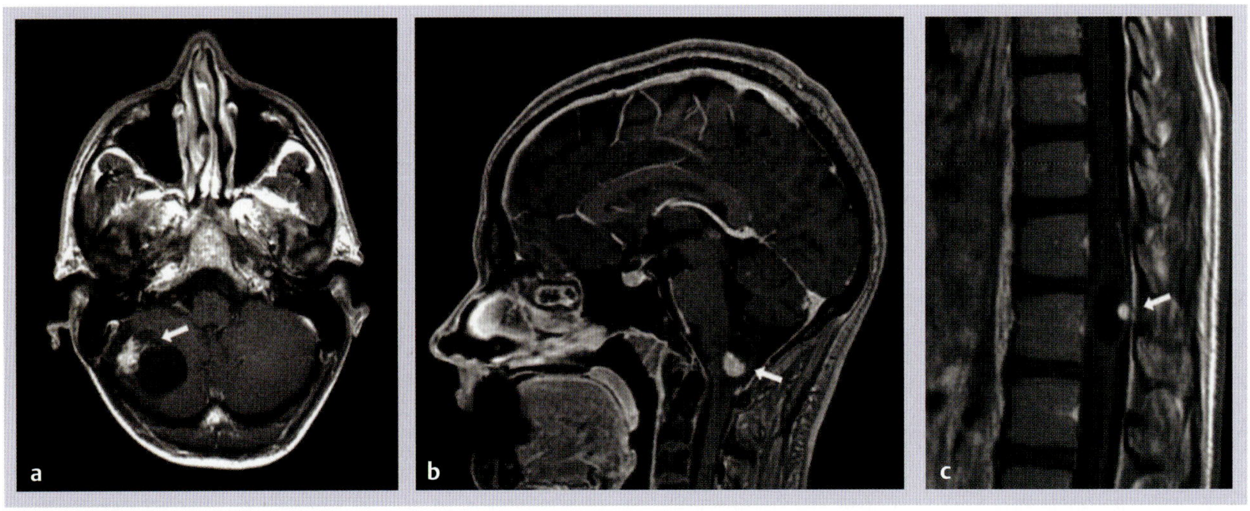

Fig. 19.1 Typical appearance of central nervous system hemangioblastomas. Postcontrast T1 images demonstrate enhancing solid tumors (mural nodule) with associated peritumoral cyst in **(a)** cerebellum, **(b)** obex, **(c)** thoracic spinal cord. (Adapted from Wind and Lonser.[36])

Less frequently, hemangioblastomas are associated with intratumoral cysts (cysts forming within the tumor substance) that are hypointense regions surrounded by enhancing tumor on contrast-enhanced T1-weighted MRI sequences (**Fig. 19.1**).

Pathological Features

Grossly, hemangioblastomas are intensely vascular benign lesions that appear bright red/orange and/or yellow. The tumors are categorized as World Health Organization grade I lesions. Hemangioblastomas are associated with large abnormal feeding vessels and draining veins. They are thinly encapsulated, and their associated cysts are formed from reactive gliosis. Microscopic inspection demonstrates endothelial cells that form extensive vascular channels and characteristic lipid-laden stromal cells (**Fig. 19.2**). Immunohistochemistry demonstrates positive staining for inhibin A, glucose transporter 1, vascular endothelial growth factor, notch receptors 1 through 4, and CD56, but negative staining for epithelial membrane antigen (EMA).[7–9] Positive staining for inhibin A and negative staining for EMA can differentiate hemangioblastomas from renal cell carcinoma, which is common in VHL patients and can metastasize to the CNS and/or CNS hemangioblastomas.[10,11]

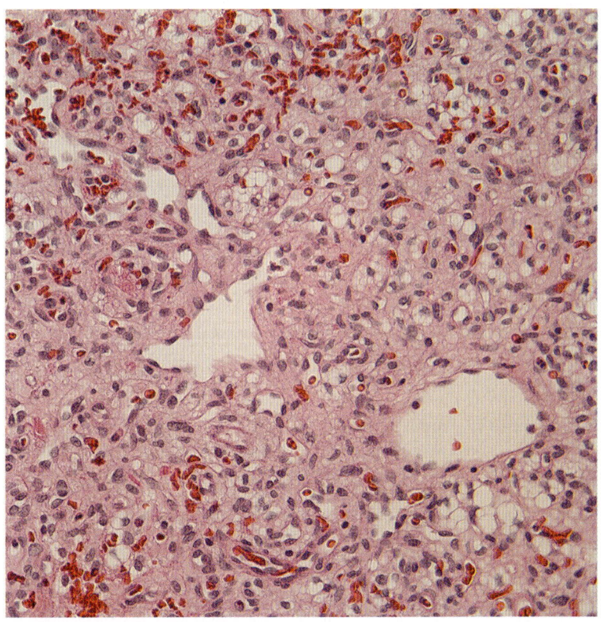

Fig. 19.2 Typical low-power hematoxylin and eosin stain of hemangioblastoma from a patient with von Hippel-Lindau disease. Note the thin-walled vascular network and the lipid-laden stromal cells.

■ Preoperative Considerations

Pheochromocytoma Evaluation

Pheochromocytomas are present in up to 30% of VHL patients.[3,12–15] Failure to recognize and manage a concurrent pheochromocytoma can result in perioperative hypertensive crises and cardiac dysfunction with significant associated morbidity and/or mortality.[16] Evaluation for pheochromocytoma includes measurement of serum metanephrines and 24-hour urine testing for catecholamines in combination with abdominal and pelvic contrast-enhanced computed tomography (CT) or MRI, with the addition of nuclear imaging in uncertain cases.[12] Surgical resection of pheochromocytomas is curative, though α- and β-adrenergic blockade may be used to ameliorate risks when CNS surgery is required before pheochromocytoma resection.[14]

Arteriography and Embolization

Although arteriography can delineate the vascular supply of large hemangioblastomas, we have not found arteriography with embolization necessary for safe, effective resection of these tumors. However, some centers have advocated preoperative embolization to help minimize intraoperative blood loss.[17] Nevertheless, embolization of hemangioblastomas has been associated with significant risk, including intratumoral hemorrhage, stroke, and death.[18,19] Thus the potential benefit of embolization must be weighed against the defined risks of this procedure.

Preoperative Evaluation in Patients with VHL Recommendations

1. All patients with VHL should be screened for the presence of a pheochromocytoma before surgery. This screening should include testing of serum metanephrines and 24-hour urine catecholamine levels along with abdominal/pelvic imaging.
2. Patients with evidence of pheochromocytomas should be managed with α- and β-adrenergic blockade when CNS surgery is required before pheochromocytoma resection.
3. Preoperative arteriography need not be routinely performed before resection of hemangioblastomas.

■ Natural History

Several studies have helped define the natural history of CNS manifestations in VHL.[3,4,13,20,21] In a retrospective review of 231 VHL patients, 160 patients (69%) were found to have CNS hemangioblastomas. Patients were found to harbor tumors in the cerebellum in 68%, spinal cord in 76%, brainstem in 31%, and supratentorial compartment in 6%. Most patients harbored multiple hemangioblastomas (79% of patients) in multiple CNS anatomical compartments (64% of patients). Increased tumor size was related to symptom development, and most symptomatic tumors harbored a cyst larger than the tumor itself.[21]

Ammerman and coworkers[20] analyzed symptom development and tumor growth rate in 19 patients with VHL followed for longer than 10 years (mean, 12.4 years). Despite growth of hemangioblastomas in all but one patient, only 42% of the tumors eventually caused symptoms. A saltatory growth pattern was demonstrated in almost all tumors, with the mean growth phase of 13 months and mean quiescent phase of 25 months. Of tumors that eventually caused symptoms, 45% were not evident on initial imaging. Because many tumors may grow for a period of time and then halt before causing symptoms, timing of resection (and waiting for early symptom/sign formation) is a critical consideration in the management of hemangioblastomas in patients with VHL. In the foregoing study, had the criterion of any radiographic growth been used as the standard for resection, four additional unnecessary surgeries per patient would have been performed.

■ Operative Technique

CNS hemangioblastomas in all compartments are resected using established microsurgical techniques and circumferential dissection.[22–26] Adequate bony exposure is performed to allow for complete identification of the solid tumor component. Once the dura is exposed and after confirmation of adequate exposure using ultrasonography, the dura and arachnoid are sequentially opened and tacked back, with care taken to minimize any blood from entering the subarachnoid space. Specific features of resection in various CNS regions are briefly described next.

Microsurgical Technique

For hemangioblastomas that present to the pial surface, the pia–tumor junction is sharply incised to develop a surgical plane at the tumor–tissue interface. Cortisectomy (cerebellum) or myelotomy (brainstem or spinal cord) may be required to reach tumors that do not present to the pial surface. After identifying the tumor–tissue interface, circumferential dissection is performed. During dissection, tumor-associated vessels are identified, bipolar coagulated, and sharply divided. For tumors with associated cysts/syringes, the solid tumor is circumscribed, and the cyst wall is maintained intact if possible to aid with dissection. Gentle retraction using a sucker tip positioned on a patty aids with deep dissection. After the tumor is completely circumscribed, it is thoroughly devascularized and can usually be safely removed en bloc without inciting any hemorrhage.

Cerebellum and Brainstem

For cerebellar and brainstem hemangioblastomas, a suboccipital *craniectomy* is generally utilized in VHL patients, given the likely need for future surgeries and to limit any imaging artifact.[22,25] C1 laminectomy is generally performed for brainstem tumors, and C2 laminectomy is added if necessary for exposure.

Spinal Cord

As is discussed here, 96% of spinal cord hemangioblastomas present dorsally.[27] For dorsal tumors, laminectomies are performed to provide adequate exposure rostral and caudal to the tumor.[23] For ventrally located spinal cord hemangioblastomas, an anterior approach with corpectomies and instrumentation may be preferential.[26]

Nerve Root

Hemangioblastomas of spinal and cauda equina nerve roots can become symptomatic and require resection. Because these tumors universally originate intrafascicularly, it is necessary to sacrifice the nerve root of origin for complete tumor resection.

■ Anatomically Specific Implications

Cerebellum

Patient and Tumor Characteristics

Cerebellar hemangioblastomas represent 40 to 50% of the CNS hemangioblastomas in patients with VHL. Jagannathan and colleagues[22] described the presentation and operative results of 80 patients with VHL who underwent resection of 164 cerebellar hemangioblastomas (mean follow-up, 8 years). Ninety-three percent of resected tumors arose in the cerebellar hemispheres and 7% arose in the vermian region. Seventy-five percent of tumors were located in the posterior half of the cerebellum. Although peritumoral cysts were present in 55% of resected tumors and intratumoral cysts were present in 21%, 4% of tumors had both intra- and peritumoral cysts. Patients were symptomatic (most commonly with headache and gait changes) in 96% of cases (**Table 19.1**). All symptomatic tumors contained either peritumoral cysts or edema, compared with only 18% of asymptomatic tumors.

Outcomes

Patients remained stable or improved at 3 months after resection in 98% of operations. Only one patient developed persistent postoperative decline in neurological function, which manifested as exacerbation of dysarthria. An additional five patients (6% of patients) subsequently experienced neurological decline as a result of disease progression. All five asymptomatic patients (6% of total surgical population) remained intact postoperatively. All tumor-related cysts were inactivated after tumor resection. There were no cases of tumor recurrence.

Brainstem

Patient and Tumor Characteristics

The brainstem is the location of ~ 10% of hemangioblastomas in patients with VHL. Brainstem hemangioblastomas arise most frequently in the medullary obex (**Fig. 19.1**). Headache, dysphagia, and hiccups are the most common symptoms (**Table 19.1**). In a retrospective analysis of brainstem hemangioblastomas in patients with VHL, Weil and coworkers demonstrated that surgery for symptomatic tumors was required in only 25% of all patients followed (the remainder of patients in the study remained asymptomatic).[25] More recently, Wind and colleagues[28] reported the long-term outcomes of a cohort of VHL patients followed at the National Institutes of Health (NIH), which included 44 patients who underwent resection of 71 brainstem hemangioblastomas (mean follow-up, 5.9 years).

Outcomes

Better understanding of the tumors and improved microsurgical technique have been associated with improvements in outcomes in the resection of brain-

Table 19.1 Symptom distribution in patients with von Hippel-Lindau disease and central nervous system hemangioblastomas by location

Symptoms at time of presentation	Location of hemangioblastoma		
	Cerebellum (%)	Brainstem (%)	Spinal cord (%)
Headache	75	59	
Gait disturbances	55	31	
Dysmetria	29		
Hydrocephalus	28		
Nausea/vomiting	28	24	
Nystagmus	13		
Dysarthria	9	20	
Dysphagia	8	33	
Hypesthesia		26	64
Hyperreflexia			57
Dysesthesia			43
Weakness		18	36
Proprioceptive changes			17
Bowel/bladder complaints			12
Spasticity			5
Ataxia		29	
Hiccups		31	
Visual changes		26	

Note: Symptoms of brainstem hemangioblastomas are noted to overlap with both cerebellar and spinal cord tumors. Headache is seen to be the most common symptom associated with brainstem and cerebellar tumors, whereas hypesthesia and hyperreflexia are most common in spinal cord tumors.

Source: Results from Jagannathan et al, Mehta et al, and Wind et al.[22,27,28]

stem hemangioblastomas. Early reports included a mortality rate up to 33%, with substantial additional morbidity.[29] By contrast, in the long-term follow-up of the NIH cohort of 44 patients, Wind and coworkers found that by 6 months postoperatively, only one (2% of operations) patient was persistently impaired.[28] There were no operative mortalities, and complete resection was universally achieved. In the early postoperative period, 18% of patients did experience impairment in functional status and 12% required tracheostomy or gastrostomy as a result of exacerbation of lower cranial nerve dysfunction. No factors were identified that significantly predicted outcome. Results from an Italian cohort were similar.[30]

Spinal Cord

Patient and Tumor Characteristics

Spinal cord hemangioblastomas represent 40 to 50% of the CNS hemangioblastomas in patients with VHL. Mehta and coworkers presented the surgical results of the NIH VHL cohort over the 25-year period from 1984 to 2008, with a focus on long-term functional outcome.[27] In this series, 108 patients underwent resection of 218 spinal cord hemangioblastomas. Symptoms, most commonly hypesthesia and hyperreflexia, were present in 94% of patients before resection (**Table 19.1**). Most tumors (95%) were located dorsal to the dentate ligament, and 54% of these were located at the dorsal root entry zone. Mean tumor volume was 0.8 cm^3, and an associated syrinx was present in 85% of operations. Others have demonstrated similar patient and tumor characteristics.[31]

Outcomes

The details of long-term surgical outcomes over an average 7-year follow-up were analyzed by Mehta and colleagues.[27] Almost all tumors (99.5%) were completely resected. Though mild and not function limiting, 61% of operations were associated with worsening of preoperative neurological signs/symptoms or development of new mild signs/symptoms immediately after surgery. By 6 months postsurgery, patients remained stable or improved clinically following 96% of operations. Following the majority of operations (71%), patients noted improvements in tumor-associated symptoms by 6 months. In all 10 operations (6%) for asymptomatic but rapidly enlarging spinal cord hemangioblastomas, patients remained asymptomatic postoperatively. Ninety-six percent of associated syringes diminished or collapsed postoperatively. Worsened functional outcome related to surgery was associated with ventral and entirely intramedullary tumor location. Some have advocated resection of asymptomatic spinal cord hemangioblastomas larger than 50 mm^3, based on the likelihood of future symptom development.[32]

Long-term spinal column stability must be considered in patients with VHL and spinal cord hemangioblastomas because many of these patients require multiple operations, including multilevel laminectomies. Asthagiri and coworkers[33] addressed this question in a study of 25 patients with VHL who underwent 34 operations involving cervical laminectomies for resection of dorsal hemangioblastomas. Only 12% of patients developed cervical spine clinical instability over the follow-up period (mean, 9.1 years). Inclusion of C2 laminectomy was a risk factor for the development of clinical instability, increased neck disability was associated with an increased number of operations.

Hemangioblastomas of the ventral half of the spinal cord can be surgically challenging. As already mentioned, this location was associated with worse functional outcome postoperatively. In a small study by Pluta et al, anterior and posterior approaches to these tumors were compared.[26] Although ambulation was significantly impaired postoperatively in four of five patients treated via a posterior approach, none of the patients treated via anterior approach declined.

Supratentorial Compartment

Although relatively rare, CNS hemangioblastomas may occur in the supratentorial compartment. Though these tumors constitute a small percentage of total CNS hemangioblastomas in patients with VHL, up to 11% of patients have been found to harbor supratentorial hemangioblastomas.[34] Peyre and coworkers[35] presented the natural history of 13 patients with VHL who harbored 18 supratentorial hemangioblastomas with a mean clinical follow-up of 9 years. The most common location for the tumors was the hippocampus/temporal lobe. Resection was performed in 10 of 13 patients for 13 of 18 total tumors, only three of which were symptomatic. The remaining tumors were resected after demonstrating asymptomatic growth. These patients represented 3.2% of all patients in the French VHL study group. Median tumor size at the time of resection was 1.38 cm^3 with a 4.4 cm^3 cyst. No patients developed permanent deficits related to the surgery. Lonser and coworkers[34] found that supratentorial hemangioblastomas in VHL patients were most often located in the pituitary stalk (29%), hippocampus (21%), and optic nerve or chiasm (14%). Of the patients with pituitary stalk tumors, none required surgery because none developed any signs or symptoms during follow-up.

Spinal Nerve Roots and Cauda Equina

Hemangioblastomas may rarely present on lumbosacral spinal nerve roots. Lonser and colleagues[24] reported on six consecutive patients with VHL who underwent resection of eight cauda equina tumors. All patients presented experienced numbness and most experienced low-back or radicular pain. All tumors originated within a single nerve root/rootlet. Complete resection required sacrificing the rootlet of tumor origin. Complete resection was performed in all patients, except one patient with tumor originating from a motor rootlet. Painful symptoms resolved and urinary retention (when present preoperatively) improved or resolved. No patients developed persistent deficits postoperatively. Numbness present preoperatively persisted in the distribution of the sacrificed nerve root.

Expert Recommendations

1. All patients with VHL should be screened for pheochromocytoma prior to surgery.
2. Preoperative arteriography need not be routinely performed.
3. Care must be taken to minimize the possibility of any blood entering the subarachnoid space.
4. Craniectomy is generally preferred to craniotomy for cerebellar hemangioblastomas given the need for frequent follow-up imaging and additional surgery.
5. Peritumoral cyst walls need not be resected as these comprise compressed, gliotic tissue and universally resolve after complete resection of the hemangioblastoma.

■ Summary and Conclusions

The characteristics of hemangioblastomas in patients with VHL and the outcomes of surgical resection have been defined through several natural history studies and large surgical series. Hemangioblastomas often demonstrate a saltatory growth pattern and can remain quiescent for indefinite periods of time. Further, features predictive of symptom formation have not been identified. Therefore, we currently maintain that surgical removal should be reserved for symptomatic and rapidly enlarging hemangioblastomas.

■ References

1. Maher ER, Iselius L, Yates JR, et al. Von Hippel-Lindau disease: a genetic study. J Med Genet 1991;28(7):443–447
2. Latif F, Tory K, Gnarra J, et al. Identification of the von Hippel-Lindau disease tumor suppressor gene. Science 1993; 260(5112):1317–1320
3. Maher ER, Yates JR, Harries R, et al. Clinical features and natural history of von Hippel-Lindau disease. Q J Med 1990; 77(283):1151–1163
4. Neumann HP, Eggert HR, Scheremet R, et al. Central nervous system lesions in von Hippel-Lindau syndrome. J Neurol Neurosurg Psychiatry 1992;55(10):898–901
5. Butman JA, Linehan WM, Lonser RR. Neurologic manifestations of von Hippel-Lindau disease. JAMA 2008;300(11): 1334–1342
6. Choyke PL, Glenn GM, Walther MM, Patronas NJ, Linehan WM, Zbar B. von Hippel-Lindau disease: genetic, clinical, and imaging features. Radiology 1995;194(3):629–642
7. Merrill MJ, Edwards NA, Lonser RR. Notch receptor and effector expression in von Hippel-Lindau disease-associated central nervous system hemangioblastomas. J Neurosurg 2011;115(3):512–517
8. North PE, Mizeracki A, Mihm MC Jr, Mrak RE. GLUT1 immunoreaction patterns reliably distinguish hemangioblas-

toma from metastatic renal cell carcinoma. Clin Neuropathol 2000;19(3):131–137
9. Ishizawa K, Komori T, Hirose T. Stromal cells in hemangioblastoma: neuroectodermal differentiation and morphological similarities to ependymoma. Pathol Int 2005;55(7):377–385
10. Hoang MP, Amirkhan RH. Inhibin alpha distinguishes hemangioblastoma from clear cell renal cell carcinoma. Am J Surg Pathol 2003;27(8):1152–1156
11. Jarrell ST, Vortmeyer AO, Linehan WM, Oldfield EH, Lonser RR. Metastases to hemangioblastomas in von Hippel-Lindau disease. J Neurosurg 2006;105(2):256–263
12. Havekes B, King K, Lai EW, Romijn JA, Corssmit EP, Pacak K. New imaging approaches to phaeochromocytomas and paragangliomas. Clin Endocrinol (Oxf) 2010;72(2):137–145
13. Maddock IR, Moran A, Maher ER, et al. A genetic register for von Hippel-Lindau disease. J Med Genet 1996;33(2):120–127
14. Pacak K. Preoperative management of the pheochromocytoma patient. J Clin Endocrinol Metab 2007;92(11):4069–4079
15. Walther MM, Reiter R, Keiser HR, et al. Clinical and genetic characterization of pheochromocytoma in von Hippel-Lindau families: comparison with sporadic pheochromocytoma gives insight into natural history of pheochromocytoma. J Urol 1999;162(3 Pt 1):659–664
16. Agarwal G, Sadacharan D, Kapoor A, et al. Cardiovascular dysfunction and catecholamine cardiomyopathy in pheochromocytoma patients and their reversal following surgical cure: results of a prospective case-control study. Surgery 2011;150(6):1202–1211
17. Horvathy DB, Hauck EF, Ogilvy CS, Hopkins LN, Levy EI, Siddiqui AH. Complete preoperative embolization of hemangioblastoma vessels with Onyx 18. J Clin Neurosci 2011;18(3):401–403
18. Cornelius JF, Saint-Maurice JP, Bresson D, George B, Houdart E. Hemorrhage after particle embolization of hemangioblastomas: comparison of outcomes in spinal and cerebellar lesions. J Neurosurg 2007;106(6):994–998
19. Montano N, Doglietto F, Pedicelli A, et al. Embolization of hemangioblastomas. J Neurosurg 2008;108(5):1063–1064, author reply 1064–1065
20. Ammerman JM, Lonser RR, Dambrosia J, Butman JA, Oldfield EH. Long-term natural history of hemangioblastomas in patients with von Hippel-Lindau disease: implications for treatment. J Neurosurg 2006;105(2):248–255
21. Wanebo JE, Lonser RR, Glenn GM, Oldfield EH. The natural history of hemangioblastomas of the central nervous system in patients with von Hippel-Lindau disease. J Neurosurg 2003;98(1):82–94
22. Jagannathan J, Lonser RR, Smith R, DeVroom HL, Oldfield EH. Surgical management of cerebellar hemangioblastomas in patients with von Hippel-Lindau disease. J Neurosurg 2008;108(2):210–222
23. Lonser RR, Oldfield EH. Microsurgical resection of spinal cord hemangioblastomas. Neurosurgery 2005;57(4, Suppl):372–376
24. Lonser RR, Wait SD, Butman JA, et al. Surgical management of lumbosacral nerve root hemangioblastomas in von Hippel-Lindau syndrome. J Neurosurg 2003;99(1, Suppl):64–69
25. Weil RJ, Lonser RR, DeVroom HL, Wanebo JE, Oldfield EH. Surgical management of brainstem hemangioblastomas in patients with von Hippel-Lindau disease. J Neurosurg 2003;98(1):95–105
26. Pluta RM, Iuliano B, DeVroom HL, Nguyen T, Oldfield EH. Comparison of anterior and posterior surgical approaches in the treatment of ventral spinal hemangioblastomas in patients with von Hippel-Lindau disease. J Neurosurg 2003;98(1):117–124
27. Mehta GU, Asthagiri AR, Bakhtian KD, Auh S, Oldfield EH, Lonser RR. Functional outcome after resection of spinal cord hemangioblastomas associated with von Hippel-Lindau disease. J Neurosurg Spine 2010;12(3):233–242
28. Wind JJ, Bakhtian KD, Sweet JA, et al. Long-term outcome after resection of brainstem hemangioblastomas in von Hippel-Lindau disease. J Neurosurg 2011;114(5):1312–1318
29. Fukushima T, Sakamoto S, Iwaasa M, et al. Intramedullary hemangioblastoma of the medulla oblongata—two case reports and review of the literature. Neurol Med Chir (Tokyo) 1998;38(8):489–498
30. Pavesi G, Berlucchi S, Munari M, Manara R, Scienza R, Opocher G. Clinical and surgical features of lower brain stem hemangioblastomas in von Hippel-Lindau disease. Acta Neurochir (Wien) 2010;152(2):287–292
31. Kanno H, Yamamoto I, Nishikawa R, et al; Clinical VHL Research Group in Japan. Spinal cord hemangioblastomas in von Hippel-Lindau disease. Spinal Cord 2009;47(6):447–452
32. Harati A, Satopää J, Mahler L, et al. Early microsurgical treatment for spinal hemangioblastomas improves outcome in patients with von Hippel-Lindau disease. Surg Neurol Int 2012;3:6
33. Asthagiri AR, Mehta GU, Butman JA, Baggenstos M, Oldfield EH, Lonser RR. Long-term stability after multilevel cervical laminectomy for spinal cord tumor resection in von Hippel-Lindau disease. J Neurosurg Spine 2011;14(4):444–452
34. Lonser RR, Butman JA, Kiringoda R, Song D, Oldfield EH. Pituitary stalk hemangioblastomas in von Hippel-Lindau disease. J Neurosurg 2009;110(2):350–353
35. Peyre M, David P, Van Effenterre R, et al; French NCI Network VHL Disease and Inherited Predisposition to Kidney Cancer. Natural history of supratentorial hemangioblastomas in von Hippel-Lindau disease. Neurosurgery 2010;67(3):577–587
36. Wind JJ, Lonser RR. Management of von Hippel-Lindau disease-associated CNS lesions. Expert Rev Neurother 2011;11(10):1433–1441

20

The Role of Radiosurgery in the Management of Hemangioblastomas

Sze Chun Ho and Ashok R. Asthagiri

Central nervous system (CNS) hemangioblastomas are World Health Organization (WHO) grade I tumors that account for ~ 1% of all central nervous system neoplasms.[4] One third of hemangioblastomas are identified in the setting of von Hippel-Lindau disease (VHL), a multiple neoplasia syndrome caused by a mutation in the VHL tumor suppressor gene located on 3p. The remainder are solitary lesions identified as sporadic tumors in the general population. Although hemangioblastomas may occur throughout the CNS, they are most frequently identified below the level of the tentorium (cerebellum, brainstem, and spinal cord).[1,24] Hemangioblastomas are benign tumors for which complete resection confers a cure, but the utility of radiosurgery has been explored as a treatment approach in three settings. First, tumors in patients who are poor surgical candidates have been treated with radiosurgery either due to (1) the location of the tumor or (2) multiple patient comorbidities that confer unacceptable operative risk. Second, in the setting of patients with VHL harboring multiple tumors, the cumulative risk and morbidity associated with multiple resections have led to radiosurgery of both symptomatic and asymptomatic tumors. Finally, in patients with tumor recurrence after prior resection, radiosurgery has been utilized as a salvage therapy. This chapter reviews the pathobiology of hemangioblastomas (sporadic and VHL-associated), the biology of radiosurgery, and the controversial role of radiosurgery in the management of hemangioblastomas in these different clinical situations.

■ Hemangioblastomas

The majority of hemangioblastomas, whether sporadic or VHL associated, share common cytogenetic alterations, histopathological and radiological appearance, and treatment challenges. Hemangioblastomas originate from embryonic hemangioblasts that develop into highly vascular lesions consisting of two separate components—proliferated endothelial capillaries and stromal cells[9,36] (**Fig. 20.1**). These tumors histologically resemble clear cell renal carcinomas but may be distinguished by immunoreactivity to nonspecific enolase (NSE) and inhibin and lack of staining with CD10 and epithelial membrane antigen (EMA) (NSE+, inhibin+, CD10−, EMA−).[11]

Cytogenetic evaluation of VHL-associated hemangioblastomas reveals that the stromal element is neoplastic and harbors mutations in the VHL tumor suppressor gene located on chromosome 3.[34] VHL tumor suppressor gene inactivation causes upregulation of vascular endothelial growth factor (VEGF) expression in the stromal compartment that leads to vascular proliferation and increased vascular permeability.[14,31] As the resultant peritumoral edema caused by plasma ultrafiltrate leakage exceeds the reabsorptive capacity of adjacent tissues, cyst formation ensues and results in the characteristic radiographic appearance of hemangioblastomas.[7,27] Although the classic appearance of hemangioblastomas on magnetic resonance imaging (MRI) is charac-

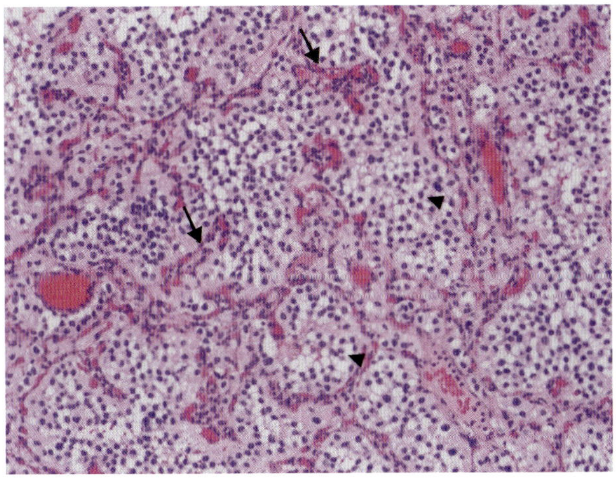

Fig. 20.1 Hematoxylin and eosin–stained, paraffin-embedded section (×40) reveals the presence of a highly vascular lesion consisting of two separate components—proliferated endothelial capillaries (*arrows*) and stromal cells (*arrowheads*).

terized by the presence of an avidly enhancing mural tumor nodule in association with a hypointense peritumoral cyst on T1-weighted sequences, tumors may also have primarily only a solid component or may harbor intratumoral cysts (**Fig. 20.2**). Hemangioblastomas with associated cysts are often symptomatic from mass effect or resultant obstructive hydrocephalus.[36] In contrast to the vascular leak etiology of the peritumoral cyst, the opaque fluid with high protein levels identified in intratumoral cysts suggests they may be a result of tumor necrosis.

Sporadic

Sporadic tumors are solitary by definition and account for two thirds of hemangioblastomas that are identified.[9] The incidence peaks in the fourth decade and is slightly greater in males. Most tumors originate within the cerebellar hemisphere (83 to 95%), but the spinal cord (3 to 13%), brainstem (2%), and supratentorial location (< 5%) may also be affected.[3] About 30% of patients with cerebellar hemangioblastomas are subsequently found to have VHL; it is thus imperative that appropriate screening be performed in this patient population.[8] Also, any patient presenting with a presumed sporadic hemangioblastoma should have a detailed family history, 24-hour urine catecholamine and metanephrine test (pheochromocytoma), abdominal contrast-enhanced computed tomography (visceral manifestations), MRI scan of the remainder of the neuroaxis (additional hemangioblastomas, endolymphatic sac tumors), and ophthalmological exam (retinal hemangioblastomas). Because these tumors are World Health Organization (WHO) grade I and complete resection is curative, first-line management remains surgical removal.

Associated with von Hippel-Lindau Disease

VHL is an autosomal dominant disorder with an incidence of 1 in 35,000.[8] VHL is caused by a germline mutation in the VHL tumor suppressor gene on chromosome 3p, and clinical penetrance is identified in

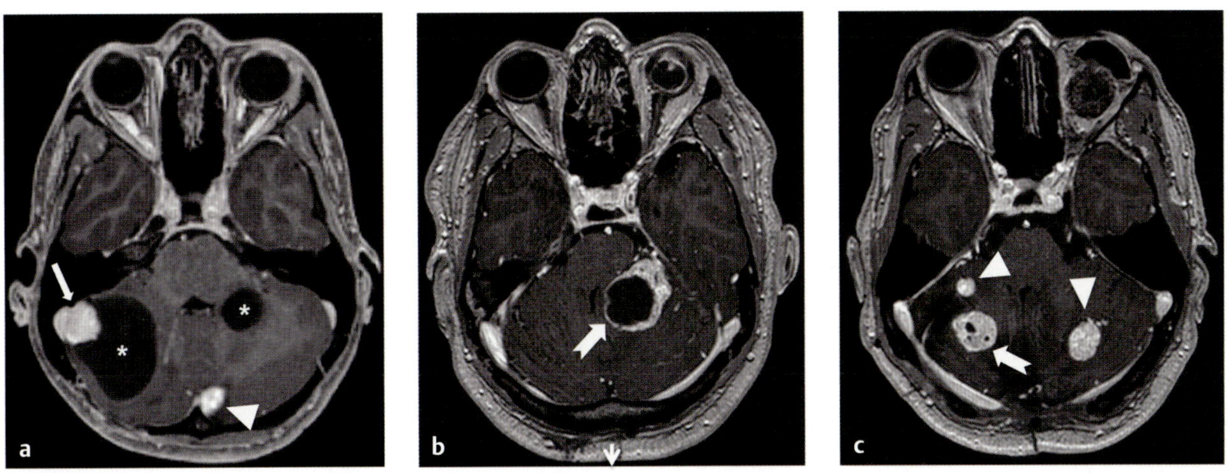

Fig. 20.2 Axial gadolinium-enhanced, T1-weighted magnetic resonance imaging of the cerebellum reveals the imaging spectrum of hemangioblastomas. **(a)** The classic appearance is characterized by an avidly enhancing mural tumor nodule (*arrow*) in association with a hypointense peritumoral cyst (*asterisk*), **(b)** but tumors may also have primarily only a solid component (*arrowhead*) or **(c)** may harbor intratumoral cyst(s) (*notched arrow*).

over 90% of patients by 60 years of age.[13,18] CNS manifestations of disease include the development of hemangioblastomas and endolymphatic sac tumors; visceral manifestations include the development of pancreatic and renal cysts, renal cell carcinoma, pheochromocytoma, and adnexal cystadenomas. Sixty to eighty percent of patients with VHL develop hemangioblastomas, and they are most often multiple.[36] Compared with sporadic hemangioblastomas, VHL-associated hemangioblastomas have a younger peak incidence of related symptom development (third decade of life), and tumors are more frequently identified within the spinal cord (40%), brainstem (12%), and supratentorial location (pituitary stalk and temporal lobe) (10%).[1,16,27]

■ Tumor Progression and Symptom Development

Given sporadic tumors are rarely followed without intervention over the long term because symptoms generally lead to their identification, much of what is known about the natural history of hemangioblastoma growth and symptom development is derived from studies based on patients with VHL. In the largest evaluation of VHL-associated hemangioblastomas, 143 tumors in 19 patients with mean follow-up duration of 12.4 ± 1.4 years revealed that virtually all (97%) tumors demonstrated measurable growth by MRI-based volumetrics over the observation period.[1] However, only 41% of patients became symptomatic over the observation period, and, further, 45% of tumors that eventually became symptomatic were not visualized on initial imaging. In addition, 97% of hemangioblastomas demonstrated a stuttering growth pattern, characterized by alternating periods of growth and quiescence (growth arrest). Individual tumors exhibited an average of 1.85 growth arrests before eventually becoming symptomatic. Tumor growth periods averaged 13 ± 15 months, and growth arrest intervals averaged 25 ± 19 months. Such unpredictability of tumor progression underscores the fundamental issue in treating hemangioblastomas based solely on radiographic progression. Indeed, over a 10-year period, if all progressive tumors were operated on, four additional procedures would have resulted per patient in this study. Therefore, the best indication for intervention with VHL-associated hemangioblastomas remains the development of early symptoms.

There are certain features of hemangioblastomas that correlate with the presence of symptoms and may help guide surveillance in asymptomatic patients. For cerebellar hemangioblastomas, symptomatic hemangioblastomas were significantly larger ($2.8\ cm^3$ vs $0.4\ cm^3$) and more frequently associated with the presence of a peritumoral cyst or edema (100% vs 18%).[9] For brainstem hemangioblastomas, rapid tumor growth (> $0.07\ mm^3/mo$) and initial tumor size (> $0.25\ cm^3$) were predictors of symptom development, whereas for spinal cord hemangioblastomas, initial tumor size (> $22\ mm^3$) was the only predictor.[1] The time to symptom development varied based on the location of the tumor. At 5 years from initial observation, 20% of spinal, 38% of cerebellar, and 60% of brainstem hemangioblastomas required treatment. At 10 years, 30% of spinal and 70% of cerebellar hemangioblastomas produced symptoms.[1]

■ Stereotactic Radiosurgery

Stereotactic radiosurgery (SRS) is a therapeutic modality pioneered in the 1950s by the Swedish neurosurgeon Lars Leksell. The principal feature of SRS is the delivery of high-dose radiation to a focal area of pathology while sparing the surrounding normal structures due to a steep decline in radiation dosage. SRS carries the appeal of being a less invasive procedure than surgery and is often performed in an outpatient or overnight observation setting.

Multiple forms of SRS have been developed utilizing different technology and sources of radiation. The Gamma Knife (GK) (Elekta, Stockholm, Sweden) system contains 192 cobalt-60 sources arranged in a conical configuration with a built-in collimator system. The ability to combine different beam sizes enables precise shaping for even complex targets. Such arrangement allows for treatment of multiple lesions in a single session. By design, GK (Elekta) is restricted to treating intracranial targets due to the need for rigid, frame-based fixation for accurate localization.

Linear accelerator (LINAC)-based systems, including the Cyberknife (CK) (Accuray, Sunnyvale, CA) and Novalis Tx (Varian Medical Systems, Palo Alto, CA) utilize a single high-energy X-ray beam shaped by collimators as the source of radiation. The single beam is repetitively fired from the LINAC head (radiation source), which moves relative to the patient, resulting in the irradiation of a common point (isocenter). Integrated LINAC systems (CK, Accuray; Novalis, Varian) combine highly accurate motorized radiation units with integrated image-guidance systems to allow stereotactic targeting. A variation of standard LINAC-based systems is the CK (Accuray), which is based on a lightweight LINAC mounted on an industrial robot with 6 degrees of freedom enabling multiple direction of movements. This design is an improvement on conventional LINACs, which allow only rotational movement of the radiation head in one plane. Orthogonal X-rays of the patient's skeletal structures can be used for "real-time" image guidance to readjust the beam in relation to the target, enabling frameless stereotaxis.[15]

Efficiency of Stereotactic Radiosurgery for Hemangioblastomas

Level I to Level II Evidence

No studies addressing the management of hemangioblastomas with SRS may be categorized as Level I or Level II evidence.

Level II to Level IV Evidence

Nonexperimental descriptive studies (comparative studies, case-control studies, expert reviews, and clinical experience) all demonstrate high local control rates of tumors with SRS (~ 70 to 100%) (**Table 20.1**). However, the majority of these studies have a limited duration of posttreatment follow-up (< 5 years). In the longest prospective follow-up of SRS-treated hemangioblastomas, Asthagiri et al evaluated 44 tumors in 12 patients with VHL with serial imaging over a mean follow-up of 8.5 years.[2] The local control rate, defined as the percentage of tumors that were either stable or regressed by volumetric analysis of MRI at 2, 5, 10, and 15 years was 91%, 83%, 61%, and 51%, respectively. This strongly suggests that the initial efficacy observed with SRS treatment diminishes over time. An observation that 25% of all treated tumors had an initial volumetric response that was different from the final outcome emphasizes the need for longitudinal evaluation in appropriately classifying treatment response (**Fig. 20.3**). Of these tumors, 18% shrank before progressing to a size larger than the initial volume, 27% grew before regressing to a size smaller than the initial volume, and 55% either grew or regressed before stabilizing and returning to the same pretreatment size. Wang et al[35] reported the largest sample of SRS-treated hemangioblastomas (93 hemangioblastomas), including both sporadic and VHL-related tumors, in 35 patients who were followed for a mean duration of 5.5 years after treatment. This study confirmed a decrease in local control rate over more extended periods of follow-up: 94% at 1 year, 85% at 2 years, 82% at 3 years, 79% at 4 years, and 71% at 5 years. These studies suggest that, although SRS may provide significant local control rates over the short term, there is diminishing marginal benefit over time compared with the natural history of these lesions.

Table 20.1 Summary of outcomes after stereotactic radiosurgery for hemangioblastomas

Study	Modality	Margin dose (Gy)	Total patients	Total tumors	Follow-up (years)	VHL vs sporadic	Control rate (%)
Page et al 1993[22]	LINAC	35 (30–75)	4	11	1.5 (0.6–2.5)	VHL	100
Chang et al 1998[5]	LINAC	23 (18–40)	13	29	3.6 (0.9–7)	VHL	97
Rajaraman et al 2004[28]	GK	20 (13–25)	13	27	2.8 (0.6–6.6)	VHL	83
Asthagiri et al 2010[2]	LINAC/GK	19 (12–24)	20	44	8.5 (3–17.6)	VHL	68
Tago et al 2005[33]	GK	20 (18–20)	12	38	2.9 (0.58–12.25)	Mixed	96
Pan et al 1998[23]	GK	18 (12–24)	13	20	2.4 (2–3)	Mixed	69
Niemelä et al 1996[21]	GK	20 (5–35)	10	11	2.2 (0.3–5.7)	Mixed	60
Jawahar et al 2000[10]	GK	16 (11.7–20)	27	29	4 (0.5–9)	Mixed	75
Park et al 2005[25]	GK	17 (12.8–29.8)	9	84	4.3 (0.7–11.8)	Mixed	96
Kano et al 2008[12]	GK	16 (11–20)	32	74	4.2 (0.5–13.8)	Mixed	92
Patrice et al 1996[26]	LINAC/GK	16 (12–20)	22	38	2.0 (0.5–6.4)	Mixed	86
Wang et al 2005[35]	GK	17 (12–24)	35	93	5.5 (2–9.5)	Mixed	71
Matsunaga et al 2007[19]	GK	14 (8–30)	22	67	5.3 (0.8–12.2)	Mixed	84
Sayer et al 2011[29]	GK	18 (10–25)	14	26	3 (0.5–12)	Mixed	69
Moss et al 2009[20]	LINAC/CK	23.4 (12–40)	28	82	4.9 (0.4–13.7)	Mixed	84

Abbreviations: CK, Cyberknife (Accuray); GK, Gamma Knife (Elekta); LINAC, linear accelerator; VHL, von Hippel-Lindau disease.

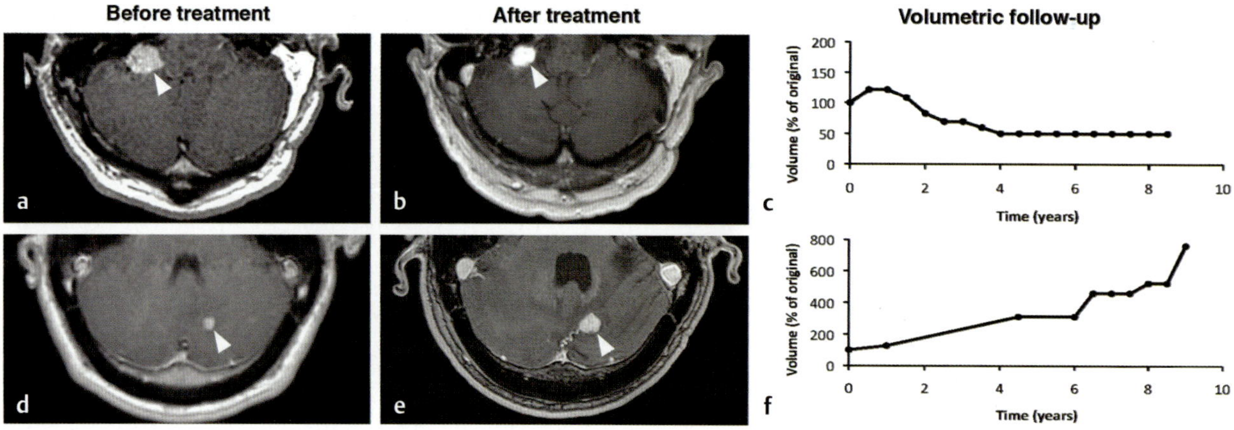

Fig. 20.3 Examples of two tumors where the initial response to stereotactic radiosurgery differed from the final outcome. **(a)** demonstrates imaging for a cerebellar peduncle lesion that underwent stereotactic radiosurgery; the immediate post-treatment response is shown in **(b)**. **(c)** demonstrates the change in tumor volume that occurs over time after treatment. Similar findings are shown for another lesion in **(d–f)**.

Factors Affecting Response to Stereotactic Radiosurgery

Tumor Size

Although many of the studies reviewed are underpowered to detect the role that pretreatment volume plays in affecting SRS response, five large studies clearly report that smaller pretreatment tumor volume is associated with a more favorable response to SRS.[10,12,25,26,33] Jawahar et al[10] showed that tumors with an initial volume of > 3.2 cm^3 have a local control rate of 56% compared with 80% for tumors < 3.2 cm^3.[3,33] Kano et al[12] identified tumor progression only in tumors with a pretreatment volume > 3.2 cm^3 (30% of these tumors progressed). The other three series showed a significant difference in mean initial tumor volume in tumors that progressed compared with those that did not.

In the prospective longitudinal study conducted by Asthagiri et al, pretreatment volume correlated with failure to respond to SRS at the 3-year interim analysis.[2] However, this association disappeared with longer follow-up periods, as a significant number of initially small tumors revealed progression. This suggests that short-term observation may skew the relationship between pretreatment volume and SRS efficiency because there may be delayed progression in smaller tumors.[2]

Presence of Cyst

Hemangioblastomas are frequently associated with peritumoral cysts accompanied by peritumoral edema.[9] It is postulated that cysts and edema develop as a result of increased tumor vasculature permeability. Convective forces drive the extracellular plasma ultrafiltrate from the interstitial space of the tumor to the interstitial space of the surrounding brain.[17] Consistent with this mechanism, surgical removal of the tumor itself universally results in rapid resolution of the peritumoral cyst.[9]

Given the aforementioned mechanism of peritumoral cyst formation, there is significant concern that SRS-induced vascular permeability may promote cyst expansion. Indeed, multiple studies have observed SRS treatment failures specific to progression of tumors with cystic components.[21,23,35] Among 67 hemangioblastomas treated with a mean follow-up period of 5.5 years, Matsunaga et al reported that 6 out of 13 (46%) tumors with a cyst exhibited progression, whereas only 5 out of 54 (9%) solid tumors exhibited progression (multivariate analysis, $p = 0.03$).[19] Kano et al also reported a higher failure rate of SRS-treated tumors with peritumoral cysts (4/9 tumors, 44.4%) versus primarily solid tumors (2/65 tumors, 3.1%). Five-year progression-free survival rates in this study were 61% and 95% for patients with cystic and solid tumors, respectively.[12]

Radiation Dose

Early series using conventional fractionated external-beam radiotherapy to treat residual or unresectable hemangioblastomas suggested a high dose of radiation (> 40 to 50 Gy) was needed to achieve tumor control and to prolong overall patient survival.[30,32] Early experience with radiosurgery for treatment of hemangioblastomas utilized high doses (40 to 75 Gy) but met with significant complications, including protracted cerebral edema and radiation necrosis.[5,22] Because 20 to 25 Gy given as a single fraction by SRS has been estimated to achieve the biological equivalence of 50 to 100 Gy given as fractionated external beam radiotherapy, a trend toward decreased dosing was employed to improve the margin of safety.[5] Hence most large SRS series have used a margin dose of 11 to 25 Gy delivered in a single fraction.

A lower margin dose, though, has also been associated with poorer tumor control in several studies. Patrice et al showed a clear difference in the dose delivered to tumors that exhibited local control (16 Gy) versus those that progressed (14 Gy) after SRS.[26] Similarly, Wang et al reported delivering a mean dosage of 18 Gy for tumors that exhibited local control and 14.2 Gy in tumors that subsequently exhibited progression.[35] Kano et al showed in univariate analysis that a marginal dose less than 15 Gy was significantly associated with decreased progression-free survival (19% of 21 tumors treated with a marginal dose of < 15 Gy exhibited progression, compared with 3.8% of 53 lesions treated with a marginal dose > 15 Gy that exhibited progression).[12] Jawahar et al also confirmed with multivariate analysis that doses greater than 18 Gy were associated with improved tumor control.[10] Contrary to the bulk of radiosurgical literature in the matter, Matsunaga et al reported *no* relation between tumor control and dosage by multivariate analysis.[19] In this study, even low marginal doses (12 to 16 Gy) were associated with local control in over 80% of cases.

Sporadic and Recurrent Hemangioblastomas Associated with von Hippel-Lindau Disease

Because hemangioblastomas are relatively rare neoplasms, most studies report VHL-associated, sporadic and recurrent tumor responses in aggregate; the difficulty in identification of matched cohorts is readily apparent. Kano et al[12] reported that, in their series of 52 VHL and 22 sporadic hemangioblastomas, only 3.8% of the SRS-treated VHL hemangioblastomas showed progression compared with 18.2% of sporadic tumors. The progression-free survival rates of VHL hemangioblastomas were 97.4% at 1, 3, and 5 years, compared with 95.5%, 88.6%, and 44.3% at 1, 3, and 5 years, respectively, for sporadic tumors. Univariate analysis performed in this study suggests that VHL hemangioblastomas are more responsive to SRS treatment, but size discrepancy between the groups (sporadic tumors, mean volume 5.04 cm^3; VHL tumors, mean volume 1.25 cm^3) is a likely significant confounder. No publications specifically address response rates of recurrent hemangioblastomas to SRS.

Complications

SRS for hemangioblastomas is generally well tolerated, with low periprocedural mortality and morbidity. Although protracted peritumoral edema and radiation necrosis were common with single-fraction marginal doses exceeding 40 Gy, current conventional dosing between 12 and 25 Gy has low incidences of either complication.[22] The most common minor symptoms reported are headache, dizziness, and diplopia, which generally respond to short-term glucocorticoid therapy. In patients with VHL, concern about the development of new tumors at an increased rate due to irradiation of haploinsufficient tissues or malignant conversion of treated tumors has not been realized.[6] Despite this, the difficulties in treatment of VHL patients, who continue to develop new tumors during the course of their lifetime, remain challenging.

Expert Recommendations

1. In all cases, because hemangioblastomas are WHO grade I, benign tumors, surgical resection is the treatment of choice (Grade 1C Recommendation, Level III Evidence).
2. The primary modality of treatment for sporadic hemangioblastomas should be surgical resection. This provides a tissue diagnosis and represents a definitive cure with complete resection. Radiosurgery should be reserved for patients who cannot tolerate surgery (Grade 1B Recommendation, Level II Evidence).
3. Given the multiplicity of tumors and unpredictability of tumor progression, intervention with SRS for management of VHL-related hemangioblastomas should be reserved for lesions that are symptomatic. There is sufficient evidence to suggest that SRS is contraindicated in symptomatic lesions that are associated with peritumoral cysts. In symptomatic solid hemangioblastomas, surgical resection should still be the mainstay of treatment. It is clear from the data presented that, although the short-term local control rate is high, the long-term durability of SRS-treated hemangioblastomas is questionable (~ 51% in 10 years) and represents diminishing marginal improvement over the long-term natural history of these tumors. Utility of SRS for VHL should therefore be limited to those patients who are unable to undergo surgery or for whom long-term control may not be required (Grade 1B Recommendation, Level II Evidence).
4. Because complete resection is curative, the treatment of choice remains surgical resection. The specific response rate to SRS for recurrent hemangioblastoma after initial resection is unknown (Grade 1C Recommendation, Level III Evidence).
5. When utilized, a marginal dose of > 16 to 18 Gy is recommended for improved tumor control. Radiation dosing and planning must take into consideration the presence of multiple tumors in patients with VHL, including those that may develop over the course of a patient's life (Grade 1B Recommendation, Level II Evidence).
6. SRS for hemangioblastomas with associated symptomatic peritumoral cysts is not recommended (Grade 1C Recommendation, Level III Evidence).

■ References

1. Ammerman JM, Lonser RR, Dambrosia J, Butman JA, Oldfield EH. Long-term natural history of hemangioblastomas in patients with von Hippel-Lindau disease: implications for treatment. J Neurosurg 2006;105(2):248–255
2. Asthagiri AR, Mehta GU, Zach L, et al. Prospective evaluation of radiosurgery for hemangioblastomas in von Hippel-Lindau disease. Neuro-oncol 2010;12(1):80–86
3. Catapano D, Muscarella LA, Guarnieri V, Zelante L, D'Angelo VA, D'Agruma L. Hemangioblastomas of central nervous system: molecular genetic analysis and clinical management. Neurosurgery 2005;56(6):1215–1221
4. Central Brain Tumor Registry of the United States. CBTRUS statistical report: primary brain and central nervous system tumors diagnosed in the United States in 2004–2008. March 23, 2012, revision. Central Brain Tumor Registry of the United States. Hinsdale, IL. www.cbtrus.org
5. Chang SD, Meisel JA, Hancock SL, Martin DP, McManus M, Adler JR Jr. Treatment of hemangioblastomas in von Hippel-Lindau disease with linear accelerator-based radiosurgery. Neurosurgery 1998;43(1):28–34
6. Evans DG, Birch JM, Ramsden RT, Sharif S, Baser ME. Malignant transformation and new primary tumours after therapeutic radiation for benign disease: substantial risks in certain tumour prone syndromes. J Med Genet 2006;43(4):289–294
7. Gläsker S, Vortmeyer AO, Lonser RR, et al. Proteomic analysis of hemangioblastoma cyst fluid. Cancer Biol Ther 2006;5(5):549–553
8. Hottinger AF, Khakoo Y. Neurooncology of familial cancer syndromes. J Child Neurol 2009;24(12):1526–1535
9. Jagannathan J, Lonser RR, Smith R, DeVroom HL, Oldfield EH. Surgical management of cerebellar hemangioblastomas in patients with von Hippel-Lindau disease. J Neurosurg 2008;108(2):210–222
10. Jawahar A, Kondziolka D, Garces YI, Flickinger JC, Pollock BE, Lunsford LD. Stereotactic radiosurgery for hemangioblastomas of the brain. Acta Neurochir (Wien) 2000;142(6):641–644
11. Jung SM, Kuo TT. Immunoreactivity of CD10 and inhibin alpha in differentiating hemangioblastoma of central nervous system from metastatic clear cell renal cell carcinoma. Mod Pathol 2005;18(6):788–794
12. Kano H, Niranjan A, Mongia S, Kondziolka D, Flickinger JC, Lunsford LD. The role of stereotactic radiosurgery for intracranial hemangioblastomas. Neurosurgery 2008;63(3):443–450
13. Latif F, Tory K, Gnarra J, et al. Identification of the von Hippel-Lindau disease tumor suppressor gene. Science 1993;260(5112):1317–1320
14. Lee JY, Dong SM, Park WS, et al. Loss of heterozygosity and somatic mutations of the VHL tumor suppressor gene in sporadic cerebellar hemangioblastomas. Cancer Res 1998;58(3):504–508
15. Levivier M, Gevaert T, Negretti L. Gamma Knife, CyberKnife, TomoTherapy: gadgets or useful tools? Curr Opin Neurol 2011;24(6):616–625
16. Lonser RR, Butman JA, Kiringoda R, Song D, Oldfield EH. Pituitary stalk hemangioblastomas in von Hippel-Lindau disease. J Neurosurg 2009;110(2):350–353
17. Lonser RR, Vortmeyer AO, Butman JA, et al. Edema is a precursor to central nervous system peritumoral cyst formation. Ann Neurol 2005;58(3):392–399
18. Maher ER, Iselius L, Yates JR, et al. Von Hippel-Lindau disease: a genetic study. J Med Genet 1991;28(7):443–447
19. Matsunaga S, Shuto T, Inomori S, Fujino H, Yamamoto I. Gamma knife radiosurgery for intracranial haemangioblastomas. Acta Neurochir (Wien) 2007;149(10):1007–1013
20. Moss JM, Choi CY, Adler JR Jr, Soltys SG, Gibbs IC, Chang SD. Stereotactic radiosurgical treatment of cranial and spinal hemangioblastomas. Neurosurgery 2009;65(1):79–85
21. Niemelä M, Lim YJ, Söderman M, Jääskeläinen J, Lindquist C. Gamma knife radiosurgery in 11 hemangioblastomas. J Neurosurg 1996;85(4):591–596
22. Page KA, Wayson K, Steinberg GK, Adler JR Jr. Stereotaxic radiosurgical ablation: an alternative treatment for recurrent and multifocal hemangioblastomas. A report of four cases. Surg Neurol 1993;40(5):424–428
23. Pan L, Wang EM, Wang BJ, et al. Gamma knife radiosurgery for hemangioblastomas. Stereotact Funct Neurosurg 1998;70(Suppl 1):179–186
24. Park DM, Zhuang Z, Chen L, et al. von Hippel-Lindau disease-associated hemangioblastomas are derived from embryologic multipotent cells. PLoS Med 2007;4(2):e60
25. Park YS, Chang JH, Chang JW, Chung SS, Park YG. Gamma knife surgery for multiple hemangioblastomas. J Neurosurg 2005;102(Suppl):97–101
26. Patrice SJ, Sneed PK, Flickinger JC, et al. Radiosurgery for hemangioblastoma: results of a multiinstitutional experience. Int J Radiat Oncol Biol Phys 1996;35(3):493–499
27. Peyre M, David P, Van Effenterre R, et al; French NCI Network VHL Disease and Inherited Predisposition to Kidney Cancer. Natural history of supratentorial hemangioblastomas in von Hippel-Lindau disease. Neurosurgery 2010;67(3):577–587
28. Rajaraman C, Rowe JG, Walton L, Malik I, Radatz M, Kemeny AA. Treatment options for von Hippel-Lindau's haemangioblastomatosis: the role of gamma knife stereotactic radiosurgery. Br J Neurosurg 2004;18(4):338–342
29. Sayer FT, Nguyen J, Starke RM, Yen CP, Sheehan JP. Gamma knife radiosurgery for intracranial hemangioblastomas—outcome at 3 years. World Neurosurg 2011;75(1):99–105
30. Smalley SR, Schomberg PJ, Earle JD, Laws ER Jr, Scheithauer BW, O'Fallon JR. Radiotherapeutic considerations in the treatment of hemangioblastomas of the central nervous system. Int J Radiat Oncol Biol Phys 1990;18(5):1165–1171
31. Stratmann R, Krieg M, Haas R, Plate KH. Putative control of angiogenesis in hemangioblastomas by the von Hippel-Lindau tumor suppressor gene. J Neuropathol Exp Neurol 1997;56(11):1242–1252
32. Sung DI, Chang CH, Harisiadis L. Cerebellar hemangioblastomas. Cancer 1982;49(3):553–555
33. Tago M, Terahara A, Shin M, et al. Gamma knife surgery for hemangioblastomas. J Neurosurg 2005;102(Suppl):171–174
34. Vortmeyer AO, Gnarra JR, Emmert-Buck MR, et al. von Hippel-Lindau gene deletion detected in the stromal cell component of a cerebellar hemangioblastoma associated with von Hippel-Lindau disease. Hum Pathol 1997;28(5):540–543
35. Wang EM, Pan L, Wang BJ, et al. The long-term results of gamma knife radiosurgery for hemangioblastomas of the brain. J Neurosurg 2005;102(Suppl):225–229
36. Wind JJ, Lonser RR. Management of von Hippel-Lindau disease-associated CNS lesions. Expert Rev Neurother 2011;11(10):1433–1441

■ SECTION V ■

Medulloblastoma

21

The Role of Surgery in the Treatment of Children with Medulloblastoma

M. Özgür Taşkapilioglu and James T. Rutka

The highly malignant glioma arising from the medullary velum and filling the cavity of the fourth ventricle was first referred to as medulloblastoma (MB) by Bailey and Cushing in 1925.[1] MB is a highly malignant embryonal tumor or primitive neuroectodermal tumor (PNET) of the cerebellum with propensity for leptomeningeal dissemination. It is classified as a World Health Organization (WHO) grade IV tumor. MBs are usually sporadic; however, they may be seen as a part of Li-Fraumeni syndrome, Turcot syndrome, Gorlin syndrome, Nijmegen and ataxia-telangiectasia, or Rubinstein-Taybi syndrome. Rare familial MBs with mutations of human *Suppressor of Fused* (SUFU) have been reported.[2]

Surgery, radiation therapy, and chemotherapy are the mainstays of treatment for MB in children. Radiation therapy is used mainly for patients who are older than 3 years of age. There was a significant improvement of survival for children diagnosed in 2000 to 2002 compared with those diagnosed in 1995 to 1999.[3] The risk of mortality from the disease has been reduced by 30%.[3] The 5-year survival rate is 70% today.[4] This chapter focuses on the role of gross total resection in MB using evidence-based medicine recommendations.

■ Epidemiology

MB is the most common malignant brain tumor in children and accounts for 40% of all posterior fossa tumors.[1] The annual incidence is 0.6 per 100,000 population in the United States and 6.5 per million children (age 0 to 14 years) for the period 1988 to 1997 in Europe, with no substantial differences between European regions.[1,5] Ten percent of the cases were diagnosed within the first year of life, and the annual incidence rate was higher in children between 1 and 9 years of age.[1,5] MB is 1.85 times more common in whites than in blacks and more common in males (60%) than in females.[1] Tumors in adults are most frequently diagnosed in the third and fourth decades of life.[6]

■ Clinical Presentation and Diagnosis

The median duration of symptoms prior to radiological diagnosis is 6 to 7 weeks.[7] The clinical presentation is generally dominated by the signs of the increased intracranial pressure (ICP) that is caused by either the tumor itself or the obstructive hydrocephalus. This effect is aggravated by the volume of the tumor and by peritumoral edema. Papilledema is characteristic for raised ICP, but in neonates and infants with open fontanelles, this symptom may not be present. Instead, these patients may present with an increasing head circumference. Half the children with brain tumors initially show no signs of increased ICP.[8] Symptoms of hyperarousal, such as loud crying for no apparent reason in neonates and infants, excessive irritability, vomiting in the morning before intake of food, "sunsetting" sign (downward deviation of the eyes), diplopia, nystagmus, and ataxia can all be symptoms of MB. In older children, morning headache is usually the first symptom. The headaches get worse when the patients are lying down and there is often some relief with vomiting. The nausea often improves during the course of the day. Parinaud syndrome, also known as dorsal midbrain syndrome, can be seen. Midline cerebellar tumors usually cause truncal ataxia and unsteady gait, whereas cerebellar hemispheric tumors may cause appendicular ataxia and dysmetria. Spinal dissemination, occurring in up to 40% of patients, may cause signs and symptoms of cord compression. Occasionally, children may present with seizures related to cerebral metastatic lesions, but this is rare.

Computed tomography (CT) is often the first imaging study performed for patients in the emergency room with the complaint of headache, vomiting, and gait disturbance. On CT, MB appears as a midline, solidly enhancing, and homogeneous mass in the posterior fossa. Magnetic resonance imaging (MRI) is the gold standard for the diagnosis of MB. A heterogeneously contrast-enhancing posterior fossa mass with hypointensity on T1-/T2-weighted images is characteristic of MB. Spinal MRI should be performed prior to lumbar puncture, if possible, because blood from a traumatic lumbar puncture in the spinal canal can give a false appearance of drop metastases. Elevated taurine on magnetic resonance spectroscopy (MRS) can be used to distinguish MB from other tumors in the posterior fossa.[9] MRS, positron-emission tomography (PET), and single-photon emission computed tomography (SPECT) can be helpful to distinguish tumor recurrence from posttherapy necrosis.

■ Pathology

MBs are made up of small, round, blue cells with little cytoplasm and hyperchromic nuclei. They usually stain positively for vimentin and synaptophysin.[10] In 2007, the World Health Organization (WHO) classified MBs in four histological subtypes: classical MB, large cell/anaplastic MB, nodular desmoplastic MB, and MB with extensive nodularity (MBEN).[11] The large-cell/anaplastic MBs have the worst outcome, whereas the nodular desmoplastic variant, including the MBEN, have the best outcome.[2] However, this survival benefit does not extend to adults with desmoplastic histology. Besides these morphological subtypes, recently four principal transcriptional profiling subgroups of MB have been described: (1) WNT, (2) SHH, (3) group 3, and (4) group 4. The prognosis for the WNT subgroup is excellent in children, whereas SHH subgroup prognosis is very good in infants, and in both groups prognosis is intermediate in adults. Group 3 MB patients have very poor prognosis, and group 4 MB patients have intermediate prognosis for all ages.[12] Although there are not sufficient data on survival rates in adults, they are in the range of 50 to 60%, similar to those in children treated with radiotherapy alone and seemingly inferior to those in patients younger than 21 years receiving adjuvant radiotherapy and chemotherapy.[13]

■ Prognostic Factors

The clinical outcome of patients with MB depends on age at diagnosis (less than or greater than 3 years of age), postoperative tumor residual, presence or absence of disseminated disease based on MRI, and cerebrospinal fluid (CSF) cytology (Chang classification system) (**Table 21.1**).[14] The risk of relapse or death was 93% lower for desmoplastic MB than for classic MB.[15] Freedom from relapse after 8 years is considered a cure by some authors.[16] Recent studies are focused on the molecular mechanisms of MB. Patients with no *MYC* oncogene amplification and positive β-catenin were determined as low risk.[17] Brainstem invasion, which was previously thought to be a high-risk feature, is no longer considered to be so, but this condition increases the chance of postoperative mutism.[18]

■ Treatment

The typical treatment strategy for MB is surgery, followed by radiotherapy and chemotherapy (**Table 21.2**). Surgery is the mainstay of treatment in posterior fossa tumors in children (**Fig. 21.1**). Neurosurgical approaches can include splitting of the inferior vermis (transvermian), supracerebellar infratentorial, telovelar, retrosigmoid, and far lateral. In recent times, the telovelar approach has been used widely and is perhaps the best choice to avoid postoperative mutism and other posterior fossa syndromes. The mortality rate from neurosurgical resection these days ranges from 1 to 5%.[7]

Hydrocephalus can be treated by insertion of a ventriculoperitoneal (VP) shunt or by endoscopic third ventriculocisternostomy (ETV). Interestingly, ETV may reveal ependymal spread of the disease otherwise not seen on preoperative MRI.[2]

Stereotactic radiosurgery is infrequently used but may be applied to residual and recurrent tumors in adults and children.[19] Presurgical chemotherapy has been suggested as beneficial in some studies. These authors report that presurgical chemotherapy makes the tumors more conducive to total or near-total resection and makes surgery safer, leading to improved survival.[20] The major drawback of this strategy would be the lack of a surgical biopsy, because up to one

Table 21.1 Chang's staging classification

T stage	
T1	Tumor < 3 cm in diameter and limited to the classic midline position in the vermis, the roof of the fourth ventricle, and less commonly to the cerebellar hemispheres
T2	Tumor > 3 cm and invading one adjacent structure or partly filling the fourth ventricle
T3a	Tumor further invading two adjacent structures or completely filling the fourth ventricle, with extension into the aqueduct of Sylvius, foramen of Magendie, or foramen of Luschka, thus producing prominent internal hydrocephalus
T3b	Tumor arising from the floor of the fourth ventricle and filling the fourth ventricle
T4	Tumor spread through the aqueduct of Sylvius to involve the third ventricle or midbrain or down into the upper cervical cord
M stage	
M0	No gross subarachnoid or hematogenous metastasis
M1	Tumor cells found in cerebrospinal fluid on microscopic analysis
M2	Gross nodular seeding in the cerebellum, cerebral subarachnoid space, or the third or fourth ventricles
M3	Gross nodular seeding in the spinal subarachnoid space
M4	Extraneuraxial metastasis

Table 21.2 Algorithm depicting the suggested course of treatment for children with medulloblastoma

Posterior fossa mass
↓
Surgery
↓
MB
↓

< 3 y
CT

> 3 y
No metastatic disease
≤ 1.5 cm²
Desmoplastic
No MYC amp
↓
24/54 Gy CSI and CT
↓
5 y survival 80%

> 3 y
Metastatic disease
> 1.5 cm²
Large cell
MYC amp
↓
Higher Rt doses and CT
↓
5 y survival 50%

Abbreviations: amp, amplification; CSI, craniospinal irradiation; CT, computed tomography; MB, medulloblastoma; Rt, radiation therapy.

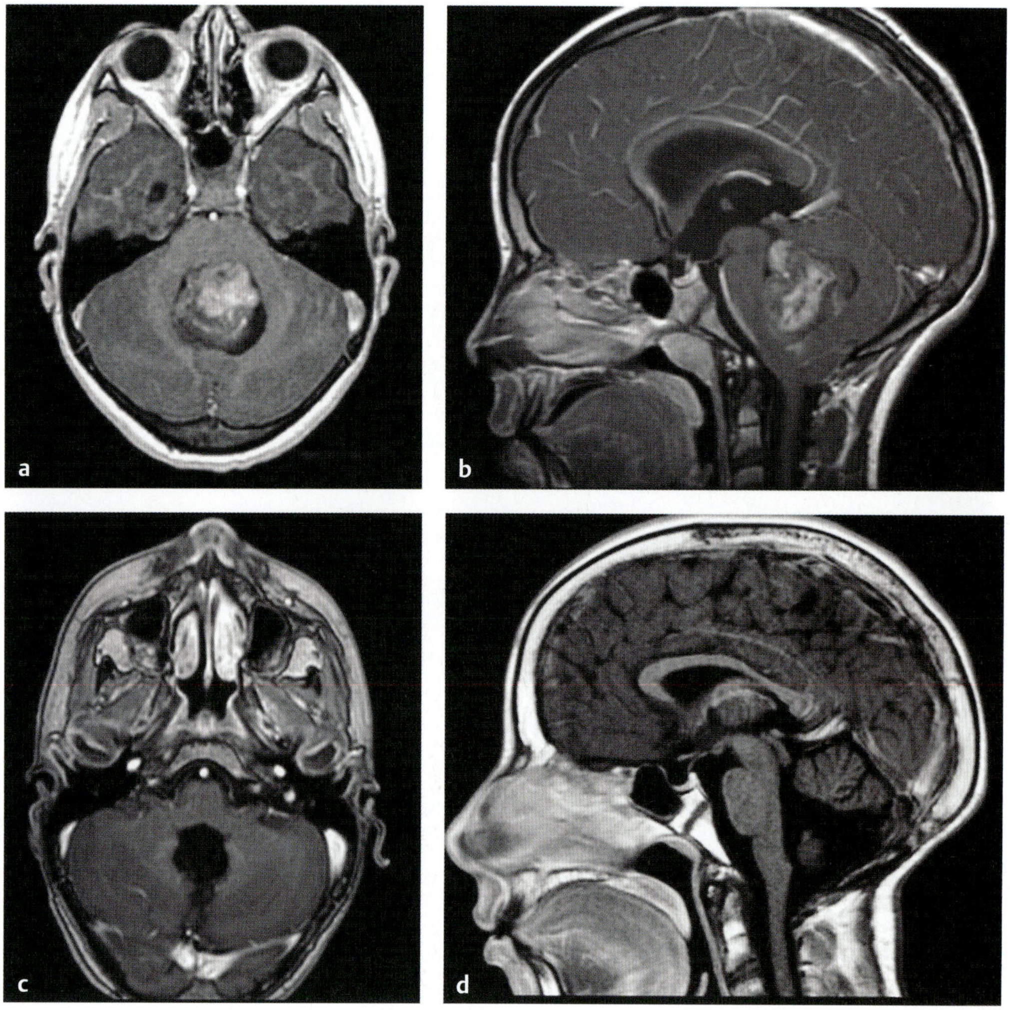

Fig. 21.1 **(a)** Preoperative axial magnetic resonance imaging (MRI) with gadolinium depicting a large midline fourth ventricular tumor that proved to be medulloblastoma (MB). **(b)** Preoperative sagittal MRI with gadolinium showing extent of tumor filling the fourth ventricle. **(c)** Postoperative axial MRI showing complete resection of the tumor. **(d)** Postoperative sagittal MRI showing complete resection of the tumor.

fourth of all embryonal tumors could be atypical teratoid/rhabdoid (ATRT) lesions, especially in children younger than 2 years of age.[21] Using a systemic chemotherapy schedule combined with intraventricular methotrexate has resulted in a 5-year progression-free survival of 83%.[22] Relapses occur in nearly 75% of pediatric cases within 2 years.

■ Surgical Controversies

The treatment of MB includes surgery, chemotherapy, and irradiation. There is no question concerning the role of surgery as first-line therapy in MB. Gross total resection is the aim of surgery, but this might not be possible in the presence of brainstem invasion or CSF dissemination.

Brainstem invasion by MB qualifies as T3b or T4 stage of disease. In a series of 19 patients with MB, Di Rocco et al showed that brainstem infiltration was one of the most significant adverse prognostic factors. Seven (77.7%) of nine patients with brainstem involvement died, whereas only four (40%) of 10 patients without brainstem invasion died in their series. In their series, metastases within the CNS occurred in five infants, associated with recurrence of tumor in two cases after total tumor resection, and progression of the residual tumor in the remaining three cases where surgical excision was incomplete.[23]

In general, progression-free survival is significantly lower in children with evidence of tumor dissemination (M stages 1 through 4). In most centers, it is advocated that neurosurgeons remove as much tumor as can be done safely, irrespective of age or M stage.[24]

Complications after Neurosurgical Resection of Medulloblastoma

The term *cerebellar mutism* refers to a specific disorder in which a complete but transient loss of speech is followed by dysarthria. It develops over 48 to 72 hours after resection of the tumor and can persist from weeks to years. Its pathophysiology is unclear. Injury of the dentate nucleus and the dentatorubrothalamic tracts to the brainstem are the most cited potential substrates of this disorder. Vermian incision, histological diagnosis of MB, extent of tumor, brainstem infiltration, and hydrocephalus are risk factors for postoperative cerebellar mutism.[25] Other common temporary postoperative complications are ataxia, hemiparesis, dysphagia, and seventh cranial nerve palsy.[26] Endocrinological deficiencies, such as growth hormone deficiency and hypothyroidism, can be seen.[2] Cerebellar mutism syndrome developed in 107 (24%) of 450 children after the MB surgery in a prospective study. Brainstem involvement was predictive for the development of mutism.[27] In their prospective study, Di Rocco et al showed that tumor infiltration of the brainstem, the severity of hydrocephalus, and a histological diagnosis of MB might be related to cognitive deficits in the preoperative as well as in the postoperative period.[28] Some case reports suggest the usage of dopamine agonists, such as bromocriptine, for the treatment of mutism, but there is no prospective study on this issue.[29] Speech therapy and supporting modalities are still the best treatment options today.

Evidence That Surgical Resection of Medulloblastomas Improves Survival

Level I Evidence

There are no Level I evidence studies demonstrating the role of gross total resection in MB (**Table 21.3**).

Level II Evidence

Since the early 1980s, studies have identified the role of extent of resection as a significant outcome predictor.[7,30] Currently, in clinical practice and clinical trials, subtotal tumor resection is defined as the presence of tumor ≥ 1.5 cm² on postoperative MRI scans, on the slice that reveals the maximum cross-section area. Kombogiorgas et al measured tumor volume and maximum cross-section area of residual MB on immediate postoperative MRI scans of 37 children operated between 1999 and 2005 and concluded that volumetric measurement of residual MB on immediate postoperative MRI scans may further improve the accuracy of the staging process.[31]

In a prospective, randomized trial, 286 patients were evaluated to assess the value of adjuvant chemotherapy. Five-year survivals were 52% in patients who were thought to have total or subtotal resections and 33% in those with partial resections or biopsies ($p < 0.05$). However, because patients were not systematically staged for tumor dissemination, this study could not be used to clarify the role of total resection.[32]

In a prospective, randomized, multicenter trial, von Hoff et al determined that the 10-year survival rate was 91% after complete resection but only 42% if macroscopic metastases were detected.[33]

Level III Evidence

The extent of initial tumor resection is a key prognostic and risk stratification factor for older children with MB.[34] In a prospective, randomized trial, the Children's Cancer Group reported the results of 203 patients and concluded that extent of tumor resection, as estimated by the neurosurgeon, does not correlate with outcome, but that extent of residual tumor (< 1.5 cm²) does correlate with prognosis in certain children (those who are > 3 years old, with no tumor dissemination).[24]

Park et al reviewed 144 MB cases. Radical excision was achieved in 31 patients, subtotal excision in 66 patients, and partial excision or biopsy in 32 patients. The 5-year survival rates were 59%, 49%, and 30%, respectively. This was a statistically significant difference in the 5-year survival rates between these three groups.[30]

Jaing et al reviewed the records of 22 infants with brain tumors retrospectively. Four of the tumors were MB and all were totally removed. The authors found significant survival benefit associated with a gross total resection.[35]

Di Rocco et al and Lang et al analyzed the data of infants with brain tumors retrospectively and concluded that prognosis is correlated with surgical resection.[23,36]

The survival of patients who had clinical and radiological complete resection of tumor at surgery was significantly better than that of patients with incomplete tumor removal.[37] However, in contrast to the literature already cited, Kombogiorgas et al showed that there is no significant difference between the 5-year survival rate of patients with total (61.1%) and subtotal (61.8%) excision of MB. The authors' explanation for this is twofold: first, because of the improvements

Table 21.3 Level of evidence supporting neurosurgical resection of medulloblastoma

Level I	
There is no Level I evidence study	
Level II	
Sutton et al 1996[7]	The guiding principle for the neurosurgeon remains removal of bulky disease, but there is no justification for removal of small amounts of tumor from critical locations
Kombogiorgas et al 2011[31]	Volumetric measurement of residual medulloblastoma on immediate postoperative MRI scans may further improve the accuracy of the staging process
Tait et al 1990[32]	Benefit for chemotherapy persists in several subgroups: partial or subtotal surgery, brainstem involvement, and stage T3 and T4 disease Several prognostic factors for medulloblastoma have emerged: subtotal resection, extent of disease, and male sex carry a poor prognosis
Von Hoff et al 2009[33]	After maintenance therapy, long-term survival was excellent in fully assessable patients with localized medulloblastoma, and favorable for M1 patients
Level III	
Belza et al 1991[16]	Freedom from relapse beyond 8 years from diagnosis can be considered as a cure in this disease
Park et al 1983[30]	Extent of surgical excision proved to be a statistically significant prognostic factor
Zeltzer et al 1999[34]	For patients with M0 tumors, residual tumor bulk (not extent of resection) is a predictor for progression-free survival Patients with M0 tumors, ≥ 3 years with ≤ 1.5 cm^2 residual tumor, had a 78% ± 6% 5-year progression-free survival rate Children < 3 years old who received a reduced radiation therapy dosage had the lowest survival rate
Albright et al 1996[24]	Extent of tumor resection does not correlate with outcome but, extent of residual tumor does correlate with prognosis in certain children (those who are > 3 years old, with no tumor dissemination) In contrast to age and M stage, the major factors associated with outcome, residual tumor is an important variable in outcome, one that neurosurgeons can control
Jaing et al 2011[35]	Because of the expandability of the skull, brain tumors in infants may have protean manifestations Although pathology categorization was quite variable in this study, three quarters of patients have survived after current therapeutic modalities
Di Rocco et al 1997[23]	The current prognosis for infants with medulloblastoma is not necessarily any worse than that for older children with the same disease, and chemotherapy can be particularly useful in this subgroup of patients, as shown by three long-term survivals obtained in children treated with this type of therapy only
Lang et al 2012[36]	Brain tumors are uncommon in children < 6 months of age
Khafaga et al 1996[37]	T stage, ventriculoperitoneal shunt, radiation doses, and extent of surgery were important prognostic factors In this study, radiation doses of more than 50 Gy to the posterior fossa and 30 Gy to the craniospinal axis resulted in improved survival
Kombogiorgas et al 2007[38]	The contribution of chemotherapy in the improvement of the overall survival appears more evident in children < 3 years or presenting with metastases The absence of significant difference in survival between patients with total or subtotal excision of medulloblastoma supports the view that total excision of medulloblastoma can be avoided when the risk for potential intraoperative damage and consequent neurological deficits is high
Muzumdar et al 2011[39]	Surgery for medulloblastoma is formidable A safe maximal resection and a good Karnofsky score are paramount to ensure compliance with adjuvant therapy and contribute to an overall survival advantage
Bhatia et al 2009[40]	The use of preresectional endoscopic third ventriculocisternostomy is an effective and safe procedure with a high success rate at up to 7.5 years of follow-up
Kombogiorgas et al 2008[41]	The rate of ventricular size reduction in response to tumor excision does not have predictive value for the later need for shunt placement because ventricular volume is related to tumor volume. It appears that the removal of cerebellar medulloblastoma converts hydrocephalus from obstructive to communicating, which requires surgical treatment if it exceeds a certain level of cerebrospinal fluid volume

in imaging and surgical techniques, the residual after surgery is considerably smaller than in the past; and second, with modern surgical techniques, surgical morbidity has been reduced. This allows the majority of patients to start early and complete adjuvant treatments in a timely manner.[38]

Belza et al found that, of 20 patients in whom gross total removal of the tumor was achieved, 63% were free of relapse at 15 years after diagnosis, in contrast to 38% of patients with subtotal resection ($p = 0.79$).[16]

A retrospective analysis of 365 patients (age < 18 years) of MB by Muzumdar et al demonstrated that hydrocephalus at presentation is not a statistically significant factor affecting the 5-year survival. Preoperative shunting or ETV is performed in few centers, but these procedures have the risk of upward herniation, hemorrhage into the tumor, and seeding or metastases.[39]

In a retrospective review of 59 cases, ETV was done in 63% of the patients, and symptoms improved in 1.5 days. The authors concluded that the procedure is effective and safe and should be considered instead of the classic CSF diversion with VP shunts.[40] Kombogiorgas et al studied the pre- and postoperative measurements of ventricular volumes in 20 MB patients. The authors concluded that removal of cerebellar MB converts hydrocephalus from obstructive to communicating and requires shunting only if it exceeds a certain level of CSF volume.[41]

■ Summary and Conclusions

As described in this chapter, the extent of neurosurgical resection correlates with overall patient survival and event-free survival primarily within retrospective studies (Level III evidence). Attempts at gross total resection should be undertaken in any child with a posterior fossa MB where the disease is focal and not metastatic. In the face of widespread metastatic disease, as much tumor as can be safely removed should be.

The real question is whether gross total resection predisposes children with MB to postoperative sequelae like posterior fossa mutism syndrome. The answer to this question is not known. But at the present time, most cooperative childhood oncology groups would advocate for gross total resection of MB if it could be performed safely and without undue morbidity.

Expert Recommendations

1. Surgery, radiation therapy, and chemotherapy are the mainstays of treatment for MBs in children.
2. The large-cell/anaplastic MBs have the worst outcome, whereas the nodular desmoplastic variant, including the MBEN, has the best outcome (Grade 1B Recommendation, Level II Evidence).
3. Data from transcriptional profiling and genetic characterization reveal four subgroups of MBs; the prognosis of the WNT subgroup is best in children whilst the prognosis for Group 3 MB patients is the worst (Grade 1B Recommendation, Level II Evidence).
4. The clinical outcome of patients with MB is based on age at diagnosis with a cut-off at 3 years, postoperative tumor residual, presence or absence of disseminated disease based on MRI, and/or CSF cytology (Grade 1B Recommendation, Level I–III Evidence).
5. Posterior fossa surgery to remove the tumor is typically the first step in the management of a child with MB. The goal of the surgery is maximum safe neurosurgical resection .
6. The goal at surgery should be to remove the tumour in its entirety so that the post-operative MRI scan shows no residual. The presence of less than 1.5 cm^2 residual tumor on postoperative MRI scans still places the child in a favorable risk category (Grade 1C Recommendation, Level II/III Evidence).
7. The telovelar approach may be the best method to avoid postoperative cerebellar mutism.
8. Following surgery, radiation therapy is typically used for patients older than 3 years of age (Grade 1B Recommendation, Level I/II Evidence).

■ References

1. Dhall G. Medulloblastoma. J Child Neurol 2009;24(11):1418–1430
2. Bourdeaut F, Miquel C, Alapetite C, Roujeau T, Doz F. Medulloblastomas: update on a heterogeneous disease. Curr Opin Oncol 2011;23(6):630–637
3. Gatta G, Zigon G, Capocaccia R, et al; EUROCARE Working Group. Survival of European children and young adults with cancer diagnosed 1995-2002. Eur J Cancer 2009;45(6):992–1005
4. Rutka JT, Kuo JS, Carter M, Ray A, Ueda S, Mainprize TG. Advances in the treatment of pediatric brain tumors. Expert Rev Neurother 2004;4(5):879–893
5. Peris-Bonet R, Martínez-García C, Lacour B, et al. Childhood central nervous system tumours—incidence and survival in Europe (1978-1997): report from Automated Childhood Cancer Information System project. Eur J Cancer 2006;42(13):2064–2080

6. Packer RJ, Vezina G. Management of and prognosis with medulloblastoma: therapy at a crossroads. Arch Neurol 2008; 65(11):1419–1424
7. Sutton LN, Phillips PC, Molloy PT. Surgical management of medulloblastoma. J Neurooncol 1996;29(1):9–21
8. Wilne S, Collier J, Kennedy C, Koller K, Grundy R, Walker D. Presentation of childhood CNS tumours: a systematic review and meta-analysis. Lancet Oncol 2007;8(8):685–695
9. Panigrahy A, Krieger MD, Gonzalez-Gomez I, et al. Quantitative short echo time ^{1}H-MR spectroscopy of untreated pediatric brain tumors: preoperative diagnosis and characterization. AJNR Am J Neuroradiol 2006;27(3):560–572
10. Klesse LJ, Bowers DC. Childhood medulloblastoma: current status of biology and treatment. CNS Drugs 2010;24(4): 285–301
11. Ellison DW, Dalton J, Kocak M, et al. Medulloblastoma: clinicopathological correlates of SHH, WNT, and non-SHH/WNT molecular subgroups. Acta Neuropathol 2011;121(3): 381–396
12. Ramaswamy V, Northcott PA, Taylor MD. FISH and chips: the recipe for improved prognostication and outcomes for children with medulloblastoma. Cancer Genet 2011;204(11):577–588
13. Packer RJ, Vezina G. Management of and prognosis with medulloblastoma: therapy at a crossroads. Arch Neurol 2008; 65(11):1419–1424
14. Gilbertson RJ. Medulloblastoma: signalling a change in treatment. Lancet Oncol 2004;5(4):209–218
15. Rutkowski S, Bode U, Deinlein F, et al. Treatment of early childhood medulloblastoma by postoperative chemotherapy alone. N Engl J Med 2005;352(10):978–986
16. Belza MG, Donaldson SS, Steinberg GK, Cox RS, Cogen PH. Medulloblastoma: freedom from relapse longer than 8 years—a therapeutic cure? J Neurosurg 1991;75(4):575–582
17. Kool M, Koster J, Bunt J, et al. Integrated genomics identifies five medulloblastoma subtypes with distinct genetic profiles, pathway signatures and clinicopathological features. PLoS ONE 2008;3(8):e3088
18. Gajjar A, Sanford RA, Bhargava R, et al. Medulloblastoma with brain stem involvement: the impact of gross total resection on outcome. Pediatr Neurosurg 1996;25(4):182–187
19. Navajas A, Giralt J. Evidence in medulloblastomas. Clin Transl Oncol 2010;12(4):271–277
20. Grill J, Lellouch-Tubiana A, Elouahdani S, et al. Preoperative chemotherapy in children with high-risk medulloblastomas: a feasibility study. J Neurosurg 2005;103(4, Suppl): 312–318
21. Packer RJ. Medulloblastoma. J Neurosurg 2005;103(4, Suppl): 299–300, discussion 300–301
22. Rutkowski S, Bode U, Deinlein F, et al. Treatment of early childhood medulloblastoma by postoperative chemotherapy alone. N Engl J Med 2005;352(10):978–986
23. Di Rocco C, Iannelli A, Papacci F, Tamburrini G. Prognosis of medulloblastoma in infants. Childs Nerv Syst 1997;13(7): 388–396
24. Albright AL, Wisoff JH, Zeltzer PM, Boyett JM, Rorke LB, Stanley P. Effects of medulloblastoma resections on outcome in children: a report from the Children's Cancer Group. Neurosurgery 1996;38(2):265–271
25. Kotil K, Eras M, Akçetin M, Bilge T. Cerebellar mutism following posterior fossa tumor resection in children. Turk Neurosurg 2008;18(1):89–94
26. Nejat F, El Khashab M, Rutka JT. Initial management of childhood brain tumors: neurosurgical considerations. J Child Neurol 2008;23(10):1136–1148
27. Robertson PL, Muraszko KM, Holmes EJ, et al; Children's Oncology Group. Incidence and severity of postoperative cerebellar mutism syndrome in children with medulloblastoma: a prospective study by the Children's Oncology Group. J Neurosurg 2006;105(6, Suppl):444–451
28. Di Rocco C, Chieffo D, Pettorini BL, Massimi L, Caldarelli M, Tamburrini G. Preoperative and postoperative neurological, neuropsychological and behavioral impairment in children with posterior cranial fossa astrocytomas and medulloblastomas: the role of the tumor and the impact of the surgical treatment. Childs Nerv Syst 2010;26(9):1173–1188
29. Adachi J, Nishikawa R, Hirose T, Matsutani M. Mixed neuronal-glial tumor of the fourth ventricle and successful treatment of postoperative mutism with bromocriptine: case report. Surg Neurol 2005;63(4):375–379
30. Park TS, Hoffman HJ, Hendrick EB, Humphreys RP, Becker LE. Medulloblastoma: clinical presentation and management. Experience at the Hospital for Sick Children, Toronto, 1950-1980. J Neurosurg 1983;58(4):543–552
31. Kombogiorgas D, Puget S, Boddaert N, et al. Appraisal of the current staging system for residual medulloblastoma by volumetric analysis. Childs Nerv Syst 2011;27(12):2101–2106
32. Tait DM, Thornton-Jones H, Bloom HJ, Lemerle J, Morris-Jones P. Adjuvant chemotherapy for medulloblastoma: the first multi-centre control trial of the International Society of Paediatric Oncology (SIOP I). Eur J Cancer 1990;26(4):464–469
33. von Hoff K, Hinkes B, Gerber NU, et al. Long-term outcome and clinical prognostic factors in children with medulloblastoma treated in the prospective randomised multicentre trial HIT'91. Eur J Cancer 2009;45(7):1209–1217
34. Zeltzer PM, Boyett JM, Finlay JL, et al. Metastasis stage, adjuvant treatment, and residual tumor are prognostic factors for medulloblastoma in children: conclusions from the Children's Cancer Group 921 randomized phase III study. J Clin Oncol 1999;17(3):832–845
35. Jaing TH, Wu CT, Chen SH, et al. Intracranial tumors in infants: a single institution experience of 22 patients. Childs Nerv Syst 2011;27(3):415–419
36. Lang SS, Beslow LA, Gabel B, et al. Surgical treatment of brain tumors in infants younger than six months of age and review of the literature. World Neurosurg 2012;78(1-2):137–144
37. Khafaga Y, Kandil AE, Jamshed A, Hassounah M, DeVol E, Gray AJ. Treatment results for 149 medulloblastoma patients from one institution. Int J Radiat Oncol Biol Phys 1996;35(3): 501–506
38. Kombogiorgas D, Sgouros S, Walsh AR, et al. Outcome of children with posterior fossa medulloblastoma: a single institution experience over the decade 1994-2003. Childs Nerv Syst 2007;23(4):399–405
39. Muzumdar D, Deshpande A, Kumar R, et al. Medulloblastoma in childhood-King Edward Memorial hospital surgical experience and review: comparative analysis of the case series of 365 patients. J Pediatr Neurosci 2011;6(Suppl 1):S78–S85
40. Bhatia R, Tahir M, Chandler CL. The management of hydrocephalus in children with posterior fossa tumours: the role of pre-resectional endoscopic third ventriculostomy. Pediatr Neurosurg 2009;45(3):186–191
41. Kombogiorgas D, Natarajan K, Sgouros S. Predictive value of preoperative ventricular volume on the need for permanent hydrocephalus treatment immediately after resection of posterior fossa medulloblastomas in children. J Neurosurg Pediatr 2008;1(6):451–455

22

The Role of Adjuvant Therapy in Medulloblastoma with and without Neuroaxis Seeding

Erin M. Dunbar

■ Epidemiology

Central nervous system (CNS) tumors are the most common solid tumor affecting the U.S. pediatric population, with an incidence exceeding 3,000 new cases annually, and with the highest mortality rate for cancer. Malignant CNS tumors affecting the pediatric population originate from within the infratentorium 60 to 70% of the time, with the most frequent histologies including medulloblastomas, astrocytomas, and ependymomas. Of these, medulloblastomas are the most common and arise exclusively from within the infratentorium, overwhelmingly from within the medullary velum. The incidence of medulloblastoma peaks between 5 and 10 years of age, with ~ 70% diagnosed by age 20, and essentially none diagnosed after 40. Although only 2 to 5% of pediatric medulloblastomas can be attributed to germline mutations of specific genes (discussed extensively in this chapter), exploration into their tumorigenesis has profoundly advanced molecular pathology, and as a result, potential adjuvant treatments of all medulloblastomas.[1]

■ Histology

Grossly, medulloblastomas are soft, friable, and often necrotic. Histologically, they are composed of small, round cells with round hyperchromatic nuclei, minimal cytoplasmic differentiation, abundant mitoses, and, in up to 40%, neuroblastic Homer Wright rosettes.[1] Immunohistochemically, the majority of medulloblastomas express markers specific for cerebellar granule cells. Markers include the neurotrophin-3 receptor, TrkC, which supports granular cells and is central to the investigations regarding tumorigenesis. Furthermore, there is emerging evidence that high expression of TrkC may correlate with superior outcome.[2] Medulloblastomas also commonly express the neuronal markers synaptophysin and neuron-specific enolase, as well as the primitive neuroepithelial cell marker nestin.[1]

■ Histopathology

The World Health Organization (WHO) currently divides medulloblastomas into five variants based predominantly on histology and immunohistochemistry, as in **Table 22.1**.[3] Histopathology is an important prognostic factor, especially in young patients (usually < 5 years old), and especially in the desmoplastic and large-cell anaplastic WHO variants. For example, Ellison et al reported on a large, prospective international study in which patients < 5 years old received one of many contemporary adjuvant regimens and whose WHO subtypes were retrospectively compared (while also accounting for other

Table 22.1 World Health Organization medulloblastoma variants

Variant	Histopathological features
Classic	– Occasional neuroblastic differentiation
Desmoplastic	– Common neurocytic differentiation – Collagen-rare and reticulin-rich extracellular matrix – Reticulin-free "pale islands" – Associated with aberrations of the patched (*PTCH*) gene (chromosome 9), which is associated with a superior prognosis and possible benefit from sonic hedgehog (SHH) pathway targeted therapies
Large-cell anaplastic	– Associated with cerebrospinal fluid dissemination and with an inferior prognosis
Melanotic	– Very uncommon
Medullomyoblastoma	– Very uncommon

prognostic variables, such as stage). Superior outcome, including progression-free survival (PFS) and overall survival (OS), was strongly correlated with desmoplasia. Inferior outcome was strongly correlated with large-cell or anaplastic variants.[4] Several other large studies have corroborated the strong correlation of desmoplasia with superior outcome, even in patients presenting with metastatic disease.[5] It is important to highlight that the wide variance in frequency of desmoplasia reported across international series brings attention to the need for more stringent criteria in its definition.

Yet we also know that histopathology does not provide a degree of classification that explains why patients with identical histopathology characteristics experience such diverse outcomes with adjuvant therapy. Thus it is important to highlight the significant limits of the current WHO classification system in optimizing both risk stratification as well as, ultimately, adjuvant therapy. With that said, advances in the understanding of tumorigenesis and related molecular pathology will profoundly improve the power of future WHO classification systems.

■ Molecular Pathology

Historically, medulloblastomas were considered a subset of primitive neuroectodermal tumors (PNETs).[6] Recently, gene expression and other techniques have defined a distinct molecular profile. Although exact tumorigenesis remains unknown, current gene expression profiling data suggest medulloblastomas originate from granule cells or multipotent progenitors within the ventricular zone.[7] Molecular profiling (often termed gene expression signatures) of medulloblastomas is providing more than insights into tumorigenesis. It is also providing an improved method for distinguishing desmoplastic and other variants of medulloblastomas, as well as other nonmedulloblastoma malignant CNS tumors, such as malignant gliomas, lymphomas, and atypical teratoid/rhabdoid tumors. Most importantly, molecular profiling of medulloblastomas is also providing advances in optimizing prognostic factors, risk stratification, design and analysis of risk-adapted adjuvant therapy, and, ultimately, outcome.[8–10] In the therapy sections that follow, prospective studies by academic centers and consortia across the United States and Europe incorporate molecular pathology studies aimed at optimizing the foregoing concepts. For example, Entz-Werle et al reported on a multicenter study that demonstrated that combining tumor ERBB2 expression data with clinical data provided improved risk stratification. Standard-risk patients who also demonstrated ERBB2 negativity demonstrated 100% 5-year PFS (5-PFS) as opposed to 54% in patients with ERBB2 positivity.[11] To date, preliminary data on numerous other molecular receptors suggest they may optimize risk stratification, including TrkC, which has been correlated with superior outcome. In contrast, ERBB2-positivity, platelet-derived growth factor receptor-α, and insulinlike growth factor receptor 1 have been correlated with inferior outcome.[12]

Molecular Pathology Most Impacting Adjuvant Therapy

The molecular pathology most impacting adjuvant therapy is discussed next. The tremendous advances in understanding of the molecular pathology of medulloblastomas are largely attributable to the continuous and arduous basic and clinical-translational research into two rare genetic disorders affecting medulloblastomas, Gorlin and Turcot syndromes. The molecular pathology less impacting adjuvant therapy is listed in **Table 22.2**.

Table 22.2 Molecular pathology

Genetic alterations	Loss of alleles on chromosome 17p	– Occurs in up to 30 to 40% of medulloblastomas (most common cytogenetic abnormality) – Implicated in pathogenesis
WNT pathway	Aberrations in the WNT signaling pathway	– Occurs in up to 15% of sporadic medulloblastomas – Is the defining feature in the rare genetic disorder known as Turcot syndrome; such patients are at risk for familial adenomatous polyposis (FAP), an autosomal dominant disorder caused by a mutation in the adenomatous polyposis coli (*APC*) gene on chromosome 5 – *APC* gene mutations raise the risk for medulloblastomas and, less so, malignant gliomas – Sporadic medulloblastomas may also contain *APC* mutations and other aberrations along the WNT pathway – Aberrations along the WNT pathway are associated with superior outcomes, both independently as well as with associated desmoplasia – Certain WNT pathway aberrations may be amenable to targeted therapy
PTCH1/SHH pathway		– 3 to 5% of patients with mutations of the PTCH1signaling pathway develop medulloblastomas – It is the defining feature of the rare autosomal dominant genetic disorder known as Gorlin syndrome; such patients are at risk for large body size, other skeletal anomalies, basal cell carcinomas, and medulloblastomas – Gorlin syndrome, due to germline mutations in the *PTCH1* gene (chromosome 9), encodes for a transmembrane protein that binds the sonic hedgehog (SHH) family of signaling proteins – Deleterious SHH activation appears to have a role in medulloblastoma tumorigenesis – Aberrations of the PTCH1/SHH pathway, including mutations of PTCH2 (chromosome 1), suppressor of fused (SUFU) (chromosome 10q) and GLI3 (chromosome 7p), have been identified in up to 10% of sporadic medulloblastomas – Aberrations of the *PTCH* gene (chromosome 9) are associated with superior outcomes, both independently, as well as with its association with desmoplasia – Certain PTCH1 aberrations may be amenable to sonic hedgehog (SHH) pathway targeted therapies
Several others of many	ERBB2-negativity	– Associated with superior outcomes (ERBB2-positivity inversely correlates)
	TrkC	– Associated with superior outcomes
	Platelet-derived growth factor receptor-α	– Associated with inferior outcomes
	Insulinlike growth factor receptor 1	– Associated with inferior outcomes

WNT Pathway

Although mutation in the wingless (Wnt, aka WNT) signaling pathway has been identified in up to 15% of sporadic medulloblastomas, it is the defining feature in the rare genetic disorder known as Turcot syndrome (glioma-colonic polyposis syndrome). Patients with Turcot syndrome are at risk for familial adenomatous polyposis (FAP), an autosomal dominant disorder caused by a mutation in the adenomatous polyposis coli (*APC*) gene on chromosome 5. *APC* is a tumor suppressor gene involved in numerous developmental functions, including the proliferation and survival of neural progenitor cells.[7] Mutations in the *APC* gene place patients at greater risk for medulloblastomas than for malignant gliomas.[13] Of note, mutations of the *APC* gene, and other aberrations along the WNT pathway, have also been identified in sporadic medulloblastomas. It is important to highlight that, across clinical-translational studies, aberrant activation of the WNT developmental pathway often correlates with an improved outcome, both independently as well as in association with desmoplasia.[4]

SHH Pathway

Although only 3 to 5% of patients with mutations of the patched-1 (PTCH1) signaling pathway develop medulloblastomas, usually the desmoplastic variant, it is the defining feature of the rare autosomal dominant genetic disorder known as Gorlin syndrome (basal cell nevus syndrome). Patients with Gorlin syndrome are at risk for large body size, other skeletal anomalies, basal cell carcinomas, and medulloblastomas. Gorlin syndrome, due to germline mutations in the *PTCH1* gene on chromosome 9, encodes for a transmembrane protein that binds the sonic hedgehog (SHH) family of signaling proteins.[14] Deleterious SHH activation appears to have a proliferative effect on granule cells, the cell theorized to be central to medulloblastoma tumorigenesis. It is important to note that aberrations of the SHH/PTCH1 pathway, including mutations of PTCH2 (chromosome 1), suppressor of fused (SUFU) (chromosome 10q) and GLI3 (chromosome 7p), have been identified in up to 10% of sporadic medulloblastomas—which are also often desmoplastic.[15,16]

Evidence-Based Diagnosis of Medulloblastoma

Level I to Level II Evidence

A diagnosis based on the combination of molecular pathology and histopathology is superior to histology alone.

The WHO histopathological variant of desmoplasia is an important positive prognostic factor.

The WHO anaplastic large-cell variant is an important negative prognostic factor.

Aberrant activation of the WNT developmental pathway often correlates with an improved outcome, both independently as well as with associated desmoplasia.

Deleterious SHH activation appears central to medulloblastoma tumorigenesis and appears to be associated with desmoplasia.

■ Clinical Presentation

Clinical symptoms and signs of malignant CNS tumors are caused by "localized" invasion and/or compression of structures, as well as "nonspecific" increased intracranial pressure (ICP), by either mass effect or obstructed cerebrospinal fluid (CSF) flow. It is important to highlight that the clinical presentation of medulloblastomas is profoundly affected by both age and duration of onset. For example, infants are unable to articulate their symptoms, as opposed to older children and adults. Furthermore, infants and children are more likely to have midline (vermian) tumors, as opposed to adults, who are more likely to have lateral cerebellar hemispheric tumors. Finally, the duration of symptoms prior to diagnosis strongly correlates with higher presenting stage and inferior outcome.[17]

■ Staging

At presentation, approximately one third of medulloblastomas have metastases throughout the CNS, often measurable radiographically or cytologically. Historically (defined as prior to the incorporation of molecular pathology), the modified Chang staging system was created to incorporate radiographic and clinical factors, as detailed in **Table 22.3.**[18]

Radiographic staging often begins with a computed tomographic (CT) scan, given CT's wide availability and unburdensome study time/techniques. A heterogeneous, contrast-enhancing tumor, which also spontaneously enhances, is most common.

Recommendations for the Diagnosis of Medulloblastoma

1. High-quality histopathologic diagnosis, inclusive of determining desmoplasia and anaplastic large-cell variant whenever possible, is essential. Pathology consultation at an academic center should be considered (Grade 1C+ Recommendation, Level I/II Evidence).
2. In all cases, one should attempt to obtain molecular pathological diagnosis if feasible. Molecular profiles of medulloblastomas are being incorporated into prognostic factors, risk stratification, and design and analysis of risk-adapted therapy. Wingless (Wnt, aka WNT) signaling pathway and the sonic hedgehog (SHH) pathway are the most clinically relevant. Pathology consultation at an academic center should be considered (Grade 1C Recommendation, Level I/II Evidence).
3. Genetic counseling and/or testing should be obtained if possible (Grade 1C Recommendation, Level I/II Evidence).
   a. Although mutation in the wingless Wnt signaling pathway has been identified in up to 15% of sporadic medulloblastomas, it is the defining feature in the rare genetic disorder known as Turcot syndrome (glioma-colonic polyposis syndrome).
   b. Although only 3 to 5% of patients with mutations of the patched-1 (PTCH1) signaling pathway develop medulloblastomas, usually the desmoplastic variant, it is the defining feature of the rare autosomal dominant genetic disorder known as Gorlin syndrome (basal cell nevus syndrome). Gorlin syndrome, due to germline mutations in the *PTCH1* gene on chromosome 9, encodes for a transmembrane protein that binds the sonic hedgehog (SHH) family of signaling proteins.

Table 22.3 Modified Chang criteria[18]

T	Tumor < 3 cm in diameter and limited to the classic position in the vermis, roof of the fourth ventricle, or cerebellar hemisphere
T2	Tumor ≥ 3 cm in diameter and further invading one adjacent structure or partially filling the fourth ventricle
T3a	Tumor further invading two adjacent structures or completely filling the fourth ventricle, with extensions into the aqueduct or foramina of Magendie or Luschka—with marked internal hydrocephalus
T3b	Tumor arising from the floor of the fourth ventricle or brainstem and filling the fourth ventricle
T4	Tumor penetrates the aqueduct to involve the third ventricle or midbrain or extends to the cervical cord
M0	No metastases
M1	Microscopic evidence of tumor cells in the cerebrospinal fluid
M2	Macroscopic metastases in the cerebellar and/or cerebral subarachnoid space and/or the supratentorial ventricular system
M3	Macroscopic metastases to the spinal subarachnoidal space
M4	Metastases outside the central nervous system

However, it is important to highlight that medulloblastomas are often missed on CT scans. Contrast-enhanced magnetic resonance imaging (MRI) of the entire neuroaxis (also termed cranial-spinal axis; e.g., brain and complete spine) are required for adequate prediction, neurosurgical planning, and determination of the extent of disease. MRI's limitations include less availability and more cumbersome times/techniques, which commonly require sedation. A heterogeneous contrast-enhancing tumor, often with areas of necrosis, hemorrhage, or cysts, is most common. However, it is important to highlight that the desmoplastic variant in adults may lack contrast enhancement. Metastases to the ventricles and leptomeninges commonly appear as enhancing nodules or linear patterns. Metastases to the bone marrow and systemic organs are sufficiently uncommon at presentation that initial systemic staging is not needed. Across series, systemic metastases occur an average of 16 months after presentation and most commonly occur in conjunction with active CNS disease.[19] Optimal timing of radiographic staging is pre-LP and preoperative, given that postprocedure blood products and other changes can mimic metastases. If preoperative imaging is not feasible, it should be postponed ~ 14 days to allow postprocedure blood products and other changes to minimize. However, it is important to highlight that postoperative imaging is important for estimating extent of resection (EoR) as well as estimating postop sequelae, such as ischemia. Relatedly, it is important to highlight the role of dedicated neuroradiologists, neuropathologists, and multidisciplinary tumor boards in optimal staging.

Cytological staging, via LP, is also important. A cluster of coarsely granulated, chromatin-rich, scant cytoplasm cells, morphologically reminiscent of lymphocytes/-blasts, and distinguished with immunohistochemistry markers, is most common. Optimal timing of cytological staging is less defined, with signs of elevated ICP, urgency of resection, degree of suspicion of medulloblastoma, and so forth, as factors. The relevance of a "positive" CSF cytology in samples obtained within the first ~ 7 to 10 days of diagnosis is undefined. The relevance of "positive" CSF cells collected at the time of resection is also undefined.[20,21] If preoperative cytology is not feasible, it should be postponed ~ 14 to 21 days to allow postprocedure blood products and other changes to minimize. Positive cells collected > 14 to 21 days postprocedure strongly correlate with increased relapse and inferior outcome. For example, in a Swiss series, 70% of patients with CSF-positive staging relapsed, as opposed to 40% of those without.[22] Regardless of timing, an advanced stage can be missed with CSF sampling.

Over all, optimal staging is more obtainable when radiographic and cytological staging are combined. For example, Terterov et al[23] retrospectively studied 150 resected patients staged by both MRI and cytology, in which 7 of 40 (18%) were discordant. It is important to highlight that perioperative MRI correlated with survival, whereas perioperative CSF cytology, regardless of whether obtained from LP or intracranially, did not.[23] Numerous similar studies exist.[20] Thus, combining staging techniques should be the goal whenever possible.

■ Prognostic Factors

Historically (defined as prior to the incorporation of molecular pathology), the most important prognostic factors, aside from the histological variant, have been clinical and radiographic, specifically—*age* and *extent of disease* at presentation.

Younger age correlates with inferior outcome, with patients < 3 to 5 years old affected the most. For example, Zeltzer et al reported on a large prospective study of 188 patients who were randomized between contemporary combined-modality therapies. Regardless of treatment arm, 5-PFS was ~ 30% in the group < 3 years old, as opposed to ~ 50% in the group ≥ 3 years old.[21] This trend appears to hold true for older children. For example, Tabori et al reported a study of patients aged 10 to 20 years whose 5-PFS was 70%.[24] Numerous studies duplicate these trends. It is important to highlight that superior outcome often occurs at the price of inferior quality of life, as discussed in the "Deleterious Sequelae of Treatment" section later in the chapter.

Greater extent of disease at presentation, which incorporates both T and M stage, also strongly correlates with inferior outcome. Across series, the impact of presenting M stage is clearly defined. For example, in the same study referenced earlier, Zeltzer et al reported 5-year PFS was 70% for M0, 57% for M1, and 40% for M2 to M4 disease.[21] Similar results are noted in other studies. It is important to highlight that the relative impact of T stage on outcome, as opposed to EoR, is undefined. For example, across series, it appears that both prognostic factors may have a similar impact.[25,26] Their relative effects in the infant population have been of particular interest to researchers and are further discussed in the section "Initial Therapy at Presentation." Given that the relative impacts of presenting T stage and EoR remain undefined, patients are recommended to receive care within academic centers, where state-of-the-art results can be incorporated into each patient's therapy plan, and where outcomes can be incorporated into the international body of literature.

■ Risk Stratification

Historically (defined as prior to the incorporation of molecular pathology), clinical and radiographic factors classified patients into one of two risk groups: *standard-risk* (also termed average-risk) medulloblastoma, defined by nonmetastatic disease treated by total or subtotal tumor resection with < 1.5 cm^3, and *high-risk* medulloblastoma, defined as disseminated disease at presentation and/or > 1.5 cm^3 postoperative residual disease. Across studies, these classifications strongly correlated with outcome and thus became risk-adjusted groups used to design and stratify subsequent international studies.[4,5] Since the incorporation of molecular pathology, a much more complex risk-stratification algorithm is evolving, promising to more powerfully contribute to the design and stratification of advanced adjuvant therapies as well as to correlate even more with outcome. However, it is also important to highlight that, during this transitional decade, it remains undefined how to incorporate or analyze the results of studies—especially when they are so divergent. Thus, for reasons already discussed, patients are recommended to receive care within academic centers and studies.

Evidence-Based Risk Stratification

Level I and Level II Evidence

Histopathological, clinical, and radiographic factors classify patients into one of two risk groups, known as the modified Chang criteria:

- Standard-risk (also termed average-risk) medulloblastoma, defined by nonmetastatic disease treated by total or subtotal tumor resection with < 1.5 cm^3
- High-risk medulloblastoma, defined as disseminated disease at presentation and/or > 1.5 cm^3 postoperative residual disease

Across studies, the modified Chang criteria classifications strongly correlated with outcome and thus became risk-adjusted groups used to design and stratify subsequent international studies.

Level I and Level II Evidence

The addition of molecular pathological diagnosis to the risk stratification of patients is proving to be an extremely powerful tool.

Recommendation for Risk Stratification

In all cases, timely and accurate diagnosis, staging, and risk stratification should be sought because they each independently correlate with outcome. Referral to an academic center should be considered as needed (Grade 1C+ Recommendation, Level I–III Evidence).

■ Initial Treatment at Presentation

Defining the goals of care, including symptom-directed and tumor-directed goals, is essential. Resection, radiation, and chemotherapy are the tools for achieving these goals of care. Optimizing adjuvant therapy requires an adequate understanding of each of the goals and tools. It is important to highlight that the optimal application of these tools remains undefined and is, thus, the emphasis of the remainder of this chapter.

The goals of initial management are largely symptom directed, including airway protection, steroids, antiemetics, pain medications, and management of obstructive hydrocephalus by either a ventriculoperitoneal (VP) shunt (CSF diversion) or endoscopic third ventriculostomy (ETV).

The goals of resection include relieving obstructive hydrocephalus, acquiring tissue for diagnosis, and maximal safe resection (MSR). Historically, a biopsy-only strategy has been clearly defined as strongly correlated with inferior outcome. For example, in the 1930s, Cushing reported a study where 3-year OS was only 1.6%.[27] Since then, the current standard of care is to attempt an MSR. A closely related term, gross total resection (GTR), is currently defined as resection of ≥ 90% of the visible tumor mass and with the least deleterious sequelae. Across studies, this can be achieved in at least 80% of patients and strongly correlates with superior outcome.[26] For example, in two studies comparing GTR/MSR to biopsy only, 5-year actuarial survival rates were mid-70% versus 40%, and local posterior fossa control rates were mid-80% versus mid-20%, respectively.[28,29] Although, across studies, it is clearly defined that biopsy-only strongly correlates with inferior outcome in patients without disseminated disease at presentation, it is important to highlight that the impact of the exact extent of aggressive resection (e.g., beyond 80 to 90%) remains undefined.[26] And, relatedly, the relative impact of T stage (extent of disease, nondisseminated [M0]), as opposed to EoR, remains undefined.

Evidence-Based Surgery as Initial Treatment

Level I Evidence

There are no randomized studies of GTR versus subtotal resection or biopsy.

Level II Evidence

GTR is superior to subtotal resection and is widely considered a very important mainstay of initial treatment.

However, these undefined issues cannot be optimized without also attending to several important realities. First, results of studies to date have not benefited from recent perioperative advances, including preoperative stabilization, intraoperative microscopically assisted miscodissection techniques, intraoperative imaging and frozen-section analysis, intraoperative neuroanesthesia monitoring, and postoperative neurocritical care. Second, results of studies to date have not benefited from recent adjuvant therapy advances, such as small-molecule targeted therapies. Third, studies to date, regardless of attempted resection, do not adequately address the profound impact that postoperative sequelae have on the selection, tolerance, and efficacy of adjuvant therapy. For example, postoperative mutism (also termed cerebellar mutism [syndrome] or posterior fossa syndrome), hypothesized to be from bilateral dentatothalamocortical pathway damage, occurs in 5 to 30% of patients undergoing resection of large midline cerebellar masses. Across studies, mutism commonly occurs suddenly, usually within 1 to several days, and may be associated with cerebellar, lower cranial nerve, or brainstem dysfunction (ataxia; emotional lability; inattention and other cognitive dysfunctions; difficulty initiating movement; difficulty producing speech and other language/communication dysfunctions; dysphagia, facial palsy and other cranial nerve dysfunctions; hypotonia; pyramidal tract signs). Commonly, recovery takes many months and is incomplete.[30] To date, the presence of brainstem invasion and associated aggressiveness at attempted resection are two of the factors most strongly correlated with both the occurrence and the severity of postoperative mutism. Relatedly, lateral cerebellar hemispheric location correlates oppositely.[30] Therefore, a balance of these issues is required and, for reasons already discussed, patients are recommended to receive care within academic centers and studies.

Recommendations for Surgical Management

1. Presentation usually requires urgent and/or emergent management. Acute hydrocephalus is common and requires emergent neurosurgical consultation. Comprehensive medical management is also essential at presentation (Grade 1C+ Recommendation, Level II/III Evidence).
2. In all cases, attempt GTR over either subtotal resection or biopsy if it can be performed with reasonable expected morbidity.
3. Extent of resection documenting < 1.5 cm^3 residual visible disease, or > 90% resected, strongly correlates with an increased overall survival. Referral to an academic medical center should be considered (Grade 1C+ Recommendation, Level I/II Evidence).
4. The relative importance of initial modified Chang T stage versus extent of resection is yet unknown (Grade 1C Recommendation, Level III Evidence).
5. Postoperative sequelae, which can be profound, affect the selection and timing of adjuvant therapy (Grade 1C+ Recommendation, Level II/III Evidence).
6. In cases where GTR is felt to be of prohibitively high risk, adjuvant treatment improves outcome (Grade 1C+ Recommendation, Level I–III Evidence).

■ Adjuvant Therapy—with and without Neuroaxis Seeding at Presentation

Patient, tumor, and initial therapy factors that lead up to adjuvant therapy profoundly impact the application of radiotherapy (RT) and chemotherapy. It is important to highlight that adjuvant therapy has evolved in conjunction with technological and methodological advances—directly resulting from rigorous studies conducted across Europe and the United States over the last 40 years. For example, across studies of children > 3 years old, the combination of RT and chemotherapy with MSR has strongly correlated with improved outcomes. Generalized 5-year OS rates currently range in the 70 to high-80% for standard-risk patients and range in the 50 to mid-70% for high-risk patients.[31] It is important to highlight that much less is known about the outcomes of several patient populations, specifically infants, adults, and patients with certain molecular pathology markers. Given that it remains undefined how to optimally treat these specific populations, individualization is needed. For reasons already discussed, such patients are recommended to receive care within academic centers whenever possible. Despite these undefined issues, the best available evidence is summarized here.

Adjuvant Radiotherapy

The goals of RT include treating residual visible tumor as well as treating microscopic disease throughout the neuroaxis (also termed the craniospinal [CS] axis). From here forward, *RT* refers to complete neuroaxis RT (also termed CSRT or CS irradiation [CSI]), unless otherwise specified. Techniques of RT include use of external beam, fractionation, and, recently, intensity-modulated RT (IMRT). Timing of RT incorporates time for adequate surgical recovery and most commonly occurs within 3 to 4 weeks after surgery. For example, Abacioglu et al reported a large retrospective review of patients > 16 years old who received RT-containing regimens. The median time interval between resection and RT was 31 days (range 12 to 69). Optimal timing for RT remains undefined and will likely always require patient individualization. With that said, several studies to date appear to correlate the time interval between resection and RT as a prognostic factor; therefore, timing is the focus of ongoing studies.[32] Distribution of RT includes the entire craniospinal axis, followed by a boost to either the tumor bed (or residual visualized tumor) or the entire posterior fossa. This is based on numerous studies reporting distribution of disease at presentation and recurrence/progression. Across studies, it is clear that higher doses of RT correlate with both superior tumor control as well as toxicity, the latter especially in those < 3 to 5 years old. Recent studies attempting to maintain or improve outcome while simultaneously minimizing toxicity through the alteration of RT dose, distribution, and other techniques are discussed in the following sections.

Adjuvant Chemotherapy

The goal of chemotherapy depends on, to a large extent, whether it uses traditional cytotoxic or small-molecule targeted agents. The goals of cytotoxic chemotherapy include radiosensitization, treating microscopic disease throughout the neuroaxis, primarily treating bulky disease not amenable to resection or RT, and attempting to minimize the sequelae of RT via minimizing, delaying, or avoiding RT. The goals of small-molecule agents are yet to be defined but will likely include adjuvant therapy that augments cytotoxic chemotherapy, maintenance therapy that minimizes the risk of recurrence/progression, and even possibly preventive therapy that minimizes the presentation of medulloblastoma in those at high risk, such as patients with Gorlin and Turcot syndromes.

Techniques include intravenous (IV) and oral agents administered in various regimens. Cytotoxic agents are most commonly administered intermittently, via IV or oral routes, and include cisplatin, vincristine, cyclophosphamide, methotrexate, and platinums. Small-molecule targeted agents are commonly administered continuously and orally and include agents yet to be discussed here. Similar to RT, across studies, it is clear that higher doses correlate with superior tumor control as well as toxicity, the latter especially in those < 3 to 5 years old. Recent studies attempting to maintain or improve outcome while simultaneously maintaining or minimizing toxicity are discussed in the following sections.

Timing of chemotherapy is variable and depends on the goal. Cytotoxic chemotherapy is most commonly given after RT and variably during RT. Small-molecule targeted therapy timing is also variable and under active investigation.

Across studies, although randomized studies do not uniformly demonstrate a statistically significant superior outcome, subset analyses have suggested that chemotherapy does improve outcomes in some patients.[33,34] It is important to highlight the nontrivial elevated risk of secondary malignancies, occurring both within and outside the CNS, in patients who have received intensive cytotoxic chemotherapy, especially younger children. Similar risk elevations occur in patients who receive intensive RT. However, the risk is undefined in those who have received small-molecule targeted therapy.

To date the optimal application of adjuvant RT and chemotherapy is best discussed within the context of historical risk-stratification groups and within the context of pivotal prospective trials conducted over the last 4 decades. When applying best-evidence therapies to a specific patient, the various undefined areas and the resultant limitations in our evidence (discussed in the preceding sections) must be attended to. Prior to discussing the best evidence regarding specific patient populations, a review of the evidence-based principles of adjuvant therapy is worthwhile.

Evidence-Based Principles of Adjuvant Therapy

Level I and Level II Evidence

Craniospinal irradiation, followed by a boost to either the tumor bed (or residual visualized tumor) or the entire posterior fossa, correlates with improved tumor control, delayed progression, and in most cases, superior outcome.

The term *chemotherapy* may refer either to traditional cytotoxic or to small-molecule targeted agents. Modern chemotherapy agents correlate to improved tumor control, delayed progression, and in most cases, superior outcome.

Intensity and distribution of RT correlate with both superior tumor control and toxicity, the latter especially in children < 3 to 5 years old.

Intensity and duration of chemotherapy regimens correlate with superior tumor control as well as toxicity, the latter at extremes of age.

The onset of toxicities ranges from acute to delayed. The toxicity profile is impacted by host (e.g., age, comorbidities) and treatment (e.g., regimen specifics) factors. The management is palliative (symptom directed).

It is clear that combination adjuvant therapy provides select patients an improved outcome. Currently, modified Chang criteria for risk stratification provide the basis for algorithms for optimal application of adjuvant RT and chemotherapy. However, molecular pathological results are rapidly being incorporated into decision making. Both modified Chang criteria and molecular pathological results correlate with outcome.

Large, prospective consortium studies performed across Europe and the United States over the past 40 years formed the basis of the current algorithm for optimal application of adjuvant RT and chemotherapy. Individualization is necessary, and patients not clearly fitting into these categories are especially encouraged to consider referral to an academic center for investigational study.

Specific Patient Populations

Infants and young children < 3 years old are the first risk groups discussed because the studies designed to address adjuvant therapy in this group have resulted in many of the "best" evidence-based paradigms subsequently applied to other risk groups.

Children < 3 Years Old, Standard-Risk Patients

When the population of children < 3 years old is discussed within the context of medulloblastoma adjuvant therapy, it is important to highlight the overlapping definitions of the term *infant* to describe the youngest patients within this special population. It is clear that intensity of adjuvant RT, whether via dose, fractionation, distribution, or the like, is strongly correlated with both tumor control and deleterious sequelae. Thus, historically, application of the term *infant* has ranged from the classic pediatric definition of patients < 24 months old without the acquisition of speech to the neuro-oncology definition of patients < 36 months (to up to < 5 to 10 years old) at higher risk for neurocognitive sequelae with RT. Over the last 4 decades, numerous infant (also termed baby brain) studies have been designed to test contemporary attempts to minimize RT's toxicity to the maturing brain. Such attempts have included various combinations of systemic chemotherapies, intrathecal chemotherapy, and high-dose myeloablative chemotherapy followed by autologous stem cell rescue to minimize, delay, or avoid adjuvant RT. These studies have also profoundly affected the current prognostic factors, risk stratification groups, and, more recently, importance of molecular pathology results, on outcomes and sequelae.

It is important to highlight the difficulty in determining the relative impacts of various RT and chemotherapy regimens within a combined modality strategy. Furthermore, it is important to highlight the difficulty in comparing diverse trials across time. Lastly, it is important to note that many studies reporting on this special population incorporated malignant CNS tumors of multiple histologies, including medulloblastomas, gliomas, and ependymomas. Therefore, for reasons already discussed, patients are recommended to receive care within academic centers and studies.

Conventional Chemotherapy-Only Regimens

Examples of conventional chemotherapy-only regimens include a study initially reported by van Eys et al and later updated by Ater et al in which patients with malignant brain tumors, including medulloblastoma, received a chemo-only regimen and demonstrated superior survival compared with resection alone. Results also demonstrated reasonable comparability to many of the contemporary RT-alone studies.[35,36]

In a French series of 79 children younger than 5 years, patients were treated with a four-drug combination chemotherapy regimen that did not include methotrexate. RT was given only if relapse occurred. Among the 47 patients who had a GTR, 14 were alive in their first complete remission, including 13 who had not received RT. In contrast, among the 32 children with either residual disease following surgery or metastases, only two were alive in their first complete remission without having received RT.[37]

Early, Extended-Duration Conventional Chemotherapy Regimens

Examples of an early, extended-duration conventional chemotherapy regimen, followed by delayed RT, include a multicenter study reported by Duffner et al on behalf of the Pediatric Oncology Group (POG), in which patients < 36 months old with malignant brain tumors, including medulloblastoma, received varying combinations of age-based, multiagent, extended-duration chemotherapy, followed by a delay of RT until they were at least 3 years old. The 5-PFS was 30% and the OS was 39.4%. Importantly, a portion of the long-term survivors were patients whose parents declined RT completely.[38] In another example, Geyer et al reported a multicenter study, on behalf of the Children's Cancer Group (CCG), in which patients with advanced stage, unresectable medulloblastomas received one of two different chemotherapy combinations, either an "intensive regimen" called 8 in 1 (eight chemotherapies in 1 day) both before and after RT, or a "standard regimen" called VCP (vincristine, CCNU, and prednisone) following RT. Interestingly, the standard regimen correlated with superior outcome, with a 5-PFS of 63%, as opposed to 45% in the 8 in 1 group.[21] These and numerous other studies demonstrated at least comparability to many of the contemporary "upfront" RT regimens.

Dose-Intensified Chemotherapy Regimens with RT Deferred until Recurrence/Progression

Examples of dose-intensified chemotherapy regimens with RT deferred until recurrence/progression include a multicenter study reported by Geyer et al, on behalf of Children's Cancer Group (CCG 9921), in which patients < 5 years old received a multiagent chemotherapy regimen, not including methotrexate, for ≥ 16 months, regardless of presenting stage and resection status. However, patients were analyzed in one of three predetermined categories: R0M0 (no residual disease, no metastasis), R1M0 (radiological residual disease alone), and RXM+ (presence of metastases). For R0M0 patients, the primary end point was 5-year OS (5-OS) and the secondary end point was 5-PFS. For R1M0 or RXM+ patients, the primary end point was best radiological response and the secondary end points were 5-OS and 5-PFS. Four of 17 R1M0 patients and, remarkably, two of 15 RXM+ patients had a complete radiological response. The 5-PFS was 29% for R0M0 patients, 6% for R1M0 patients, and 13% for RXM+ patients. The 5-OS was 73% for R0M0 patients, 41% for R1M0 patients, and 13% for RXM+ patients. Interestingly, the 5-PFS was 41% for the R0M0 patients who underwent GTR as opposed to 0% for the R0M0 patients who underwent subtotal resection. These overall study results demonstrated at least comparability, in both 5-PFS and OS, to OS in contemporary "routine" RT studies. Importantly, 58% of the long-term survivors (OS > 5 years) were patients who never received RT. If these patients recurred/progressed, they received myeloablative chemotherapy followed by autologous stem cell transplant.[39] Collectively, these and numerous other studies demonstrated at least comparability to many of the contemporary regimens focusing on RT as the curative tool. Furthermore, this study demonstrated that conventional chemotherapy-alone regimens can be curative in patients without metastasis at presentation and who undergo a GTR, yet are insufficient for patients with metastasis and less than GTR.

In another example of a dose-intensified chemotherapy regimen with deferred RT until recurrence/progression, Rutkowski et al reported a multicenter study on behalf of the German Society of Pediatric Oncology and Hematology (GPOH), in which predominantly patients < 36 months old received the addition of up to 36 doses of intrathecal methotrexate chemotherapy (2 mg each) to an intensive (5 g/m^2) methotrexate-based chemotherapy regimen, which ended if patients achieved complete remission within 6 months. Patients experiencing subsequent recurrence/progression received repeat resection, RT, or investigational therapies. The patients were analyzed in three predetermined groups after resection: those with complete resection and without metastases, those with residual disease and without metastases, and those with macroscopic metastatic disease (M2 and M3) regardless of initial resection status. For the M0/GTR group, the PFS was 82% and the OS was 93%. For the M2 group, the PFS was 50% and the OS was 56%. For the M3 group, the PFS was 33% and the OS was 38%. Similar to the previous example, the overall study results demonstrated comparability, and in many ways, favorability over contemporary "routine" RT studies, especially in very young patients without metastasis at presentation. Furthermore, this study demonstrated two important paradigms: first, that the duration of chemotherapy could successfully be shortened; second, that methotrexate-containing regimens (with methotrexate being a known neurotoxin), were similar to contemporary nonmethotrexate regimens in terms of outcome and sequelae. To generalize greatly, patients receiving methotrexate subsequently scored significantly lower than healthy children of the same age, yet significantly higher than comparable patients from other studies having received upfront RT as part of their adjuvant therapy regimen.[40]

In another example of dose-intensified chemotherapy regimen with deferred RT until recurrence/progression, Mason et al reported a "Head Start" regimen involving numerous cycles of multiagent "induction" chemotherapy, repeat resection for residual disease (if needed), and "consolidation" myeloablative chemotherapy followed by autologous stem cell rescue. The 5-OS for all patients < 3 years old was 52%. Importantly, 71% of the long-term survivors never received RT. However, it is also important to highlight the extreme sequela of 19% mortality. As expected, this became a dominant area for improvement in subsequent international studies.[41,42]

In a last example, Grundy et al, on behalf of the Children's Cancer and Leukemia Group, reported a multicenter study in which children < 3 years old with malignant brain tumors, including medulloblastoma, received MSR followed by multiagent chemotherapy every 14 days for up to 1 year. RT was deferred until recurrence/progression. Importantly, 89% of the medulloblastoma patients had residual postoperative disease and/or metastasis at presentation. In these high-risk patients, outcome correlated to histology, with a 5-OS of 53% for the desmoplastic variant as opposed to 33% for the classic variant. The 5-year PFS was 35% and 33%, respectively. Importantly, superior outcome correlated to the desmoplastic variant, despite having a heavier burden of deleterious prognostic factors, specifically metastatic disease and subtotal resection. Of the large-cell/anaplastic variant, 100% died within 2 years of presentation, regardless of therapy. Overall study results, including multiple histologies, did not demonstrate a correlation of outcome with intensified-dose chemotherapy, yet no generalizations can be made to medulloblastoma.[43]

High-Risk Patients < 3 Years Old

Optimal adjuvant therapy for patients with presenting metastatic disease and/or subtotal resections remains undefined. Subset analyses of this special subpopulation are found within the previous section's studies. Given these realities, for reasons already discussed, patients are recommended to receive care within academic centers and studies.

Standard-Risk Patients > 3 Years Old

When the population of patients > 3 years old is discussed within the context of medulloblastoma adjuvant therapy, it is important to highlight that studies over the last 4 decades have variably included patients ranging from 3 years old to the mid-20s. As expected, it is clear that intensity of adjuvant RT, whether via dose, fractionation, distribution, or other factors, is strongly correlated with both tumor control and deleterious sequelae. Importantly, the sequelae in this special population are distinct from those of younger patients, ranging from unique organ toxicities to social and emotional dysfunction. Over the last 4 decades, numerous studies have been designed to test contemporary attempts to minimize the sequelae. Such attempts have included various combinations of systemic chemotherapies, intrathecal chemotherapy, and high-dose myeloablative chemotherapy followed by autologous stem cell rescue to minimize, delay, or avoid adjuvant RT. These studies have also profoundly affected the current prognostic factors, risk stratification groups, and, more recently, importance of molecular pathology results, on outcomes and sequelae.

The current U.S. standard of care includes reduced-dose RT (defined as compared with historical regimens) in combination with multiagent chemotherapy. Packer et al, on behalf of the Children's Oncology Group, reported a study wherein, after maximal safe resection, standard-risk patients (< 1.5 cm^2 residual disease and M0 by MRI/CSF) received 23.4 Gy to the craniospinal axis, with a posterior fossa boost of 32.4 Gy, to a total dose of 55.8 Gy to the tumor bed, along with weekly vincristine. This was followed by randomization to one of two chemotherapy regimens for eight cycles of multiagent chemotherapy (vincristine, cisplatin, plus CCNU, or vincristine, cisplatin, plus cyclophosphamide). At a median follow-up of > 5 years, the 5-PFS was 81% and the 5-OS was 86%. No significant differences were reported between the two chemotherapy regimens.[44] It is important to highlight several outcomes of this trial that established new paradigms for this population. First, this study demonstrated that improved outcomes were achievable with the addition of conventional chemotherapy to RT, as opposed to RT-alone, even more intensive RT regimens. Second, this study demonstrated at least comparable outcomes, as well as comparable deleterious sequelae, to many of the contemporary studies using more intensive chemo regimens.

High-Risk Patients > 3 Years Old

Optimal adjuvant therapy for patients with presenting metastatic disease and/or subtotal resections remains undefined. Subset analyses of this special subpopulation are found within the previous section's studies. Given these realities, for reasons already discussed, patients are recommended to receive care within academic centers and studies. With that said, studies to date demonstrate trends suggesting the possibility of comparable to superior outcomes with intensified-dose and/or durations of multiagent chemotherapy regimens. Some studies suggest similar results for intensified RT localized to visible disease.[45]

Adult Standard-Risk Patients

When the adult population is discussed within the context of medulloblastoma adjuvant therapy, it is important to highlight that studies over the last 4 decades have variably included patients ranging from age 18 years to, albeit less commonly, the mid-40s. Medulloblastoma are much less common in this age group; thus the paradigms for initial therapy and adjuvant therapy are modeled after the younger populations. Importantly, in addition to their rarity, adults have a unique presentation that profoundly impacts their adjuvant therapy, including laterally located tumors, greater likelihood of a desmoplastic variant (over large-cell/anaplastic cell variants), more dissemination at presentation, and more likelihood to have delayed recurrence/progressions. Regarding the latter, it is important to highlight that patients with a good response to adjuvant therapy require close follow-up for the remainder of their lifetime.[7,46] In another example, Abacioglu et al reported a retrospective review of patients > 16 years old (median 27), who received RT-containing regimens. After a follow-up of > 8 years, of those who relapsed/progressed, > 50% occurred after 2 years and 17% after 5 years.[32] Other examples are also discussed in this chapter.

Also importantly, the sequelae in this special population are distinct from those of the "< 3 years old and > 3 years old" patients, ranging from unique comorbid toxicities to educational and work dysfunction. Over the last 4 decades, numerous studies have been designed to test strategies designed to minimize the sequelae.[8,32,47] As expected, it is clear that intensity of adjuvant RT, whether via dose, fractionation, distribution, or other factors, strongly correlates with both tumor control and deleterious sequelae.

Optimal adjuvant therapy in adults is undefined. Therefore, for reasons already discussed, patients are recommended receive care within academic centers and studies. With that said, studies to date demonstrate trends suggesting the possibility of comparable to superior outcomes with combined-modality therapy regimens, including the possibility of long-term survival in subpopulations. To date, this regimen has demonstrated clear superiority.[32,46,47] For example, Riffaud et al reported a study in which patients > 16 years old (median age of 20), of various risk stratifications and histological variants, received RT. Of note, some had also received chemotherapy before RT. The 5-PFS was 72% and the 10-PFS was 57%. The 5-OS was 81% and the 10-OS was 62%. Reinforcing the age-specific trend for delayed recurrence/progression, the median time to recurrence was 4.2 years, and in those, the median PFS was 17.9 years and the median OS was 17.7 years. Multivariate analysis identified gender, precipitousness of symptom progression leading to diagnosis, and presenting M stage as independent prognostic factors for OS and PFS.[47]

In another example, Brandes et al reported a study in which patients > 18 years old received treatment based on risk stratification. Standard-risk patients (no postoperative residual disease) received RT to 36 Gy, followed by an RT boost to the tumor site of 18.8 Gy, for a total of 54.8 Gy. High-risk patients (residual disease or disseminated metastases at presentation) received two cycles of pre-RT multiagent chemotherapy, including cisplatin, etoposide, and cyclophosphamide, followed by the foregoing RT regimen. For standard-risk patients, the 10-PFS was 46% and the 10-OS was 65%. For high-risk patients, the 10-PFS was 36% and the 10-OS was 45%. It is important to highlight that, although this is one of the most robust prospective studies within this age-specific subpopulation, the resultant accrual time period of > 20 years introduced unintended variations in therapy technologies.[48]

In another example, Greenberg et al reported a retrospective multicenter study in which patients > 17 years old received maximal safe resection, followed by RT, and then followed by one of two multiagent chemotherapy regimens originally designed for younger children. Specifically, the regimens used were either the Children's Oncology Group (COG) or Packer protocol, which includes RT with weekly vincristine followed by eight cycles of cisplatin, lomustine, and vincristine, or the Pediatric Oncology Group (POG) protocol, which includes alternating cycles of cisplatin/etoposide and cyclophosphamide/vincristine doublets, then followed by RT. The median PFS was 26 months for the Packer protocol, as opposed to 48 months for the POG protocol. The median OS was 36 months, as opposed to 57 months for the POG protocol. It is important to highlight that, given the small sample size, statistically significant differences in PFS and OS were unobtainable. With that said, adult patients on the Packer protocol appeared to have inferior outcomes and higher toxicity than the adults on the POG protocol as well as the children receiving these protocols (albeit acknowledging the inherent limitations in cross-study analyses).[49] In a last example, Lai reported a large Surveillance, Epidemiology, and End Results (SEER) database study demonstrating outcomes generally comparable to the foregoing studies.[50]

Recommendations for Adjuvant Therapy

1. For standard-risk patients < 3 years old, a chemotherapy-alone approach is considered the mainstay of adjuvant treatment. The addition of multiagent chemotherapy to resection has strongly correlated with improved tumor control, delayed progression, and, in many cases, improved outcome. The optimal regimen and duration of chemotherapy are unknown and are thus the subject of ongoing investigation. Because of devastating toxicity to the developing brain, cranial-spinal irradiation is traditionally delayed until either recurrence/progression or the patient is ≥ 3 years old. It is important to note that "< 3 years old" requires individualization, and often patients ≥ 5 years old are treated under this paradigm (Grade 1C+ Recommendation, Level I/II Evidence).
2. For high-risk patients (i.e., patients presenting with metastatic disease and/or subtotal resections) < 3 years old, the optimal adjuvant therapy is unknown. Subset analyses of this special subpopulation can often be found within other studies and thus used for extrapolation. Whenever possible, patients should be referred to academic medical centers and enrolled in investigational studies (Grade 2B Recommendation, Level III/IV Evidence).
3. For standard-risk patients > 3 years old, the addition of RT and multiagent chemotherapy to MSR has strongly correlated with improved outcomes. This is the mainstay of initial treatment (Grade 1C+ Recommendation, Level I/II Evidence).
   a. Based on numerous studies reporting distribution of disease at presentation and recurrence/progression. Distribution of RT includes the entire craniospinal axis.
   b. Irradiation (CSI), followed by a boost to either the tumor bed (or residual visualized tumor) or the entire posterior fossa
   c. The timing of radiation (cranial-spinal irradiation) incorporates time for adequate surgical recovery and most commonly occurs within 3 to 4 weeks.
   d. The current U.S. standard of care includes postoperative "reduced-dose" RT in combination with multiagent chemotherapy—the Packer protocol. Standard-risk patients (< 1.5 cm^2 residual disease and M0) receive 23.4 Gy to the craniospinal axis, with a posterior fossa boost of 32.4 Gy, to a total dose of 55.8 Gy to the tumor bed, along with weekly vincristine. This was followed by randomization to one of two chemotherapy regimens for eight cycles of multiagent chemotherapy (vincristine, cisplatin, plus CCNU, or vincristine, cisplatin, plus cyclophosphamide). The addition of multiagent chemotherapy strongly correlated with prolonged PFS as well as superior survival.
4. For high-risk patients (i.e., patients presenting with metastatic disease and/or subtotal resections) > 3 years old, the optimal adjuvant therapy is unknown. Subset analyses of this special subpopulation can often be found within other studies and thus used for extrapolation. Whenever possible, patients should be referred to academic medical centers and enrolled in investigational studies (Grade 2B Recommendation, Level III/IV Evidence).

■ Small-Molecule Targeted Therapy

Despite a relentless, scientifically rigorous, international effort, medulloblastomas are not routinely cured with combined modality therapy. Historically, basic and clinical-translational studies have implicated inherent invasiveness, tumor and native CNS stem cells, clinicoradiographic details, toxicity ceilings of contemporary therapies, and many other variables as potential factors affecting outcome. More recently, advances in molecular pathology have profoundly broadened the potential influences. To date, molecular pathological factors have demonstrated their impact on timely/accurate diagnoses, risk-stratification, prognostic factors, design of therapies, risk-adjusted stratification of therapies across populations, and more robust analyses of study data.[14] For example, atypical teratoid/rhabdoid tumor was delineated as an embryonal tumor with poor prognosis and linked with mutations of the *INI1/SNF5* gene.[14]

Given their unique and diverse mechanisms, it is clear that the goals of small-molecule targeted agents are distinct from those of cytotoxic chemotherapy. Numerous agents are currently under investigation for their potential to provide superior outcomes with less deleterious sequelae. Optimal agents and their therapeutic applications remain undefined. Given these realities, and for reasons already discussed, patients are recommended to receive care within academic centers and studies. With that said, agents targeting some of the most well-defined molecular-genetic aberrations, as summarized in a recent review by Rossi et al are discussed here.[31]

Evidence-Based Use of Small-Molecule Targeted Agents as Adjuvant Therapy

Level I and Level II Evidence

There are currently no randomized studies of cytotoxic chemotherapies versus small-molecule targeted therapies nor of combinations of small-molecule targeted agents.

Level III and Level IV Evidence

There is strong circumstantial evidence that small-molecule targeted therapies may soon become a mainstay of initial therapy, yet the details and timing remain unclear.

Examples of agents targeting the SHH pathway include cyclopamine and HhAntag. Cyclopamine is a plant-derived teratogen that selectively targets SHH-dependent gene expression and, eventually the initiation of neuronal differentiation and/or loss of neuronal stem cell–like characteristics in medulloblastoma cells. HhAntag, another inhibitor of the SHH pathway, is undergoing preclinical studies. Examples of drugs capable of reducing invasiveness include inhibitors of receptor tyrosine kinases. More specifically, dual-specific inhibitors of ERBB1 or ERBB2 activity, such as OSI-774, regulate other factors and ultimately reduce invasiveness of medulloblastomas in vitro and in vivo. Numerous inhibitors of ERBB1 or ERBB2 activity are undergoing both preclinical and clinical studies, including many within U.S. consortia. Examples of drugs targeting the deleterious activation of Wnt signaling, given its role in tumorigenesis, include the Wnt signaling antagonists Dkk-3 and FRPs. Agents inhibiting neural promoters and/or neural progenitor cells include the neuronal repressor REST/NRSF, whose activities ultimately lead to apoptosis. Agents inhibiting endogenous reverse transcriptases include nevirapine and efavirenz. They demonstrate ability to reduce proliferation, induce morphological differentiation, and reprogram gene expression in many tumor histologies. They also have the added benefit of being lipophilic, so it is potentially easier for them to cross the blood–brain barrier. Agents inhibiting the Notch pathway include ADAM10, a disintegrin-metalloproteinase. Lastly, agents that inhibit neovascularization include halofuginone, a small molecule inhibitor of collagen I synthesis. Halofuginone has demonstrated inhibition of neovascularization both in vitro and in tumor-bearing animal models.

Recommendation for Small-Molecule Targeted Adjuvant Treatment

Currently, this is considered an emerging therapy, and evidence is insufficient for mainstay therapy. Routine molecular pathological testing will likely tightly correlate with the clinical utility of these agents and vice versa. Whenever possible, patients are encouraged to consider referral to an academic medical center and enrollment in an investigational study (Grade 1C Recommendation, Level II/III Evidence).

■ Deleterious Sequelae of Treatment

Deleterious sequelae of adjuvant therapy have profoundly impacted the evolution of sequential studies and resultant treatment paradigms. When deleterious sequelae of adjuvant therapy are discussed, several important limitations must be acknowledged. First, it is impossible to dissect the individual impacts, whether direct or indirect, of the inherently invasive tumor or the resection. Second, it is impossible to dissect the effects of individual modalities in combined therapy, whether RT or chemotherapy.[51] Third, it is impossible to compare results across 4 decades of trials—whether it is the diversity of treatment/techniques or the diversity of patient ages/risk groups. Lastly, advances in molecular pathology and small molecular targeted agents provide an unprecedented opportunity to overcome the foregoing limitations.

With those limitations acknowledged, numerous general trends have emerged.[52] Sequelae are commonly divided arbitrarily into acute (also termed early), subacute (early-delayed), and chronic (delayed or late). The intensity of sequelae usually correlates with the intensity of adjuvant therapy and extremes of age. The intensity of sequelae also usually correlates with the areas of the CNS receiving the most intensive treatment, but not always. In other words, sequelae can affect distal CNS areas and distal systemic organs profoundly as well. Lastly, RT and cytotoxic chemotherapy demonstrate general trends important to attend to when treating medulloblastoma.

Sequelae Commonly Attributed to Combined-Modality Adjuvant Therapy

Secondary cancers and endocrine dysfunction occur with higher frequency in medulloblastoma patients, regardless of the specifics of their adjuvant therapy, and are detailed in **Table 22.4**.[52,53] It is important to highlight that the occurrence of secondary cancers and endocrine dysfunction can be delayed and can involve non-CNS organs. For example, Duffner et al, on behalf of POG, reported on 198 patients < 3 years old whose occurrence of secondary malignancies ranged from 33 to 92 months and included myelodysplastic syndromes, acute myeloid leukemia, sarcoma, and meningioma.[53] Given these realities, yearly cancer screening, at least via H&P, is recommended for the remainder of the patient's life. Similarly, screening for endocrine dysfunction is also recommended for the remainder of the patient's life—specifically, at least every 3 to 6 months during adjuvant therapy, at least yearly thereafter, and including assessments of musculoskeletal growth, puberty, and so forth.[54,55]

Sequelae Commonly Attributed to Cytotoxic Chemotherapy

Cytotoxic chemotherapy most commonly impacts rapidly dividing cells preferentially. Examples include the mucosa, gonads, hair follicles, bone marrow, and other stem/progenitor cells. Similarly to RT, effects can be quite delayed, yet even more so than with RT, effects outside the CNS can be profound. For example, Bull et al, on behalf of the CCLG Consortium, reported a study in which 108 long-term survivors had previously received either RT alone or combined-modality therapy at presentation. At a mean follow-up of 7 years, those who received combined-modality therapy reported a significantly inferior overall health status as opposed to those who received only RT.[56] It is important to highlight that specific chemotherapy agents produce specific sequelae. It is essential for prescribers to have a thorough working knowledge of these agents, whether they are used as single agents or are combined with RT, other therapeutic agents, or concomitant medicines.

Sequelae Commonly Attributed to Radiotherapy

It is clear that sequelae of RT correlate with the volume/distribution treated, the total dose, the fractionation schedule, the patient's age and comorbidities, the use of concurrent chemotherapy, and possibly factors of histological, molecular, and even genetic pathology. Acute effects are defined as those that occur during RT, early-delayed effects appear 2 to 4 months after RT, and late effects develop > 90 days after the initiation of RT. Importantly, the Radiation Therapy Oncology Group (RTOG) has established specific grading criteria for toxicities.[57] As with chemotherapy, effects can be quite delayed and can affect the CNS and beyond. When discussing studies to date reporting deleterious sequelae of RT, it is important to highlight that many incorporated diverse CNS or head and neck cancers. Similarly, many data are extrapolated from other tumors receiving similar RT regimens, including gliomas, lymphomas, and, in adults, metastases. Acknowledging these limitations, numerous general trends have emerged.

Nonneurocognitive sequelae are detailed in **Table 22.4**. Directly correlated to their profound impact on outcomes, and thus, sequential studies and resultant treatment paradigms, neurocognitive sequelae are discussed in detail. Neurocognitive sequelae affect intellect, attention, emotion, mood, and personality, and are intensified by age, neurological deficits (hearing, seeing, motor, sensory, etc.), endocrine milestones, psychosocial challenges, and demands from family, school, and work.[58] Minimizing neurocognitive sequelae has been a dominant focus of the last 4 decades of sequential studies. Studies reducing the RT dose and/or distribution (while maintaining RT as the primary adjuvant therapy) are best reviewed with respect to the age-specific subpopulation in which they were conducted.

For patients < 3 years old, examples include a study reported by Fouladi et al in which patients with malignant brain tumors, including medulloblastomas, had their prospectively collected, longitudinally assessed, neurocognitive functions retrospectively reviewed. Neuroaxis RT was strongly correlated with greater progressive impairment of intelligence quotient (IQ), as opposed to either local RT only or no RT. Furthermore, neuroaxis RT was strongly associated with severe impairment (IQ < 70), as opposed to either local RT only or no RT (71% vs 24% vs 20%, respectively).[59] In another example reported by Mulhern et al, patients received risk-adapted RT and were assessed longitudinally for both IQ and academic achievement, including reading, spelling, and mathematics. High-risk patients (either metastatic disease or residual tumor > 1.5 cm^3) received craniospinal RT (36 to 39.6 Gy) followed by conformal boost to the primary site. Standard-risk patients received a lower dose of craniospinal RT (23 Gy) followed by boosts to the tumor bed and posterior fossa. The patients were evaluated for both IQ and academic achievement at baseline and 1, 2, and 5 years. Although multivariate analysis demonstrated statistically significant declines in both groups, they were more pronounced in the high-risk group, which had received the higher dose of irradiation. However, the factor correlating most strongly with decline was age at diagnosis, especially for future impairment of reading skills.[58]

Table 22.4 Deleterious sequelae

		Radiation		
Time course	**Surgery**	**Endocrine**	**Neurological**	**Other**
Acute or early	- Posterior fossa syndrome		- Acute encephalopathy - Cerebral edema - Nausea and vomiting - Dermatitis - Alopecia - Serous otitis media - Conductive hearing loss	- Myelosuppression—especially with chemotherapy - Mucositis
Subacute or early-delayed		- Somnolence and the somnolence syndrome	- Ototoxicity - Transient focal neurological symptoms - Reversible defects in memory	
Delayed		- Cortisol deficiency, growth hormone deficiency, hypothyroidism - RT to the thyroid may also cause primary hypothyroidism	- Sensorineural hearing loss - Ataxia - Asymptomatic diffuse white matter injury (gliomatosis) - Leukoencephalopathy syndrome (symptomatic) - Headache, including strokelike migraine attacks after radiation therapy (SMART)	- Secondary malignancies, including meningiomas, malignant gliomas, etc. (risk correlates to the intensity and locations of RT) - Scoliosis - Radiation necrosis - Radiation-induced vasculopathy and other cerebrovascular diseases (e.g., ischemic stroke) - Cataracts - Optic neuropathy, cortical blindness - Cataracts - Retinopathy, vasculopathy

For patients < 5 to 7 years old, examples include a study reported by Jenkin et al in which patients received RT-containing regimens at < 4 years of age and subsequently survived to adulthood. Only one third reported full-time employment and/or a "normal" lifestyle.[60] In another example, Goldwein et al reported a study in which patients < 5 years old received reduced-dose RT (18 Gy CSI, with a posterior fossa boost to 50.4 Gy) followed by chemotherapy. Acknowledging the limitations of a small sample size ($n = 10$), outcomes appeared generally comparable to contemporary combined-modality therapies, yet IQ scores remained in the normal range over many longitudinal assessments.[61] In a final example, Dufour et al preliminarily reported a pilot study of patients < 7 years old with metastatic disease who received five sequential courses of high-dose chemotherapy followed by autologous stem cell rescue, and then followed by age-adapted RT (doses ranged from 18 to 35 Gy). In this poor prognostic group, the OS at 30 months was 50%, and the toxicity, including neurocognitive, was manageable. Longitudinal assessments are still under way.[62]

■ Life-Long Surveillance

Specific long-term follow-up guidelines for survivors of childhood CNS tumors are available through many organizations, including the National Cancer Institute (www.cancer.gov) and the Children's Oncology Group (www.survivorshipguidelines.org). They are also available through many recent publications cit-

Chemotherapy		
Endocrine	**Neurological**	**Other**
– Cortisol deficiency, growth hormone deficiency, hypothyroidism may cause – Nausea, anorexia, weight loss – Slow growth – Fatigue, weakness – Alopecia – Symptoms may also simply be related to the tumor and/or therapies.	– Seizures, tremor – Headache – Transient paresthesias, neuropathies	– Myelosuppression—especially with RT – Mucositis—especially with RT
– Ototoxicity – Abnormal pubertal development and gonadal function – Growth catch-up (or failure to do so), osteopenia, fractures – Failure to thrive, underweight, obesity – Deconditioning, weakness, fatigue – Anorexia, obesity – Gastroparesis, constipation – Dry skin, thin/brittle hair – Symptoms may also simply be related to the tumor and/or therapies.	– Sensory peripheral neuropathies – Conductive hearing loss	
– Gonads or the hypothalamus permanently: failure to show catch-up growth, slow growth rate – Failure to thrive – Obesity – Persistent fatigue – Anorexia – Dry skin and thin, brittle hair – Constipation – Osteopenia, fractures – Abnormal puberty (e.g., precocious, persistent, or delayed)	– Sensory peripheral neuropathies – Sensorineural hearing loss, especially with cisplatin	– Secondary malignancies (risk correlates to the intensity)

ed within this chapter, including one by lead author Landier and colleagues.[63]

■ Therapy at Recurrence/Progression

Evidence-Based Use of Agents at Recurrence/Progression

Level I and Level II Evidence

Attempts at prospective studies in this setting, albeit inherently difficult, have not defined an optimal therapy.

Despite the improved outcomes for some patients with medulloblastoma, an estimated 20 to 30% will relapse/progress. Optimal therapy at recurrence/progression is undefined and is thus a major focus of ongoing studies. Investigational strategies involve single- or multiagent conventional chemotherapy; high-dose consolidative multiagent chemotherapy followed by autologous stem cell rescue; re-resection; or, most recently, small molecular targeted agents. Examples of single-agent chemotherapies demonstrating activity include platinums, methotrexate, etoposide, and, in particular, cyclophosphamide. Combination chemotherapies, commonly in the setting of myeloablative chemotherapy followed by autologous stem cell transplant, have also shown activity. Examples include those presented in the previous sections, as well as many others.[5,64] Lastly, pilot studies with small-molecule targeted agents, including inhibitors of the SHH pathway, are beginning to report preliminary results.[65] For reasons already discussed, patients are recommended to receive care within academic centers and studies. Available studies can be identified via the National Cancer Institute's search engine (www.clinicaltrials.gov).

Expert Recommendation

Currently, there is no optimal therapy; thus, this is a major focus of ongoing studies. Treatments vary widely. Whenever possible, patients are encouraged to consider referral to an academic medical center and enrollment in an investigational study (Grade 1C Recommendation, Level II/III Evidence).

■ Unmet Needs and Resultant Future Strategies

Unmet needs exist in several areas, including optimal adjuvant therapy for many age-specific subpopulations, optimal therapy at recurrence/progression, and optimal strategies to minimize deleterious sequelae of all therapeutic tools. Continual, rigorous, international studies, investigating the "right" next question, and collecting both provider- and patient-generated outcomes, is essential. General topics include further minimizing RT dose/distribution, alternative chemotherapy regimens, and increasing aggressiveness in preventing and ameliorating deleterious sequelae (especially neurocognitive and endocrine) in "real time." Furthermore, improvements in the classification system, risk-stratification system, prognostic factors, and therapeutic agents are needed to optimally design, conduct, and analyze studies. Advances in molecular pathology have the potential to make profound contributions.

■ Summary and Conclusions

Medulloblastomas represent the most common malignant solid tumor affecting the CNS in the pediatric population. Clinicoradiographic presentation varies with age. Factors correlated with superior outcome include age and extent of disease at presentation, desmoplastic variant, and, possibly, certain molecular pathology markers. Risk stratification, which incorporates the modified Chang stage, determines adjuvant therapy selection. As a direct result of 4 decades of sequential international studies, a certain age-specific subpopulation has demonstrated significantly improved outcomes with combined-modality adjuvant therapy following attempts at maximal safe resection (specifically, standard-risk patients < 3 to 5 years old). In the remainder, combined-modality adjuvant therapy is considered investigational. In addition, optimal therapies for all patients at recurrence/progression remain unkown. Despite this, ongoing scientific efforts continue to result in incremental progress. Recent advances in molecular pathology are at the forefront of efforts to improve classification systems, risk-stratification systems, prognostic factors, and therapeutic agents. More robust attempts to prevent, minimize, and follow deleterious sequelae of treatment are essential. Whenever possible, patients are recommended to receive care within academic centers and studies.

■ References

1. Mueller S, Chang S. Pediatric brain tumors: current treatment strategies and future therapeutic approaches. Neurotherapeutics 2009;6(3):570–586
2. Kim JY, Sutton ME, Lu DJ, et al. Activation of neurotrophin-3 receptor TrkC induces apoptosis in medulloblastomas. Cancer Res 1999;59(3):711–719
3. Giangaspero F, Eberhart CG, Haapasalo H, et al. Medulloblastoma. In: WHO Classification of Tumours of the Central Nervous System. 4th ed. Louis DN, Ohgaki H, Wiestler OD, Cavenee WK, eds. Lyon: IARC; 2007:132
4. Ellison DW, Kocak M, Dalton J, et al. Definition of disease-risk stratification groups in childhood medulloblastoma using combined clinical, pathologic, and molecular variables. J Clin Oncol 2011;29(11):1400–1407
5. Rutkowski S, von Hoff K, Emser A, et al. Survival and prognostic factors of early childhood medulloblastoma: an international meta-analysis. J Clin Oncol 2010;28(33):4961–4968
6. Bigner DD, McLendon RE, Bruner JM. Russell and Rubenstein's Pathology of Tumors of the Nervous System. London: Arnold; 1998
7. Polkinghorn WR, Tarbell NJ. Medulloblastoma: tumorigenesis, current clinical paradigm, and efforts to improve risk stratification. Nat Clin Pract Oncol 2007;4(5):295–304
8. Ellison DW, Kocak M, Dalton J, et al. Definition of disease-risk stratification groups in childhood medulloblastoma using combined clinical, pathologic, and molecular variables. J Clin Oncol 2011;29(11):1400–1407
9. Korshunov A, Remke M, Werft W, et al. Adult and pediatric medulloblastomas are genetically distinct and require different algorithms for molecular risk stratification. J Clin Oncol 2010;28(18):3054–3060
10. Pomeroy SL, Tamayo P, Gaasenbeek M, et al. Prediction of central nervous system embryonal tumour outcome based on gene expression. Nature 2002;415(6870):436–442
11. Entz-Werle N, Velasco V, Neuville A, et al. Do medulloblastoma tumors meet the Food and Drug Administration criteria for anti-erbB2 therapy with trastuzumab? Pediatr Blood Cancer 2008;50(1):163–166
12. Gajjar A, Hernan R, Kocak M, et al. Clinical, histopathologic, and molecular markers of prognosis: toward a new disease risk stratification system for medulloblastoma. J Clin Oncol 2004;22(6):984–993
13. Attard TM, Giglio P, Koppula S, Snyder C, Lynch HT. Brain tumors in individuals with familial adenomatous polyposis: a cancer registry experience and pooled case report analysis. Cancer 2007;109(4):761–766
14. Raffel C. Medulloblastoma: molecular genetics and animal models. Neoplasia 2004;6(4):310–322

15. Taylor MD, Liu L, Raffel C, et al. Mutations in SUFU predispose to medulloblastoma. Nat Genet 2002;31(3):306–310
16. Erez A, Ilan T, Amariglio N, et al. GLI3 is not mutated commonly in sporadic medulloblastomas. Cancer 2002;95(1):28–31
17. Halperin EC, Friedman HS. Is there a correlation between duration of presenting symptoms and stage of medulloblastoma at the time of diagnosis? Cancer 1996;78(4):874–880
18. Chang CH, Housepian EM, Herbert C Jr. An operative staging system and a megavoltage radiotherapeutic technic for cerebellar medulloblastomas. Radiology 1969;93(6):1351–1359
19. Mazloom A, Zangeneh AH, Paulino AC. Prognostic factors after extraneural metastasis of medulloblastoma. Int J Radiat Oncol Biol Phys 2010;78(1):72–78
20. Fouladi M, Gajjar A, Boyett JM, et al. Comparison of CSF cytology and spinal magnetic resonance imaging in the detection of leptomeningeal disease in pediatric medulloblastoma or primitive neuroectodermal tumor. J Clin Oncol 1999; 17(10):3234–3237
21. Zeltzer PM, Boyett JM, Finlay JL, et al. Metastasis stage, adjuvant treatment, and residual tumor are prognostic factors for medulloblastoma in children: conclusions from the Children's Cancer Group 921 randomized phase III study. J Clin Oncol 1999;17(3):832–845
22. Perek D, Perek-Polnik M, Drogosiewicz M, Dembowska-Bagińska B, Roszkowski M, Barszcz S. Risk factors of recurrence in 157 MB/PNET patients treated in one institution. Childs Nerv Syst 1998;14(10):582–586
23. Terterov S, Krieger MD, Bowen I, McComb JG. Evaluation of intracranial cerebrospinal fluid cytology in staging pediatric medulloblastomas, supratentorial primitive neuroectodermal tumors, and ependymomas. J Neurosurg Pediatr 2010; 6(2):131–136
24. Tabori U, Sung L, Hukin J, et al; Canadian Pediatric Brain Tumor Consortium. Medulloblastoma in the second decade of life: a specific group with respect to toxicity and management: a Canadian Pediatric Brain Tumor Consortium Study. Cancer 2005;103(9):1874–1880
25. Jenkin D, Goddard K, Armstrong D, et al. Posterior fossa medulloblastoma in childhood: treatment results and a proposal for a new staging system. Int J Radiat Oncol Biol Phys 1990;19(2):265–274
26. Albright AL, Wisoff JH, Zeltzer PM, Boyett JM, Rorke LB, Stanley P. Effects of medulloblastoma resections on outcome in children: a report from the Children's Cancer Group. Neurosurgery 1996;38(2):265–271
27. Cushing H. Experience with cerebellar medulloblastoma: a critical review. Acta Pathol Microbiol Scand 1930;7:1–86
28. Hughes EN, Shillito J, Sallan SE, Loeffler JS, Cassady JR, Tarbell NJ. Medulloblastoma at the Joint Center for Radiation Therapy between 1968 and 1984. The influence of radiation dose on the patterns of failure and survival. Cancer 1988; 61(10):1992–1998
29. del Charco JO, Bolek TW, McCollough WM, et al. Medulloblastoma: time-dose relationship based on a 30-year review. Int J Radiat Oncol Biol Phys 1998;42(1):147–154
30. Robertson PL, Muraszko KM, Holmes EJ, et al; Children's Oncology Group. Incidence and severity of postoperative cerebellar mutism syndrome in children with medulloblastoma: a prospective study by the Children's Oncology Group. J Neurosurg 2006;105(6, Suppl):444–451
31. Rossi A, Caracciolo V, Russo G, Reiss K, Giordano A. Medulloblastoma: from molecular pathology to therapy. Clin Cancer Res 2008;14(4):971–976
32. Abacioglu U, Uzel O, Sengoz M, Turkan S, Ober A. Medulloblastoma in adults: treatment results and prognostic factors. Int J Radiat Oncol Biol Phys 2002;54(3):855–860
33. Evans AE, Jenkin RD, Sposto R, et al. The treatment of medulloblastoma. Results of a prospective randomized trial of radiation therapy with and without CCNU, vincristine, and prednisone. J Neurosurg 1990;72(4):572–582
34. Tait DM, Thornton-Jones H, Bloom HJ, Lemerle J, Morris-Jones P. Adjuvant chemotherapy for medulloblastoma: the first multi-centre control trial of the International Society of Paediatric Oncology (SIOP I). Eur J Cancer 1990;26(4):464–469
35. van Eys J, Cangir A, Coody D, Smith B. MOPP regimen as primary chemotherapy for brain tumors in infants. J Neurooncol 1985;3(3):237–243
36. Ater JL, van Eys J, Woo SY, Moore B III, Copeland DR, Bruner J. MOPP chemotherapy without irradiation as primary postsurgical therapy for brain tumors in infants and young children. J Neurooncol 1997;32(3):243–252
37. Grill J, Sainte-Rose C, Jouvet A, et al; French Society of Paediatric Oncology. Treatment of medulloblastoma with postoperative chemotherapy alone: an SFOP prospective trial in young children. Lancet Oncol 2005;6(8):573–580
38. Duffner PK, Horowitz ME, Krischer JP, et al. Postoperative chemotherapy and delayed radiation in children less than three years of age with malignant brain tumors. N Engl J Med 1993;328(24):1725–1731
39. Geyer JR, Sposto R, Jennings M, et al; Children's Cancer Group. Multiagent chemotherapy and deferred radiotherapy in infants with malignant brain tumors: a report from the Children's Cancer Group. J Clin Oncol 2005;23(30):7621–7631
40. Rutkowski S, Bode U, Deinlein F, et al. Treatment of early childhood medulloblastoma by postoperative chemotherapy alone. N Engl J Med 2005;352(10):978–986
41. Mason WP, Grovas A, Halpern S, et al. Intensive chemotherapy and bone marrow rescue for young children with newly diagnosed malignant brain tumors. J Clin Oncol 1998;16(1): 210–221
42. Dhall G, Grodman H, Ji L, et al. Outcome of children less than three years old at diagnosis with non-metastatic medulloblastoma treated with chemotherapy on the "Head Start" I and II protocols. Pediatr Blood Cancer 2008;50(6):1169–1175
43. Grundy RG, Wilne SH, Robinson KJ, et al; Children's Cancer and Leukaemia Group (formerly UKCCSG) Brain Tumour Committee. Primary postoperative chemotherapy without radiotherapy for treatment of brain tumours other than ependymoma in children under 3 years: results of the first UKCCSG/SIOP CNS 9204 trial. Eur J Cancer 2010;46(1):120–133
44. Packer RJ, Gajjar A, Vezina G, et al. Phase III study of craniospinal radiation therapy followed by adjuvant chemotherapy for newly diagnosed average-risk medulloblastoma. J Clin Oncol 2006;24(25):4202–4208
45. Freeman CR, Taylor RE, Kortmann RD, Carrie C. Radiotherapy for medulloblastoma in children: a perspective on current international clinical research efforts. Med Pediatr Oncol 2002;39(2):99–108
46. Nieder C, Mehta MP, Jalali R. Combined radio- and chemotherapy of brain tumours in adult patients. Clin Oncol (R Coll Radiol) 2009;21(7):515–524
47. Riffaud L, Saikali S, Leray E, et al. Survival and prognostic factors in a series of adults with medulloblastomas. J Neurosurg 2009;111(3):478–487
48. Brandes AA, Franceschi E, Tosoni A, et al. Efficacy of tailored treatment for high- and low-risk medulloblastoma in adults: a large prospective phase II trial (abstract #2003). J Clin Oncol 2010;28:182s
49. Greenberg HS, Chamberlain MC, Glantz MJ, Wang S. Adult medulloblastoma: multiagent chemotherapy. Neuro-oncol 2001;3(1):29–34
50. Lai R. Survival of patients with adult medulloblastoma: a population-based study. Cancer 2008;112(7):1568–1574
51. Kiehna EN, Mulhern RK, Li C, Xiong X, Merchant TE. Changes in attentional performance of children and young adults with localized primary brain tumors after conformal radiation therapy. J Clin Oncol 2006;24(33):5283–5290
52. Landier W, Kinahan KE, Shaw S, Bhatia S. Screening for late effects in brain tumor survivors. Cancer Treat Res 2009; 150:389–409

53. Duffner PK, Krischer JP, Horowitz ME, et al. Second malignancies in young children with primary brain tumors following treatment with prolonged postoperative chemotherapy and delayed irradiation: a Pediatric Oncology Group study. Ann Neurol 1998;44(3):313–316
54. Rose SR. Endocrinopathies after childhood cancer. Endocrinologist 2003;13:488
55. Hameed R, Zacharin MR. Long-term endocrine effects of cancer treatment: experience of the Royal Children's Hospital, Melbourne. J Paediatr Child Health 2005;41(1-2):36–42
56. Bull KS, Spoudeas HA, Yadegarfar G, Kennedy CR; CCLG. Reduction of health status 7 years after addition of chemotherapy to craniospinal irradiation for medulloblastoma: a follow-up study in PNET 3 trial survivors on behalf of the CCLG (formerly UKCCSG). J Clin Oncol 2007;25(27):4239–4245
57. RTOG Acute Radiation Morbidity Scoring Criteria. www.rtog.org/members/toxicity/acute.html. Accessed June 8, 2012
58. Mulhern RK, Palmer SL, Merchant TE, et al. Neurocognitive consequences of risk-adapted therapy for childhood medulloblastoma. J Clin Oncol 2005;23(24):5511–5519
59. Fouladi M, Gilger E, Kocak M, et al. Intellectual and functional outcome of children 3 years old or younger who have CNS malignancies. J Clin Oncol 2005;23(28):7152–7160
60. Jenkin D, Danjoux C, Greenberg M. Subsequent quality of life for children irradiated for a brain tumor before age four years. Med Pediatr Oncol 1998;31(6):506–511
61. Goldwein JW, Radcliffe J, Johnson J, et al. Updated results of a pilot study of low dose craniospinal irradiation plus chemotherapy for children under five with cerebellar primitive neuroectodermal tumors (medulloblastoma). Int J Radiat Oncol Biol Phys 1996;34(4):899–904
62. Dufour C, Couanet D, Figarella-Branger D, et al. Sequential high-dose chemotherapy and reduced craniospinal irradiation in young children with metastatic medulloblastoma [abstract]. Neuro-oncol 2008;10:423
63. Landier W, Bhatia S, Eshelman DA, et al. Development of risk-based guidelines for pediatric cancer survivors: the Children's Oncology Group Long-Term Follow-Up Guidelines from the Children's Oncology Group Late Effects Committee and Nursing Discipline. J Clin Oncol 2004;22(24):4979–4990
64. Kadota RP, Mahoney DH, Doyle J, et al. Dose intensive melphalan and cyclophosphamide with autologous hematopoietic stem cells for recurrent medulloblastoma or germinoma. Pediatr Blood Cancer 2008;51(5):675–678
65. Wlodarski PK, Jozwiak J. Therapeutic targets for medulloblastoma. Expert Opin Ther Targets 2008;12(4):449–461
66. Dunkel IJ, Gardner SL, Garvin JH Jr, Goldman S, Shi W, Finlay JL. High-dose carboplatin, thiotepa, and etoposide with autologous stem cell rescue for patients with previously irradiated recurrent medulloblastoma. Neuro-oncol 2010;12(3):297–303

▪ SECTION VI ▪

Metastases

23

Surgery, Radiosurgery, or Whole Brain Radiotherapy for One to Three Asymptomatic Intracranial Metastases

Ganesh M. Shankar and Daniel P. Cahill III

A significant portion of patients with cancer will manifest with intracranial metastasis, with prevalence ranging from 10 to 40%[1] and an incidence of ~ 170,000 new cases per year.[2] Given changes in the pattern of surveillance brain imaging and more successful treatments of systemic disease, the detection of asymptomatic metastases is progressively increasing,[3] and the management of asymptomatic brain metastases is an area of controversy in modern clinical decision making.

The treatment of intracranial metastasis in any individual patient will often incorporate surgical resection, stereotactic radiosurgery (SRS), and whole brain radiation therapy (WBRT) over the course of the illness (**Figs. 23.1, 23.2**). Given the common utilization of multiple modalities in individual patients, and the attendant difficulties associated with performing randomized, controlled trials (RCTs) to compare these modalities in isolation,[4] the availability of Level I evidence to guide therapeutic decision making in asymptomatic cases is limited. To help address this gap, the American Association of Neurological Surgeons (AANS) and Congress of Neurological Surgeons (CNS) have developed guidelines for the use of these modalities through a systematic review of the literature.[5–7]

This chapter reviews the role for surgery and SRS for local control of one to three asymptomatic intracranial metastases. Furthermore, data on the role of WBRT for local and distant intracranial control are evaluated given the associated consequences for cognitive function, which have been of increasing concern for patients with asymptomatic intracranial metastases. Like many areas of cancer treatment, treatment of brain metastases is an actively evolving field, with multiple factors contributing to the individualization of treatment. These factors include the functional localization of lesions within the brain, as well as the increasing availability of molecularly targeted chemotherapeutic treatments for clearance of widely metastatic systemic disease. Thus, thoughtfully aggressive approaches can result in long-term survivors with good neurocognitive outcome.

■ Literature Review

Identifying Patients Suitable for Local Control Modalities (Surgery or Stereotactic Radiosurgery)

Framing all decision making in patients with brain metastases is the prognostication of expected overall survival in a patient with disseminated metastatic cancer. Will this patient live long enough that control of metastatic disease foci in the brain will contribute to an improvement in overall outcome?

Recursive partitioning analysis (RPA) of the Radiation Therapy Oncology Group (RTOG) aggregate brain metastases clinical datasets demonstrated that Karnofsky performance scale (KPS) score, control of the

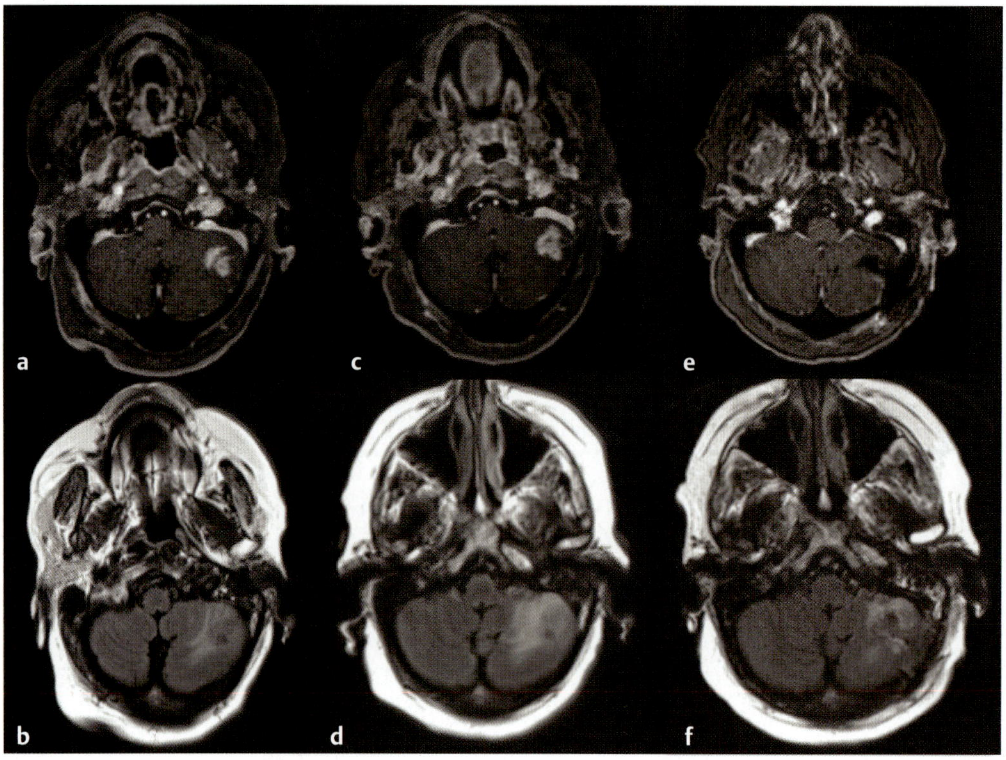

Fig. 23.1 76-year-old female with history of a previous resection of a squamous cell carcinoma of the neck, resection of left-sided breast cancer, and chemo and radiation therapy for a right lung small cell carcinoma. During the oncological assessment, a left paragittal lesion was incidentally found. Craniotomy and resection with gross total resection was achieved. Pathology diagnosed lung metastasis from a poorly differentiated small cell carcinoma. Two years postcraniotomy, the patient presented with a new small left hemispheric cerebellar metastasis that was treated with radiosurgery with a good postradiation response. Two years later, the residual lesion showed increasing cerebral edema in the follow-up MRI with absence of symptoms or neurological deficits. **(a)** T1 with gadolinium axial and **(b)** T2 FLAIR axial MRIs show postradiotherapy effect with a left hemispheric enhancing cerebellar lesion with mild surrounding edema. In **(c)** T1 with gadolinium axial and **(d)** T2 FLAIR axial MRIs, there is a significant increase in the cerebral edema. Enhancement and minimal enlargement of the left cerebellar lesion are concerns for either radiation necrosis versus tumor progression. The patient underwent left occipital craniotomy resection of tumor. **(e)** T1 with gadolinium axial and **(f)** T2 FLAIR axial MRIs show gross total resection. (Figures courtesy of Dr. A. Quiñones-Hinojosa.)

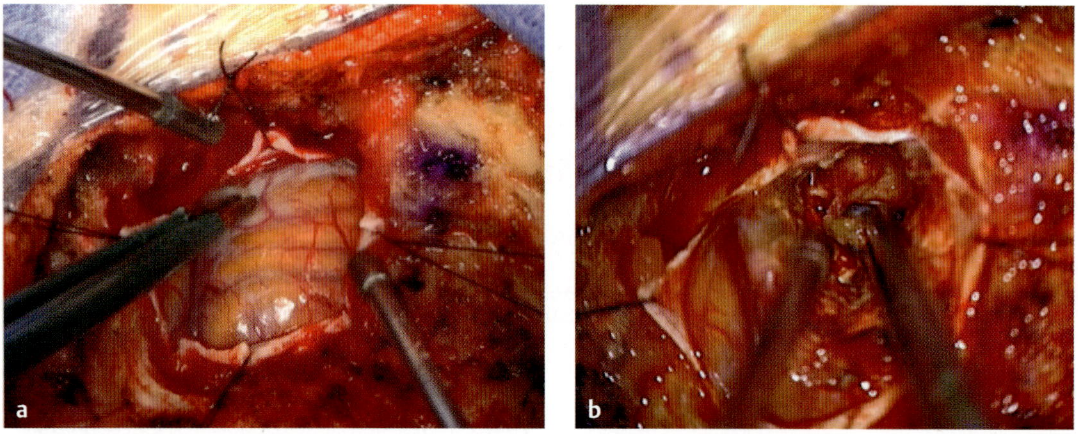

Fig. 23.2 **(a)** Gliotic cerebellar hemisphere cortex after dural opening. **(b)** Detail of the tumor resection. The pathology was reported as cerebellar tissue with extensive coagulative necrosis, compatible with radionecrosis or pseudoprogression. (Figures courtesy of Dr. A. Quiñones-Hinojosa.)

primary site of systemic disease, age, and extent of extracranial metastases segregated patients by median overall survival. Patients who were younger than 65 years with a KPS score > 70, controlled systemic disease, and metastasis limited to the brain (class 1) fared best, with a median survival of 7.1 months, whereas class 2 and class 3 patients had shorter survival times of 4.2 and 2.3 months, respectively.[8] This finding has guided the recommendation for surgical resection for RPA class 1 or 2 patients who have an expected survival that can be balanced against the postoperative risks of neurological morbidity (3.9 to 6.0%), and systemic complications (13.9%).[9]

More recently, histological diagnosis-specific graded prognostic assessment (DS-GPA) groups have been developed.[10] The DS-GPA system accounts for the inherent differences in median survival for each primary malignancy; for instance, median survival for patients with breast cancer was 11.9 months and melanoma was 6.7 months. This system provides for a calculated estimate of expected survival for a patient when histology is considered together with additional factors, such as number of intracranial and extracranial metastases, age, and KPS score.

Due to the increasing early detection of small metastases on screening brain magnetic resonance imaging (MRI) in cancer patients, the use of SRS has been increasing. SRS is minimally invasive and can be administered on an outpatient basis and thus is often recommended as frontline treatment, especially when a lesion is small (< 1 cm^3). However, surgical resection continues to have a specific role in the management of lesions causing mass effect, for those resulting in significant surrounding edema and obstructive hydrocephalus, and especially for those in the posterior fossa. Controversy remains when one is addressing the management of asymptomatic lesions for which local control can be achieved by either surgery or SRS. Specifically, these are lesions measuring > 1 cm^3 but < 3 cm^3 (~ 10 cm^3), with minimal mass effect (< 1 cm midline shift).

Surgical Resection

The central goal for management of intracranial metastasis is to achieve control of recurrence at existing sites of metastasis (local control) as well as to prevent new lesions (distal or regional control), with the implication that this control will contribute, in combination with systemic treatments, to improved overall survival. This section addresses two questions:

- Does surgical resection of asymptomatic intracranial metastasis improve median survival?
- Does adjuvant WBRT improve intracranial recurrence and overall survival?

Level I Evidence

Two RCTs[11,12] demonstrate survival benefit with surgical resection and WBRT as compared with WBRT alone for the management of a single metastasis. In the study by Patchell et al,[11] patients had KPS scores ≥ 70 and were ineligible if the known primary was relatively radiosensitive (lymphoma, germ cell tumor, small cell). Patients randomized to undergo complete surgical resection had a median survival of 40 weeks, whereas patients receiving 36 Gy alone had a median survival of 15 weeks. The multicenter trial by Vecht et al[12] similarly found a survival benefit for patients randomized to surgical resection (10 months vs 6 months) who were younger than 60 years old and had controlled extracranial disease. Another randomized trial performed by Mintz et al[13] did not find benefit; however, they included patients with lower KPS scores and poorly controlled systemic disease.

A study by Patchell et al[14] represents the single RCT examining the role of postsurgical WBRT for the management of a single brain metastasis. This study revealed decreased local (46% vs 10%) and distant (70% vs 18%) recurrence of tumor when patients received WBRT. Fewer patients died from neurological causes when receiving adjuvant WBRT (14% vs 44%). Importantly, this study was not powered to assess for effects on the secondary end point of overall survival.

Level II Evidence

A retrospective cohort study by Ampil et al[15] reported survival benefit with initial surgical resection compared with WBRT alone (15 vs 3 months) for patients with metastasis in the cerebellum.

Three retrospective cohort studies[16–18] similarly reveal improved local and distant recurrence rates when WBRT is used postoperatively. However, there is no clear benefit for median survival. Nonetheless, there is general concern about carrying forward these data into the newer era of systemic cancer treatment modalities, where extension of survival from systemic treatment is increasingly seen in targeted populations, such as trastuzumab for patients with HER2-positive breast cancer, or vemurafenib for patients with BRAF-mutant melanoma.

Consensus Statement

Level I data support surgical resection and WBRT as opposed to WBRT alone for management of intracranial metastases for patients with KPS scores ≥ 70 and controlled extracranial disease. There are insufficient data to guide management for patients who have lower performance status. This subgroup may have decreased overall survival time secondary to systemic progression, and thus local control of asymptomatic brain lesions may not contribute to their overall outcome.

The current guideline is for surgical resection of amenable lesions in patients with KPS scores ≥ 70, with adjuvant WBRT for control of intracranial recurrence. Level II evidence suggests that lesions > 3 cm^3 or those resulting in mass effect may have improved outcomes with surgical resection rather than SRS.

However, given the lack of clear benefit on survival and effects on cognitive functioning with adjuvant WBRT, an alternate treatment paradigm is for postoperative surveillance with WBRT reserved as salvage therapy. The cooperative group trial Japan Clinical Oncology Group (JCOG) 0504 is ongoing, designed to investigate the role of adjuvant WBRT versus salvage SRS for management of recurrence.

Stereotactic Radiosurgery

Although open resection is recommended for lesions > 3 cm^3 in locations amenable to surgery, SRS appears to be equivalent for the management of a smaller single lesion in terms of local control and survival. No Level I evidence exists for addressing whether SRS or WBRT alone is superior for tumor control and survival. However, retrospective[19–22] and prospective[23] cohort studies provide the basis for Level III recommendation that SRS is superior, especially for radioresistant tumors such as colon cancer, melanoma, and renal cell tumors. Ongoing investigations continue to define the optimal integration of SRS into the treatment plan for a patient with brain metastasis. This section addresses the following two questions:

- Is there a benefit to SRS compared with WBRT alone?
- Is there a difference in outcome between SRS and surgical resection?

Level I Evidence

The RCT by Andrews et al[24] revealed survival benefit for patients with a single intracranial lesion who received SRS and WBRT (6.5 months, n = 164 patients) as opposed to WBRT alone (4.9 months, n = 167 patients). One critique of this study is the large crossover between the two arms; 19% in the former did not receive the planned SRS, and 17% in the latter received salvage SRS. The RCT by Kondziolka et al[25] reported decreased local failure rates with SRS compared with WBRT alone for patients with two to four metastases (8% vs 100%). Because this trial included a total of 27 patients, it was not powered to address the secondary outcome of median survival, but a nonsignificant trend toward increased survival was noted with SRS (11.0 vs 7.5 months).

Level II Evidence

The prospective cohort study by Li et al[23] revealed improved survival (10.3 vs 5.7 months) and longer time to local recurrence (8.6 vs 4.0 months) for patients with a single lung cancer metastasis undergoing SRS and WBRT as opposed to WBRT alone. Similarly, the retrospective cohort studies by Wang et al[22] and Sanghavi et al[26] revealed a survival benefit for patients when SRS and WBRT were used in conjunction. Of note, the study by Sanghavi et al[26] reported improved survival even for patients categorized as RPA class 2 (10.3 vs 4.2 months) and class 3 (8.7 vs 2.3 months).

Retrospective cohort studies[27,28] have compared surgical resection and WBRT against SRS and WBRT. Bindal et al[27] revealed equivalence in median survival with surgical resection and SRS for patients with one or two intracranial lesions. The SRS + WBRT arm in Bindal et al[27] was noted to have higher rates of radiation necrosis and adverse events than those reported by other studies; accordingly, this group had a lower than expected length of survival. The RCT by Muacevic et al,[29] which was ended prematurely due to low patient accrual, negated the overwhelmingly positive benefit of surgery compared with SRS reported by Bindal et al.[27]

Consensus Statement

There is Level I recommendation for the use of both SRS and WBRT for single metastatic lesions in patients with a KPS score ≥ 70. The Level II recommendation is that SRS and WBRT is superior to WBRT alone for patients with one to four metastatic lesions. With regard to lesions < 3 cm^3, class 2 data suggest equivalence of surgical resection and SRS when used together with WBRT in terms of recurrence and survival rates. It is important to note that no trial has been appropriately powered to detect a small difference in survival, should one exist. However, in practice, this lack of evidence has resulted in a consideration of equivalency between surgery and SRS with regard to survival in upfront decision making for patients presenting with brain metastases.

The role of SRS in management of intracranial metastasis is an evolving domain. First, ongoing trials will aim to elucidate whether single-dose SRS is equivalent to WBRT for local control of a cavity following surgical resection. Second, a formal RCT comparing surgical resection and SRS will provide further clarity on existing class 2 evidence suggesting equivalence with regard to overall survival.

Third, although the RCT by Aoyama et al[30] observed no difference in survival between patients receiving SRS alone compared with SRS and WBRT, there was a significant difference in local and distant recurrence. However, the accompanying commentary by Patchell et al[31] noted a sample size of 2,250 patients would be required to adequately power a study to detect a difference in survival. This clinical scenario has proven controversial, and further data are needed to clarify the implications of upfront WBRT for management of systemic disease and neurocognitive functioning. Patients with asymptomatic intracranial lesions but with extensive systemic disease are able to initiate chemotherapy sooner if the intracranial disease is treated with SRS upfront and WBRT is withheld until distal failure.[32] Furthermore, withholding of WBRT may have a neurocognitive benefit, as shown in an RCT by Chang et al.[33] of 58 patients randomly assigned to treatment with SRS and WBRT or SRS alone. These investigators found that the addition of WBRT resulted in greater functional decline on the Hopkins Verbal Learning Test over 4 months. Two ongoing RCTs (National Clinical Trials [NCT] 00548756 and 00377156) aim to clarify further whether withholding upfront WBRT affects intracranial recurrence, survival, and neurocognitive functioning.

Expert Recommendations

1. Surgical resection and WBRT afford improved survival compared with either alone for a single lesion (Grade 1A Recommendation, Level I Evidence).
2. SRS and WBRT afford improved survival compared with WBRT alone for single lesions (Grade 1A Recommendation, Level I Evidence) and improved performance status for one through four lesions (Grade 1B Recommendation, Level II Evidence).
3. Surgical resection and SRS are equivalent in survival rates when used together with WBRT for lesions < 3 cm^3 (Grade 1B Recommendation, Level II Evidence).

■ Summary and Conclusions

The goal of brain metastasis management is to achieve local and regional control as a means to improve overall survival. Local control has traditionally been achieved by surgical resection, especially for RPA class 1 patients or DS-GPA patients with a longer expected survival. However, more recent studies have revealed SRS to be a useful treatment modality that may be able to achieve near-equivalent outcomes to surgical resection in terms of survival and intracranial control. For asymptomatic brain metastasis patients, surgery and SRS are modalities that are important for the local control of traditionally radioresistant histologies, such as melanoma, renal cell carcinoma, or sarcoma.

Although WBRT affects recurrence rates when applied after resection or SRS, the effect on overall survival has been less robust. Taken together with the potential negative effects of WBRT on neurocognitive function, this has led to the proposal that WBRT may be reserved as salvage therapy when more extensive brain recurrence is appreciated on surveillance imaging. The survival benefit of WBRT as an adjunct to SRS will be further clarified with ongoing RCTs. These data will be particularly helpful to guide the management of patients with asymptomatic brain metastases, which are increasingly common in the modern era.

■ References

1. Gavrilovic IT, Posner JB. Brain metastases: epidemiology and pathophysiology. J Neurooncol 2005;75(1):5–14
2. Brem S, Panattil JG. An era of rapid advancement: diagnosis and treatment of metastatic brain cancer. Neurosurgery 2005;57(5, Suppl):S5–S9, S1–S4
3. Soffietti R, Rudà R, Trevisan E. Brain metastases: current management and new developments. Curr Opin Oncol 2008;20(6):676–684
4. Roos DE, Smith JG, Stephens SW. Radiosurgery versus surgery, both with adjuvant whole brain radiotherapy, for solitary brain metastases: a randomised controlled trial. Clin Oncol (R Coll Radiol) 2011;23(9):646–651
5. Gaspar LE, Mehta MP, Patchell RA, et al. The role of whole brain radiation therapy in the management of newly diagnosed brain metastases: a systematic review and evidence-based clinical practice guideline. J Neurooncol 2010;96(1):17–32
6. Kalkanis SN, Kondziolka D, Gaspar LE, et al. The role of surgical resection in the management of newly diagnosed brain metastases: a systematic review and evidence-based clinical practice guideline. J Neurooncol 2010;96(1):33–43
7. Linskey ME, Andrews DW, Asher AL, et al. The role of stereotactic radiosurgery in the management of patients with newly diagnosed brain metastases: a systematic review and evidence-based clinical practice guideline. J Neurooncol 2010;96(1):45–68
8. Gaspar LE, Qian C, Kocha WI, Coia LR, Herskovic A, Graham M. A phase I/II study of external beam radiation, brachytherapy and concurrent chemotherapy in localized cancer of the esophagus (RTOG 92-07): preliminary toxicity report. Int J Radiat Oncol Biol Phys 1997;37(3):593–599
9. Sawaya R, Hammoud M, Schoppa D, et al. Neurosurgical outcomes in a modern series of 400 craniotomies for treatment of parenchymal tumors. Neurosurgery 1998;42(5): 1044–1055
10. Sperduto PW, Chao ST, Sneed PK, et al. Diagnosis-specific prognostic factors, indexes, and treatment outcomes for patients with newly diagnosed brain metastases: a multi-institutional analysis of 4,259 patients. Int J Radiat Oncol Biol Phys 2010;77(3):655–661
11. Patchell RA, Tibbs PA, Walsh JW, et al. A randomized trial of surgery in the treatment of single metastases to the brain. N Engl J Med 1990;322(8):494–500

12. Vecht CJ, Haaxma-Reiche H, Noordijk EM, et al. Treatment of single brain metastasis: radiotherapy alone or combined with neurosurgery? Ann Neurol 1993;33(6):583–590
13. Mintz AH, Kestle J, Rathbone MP, et al. A randomized trial to assess the efficacy of surgery in addition to radiotherapy in patients with a single cerebral metastasis. Cancer 1996; 78(7):1470–1476
14. Patchell RA, Tibbs PA, Regine WF, et al. Postoperative radiotherapy in the treatment of single metastases to the brain: a randomized trial. JAMA 1998;280(17):1485–1489
15. Ampil FL, Nanda A, Willis BK, Nandy I, Meehan R. Metastatic disease in the cerebellum. The LSU experience in 1981-1993. Am J Clin Oncol 1996;19(5):509–511
16. Armstrong JG, Wronski M, Galicich J, Arbit E, Leibel SA, Burt M. Postoperative radiation for lung cancer metastatic to the brain. J Clin Oncol 1994;12(11):2340–2344
17. Hagen NA, Cirrincione C, Thaler HT, DeAngelis LM. The role of radiation therapy following resection of single brain metastasis from melanoma. Neurology 1990;40(1):158–160
18. Skibber JM, Soong SJ, Austin L, Balch CM, Sawaya RE. Cranial irradiation after surgical excision of brain metastases in melanoma patients. Ann Surg Oncol 1996;3(2):118–123
19. Kocher M, Maarouf M, Bendel M, Voges J, Müller RP, Sturm V. Linac radiosurgery versus whole brain radiotherapy for brain metastases: a survival comparison based on the RTOG recursive partitioning analysis. Strahlenther Onkol 2004;180(5):263–267
20. Lee SS, Ahn JH, Kim MK, et al. Brain metastases in breast cancer: prognostic factors and management. Breast Cancer Res Treat 2008;111(3):523–530
21. Rades D, Bohlen G, Pluemer A, et al. Stereotactic radiosurgery alone versus resection plus whole-brain radiotherapy for 1 or 2 brain metastases in recursive partitioning analysis class 1 and 2 patients. Cancer 2007;109(12):2515–2521
22. Wang LG, Guo Y, Zhang X, et al. Brain metastasis: experience of the Xi-Jing hospital. Stereotact Funct Neurosurg 2002; 78(2):70–83
23. Li B, Yu J, Suntharalingam M, et al. Comparison of three treatment options for single brain metastasis from lung cancer. Int J Cancer 2000;90(1):37–45
24. Andrews DW, Scott CB, Sperduto PW, et al. Whole brain radiation therapy with or without stereotactic radiosurgery boost for patients with one to three brain metastases: phase III results of the RTOG 9508 randomised trial. Lancet 2004;363(9422):1665–1672
25. Kondziolka D, Patel A, Lunsford LD, Kassam A, Flickinger JC. Stereotactic radiosurgery plus whole brain radiotherapy versus radiotherapy alone for patients with multiple brain metastases. Int J Radiat Oncol Biol Phys 1999;45(2):427–434
26. Sanghavi SN, Miranpuri SS, Chappell R, et al. Radiosurgery for patients with brain metastases: a multi-institutional analysis, stratified by the RTOG recursive partitioning analysis method. Int J Radiat Oncol Biol Phys 2001;51(2):426–434
27. Bindal AK, Bindal RK, Hess KR, et al. Surgery versus radiosurgery in the treatment of brain metastasis. J Neurosurg 1996;84(5):748–754
28. Schöggl A, Kitz K, Reddy M, et al. Defining the role of stereotactic radiosurgery versus microsurgery in the treatment of single brain metastases. Acta Neurochir (Wien) 2000; 142(6):621–626
29. Muacevic A, Wowra B, Siefert A, Tonn JC, Steiger HJ, Kreth FW. Microsurgery plus whole brain irradiation versus Gamma Knife surgery alone for treatment of single metastases to the brain: a randomized controlled multicentre phase III trial. J Neurooncol 2008;87(3):299–307
30. Aoyama H, Shirato H, Tago M, et al. Stereotactic radiosurgery plus whole-brain radiation therapy vs stereotactic radiosurgery alone for treatment of brain metastases: a randomized controlled trial. JAMA 2006;295(21):2483–2491
31. Patchell RA, Regine WF, Renschler M, et al. Comments about the prospective randomized trial by Aoyama et al. Surg Neurol 2006;66(5):459–460
32. Robinet G, Thomas P, Breton JL, et al. Results of a phase III study of early versus delayed whole brain radiotherapy with concurrent cisplatin and vinorelbine combination in inoperable brain metastasis of non-small-cell lung cancer: Groupe Français de Pneumo-Cancérologie (GFPC) Protocol 95-1. Ann Oncol 2001;12(1):59–67
33. Change EL, Wefel JS, Hess KR, Allen PK, et al. Neurocognition in patients with brain metastases treated with radiosurgery or radiosurgery plus whole brain irradiation: a randomized controlled trial. Lancet Oncol 2009;10(11):1037–1044

24

Surgery Followed by Radiosurgery Boost for Metastases

Christopher Jackson, James K. C. Liu, Pablo F. Recinos, and Michael Lim

Cerebral metastases are a common and devastating complication of advanced cancer. With 20 to 40% of cancer patients developing one or more brain metastases, metastatic brain tumors are the most commonly diagnosed brain tumor in adults,[1] and the majority of patients harbor multiple lesions at the time of diagnosis.[2] The incidence of brain metastases has increased over the past decade, likely due to more sensitive screening methods and improved overall survival of patients with advanced cancer.[3,4] Despite advances in screening and systemic disease control, however, the development of brain metastases continues to portend a poor prognosis, with a median survival of 1 to 2 months when treated with steroid therapy alone[5] and 3 to 6 months with the addition of whole brain radiotherapy (WBRT).[6,7] Brain metastases not only represent a significant threat to overall life expectancy, they also frequently result in considerable morbidity and decreased quality of life for patients and increased stress for caregivers.[8]

The risk of developing one or more brain metastases is related to the histology of the primary tumor, with lung cancer, breast cancer, melanoma, and colon cancer most frequently metastasizing to the CNS.[1] Metastatic tumors are classically encountered along the gray–white junction of the cerebral hemispheres, reflecting seeding via hematologic spread. The frequency of metastases at other locations similarly correlates with the relative size and vascularity of these regions, with 15% of metastases occurring in the cerebellum and 5% occurring in the brain stem.[1,9]

Surgical resection followed by WBRT has been the standard of care for patients with symptomatic brain metastases for over 20 years.[10] Postoperative WBRT enhances local control rates within the resection cavity and inhibits development of additional intracranial tumors. Despite these benefits and a clear reduction in the risk of death from neurological causes, WBRT has not been demonstrated to improve overall survival because the majority of patients ultimately succumb to progression of their systemic disease.[11] The treatment of intracranial lesions should, therefore, be focused on palliation of neurological symptoms and maximizing quality of life.

A growing body of literature suggests that, although WBRT improves disease control within the CNS, it may also result in significant neurocognitive sequelae.[12–14] Accordingly, new treatment paradigms strive for durable control of intracranial disease while preserving cognitive function and quality of life. Stereotactic radiosurgery (SRS) allows for delivery of a high dose of conformal radiation therapy in one to five sessions (**Fig. 24.1**). Although there is no Level I evidence available, several groups have retrospectively examined the effectiveness of up-front SRS with deferment of WBRT for salvage therapy. The optimal use of surgical resection, WBRT, and SRS for patients with brain metastases has not yet been determined. This chapter reviews the evidence for select combinations of surgery, WBRT, and SRS, then focuses specifically on the emerging, but controversial, paradigm of surgery followed by SRS boost to the resection cavity.

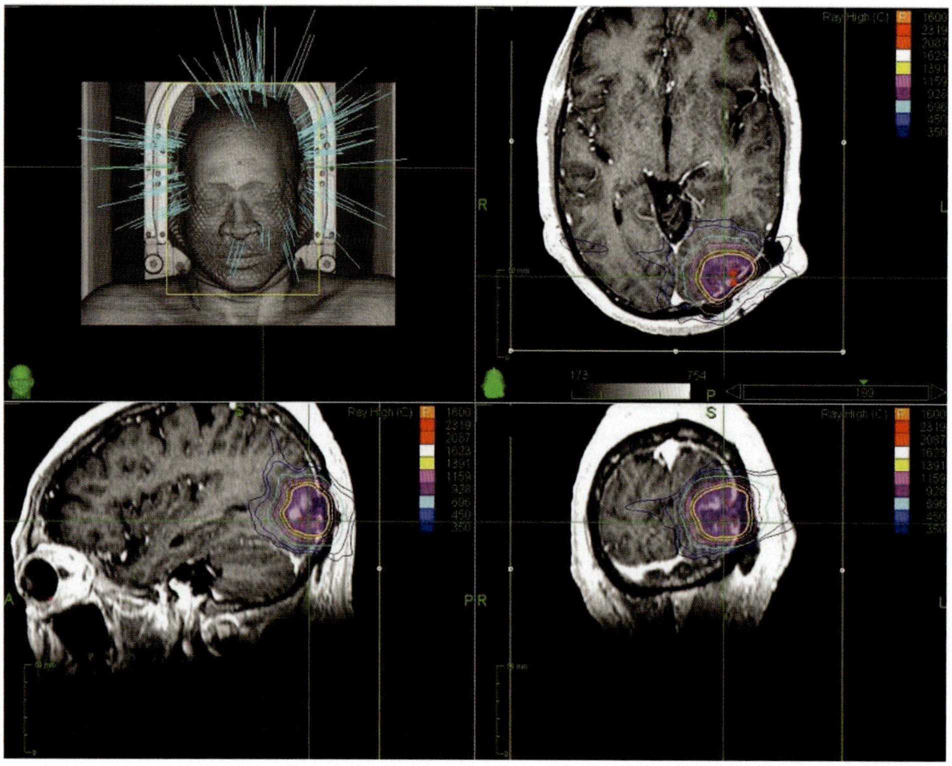

Fig. 24.1 Sample CyberKnife (Accuray, Sunnyvale, CA) plan.

■ Literature Review

Surgical Resection plus WBRT versus WBRT Alone

Even predating the inclusion of surgery, WBRT has been considered the standard of care for patients with brain metastases. The rationale for this practice is based on the principle that, even in the setting of a solitary identifiable lesion, the brain is seeded with multiple micrometastases.[15] Although no fractionation schedule has been reported to increase overall survival, a trend toward improved survival is observed with hyperfractionation.[5] Thus the standard fractionation schedules currently in use are 30 Gy in 10 fractions or 37.5 Gy in 15 fractions.[5,16,17]

Level I Evidence

In 1990, Patchell and colleagues evaluated whether surgical resection followed by WBRT provided superior intracranial disease control compared with WBRT alone.[10] This prospective, randomized trial included 48 patients with histologically confirmed brain metastases. Twenty-five patients received surgery followed by WBRT, whereas 23 patients received a stereotactic biopsy followed by WBRT. Patients with radiosensitive tumors (small-cell lung cancer, germ cell tumors, lymphoma, leukemia, and multiple myeloma) were excluded, as were patients who had received prior radiation therapy or had a poor performance status, that is, a Karnofsky performance scale (KPS) score < 70. The authors reported that surgical resection followed by WBRT improved local control, decreased the incidence of neurological death, and extended overall survival as compared with WBRT alone. In addition, patients receiving surgery maintained a higher performance status (KPS score > 70) longer than patients receiving WBRT alone.

Two subsequent prospective, randomized trials have compared surgical resection followed by WBRT versus WBRT alone. In a trial of 63 patients, Vecht and colleagues reported improved survival with surgical resection followed by WBRT as compared with WBRT alone for patients with a single brain metastasis.[18] Of note, a survival benefit was only observed in patients with stable extracranial disease (median survival 12 months vs 7 months). A third trial by

Mintz and colleagues did not find a difference in survival between the two treatment groups; however, it should be noted that this trial included patients with low KPS scores and extensive extracranial disease.[19] These studies provide Level I evidence for improved outcomes with surgery followed by WBRT versus WBRT alone in patients with good performance status and limited systemic disease (**Table 24.1**).

Level II Evidence

Sause et al initiated a randomized prospective trial comparing radiation alone to surgery plus radiation, but due to difficulty with accruing patients the authors were forced to convert to a nonrandomized trial. The study ultimately consisted of 55 patients receiving radiation alone and 25 patients receiving surgery plus radiation. Despite the loss of randomization, patient characteristics in both populations were generally evenly distributed except for a greater percentage of patients with uncontrolled extracranial disease in the radiation only arm. The authors showed that there was a survival advantage with the addition of surgical intervention. This held true in subset analyses among patients with or without advanced disease, although the difference was not statistically significant in the controlled disease patient population.[20]

Level III Evidence

There are two Level III studies evaluating WBRT as an adjunctive therapy to surgery compared with WBRT alone. Rades et al studied a cohort of 195 patients who received surgery with WBRT (99 patients) or WBRT alone (96 patients). Their study showed a significant survival increase as well as improved local tumor control with the addition of surgical intervention to WBRT.[21] Ampil et al published a similar retrospective study focusing on cerebellar metastases. Their data showed a significant survival advantage with surgical resection in addition to WBRT for metastases that did not originate from the lung.[22]

Surgical Resection plus WBRT versus Surgical Resection Alone

Level I Evidence

A follow-up study by Patchell and colleagues evaluated the role of WBRT in patients undergoing surgery for brain metastases.[11] The study included 95 patients with a single brain metastasis in whom a radiographic gross total resection was achieved. These patients were randomized postoperatively to WBRT (49 patients) or observation (46 patients). The primary end point was recurrence within the resection cavity. Secondary end points included overall survival, cause of death, and functional status. This study found that patients receiving surgery followed by WBRT had a lower incidence of recurrence within the resection cavity, were at a lower risk of forming additional brain metastases, and died less frequently from neurological causes; however, there was no difference observed in overall survival or the length of time that patients remained functionally independent. Subsequent studies have similarly failed to demonstrate a survival benefit of WBRT versus surgery alone despite consistently reporting improved control of local and distant CNS disease.[23]

Table 24.1 Surgery followed by WRBT versus surgery alone

Study	No. patients	Treatment	Local control	Distant intracranial metastases	Median survival
Patchell et al 1998[11]	95	Surgery + WBRT vs surgery	10% vs 46%	18% vs 70%	48 wk vs 43 wk
Mintz et al 1996[23]	84	Surgery + WBRT vs WBRT	NA	NA	5.6 mo vs 6.3 mo
Vecht et al 1993[18]	63	Surgery + WBRT vs WBRT	NA	NA	7 mo vs 12 mo
Patchell et al 1990[10]	48	Surgery + WBRT vs WBRT	20% vs 52%	NA	40 wk vs 15 wk

Abbreviations: NA, not applicable; WBRT, whole brain radiotherapy.

Level II Evidence

There is no Level II evidence comparing surgical resection plus WBRT to surgery alone.

Level III Evidence

Three retrospective cohort studies have been published examining the effects of adding WBRT to surgical resection for brain metastasis. All three studies showed increased median survival with the addition of WBRT,[24,25] although clinical significance was only present in one of the studies.[26]

Recommendations for Surgery and WBRT

1. The addition of surgery to WBRT improves local tumor control compared with WBRT alone (Grade 1A Recommendation, Level I Evidence).
2. The addition of WBRT to surgery improves local tumor control compared with surgery alone (Grade 1A Recommendation, Level I Evidence).
3. The addition of surgery to WBRT improves overall survival in patients with limited extracranial disease (Grade 1C Recommendation, Level III Evidence).
4. The addition of WBRT to surgery improves overall survival in patients with limited extracranial disease (Grade 1C Recommendation, Level III Evidence).

Surgical Resection plus Adjuvant Stereotactic Radiosurgery

Several groups have evaluated the effectiveness of WBRT plus SRS as compared with SRS alone in the absence of surgery. A randomized trial of 132 patients with one to four brain metastases by Aoyama and colleagues found that the addition of up-front WBRT to SRS did not improve overall survival compared with SRS alone.[15] More importantly, the authors reported no difference in local control rate, functional status, or incidence of neurological death between the two groups. Corroborating previous studies of surgery and WBRT, patients in the SRS only arm were at a greater risk of developing additional intracranial metastases, and 29/67 patients in the SRS only arm required WBRT salvage therapy.

Given the lack of a survival benefit with up-front WBRT and the cognitive sparing afforded by SRS, a growing number of institutions have transitioned to SRS boost to the resection cavity in lieu of postoperative WBRT for patients undergoing surgery for brain metastases. This approach has the theoretical benefit of harnessing the enhanced local control afforded by postoperative radiation therapy while sparing—or at least delaying—exposure of healthy brain tissue to high doses of radiation. As previously noted, the primary drawback of withholding up-front WBRT is an increased risk of new, additional intracranial metastases; however, it is unclear whether these lesions, which frequently can be controlled with SRS ± salvage WBRT, negatively impact quality of life or overall survival. Currently, there are no prospective trials comparing surgery plus WBRT to surgery plus SRS. There are, however, several retrospective studies reporting outcomes for patients receiving surgery followed by SRS boost to the resection cavity.

Level I and Level II Evidence

There is no Level I or Level II evidence comparing SRS boost to WBRT.

Level III Evidence

In 2008, Mathieu and colleagues reported on a series of 40 patients with one to seven brain metastases who underwent surgery of a single lesion due to large tumor size (> 3 cm), to obtain a histological diagnosis, or to relieve neurological symptoms.[27] Gross total resection was achieved in 80% of patients based on postoperative MRI, and systemic disease was active in 58% of patients, with the remainder considered inactive or in remission at the time of surgery. At a median of 4 weeks postresection, patients received SRS to the resection cavity as well as any additional lesions identified at the time of SRS planning. Local control was reported for 73% of patients, with a median follow-up of 13 months. New metastases were reported in 54% of patients, and median overall survival was 13 months. No variables were found to be associated with improved local control or increased survival. Although the authors concluded that these findings support SRS boost to the resection cavity as a viable option for controlling local disease, they also noted that surgical resection followed by SRS did not improve local control rates compared with those previously reported for SRS alone.[28–30] Of note, there are no published studies comparing SRS alone versus surgery followed by SRS. Based on the results of this study, however, it is reasonable to conclude that, although SRS to the resection cavity enhances local control in patients in whom surgery is indicated, surgery should not be undertaken with the expectation of improving local control rates beyond SRS alone.

In the same year that Mathieu and colleagues reported their series, Soltys and colleagues reported on 72 patients (76 resection cavities) treated with SRS boost.[31] The patients in this series had one to four brain metastases, and gross total resection was achieved in 85%. The primary tumor was under control in 72% of patients and 51% had active extracranial disease. A single SRS session was used to treat 78% of targets, whereas 9% were treated in two sessions, 12% were treated in 3 sessions, and 1% were treated in five sessions. Lesions were treated with a median of 16 Gy or biological equivalent dose. In this study, local control was reported in 79% of patients at 12 months. Additional lesions developed in 49% of patients, and 31% of these received WBRT salvage either alone or in combination with surgery or SRS. Of note, the remaining 56% of patients with distant recurrence achieved intracranial disease control with SRS salvage alone. Median survival was 15 months for these patients. Improved local control was found to be associated with conformality index. Based on these findings, the authors recommended including a 2 mm margin around the resection cavity.

The following year, Karlovits and colleagues updated their series of 52 patients with one to four lesions who received SRS boost to a single resection cavity.[32] A median dose of 15 Gy was delivered to the resection cavity. Local control was achieved in 92% of lesions, whereas 44% of patients developed additional intracranial metastases and 31% ultimately received WBRT salvage. No factors were associated with an increased risk of local recurrence or WBRT salvage; however, the conformality index was not included in the analysis. Median survival for this cohort was 15 months.

Jagannathan and colleagues reported on a series of 47 patients who underwent SRS boost to the resection cavity following gross total resection in 2009.[33] End points for this study were defined as radiographic control of treated tumors, KPS performance status, and overall survival. Median follow-up was 10 months. Local tumor control was achieved in 94% of patients, with a median of 19 Gy delivered to the resection cavity. Seventy-two percent of patients developed additional intracranial lesions. These lesions were initially treated with SRS and 28% ultimately required WBRT. Median overall survival was 10 months and the median KPS score was 80 (range 40 to 100) at the time of last clinical evaluation. Recurrence within the resection cavity was associated with larger tumor volumes, and control of systemic disease was the only variable associated with improved survival.

Also in 2009, Do and colleagues reported on a series of 30 patients treated either with SRS in a single session or stereotactic radiotherapy (SRT) in four to six fractions.[34] A dose of 15 to 18 Gy was delivered with SRS, and a cumulative dose of 22.0 to 27.5 Gy was delivered for SRT using a linear accelerator-based system. Margins of 1 and 3 mm were included for SRS and SRT, respectively. Using these techniques, control within the resection cavity was achieved in 87% of targets, and 63% of patients developed additional intracranial metastases. WBRT salvage therapy was required in 47% of patients, and the median survival was 12 months.

The highest reported local control rate comes from a small series by Hwang and colleagues.[35] These authors reported no recurrences within the resection cavity and a median survival of 15 months. The authors compared their cohort to a small number of case-matched controls receiving surgery followed by WBRT and noted a trend toward longer survival in the SRS group. Although severely limited by a lack of follow-up and failure to account for known prognostic factors, including control of systemic disease, this study is nevertheless notable for its high local control rate and the association of regional recurrence with worse survival outcomes.

Jensen and colleagues reported on their experience with a series of 106 patients (112 targets).[36] Lesions were treated with a median dose of 17 Gy. The local tumor control rate at 12 months was 80%. WBRT salvage therapy was required in 37% of patients due to either local or distant failure. Median overall survival was 11 months. Large tumor size (> 3 cm) was the only variable associated with an increased risk of local disease recurrence. A recent study by Hartford and colleagues also reported an increased risk of local recurrence for tumors > 3 cm in diameter.[37] Additionally, these authors found that larger tumor size was associated with an increase of distant failure, but not difference in overall survival, suggesting effective salvage therapy even in the setting of large lesions. Perhaps not surprisingly, another recent study found that a larger number of brain metastases at the time of treatment and melanoma histology carried a greater risk of distant failure.[38] Studies providing Level III evidence for surgery followed by SRS are summarized in **Table 24.2**.

Whole-Brain Radiotherapy versus Stereotactic Radiosurgery: Cognitive Function

The aforementioned studies provide a case for utilizing SRS as an adjunct to surgical resection, given available close monitoring for required boost treatments. One of the major drawbacks of WBRT is neurocognitive decline, which has been noted in several studies.[12,13] Furthermore, studies have correlated diminished quality of life with decreases in neurocognition, and as median survival increases with more effective therapy, this important sequela of treatment warrants careful consideration.[39]

The clinically significant effects of WBRT on neurocognition, however, remain controversial. It appears that neurocognitive decline as a result of WBRT primarily affects memory,[40,41] which needs to be weighed against an increased risk for recurrence of disease and the need for further treatment. One of the major difficulties in assessing cognitive decline is that

Table 24.2 Level III evidence for surgery followed by SRS boost

Authors	Number of patients	Local control	Development of additional metastases	WBRT salvage	Median survival (months)
Hartford et al 2012[37]	47	86%	63%	45%	>12
Robbins et al 2012[44]	85	81%	55%	35%	12.1
Choi et al 2012[38]	112	92%	54%	28%	17
Jensen et al 2011[36]	106	80%	65%	37%	11
Hwang et al 2010[35]	25	100%	28%	Not Reported	15
Do et al 2009[34]	30	87%	63%	47%	12
Jagannathan et al 2009[33]	47	94%	72%	28%	10
Karlovits et al 2009[32]	52	92%	44%	31%	15
Soltys et al 2008[31]	72	79%	49%	21%	15
Mathieu et al 2008[27]	40	73%	54%	16%	13

Expert Recommendations

Number of metastases	Tumor size (cm)	Symptoms and/or edema	Recommendations
1	< 3	No	SRS alone
1	< 3	Yes	Surgery + SRS
1	> 3	No	Surgery + SRS
1	> 3	Yes	Surgery + SRS
2–4	> 2.5	Yes	Surgery for symptomatic or large lesions followed by SRS for resected and unresected lesions
2–4	< 2.5	No	SRS alone
> 4	–	–	Whole brain radiation

patients receiving radiation treatments often have reduced neurocognition at baseline, which can skew future testing.[41,42] This likely is attributable to systemic therapeutic interventions such as chemotherapy and steroid use, or other malignancy-associated medical comorbidities, including paraneoplastic syndromes.[42]

Although early studies focused on the oncological benefits of WBRT, the cognitive effects of exposing healthy brain tissue to high doses of radiation have recently become a point of growing concern. Manifestations of neurotoxicity from WBRT range from mild inattention, memory loss, and emotional disturbances to dementia, stupor, and coma.[5] These effects are frequently progressive and irreversible, leading to a significant detriment to quality of life, especially in patients with otherwise good functional status and systemic disease control at the time of diagnosis of a brain metastasis. In 1989, DeAngelis and colleagues reported on 12 patients who developed progressive cognitive decline after receiving WBRT alone or WBRT following surgical resection.[13] Of note, the authors used higher dose fractions (3 to 6 Gy) than the current standard of care. A more recent trial including 58 patients who received lower WBRT doses in combination with SRS, however, was stopped early due to a significant decline in learning and memory 4 months after WBRT.[12] In a third study that compares neurocognition before and after WBRT, Welzel et al report a significant decline only in verbal memory 6 to 8 weeks following radiation treatment.[41]

A variety of alternative regimens have been developed in an attempt to improve cognitive outcomes without compromising intracranial disease control. For example, hippocampal-sparing WBRT with or without SRS boost, intensity-modulated radiotherapy (IMRT), radiosensitizing agents, and altered dose fractionation schemes have all shown promise and are currently under investigation in clinical trials.[43]

Summary and Conclusions

There is currently no Level I evidence comparing SRS boost to the resection cavity versus WBRT after surgery in the treatment of brain metastases. Until such evidence is available, up-front WBRT should be considered the standard of care for the majority of patients with brain metastases. Several retrospective series (Level III), however, indicate that SRS boost to the resection cavity with WBRT reserved for salvage therapy may provide local control and overall survival equivalent to that with up-front WBRT in select patients. The patients most likely to benefit from this strategy have limited intracranial disease, high functional status, and good systemic disease control. In these patients, deferring WBRT may spare radiation-associated neurotoxicity, preserving cognitive function and quality of life. It should be noted, however, that deferring up-front WBRT places these patients at an increased risk of developing intracranial lesions at distant sites. In this light, it should be noted that the cognitive effects of increased intracranial disease burden have not been directly compared with the cognitive effects of WBRT. Nevertheless, available evidence suggests that SRS boost to the resection cavity is a viable option for select patients who wish to delay or avoid WBRT. Future prospective, randomized studies will be necessary to formally evaluate the effectiveness of this approach versus standard of care and determine how SRS, WBRT, and surgery can best be employed to achieve optimal disease control while preserving cognitive function.

References

1. Patchell RA. The management of brain metastases. Cancer Treat Rev 2003;29(6):533–540
2. Sze G, Milano E, Johnson C, Heier L. Detection of brain metastases: comparison of contrast-enhanced MR with unenhanced MR and enhanced CT. AJNR Am J Neuroradiol 1990; 11(4):785–791
3. Weil RJ. Does trastuzumab increase the risk of isolated central nervous system metastases in patients with breast cancer? Nat Clin Pract Oncol 2006;3(5):236–237
4. Gondi V, Mehta MP. Novel insights into the management of brain metastases. Curr Opin Neurol 2010;23(6):556–562
5. Abe E, Aoyama H. The role of whole brain radiation therapy for the management of brain metastases in the era of stereotactic radiosurgery. Curr Oncol Rep 2012;14(1):79–84
6. Bradley KA, Mehta MP. Management of brain metastases. Semin Oncol 2004;31(5):693–701
7. Gaspar LE, Mehta MP, Patchell RA, et al. The role of whole brain radiation therapy in the management of newly diagnosed brain metastases: a systematic review and evidence-based clinical practice guideline. J Neurooncol 2010;96(1):17–32
8. Koay E, Sulman EP. Management of brain metastasis: past lessons, modern management, and future considerations. Curr Oncol Rep 2012;14(1):70–78
9. Delattre JY, Krol G, Thaler HT, Posner JB. Distribution of brain metastases. Arch Neurol 1988;45(7):741–744
10. Patchell RA, Tibbs PA, Walsh JW, et al. A randomized trial of surgery in the treatment of single metastases to the brain. N Engl J Med 1990;322(8):494–500
11. Patchell RA, Tibbs PA, Regine WF, et al. Postoperative radiotherapy in the treatment of single metastases to the brain: a randomized trial. JAMA 1998;280(17):1485–1489
12. Chang EL, Wefel JS, Hess KR, et al. Neurocognition in patients with brain metastases treated with radiosurgery or radiosurgery plus whole-brain irradiation: a randomised controlled trial. Lancet Oncol 2009;10(11):1037–1044
13. DeAngelis LM, Delattre JY, Posner JB. Radiation-induced dementia in patients cured of brain metastases. Neurology 1989; 39(6):789–796
14. Crossen JR, Garwood D, Glatstein E, Neuwelt EA. Neurobehavioral sequelae of cranial irradiation in adults: a review of radiation-induced encephalopathy. J Clin Oncol 1994; 12(3):627–642
15. Aoyama H, Shirato H, Tago M, et al. Stereotactic radiosurgery plus whole-brain radiation therapy vs stereotactic radiosurgery alone for treatment of brain metastases: a randomized controlled trial. JAMA 2006;295(21):2483–2491
16. Epstein BE, Scott CB, Sause WT, et al. Improved survival duration in patients with unresected solitary brain metastasis using accelerated hyperfractionated radiation therapy at total doses of 54.4 gray and greater. Results of Radiation Therapy Oncology Group 85-28. Cancer 1993;71(4):1362–1367
17. Murray KJ, Scott C, Greenberg HM, et al. A randomized phase III study of accelerated hyperfractionation versus standard in patients with unresected brain metastases: a report of the Radiation Therapy Oncology Group (RTOG) 9104. Int J Radiat Oncol Biol Phys 1997;39(3):571–574
18. Vecht CJ, Haaxma-Reiche H, Noordijk EM, et al. Treatment of single brain metastasis: radiotherapy alone or combined with neurosurgery? Ann Neurol 1993;33(6):583–590
19. Ellis TL, Neal MT, Chan MD. The role of surgery, radiosurgery and whole brain radiation therapy in the management of patients with metastatic brain tumors. Int J Surg Oncol 2012; 2012:952345. doi: 10.1155/2012/952345. Epub 2011 Oct 16
20. Sause WT, Crowley JJ, Morantz R, et al. Solitary brain metastasis: results of an RTOG/SWOG protocol evaluation surgery + RT versus RT alone. Am J Clin Oncol 1990;13(5):427–432
21. Rades D, Kueter JD, Pluemer A, Veninga T, Schild SE. A matched-pair analysis comparing whole-brain radiotherapy plus stereotactic radiosurgery versus surgery plus whole-brain radiotherapy and a boost to the metastatic site for one or two brain metastases. Int J Radiat Oncol Biol Phys 2009; 73(4):1077–1081
22. Ampil FL, Nanda A, Willis BK, Nandy I, Meehan R. Metastatic disease in the cerebellum. The LSU experience in 1981-1993. Am J Clin Oncol 1996;19(5):509–511
23. Mintz AH, Kestle J, Rathbone MP, et al. A randomized trial to assess the efficacy of surgery in addition to radiotherapy in patients with a single cerebral metastasis. Cancer 1996;78(7):1470–1476

24. Armstrong JG, Wronski M, Galicich J, Arbit E, Leibel SA, Burt M. Postoperative radiation for lung cancer metastatic to the brain. J Clin Oncol 1994;12(11):2340–2344
25. Hagen NA, Cirrincione C, Thaler HT, DeAngelis LM. The role of radiation therapy following resection of single brain metastasis from melanoma. Neurology 1990;40(1):158–160
26. Skibber JM, Soong SJ, Austin L, Balch CM, Sawaya RE. Cranial irradiation after surgical excision of brain metastases in melanoma patients. Ann Surg Oncol 1996;3(2):118–123
27. Mathieu D, Kondziolka D, Flickinger JC, et al. Tumor bed radiosurgery after resection of cerebral metastases. Neurosurgery 2008;62(4):817–823
28. Gerosa M, Nicolato A, Foroni R, et al. Gamma knife radiosurgery for brain metastases: a primary therapeutic option. J Neurosurg 2002;97(5, Suppl):515–524
29. Hasegawa T, Kondziolka D, Flickinger JC, Germanwala A, Lunsford LD. Brain metastases treated with radiosurgery alone: an alternative to whole brain radiotherapy? Neurosurgery 2003;52(6):1318–1326
30. Petrovich Z, Yu C, Giannotta SL, O'Day S, Apuzzo ML. Survival and pattern of failure in brain metastasis treated with stereotactic gamma knife radiosurgery. J Neurosurg 2002;97(5, Suppl):499–506
31. Soltys SG, Adler JR, Lipani JD, et al. Stereotactic radiosurgery of the postoperative resection cavity for brain metastases. Int J Radiat Oncol Biol Phys 2008;70(1):187–193
32. Karlovits BJ, Quigley MR, Karlovits SM, et al. Stereotactic radiosurgery boost to the resection bed for oligometastatic brain disease: challenging the tradition of adjuvant whole-brain radiotherapy. Neurosurg Focus 2009;27(6):E7
33. Jagannathan J, Yen CP, Ray DK, et al. Gamma Knife radiosurgery to the surgical cavity following resection of brain metastases. J Neurosurg 2009;111(3):431–438
34. Do L, Pezner R, Radany E, Liu A, Staud C, Badie B. Resection followed by stereotactic radiosurgery to resection cavity for intracranial metastases. Int J Radiat Oncol Biol Phys 2009;73(2):486–491
35. Hwang SW, Abozed MM, Hale A, et al. Adjuvant Gamma Knife radiosurgery following surgical resection of brain metastases: a 9-year retrospective cohort study. J Neurooncol 2010;98(1):77–82
36. Jensen CA, Chan MD, McCoy TP, et al. Cavity-directed radiosurgery as adjuvant therapy after resection of a brain metastasis. J Neurosurg 2011;114(6):1585–1591
37. Hartford AC, Paravati AJ, Spire WJ, et al. Postoperative stereotactic radiosurgery without whole-brain radiation therapy for brain metastases: potential role of preoperative tumor size. Int J Radiat Oncol Biol Phys 2012;(Jul):12
38. Choi CY, Chang SD, Gibbs IC, et al. Stereotactic radiosurgery of the postoperative resection cavity for brain metastases: prospective evaluation of target margin on tumor control. Int J Radiat Oncol Biol Phys 2012;84(2):336–342
39. Li J, Bentzen SM, Li J, Renschler M, Mehta MP. Relationship between neurocognitive function and quality of life after whole-brain radiotherapy in patients with brain metastasis. Int J Radiat Oncol Biol Phys 2008;71(1):64–70
40. Sun A, Bae K, Gore EM, et al. Phase III trial of prophylactic cranial irradiation compared with observation in patients with locally advanced non-small-cell lung cancer: neurocognitive and quality-of-life analysis. J Clin Oncol 2011;29(3):279–286
41. Welzel G, Fleckenstein K, Mai SK, Hermann B, Kraus-Tiefenbacher U, Wenz F. Acute neurocognitive impairment during cranial radiation therapy in patients with intracranial tumors. Strahlenther Onkol 2008;184(12):647–654
42. Grosshans DR, Meyers CA, Allen PK, Davenport SD, Komaki R. Neurocognitive function in patients with small cell lung cancer: effect of prophylactic cranial irradiation. Cancer 2008;112(3):589–595
43. Chargari C, Campana F, Pierga JY, et al. Whole-brain radiation therapy in breast cancer patients with brain metastases. Nat Rev Clin Oncol 2010;7(11):632–640
44. Robbins JR, Ryu S, Kalkanis S, et al. Radiosurgery to the surgical cavity as adjuvant therapy for resected brain metastasis. Neurosurgery 2012;71(5):937–943

25

The Role of Surgery in Patients Presenting with Multiple Metastases

J. Bradley Elder and E. Antonio Chiocca

Brain metastases represent up to 50% of all newly diagnosed intracranial neoplasms and are the most common type of brain tumor in adults.[1,2] Approximately 1.4 million patients are diagnosed with cancer per year in the United States.[3] Ten to forty percent of cancer patients will be diagnosed with brain metastases at some point during the course of their disease, and metastasis to the brain is the most common neurological manifestation of cancer.[4,5] Introductory comments in papers from 1993 and 2011 describe an incidence of brain metastasis in the United States of 82,000, and 170,000, respectively.[6,7] Currently, between 150,000 and 200,000 patients per year in the United States are diagnosed with brain metastases, and the incidence is likely to continue to rise in the future due to multiple factors, such as the overall aging of our population.[8] Patients with many types of cancer are living longer due to improved treatment of their primary disease. Novel therapeutic agents and improved surveillance and neurological imaging, as well as an improving understanding of cancer biology, have improved both quality and quantity of life for many patients. Unfortunately, the blood–brain barrier may continue to hinder brain penetrance of systemic therapies. A better understanding of the variables important for managing brain metastases is key to optimizing care for these patients and determining which patients will benefit from surgery.

The mainstays of treatment for cerebral metastases are radiation and surgery. Other chapters review the role of radiation and/or surgery for metastases in other clinical scenarios, such as solitary metastasis. There is a great deal of debate but a paucity of literature on the role of surgery in patients presenting with multiple metastases. A brief discussion is presented as a preface for understanding the basis for current concepts in surgical intervention for multiple brain metastases. This chapter presents literature that documents the evolution of surgery as a treatment for brain metastases. The focus is published evidence that specifically evaluates surgery for multiple cerebral metastases, with an emphasis on factors important to making clinical decisions. The primary goal is to present the most current and relevant evidence regarding the utility of surgery in patients with multiple cerebral metastases.

Presentation

Brain metastases are typically a late development in the course of a patient's disease. Approximately 80% of brain metastases are diagnosed in patients with known cancer, whereas 20% are diagnosed either synchronously (within 2 months of diagnosis of the primary cancer) or precociously (found in patients with no known primary cancer).[7] Clinically, patients with brain metastases typically present with headache. Other common presenting symptoms include seizure and new neurological deficit, such as visual changes, motor weakness, and aphasia.[9] Magnetic resonance imaging (MRI) with contrast is the gold standard for diagnosing brain lesions because computed tomography (CT) misses up to one third of brain lesions, and evaluation of the number of lesions is an important component in determining optimal therapy.[4] Hemispheric lesions are most common, and the frontal lobe is the most frequently affected anatomical location.[9]

■ Background

Historically, patients diagnosed with brain metastases survived only 4 to 6 weeks after diagnosis. The use of corticosteroids may improve survival to ~ 2 months. Adding whole-brain radiation therapy (WBRT) can increase overall survival to ~ 4 to 6 months, and the regimen of corticosteroids and WBRT was the standard of care for many years.[10,11] Over the last few decades, widespread implementation of CT and MRI has allowed for improved diagnosis of patients with brain metastases. At the same time, improved microsurgical techniques allowed surgery to become a safer and increasingly viable option for patients with brain metastases.[12] Initial studies focused on patients with solitary metastases. More recently, surgery in patients with multiple metastases has been evaluated. Advances in radiation techniques have also impacted treatment strategies in patients with brain metastases.

Solitary Metastases

Studies describing surgical treatment of metastatic tumors initially described resection of solitary metastases followed by WBRT.[13–15] After multiple case series demonstrated increased overall survival in a subset of patients who underwent surgery for solitary brain metastasis, prospective clinical trials were performed that further investigated the role of surgery prior to radiation for solitary brain metastases (**Table 25.1**). One study demonstrated improved local tumor control (20% vs 52%) and overall survival (40 weeks vs 15 weeks), as well as prolonged functional independence (38 weeks vs 8 weeks) in the surgical group compared with the radiation group.[16] A different study found that patients with stable extracranial disease who underwent surgical resection of a solitary metastasis followed by WBRT had prolonged overall survival (12 months vs 7 months) and functional independence (9 months vs 4 months) compared with patients who received only WBRT. Differences in overall survival and functional independence were not significantly different among patients with progressive systemic disease.[17] In a third randomized trial, Mintz et al demonstrated

Table 25.1 Prospective clinical trials comparing surgery + WBRT with WBRT alone for patients with solitary metastases

Study	No. patients	Median survival benefit surgery + WBRT vs WBRT
Patchell et al 1990[16]	47	40 wk vs 15 wk
Vecht et al 1993[17]	63	12 mo vs 7 mo (stable systemic disease)
Mintz et al 1996[18]	84	None

Abbreviation: WBRT, whole-brain radiotherapy.

no differences in overall survival.[18] One difference in this study was that patients with a Karnofsky performance scale (KPS) score of 50 and higher were included, whereas the other two trials excluded patients with KPS scores < 70. Another possible reason for the different results was that 73% of patients in the third trial had extracranial metastases or uncontrolled systemic disease.

The results from the first two randomized, prospective trials seemed to reaffirm results from retrospective studies by eliminating selection bias and clearly demonstrated a survival benefit for surgical resection of solitary metastasis. On the basis of this Level I evidence, surgical resection is considered the best management of patients with solitary, surgically accessible metastases and a KPS score of at least 70 (**Fig. 25.1**).[11] These studies also served as a basis for subsequent work investigating an expanded role of surgery in patients with recurrent and multiple metastases.

Stereotactic Radiosurgery

In recent years, stereotactic radiosurgery (SRS) has increasingly replaced WBRT for treating brain metastases. Efficacy of this technique has been demonstrated in multiple studies, and the utility of SRS alone in treating solitary, small metastases has been postulated. SRS with or without WBRT is described in the up-front treatment of tumors up to 3 cm in size.[4] Studies have compared SRS to surgical resection for solitary metastases, with mixed results. For example, Auchter et al described similar overall survival, local recurrence rates, and neurological causes of death when comparing SRS to surgery followed by WBRT. The authors concluded that SRS alone as treatment for small, solitary metastases was potentially a safer and more cost-effective method of tumor control.[19] Bindal et al included patients with

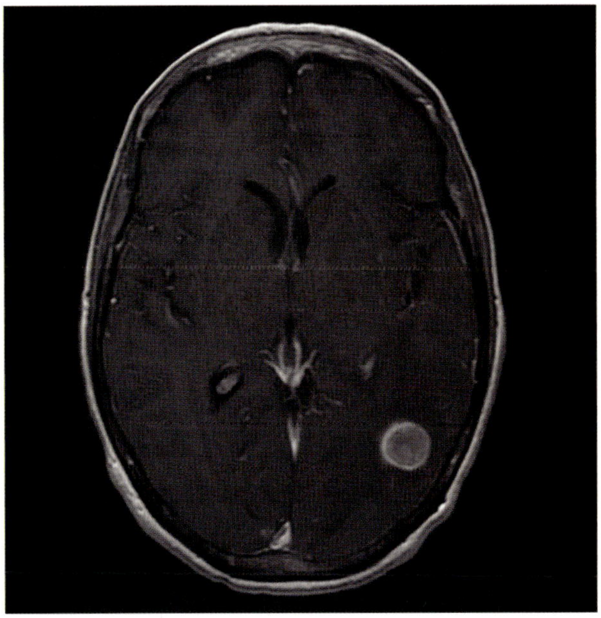

Fig. 25.1 Axial, T1-weighted, contrast-enhanced magnetic resonance imaging demonstrating a left posterior temporal lesion. The patient was neurologically intact and underwent surgical resection of the non-small-cell lung cancer metastasis.

multiple metastases in their analysis and found improved local tumor control and prolonged overall survival (16.4 months vs 7.5 months) in patients treated with surgical resection followed by WBRT compared with patients treated with SRS alone. The higher mortality rate noted in the SRS group was due to progression of brain metastases rather than progression of systemic disease.[20] A recent prospective trial compared resection followed by WBRT with SRS alone in patients with solitary, resectable metastases < 3 cm. The authors found no significant differences in overall survival or local tumor control between the groups. SRS was associated with a lower rate of complications compared with surgery, but significantly more distant recurrences requiring salvage radiation treatment were seen with SRS.[21] However, a different prospective study described higher local recurrences in patients treated with SRS alone.[4] SRS is also used in patients with multiple lesions, although the data are less robust and there are no randomized, prospective trials focusing on SRS in patients with multiple brain metastases. SRS in the up-front treatment of multiple lesions, re-treatment of recurrent lesions, and use of postoperative radiation of resection cavities are also described.[22–24] Other chapters contain detailed analyses of these clinical scenarios, and understanding this literature is important when one is weighing the risks and benefits of surgical resection of one or more brain metastases.

■ Clinical Considerations

Recursive Partitioning Analysis Classification System

There are several factors to consider when evaluating a patient for surgery. Risk stratification and outcome analysis depend on identifying important prognostic variables. Previous work identified variables such as KPS scores < 70, neurological or cognitive deficits, other sites of metastasis, and short interval from diagnosis of primary tumor to brain metastases as significant negative prognostic indicators.[19,25,26] A review of the Radiation Therapy Oncology Group (RTOG) database published in 1997 retrospectively evaluated 1,200 patients with brain metastases to determine variables important for predicting outcome. The authors used statistical methodology called recursive partitioning analysis (RPA) and ultimately organized patients into three classifications based on outcome (**Table 25.2**).[9] A patient's age, KPS score, extracranial disease status (controlled or progressing), and the presence of metastases outside of the brain were found to be important prognostic variables. KPS scores < 70 automatically placed patients into RPA class 3, in which median survival was 2.3 months. Younger patients (< age 65) with KPS scores of at least 70, controlled systemic disease, and no tumor other than the primary lesion and the brain metastases had a median survival of 7.1 months. All other patients were RPA class 2. Use of the RPA classification system has become widespread and an important consideration when one is evaluating a patient's surgical candidacy.[27]

Anatomical Location

Another primary factor in weighing surgical options is the anatomical location of the lesion. The vast majority of metastases are located in surgically accessible areas, such as the frontal, temporal, parietal, and

Table 25.2 Recursive partitioning analysis (RPA) classification[9]

RPA class	1	2	3
Median survival	7.1 mo	4.2 mo	2.3 mo
Karnofsky performance scale score	≥ 70	All other patients	≤ 70
Age	< 65		
Extracranial disease	Controlled		
Metastases	Brain only		

occipital lobes and the cerebellum. Approximately 2% are located in deeper structures, such as the brainstem (**Fig. 25.2**) or basal ganglia.[9] Although microsurgical approaches have improved significantly over the last few decades, surgery for lesions in or near eloquent areas, or deep structures such as the basal ganglia and brainstem, is associated with higher morbidity.[28] However, alternative options, such as WBRT or chemotherapy, may be less effective, and SRS may incur radiation injury or delay resolution of associated mass effect and edema.

Primary Tumor

Among adult patients with brain metastases, the most common primary cancers are lung (50 to 60%), breast (10 to 20%), melanoma (5 to 15%), kidney, and colon.[9,29,30] Melanoma has the highest tendency to metastasize to the brain.[4] The histology of the primary tumor impacts decisions regarding surgery largely in relation to its sensitivity to radiation. Some tumor types, such as lymphoma and small-cell lung cancer, are exquisitely sensitive to radiation, and surgical intervention is largely limited to biopsy. Tumors that are considered radiation resistant include renal cell carcinoma, melanoma, and sarcomas, and aggressive surgical management is ideal if possible. In fact, progressive brain disease is closely associated with mortality in patients with melanoma and sarcoma treated with SRS alone.[23] Tumors with intermediate radiation sensitivity include breast and non-small-cell lung cancers and are commonly managed with a combined surgical and radiation approach.[11]

Recurrent Metastases

Patients with recurrent metastases have likely been through both surgery and adjuvant radiation. In these cases, surgical intervention may be warranted for solitary recurrent disease, either recurrence of a solitary tumor or progression of only one of multiple metastases (**Fig. 25.3**). Recurrence at the original surgical site accounts for approximately two thirds of cases, whereas new or progressive lesions at other sites account for the remaining one third. Patients who are candidates for repeat surgery may have improved survival compared with patients managed nonsurgically.[31] Surgery may also help in differentiating radiation necrosis from recurrent disease.[4] Bindal et al retrospectively evaluated 48 patients who underwent surgery for recurrent brain metastases.[32] The average time from first surgery to recurrence was 6.7 months. Pattern of recurrence was local (n = 30), distant (n = 16), or both (n = 2). Median survival after the second surgery was 11.5 months. Multivariate analysis revealed negative prognostic factors, such as KPS scores ≤ 70, time to recurrence < 4 months, age < 40 years, and a primary tumor that was breast cancer or melanoma. Of the 48 patients, 26 developed a second recurrence, and 17 underwent another operation. The median survival for these patients was 8.6 months, compared with 2.8 months for patients who did not undergo surgery. The authors concluded that reoperation represented a safe and effective treatment strategy. As with other studies, similar prognostic variables helped predict which patients were good candidates for surgery.

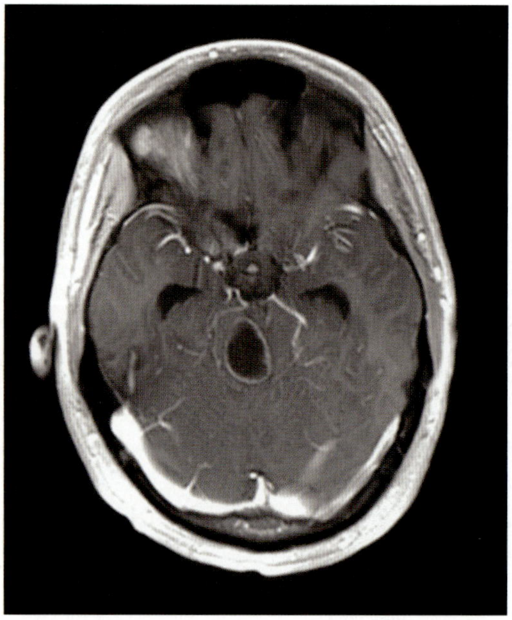

Fig. 25.2 Magnetic resonance imaging demonstrates cystic, non-small-cell lung cancer metastasis in the brainstem.

Multiple Metastases

Although the preceding evidence documents current concepts regarding treatment of solitary lesions, around 50% of patients present with multiple brain metastases. Autopsy studies indicate that 60 to 85% of patients with brain metastases have multiple lesions.[6] In the past, multiple brain lesions represented a relative contraindication to surgery due to the presumed poor survival of these patients. However, application of principles learned in studies regarding surgery for solitary lesions has yielded evidence suggesting that patients with multiple tumors may derive similar benefit from surgical resection as patients with solitary lesions. Currently, there is no Level I evidence regarding the surgical treatment of patients with multiple brain metastases.[11] However, some retrospective reviews have indicated a role for surgery in select patients.

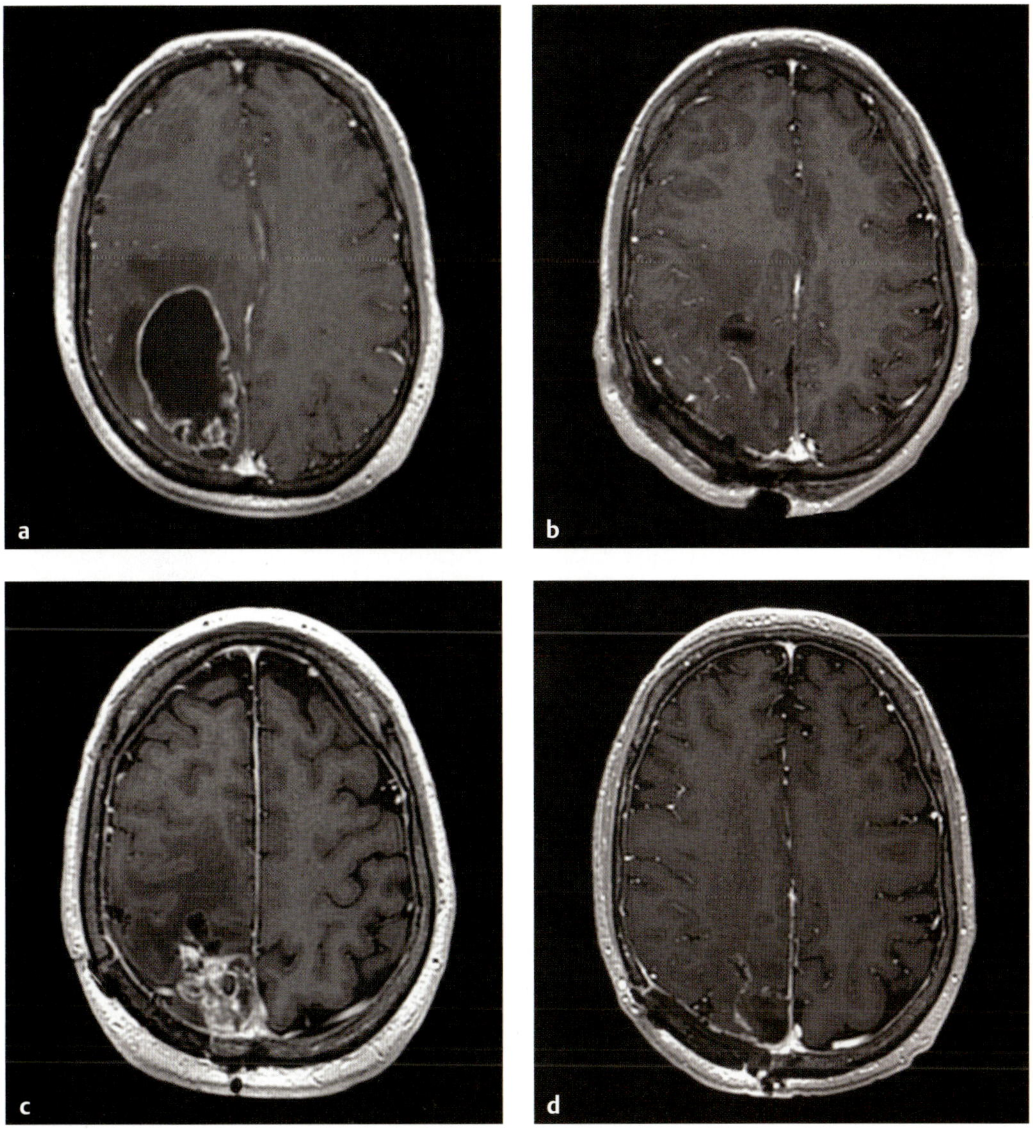

Fig. 25.3 Recurrent tumor. **(a)** Magnetic resonance imaging (MRI) demonstrates a solitary lesion in the right frontoparietal region. The patient was recursive partitioning analysis (RPA) class 1 and underwent gross total resection of the lesion. **(b)** Postoperative MRI demonstrating a small residual resection cavity with no evidence of residual enhancing tumor. **(c)** Surveillance MRI obtained 9 months after surgery demonstrated a recurrent lesion. The patient at this point was RPA class 2 due to progressive systemic disease but was otherwise doing well with a Karnofsky performance scale (KPS) score of 90, age 55, and no other brain lesions. **(d)** Repeat surgery was performed and gross total resection was achieved.

One of the first larger studies to review surgery for patients with multiple brain metastases was published in 1993. Bindal et al retrospectively reviewed 56 patients with multiple brain metastases.[6] In 30 patients (group A), one or more lesions were not surgically removed, and in 26 patients (group B) all lesions were resected. Among the 30 group A patients, 25 underwent one craniotomy, 4 underwent two craniotomies and 1 underwent three craniotomies, all in a single operation. Among the 26 group B patients, 23 patients had two tumors resected and 3 had three tumors removed. Ten patients underwent a single craniotomy, 14 underwent two craniotomies, and 2 patients underwent three craniotomies, all in a single operation. Patients in group B were compared with a cohort of patients with solitary lesions who underwent surgical resection matched by primary tumor, time from cancer diagnosis to brain metastasis, and status of systemic disease at the time of surgery (group C) (**Table 25.3**). Variables such as KPS score, age, primary tumor, and systemic disease were similar among all three groups. All patients underwent postoperative WBRT. Median overall survival was 6 months for group A and 14 months for

Table 25.3 Surgery for multiple brain metastases[6]

Group	A—Multiple lesions, one or more known lesion not resected + WBRT	B—Multiple lesions, all resected + WBRT	C—Solitary lesion, resected + WBRT
Karnofsky performance scale score (mean)	77	76	79
Age (median)	54	51	56
Craniotomies			
1	25	10	26
2	4	14	0
3	1	2	0
Lesions removed			
1	22	0	26
2	6	23	0
3	2	3	0
Lesions remaining	Yes	No	No
Median survival	6 mo	14 mo	14 mo

Abbreviation: WBRT, whole-brain radiotherapy.

both group B and group C. Rates of surgical morbidity and mortality were similar among all groups, and a higher number of craniotomies per surgery was not associated with increased complication rate. Thus, surgery for resection of all lesions in patients with multiple tumors, up to three total, was determined to be as safe and effective as surgery for solitary tumors and provided significant survival benefit in patients amenable to surgical resection of all lesions.

Since this study nearly 20 years ago, subsequent retrospective reviews have evaluated SRS as the adjuvant radiation technique. Pollock et al retrospectively evaluated 52 patients with 2 to 10 (median 3) brain metastases.[25] The median age was 58 and the median KPS score was 90. Twenty patients had received prior radiation. Treatment included surgery via multiple craniotomies (n = 5), surgery and SRS (n = 16), and radiosurgery alone (n = 31). Thus 21 patients underwent craniotomy, and 16 of these had postoperative radiosurgery. For all patients, median overall survival was 15.5 months, and median progression-free survival was 8 months. One- and 2-year survival rates were 63% and 27%, respectively. Median survival based on RPA class was 19 months for RPA class 1 patients, 13 months for RPA class 2, and 8 months for RPA class 3. The authors concluded that aggressive intervention was warranted in RPA class 1 patients and RPA class 2 patients with stable systemic disease with a low number of brain metastases.

Paek et al retrospectively reviewed patients who underwent surgery for brain metastases. Of 208 cases reviewed, 76 patients had multiple lesions, and 17 of these 76 underwent resection of two or more metastases. No differences in overall survival were seen comparing patients with solitary metastases to those with two or three metastases. Evaluation of subgroups based on RPA class was performed. The authors concluded that surgical resection should be considered in patients with solitary and multiple brain metastases, but that RPA class 3 solitary lesions and RPA class 2 multiple lesions may benefit more from SRS alone.[33]

Based on the literature available, surgical resection for patients with multiple metastases is indicated in a select group of patients. These patients have a low number of lesions (two or three), which are surgically accessible. They have stable systemic disease, high performance status, and are younger than 65. Essentially, these are RPA class 1 patients (**Fig. 25.4**). However, patients that meet these criteria represent a relatively small subset of all patients who present with multiple metastases. Only approximately one third of patients diagnosed with brain metastases will be possible surgical candidates.[3] Extrapolation of the existing evidence reveals other subsets of patients that may realize survival benefit from surgery.

Surgical decisions may be difficult in certain clinical scenarios. Patients may present with negative prognostic factors, such as uncontrolled systemic disease or a large number of brain lesions, but otherwise may be good surgical candidates based on their age, KPS score, and anatomical location of their lesion(s). Patients with progressive extracranial disease but who are naive to systemic therapy may have a more favorable prognosis than patients who have failed systemic therapy. Surgical resection of multiple brain metastases may prolong survival for patients with primary tumors like breast cancer, which may respond well to chemotherapy.

Patients with a large number of brain metastases are often not considered surgical candidates. In the retrospective reviews evaluating surgery in patients with multiple metastases described earlier in the chapter, most patients underwent one or two craniotomies to access one to three tumors.[6,33] In general, better outcomes

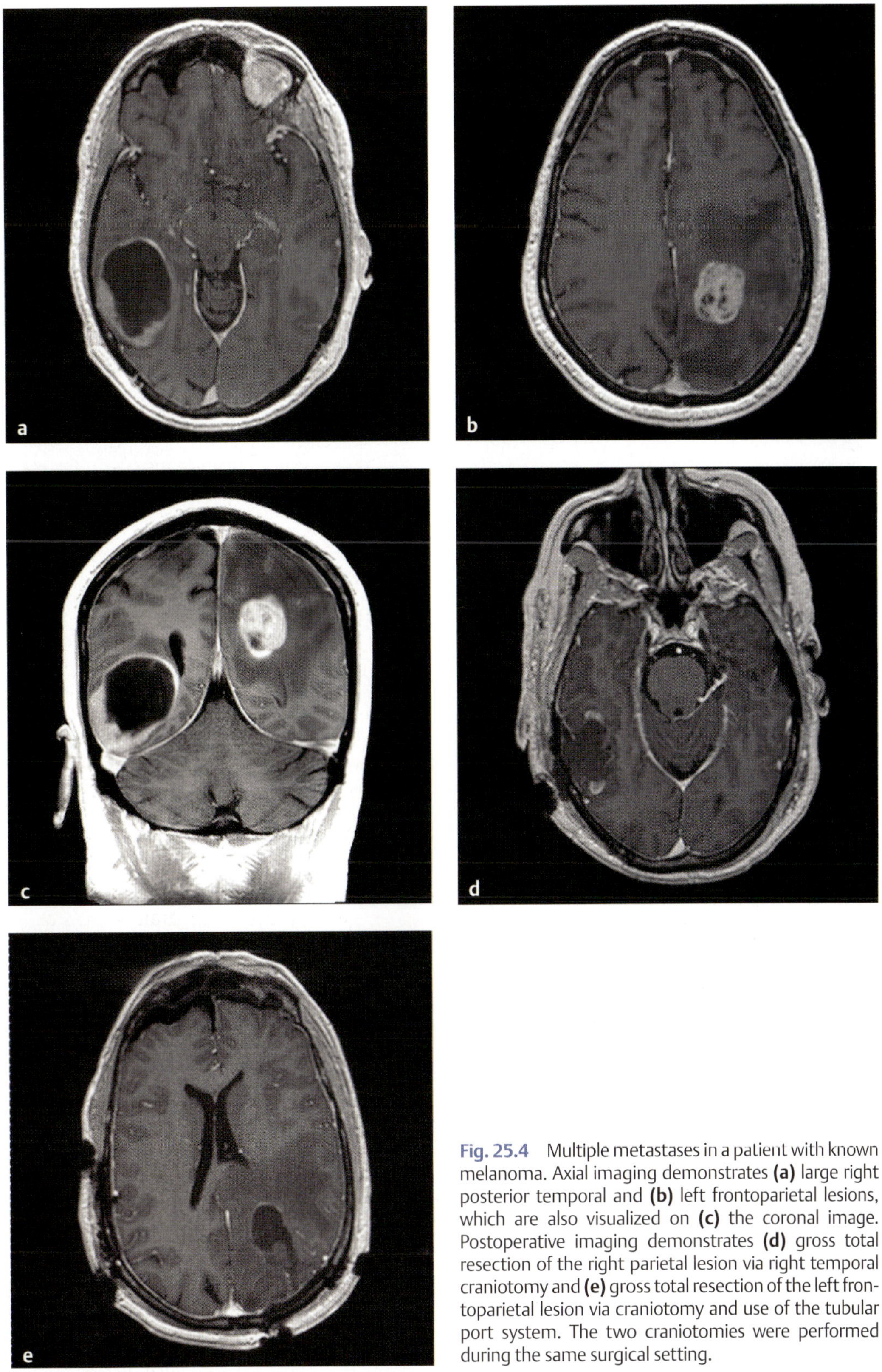

Fig. 25.4 Multiple metastases in a patient with known melanoma. Axial imaging demonstrates **(a)** large right posterior temporal and **(b)** left frontoparietal lesions, which are also visualized on **(c)** the coronal image. Postoperative imaging demonstrates **(d)** gross total resection of the right parietal lesion via right temporal craniotomy and **(e)** gross total resection of the left frontoparietal lesion via craniotomy and use of the tubular port system. The two craniotomies were performed during the same surgical setting.

were observed in cases where all tumors were resected, and no patient had more than three craniotomies. However, certain clinical scenarios may warrant consideration for surgical intervention in these patients. For example, patients who present with poor or declining functional status and one or more poor prognostic indicators in the setting of numerous brain metastases may have a dominant lesion or a specific lesion suspected of being the primary cause of the neurological decline. If the culprit lesion is removed, the patient's functional status may improve rapidly. Examples include lesions causing hydrocephalus or lesions with significant edema causing mass effect with midline shift and resulting altered mental status. Lesions affecting eloquent structures, such as primary motor or speech areas, may also cause significant neurological impairment either directly or indirectly, and surgical resection may allow significant rapid improvement in performance status (**Fig. 25.5**). In these clinical settings, resection of a limited number of lesions thought to be directly responsible for neurological decline may allow for restoration of higher functional status and improved survival.

Expert Recommendations

1. The best evidence regarding surgery for multiple metastases consists primarily of retrospective reviews. There are shortcomings associated with retrospective reviews that must be considered. These studies suggest a role for surgery in patients with multiple lesions whose tumors are surgically accessible. However, there is likely significant selection bias in analyzing patients who were screened for aggressive surgical management (Grade 1C Recommendation, Level II Evidence).
2. Only approximately one third of patients diagnosed with brain metastases will be possible surgical candidates.[3] Surgical patients in such literature represent a small subset of patients with brain metastases who are likely younger, with higher KPS scores, and limited, controlled systemic disease (i.e., RPA Level I) (**Table 25.4**) (Grade 1C Recommendation, Level II Evidence).
3. In general, current evidence most strongly suggests that patients with multiple lesions who are RPA Level I are likely to realize the same benefits from surgery as patients with a solitary lesion (Grade 1C Recommendation, Level II Evidence).
4. Evidence is not as clear for patients in RPA Level II or III who present with multiple brain metastases, and the role for surgery in these patients remains controversial. Based on the literature available, surgical resection for patients with multiple metastases is indicated in a select group of patients. These patients have a low number of lesions (two or three), which are surgically accessible (Grade 2B Recommendation, Level II Evidence).
5. Patients classified as RPA class 2 with large lesions (> 3 cm) or lesions causing mass effect or neurological symptoms may benefit from surgery to optimize neurological outcome (Grade 1C Recommendation, Level II Evidence).[25]
6. RPA class 2 patients with smaller lesions or patients with a large number of lesions (> 3) may benefit more from SRS and/or WBRT (Grade 1C Recommendation, Level II Evidence).
7. Optimal management of RPA class 3 patients is difficult to determine due to a lack of evidence in the literature and poor overall survival, which limits evaluation of outcomes (Grade 2C Recommendation, Level III Evidence).

■ Surgery

Surgical Adjuncts

Preoperative imaging consists primarily of CT and contrast-enhanced MR and is typically incorporated with frameless stereotaxy systems for intraoperative navigation. This technique improves the accuracy at each step of surgery from incision to selecting the cortical entry point to ensuring tumor margins have been reached circumferentially. Intraoperative imaging modalities include two-dimensional ultrasonography, CT, and MRI. Each may be used to evaluate for residual tumor after tumor resection to improve extent of resection. For lesions located near eloquent cortex, additional MRI techniques, such as functional MRI and diffusion tensor imaging (DTI), may be useful to better understand the relationship between the tumor and surrounding neural structures and to plan the operative approach. In some cases, intraoperative mapping of structures, such as speech and motor areas, during an awake craniotomy, or mapping of the central sulcus with an electrode grid, may be useful for intraoperative determination of the optimal surgical approach.

Surgical Techniques

Microsurgical techniques have evolved over the last few decades. The operative microscope may be registered with the neuronavigation system to assist with targeting the lesion. Tumors may have a pseudocapsule, which facilitates resection. Metastatic lesions tend to displace rather than invade brain, although infiltration can occur, and wider resection is preferred if possible. In recent work, microscopic total resection to a depth of up to 5 mm into adjacent brain reduced local recurrence compared with gross total resection, which did not involve resecting invading cells.[34]

Tumors are ideally resected en bloc (**Fig. 25.6**), although variables such as tumor size and location may preclude this technique. Recent work has demonstrated an increased risk of leptomeningeal dissemination in patients undergoing piecemeal tumor

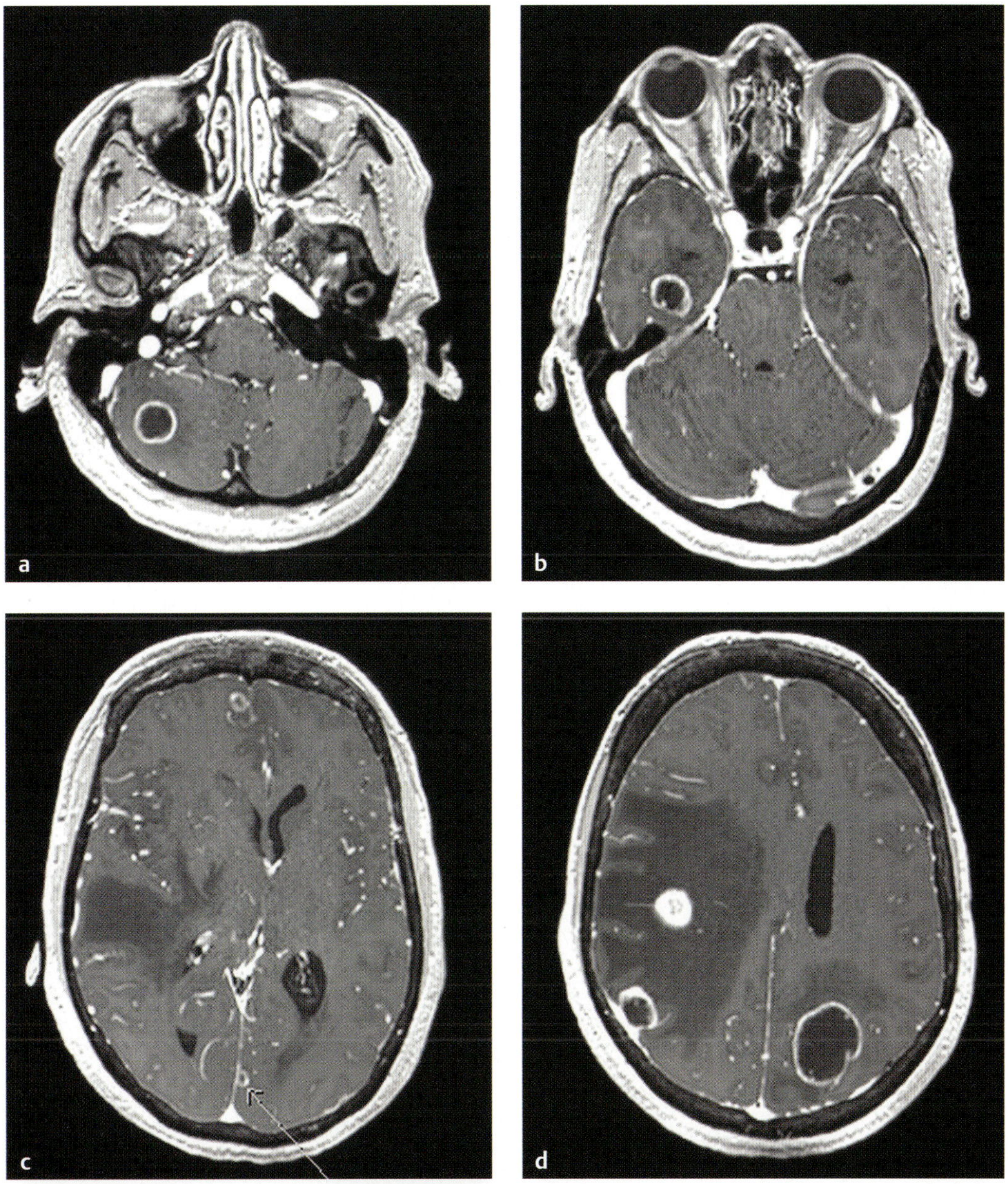

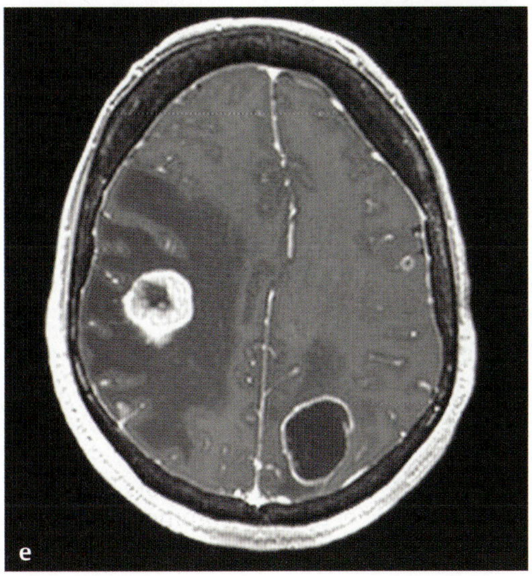

Fig. 25.5 Numerous breast cancer metastases in a patient with newly diagnosed, treatment-naive breast cancer who presented with headaches and left arm weakness. **(a)** Right cerebellar lesion, **(b)** right temporal lesion, **(c)** small right frontal and left occipital (*arrow*) lesions. Additional lesions are noted: **(d)** right frontal, right parietal, and left parietal lesions. **(e)** Another view of the two larger lesions in **(d)** as well as a smaller left frontal lesion. The patient had 11 total lesions, and not all lesions are pictured. The right frontal lesion was associated with severe edema and mass effect **(d,e)** and was felt to be causing her neurological deficit. It was surgically removed, and the patient regained full use of her arm within 2 weeks.

Table 25.4 Possible indications or contraindications for surgical resection of metastatic brain tumor

Surgical resection	Indication	Possible contraindication
Cancer	Renal, melanoma, breast, colon, lung, unknown	Lymphoma, small-cell lung cancer, germ cell, choriocarcinoma
Anatomical location	Eloquent/noneloquent hemispheric, cerebellar, superficial, ventricle	Deep nuclei, brainstem
Systemic disease	Stable	Progressive
RPA class	1 2 with stable systemic disease, low number of lesions	3 2 with uncontrolled systemic disease, large number of brain lesions
Size	Large (> 3 cm)	Very small (< 1 cm)
Other findings	Associated shift, edema, hydrocephalus	Medical comorbidities, patient declines

Abbreviation: RPA, recursive partitioning analysis.

resection compared with those who had en bloc resection of their tumors, for both posterior fossa lesions[35] and supratentorial tumors.[36] Surgical resection was also associated with increased risk of leptomeningeal dissemination compared with SRS.

Certain surgical nuances may offer value in resection of brain metastases. For example, deep tumors may benefit from use of a tubular port to minimize brain retraction during surgery. Tubular access devices can be placed into the tumor using stereotactic guidance, and held in position using standard devices such as a snake retractor system. Microscopically or endoscopically assisted resection then proceeds. An example of a tumor resected using this method at our institution is illustrated in **Fig. 25.4**.

■ Summary and Conclusions

Outcomes of patients with brain metastases have improved significantly over the past few decades. Surgical intervention has played a significant role due to advances in surgical techniques as well as an evidence-based approach to evaluating clinical data. As the population ages and patients with cancer live longer, the incidence of brain metastases is likely to rise.

The best management of patients with brain metastases employs a multidisciplinary approach involving the patient's clinical oncology team as well as neurosurgeons, neuro-oncologists, neuroradiologists, and radiation oncologists.[7] Patients with a low number of negative prognostic indicators, as possibly

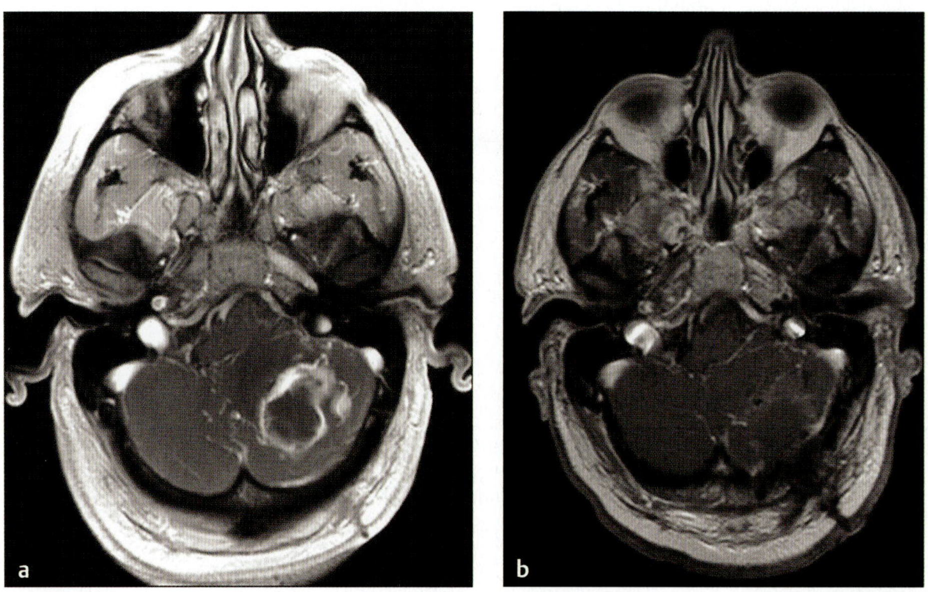

Fig. 25.6 Patient with solitary cerebellar metastasis from non-small-cell lung cancer. **(a)** Preoperative and **(b)** postoperative imaging after en bloc resection of the lesion.

reflected in being RPA class 1, represent ideal candidates for aggressive management, including surgery. Multiple craniotomies and repeat operations likely improve survival and quality of life for these patients.

Ultimately, most patients are unlikely to present as optimal surgical candidates. Until further evidence is available, decisions regarding surgical intervention must be individualized based on variables such as age, functional status, systemic disease status, extracranial metastases, medical comorbidities, neurological deficits, radiographic findings, and radiosensitivity of the primary tumor. The next step is likely prospective, randomized trials for increasingly complex patients, such as those with multiple brain metastases.

■ References

1. Gavrilovic IT, Posner JB. Brain metastases: epidemiology and pathophysiology. J Neurooncol 2005;75(1):5–14
2. Mut M. Surgical treatment of brain metastasis: a review. Clin Neurol Neurosurg 2012;114(1):1–8
3. Kalkanis SN, Kondziolka D, Gaspar LE, et al. The role of surgical resection in the management of newly diagnosed brain metastases: a systematic review and evidence-based clinical practice guideline. J Neurooncol 2010;96(1):33–43
4. Al-Shamy G, Sawaya R. Management of brain metastases: the indispensable role of surgery. J Neurooncol 2009;92(3): 275–282
5. Soffietti R, Rudā R, Mutani R. Management of brain metastases. J Neurol 2002;249(10):1357–1369
6. Bindal RK, Sawaya R, Leavens ME, Lee JJ. Surgical treatment of multiple brain metastases. J Neurosurg 1993;79(2): 210–216
7. Jenkinson MD, Haylock B, Shenoy A, Husband D, Javadpour M. Management of cerebral metastasis: evidence-based approach for surgery, stereotactic radiosurgery and radiotherapy. Eur J Cancer 2011;47(5):649–655
8. Brem S, Panattil JG. An era of rapid advancement: diagnosis and treatment of metastatic brain cancer. Neurosurgery 2005;57(5, Suppl):S5–S9
9. Gaspar L, Scott C, Rotman M, et al. Recursive partitioning analysis (RPA) of prognostic factors in three Radiation Therapy Oncology Group (RTOG) brain metastases trials. Int J Radiat Oncol Biol Phys 1997;37(4):745–751
10. Kurtz JM, Gelber R, Brady LW, Carella RJ, Cooper JS. The palliation of brain metastases in a favorable patient population: a randomized clinical trial by the Radiation Therapy Oncology Group. Int J Radiat Oncol Biol Phys 1981;7(7):891–895
11. Siu TL, Jeffree RL, Fuller JW. Current strategies in the surgical management of cerebral metastases: an evidence-based review. J Clin Neurosci 2011;18(11):1429–1434
12. Grossman R, Mukherjee D, Chang DC, et al. Predictors of inpatient death and complications among postoperative elderly patients with metastatic brain tumors. Ann Surg Oncol 2011;18(2):521–528
13. Sundaresan N, Galicich JH. Surgical treatment of single brain metastases from non-small-cell lung cancer. Cancer Invest 1985;3(2):107–113
14. Sundaresan N, Galicich JH, Beattie EJ Jr. Surgical treatment of brain metastases from lung cancer. J Neurosurg 1983;58(5):666–671
15. White KT, Fleming TR, Laws ER Jr. Single metastasis to the brain. Surgical treatment in 122 consecutive patients. Mayo Clin Proc 1981;56(7):424–428
16. Patchell RA, Tibbs PA, Walsh JW, et al. A randomized trial of surgery in the treatment of single metastases to the brain. N Engl J Med 1990;322(8):494–500
17. Vecht CJ, Haaxma-Reiche H, Noordijk EM, et al. Treatment of single brain metastasis: radiotherapy alone or combined with neurosurgery? Ann Neurol 1993;33(6):583–590
18. Mintz AH, Kestle J, Rathbone MP, et al. A randomized trial to assess the efficacy of surgery in addition to radiotherapy in patients with a single cerebral metastasis. Cancer 1996; 78(7):1470–1476
19. Auchter RM, Lamond JP, Alexander E, et al. A multiinstitutional outcome and prognostic factor analysis of radiosurgery for resectable single brain metastasis. Int J Radiat Oncol Biol Phys 1996;35(1):27–35
20. Bindal AK, Bindal RK, Hess KR, et al. Surgery versus radiosurgery in the treatment of brain metastasis. J Neurosurg 1996;84(5):748–754
21. Muacevic A, Wowra B, Siefert A, Tonn JC, Steiger HJ, Kreth FW. Microsurgery plus whole brain irradiation versus Gamma Knife surgery alone for treatment of single metastases to the brain: a randomized controlled multicentre phase III trial. J Neurooncol 2008;87(3):299–307
22. Ammirati M, Cobbs CS, Linskey ME, et al. The role of retreatment in the management of recurrent/progressive brain metastases: a systematic review and evidence-based clinical practice guideline. J Neurooncol 2010;96(1):85–96
23. Chang EL, Selek U, Hassenbusch SJ III, et al. Outcome variation among "radioresistant" brain metastases treated with stereotactic radiosurgery. Neurosurgery 2005;56(5):936–945
24. Ewend MG, Morris DE, Carey LA, Ladha AM, Brem S. Guidelines for the initial management of metastatic brain tumors: role of surgery, radiosurgery, and radiation therapy. J Natl Compr Canc Netw 2008;6(5):505–513, quiz 514
25. Pollock BE, Brown PD, Foote RL, Stafford SL, Schomberg PJ. Properly selected patients with multiple brain metastases may benefit from aggressive treatment of their intracranial disease. J Neurooncol 2003;61(1):73–80
26. Smalley SR, Laws ER Jr, O'Fallon JR, Shaw EG, Schray MF. Resection for solitary brain metastasis. Role of adjuvant radiation and prognostic variables in 229 patients. J Neurosurg 1992;77(4):531–540
27. Gaspar LE, Scott C, Murray K, Curran W. Validation of the RTOG recursive partitioning analysis (RPA) classification for brain metastases. Int J Radiat Oncol Biol Phys 2000;47(4): 1001–1006
28. Sawaya R, Hammoud M, Schoppa D, et al. Neurosurgical outcomes in a modern series of 400 craniotomies for treatment of parenchymal tumors. Neurosurgery 1998;42(5): 1044–1055
29. Johnson JD, Young B. Demographics of brain metastasis. Neurosurg Clin N Am 1996;7(3):337–344
30. Sundaresan N, Galicich JH. Surgical treatment of brain metastases: clinical and computerized tomography evaluation of the results of treatment. Cancer 1985;55(6):1382–1388
31. Arbit E, Wroński M, Burt M, Galicich JH. The treatment of patients with recurrent brain metastases: a retrospective analysis of 109 patients with nonsmall cell lung cancer. Cancer 1995;76(5):765–773
32. Bindal RK, Sawaya R, Leavens ME, Hess KR, Taylor SH. Reoperation for recurrent metastatic brain tumors. J Neurosurg 1995;83(4):600–604
33. Paek SH, Audu PB, Sperling MR, Cho J, Andrews DW. Reevaluation of surgery for the treatment of brain metastases: review of 208 patients with single or multiple brain metastases treated at one institution with modern neurosurgical techniques. Neurosurgery 2005;56(5):1021–1034
34. Yoo H, Kim YZ, Nam BH, et al. Reduced local recurrence of a single brain metastasis through microscopic total resection. J Neurosurg 2009;110(4):730–736
35. Suki D, Abouassi H, Patel AJ, Sawaya R, Weinberg JS, Groves MD. Comparative risk of leptomeningeal disease after resection or stereotactic radiosurgery for solid tumor metastasis to the posterior fossa. J Neurosurg 2008;108(2):248–257
36. Suki D, Hatiboglu MA, Patel AJ, et al. Comparative risk of leptomeningeal dissemination of cancer after surgery or stereotactic radiosurgery for a single supratentorial solid tumor metastasis. Neurosurgery 2009;64(4):664–674

26

Stereotactic Radiosurgery (SRS) versus Whole-Brain Radiation Therapy (WBRT) in the Management of Multiple Brain Metastases

Usama Mahmood, Zain A. Husain, Young Kwok, and William F. Regine

Brain metastases represent a significant cause of morbidity and mortality among cancer patients. There are over 200,000 cases of brain metastases annually, afflicting 10 to 30% of all cancer patients and outnumbering primary brain tumors by a ratio of 10:1.[1,2] Whether the result of improved detection via novel imaging techniques or improved control of extracranial disease due to more potent systemic therapies (which less effectively traverse the blood–brain barrier), the incidence of brain metastases is increasing.[3]

Historically, brain metastases were rapidly fatal, with most patients surviving approximately 1 month. The use of steroids to decrease mass effect and peritumoral edema nearly doubled survival to about 2 months. Over the last several decades, advancements in surgery and radiotherapy, combined with other strides in the general management of cancer patients, have significantly improved these results. In fact, there have even been some reports of cure among select patients with solitary metastases who undergo aggressive treatment to both their intracranial and extracranial disease sites.[4]

The initial approach to the patient with brain metastases must take into account not only the status of disease within the brain but also the status of the patient as a whole. The number and location of metastases within the brain, associated symptoms, the site and histology of the primary, the presence of other extracranial metastases, and the patient's overall performance status and comorbidities all need to be taken into account when treatment decisions are being made. Several prognostic systems for patients with brain metastases have been created that incorporate such factors and can help tailor treatment to an appropriate level of aggressiveness.[1,5,6]

Ultimately, the primary goals of the management of the patient with brain metastases are to provide effective palliation, improved quality of life and, if at all possible, extended survival. To these ends, stereotactic radiosurgery (SRS) and whole-brain radiation therapy (WBRT) are effective treatment modalities that often play a significant role in the management of brain metastases. Although sometimes thought to be competing modalities, they are, in fact, quite complementary; SRS delivers ablative radiation doses with a high degree of precision (typically in one fraction), whereas WBRT delivers lower amounts of radiation to the entire brain parenchyma (typically over the course of weeks). The former is more effective in treating clinically visible tumor deposits, whereas the latter treats microscopic foci of disease, and each has been shown to improve outcomes in specific settings. This review discusses the role of SRS and WBRT in the management of brain metastases, with a focus on Level I evidence from randomized, controlled trials.

■ Literature Review

Adjuvant (Postoperative) WBRT/SRS in Patients with a Single Brain Metastasis

Surgical resection potentially serves many functions in the patient with brain metastases. It can provide histological confirmation of metastatic disease, relieve mass effect if present, and improve local tumor control. As demonstrated in a randomized trial by Patchell et al, this improvement in local control can translate into a survival advantage for a select group of patients (Level I evidence).[7] These authors randomized 48 patients with a single, resectable brain metastasis to biopsy versus surgical resection followed by 36 Gy WBRT. Patients who underwent surgical resection in addition to WBRT had an improved median survival (40 vs 15 weeks, $p < 0.01$) and, also important, a longer mean duration of functional independence (38 vs 8 weeks, $p < 0.005$).

Given these improvements with the addition of surgery to WBRT, a logical follow-up study by Patchell et al examined the role of WBRT following surgical resection of single brain metastases (Level I evidence).[8] In this trial, 146 patients were randomized following gross total resection of a single brain metastasis to observation versus 50.4 Gy WBRT. Patients receiving WBRT had decreased intracranial recurrence rates (18% vs 70%, $p < 0.001$), including lower rates of both local (10% vs 46%, $p < 0.001$) and elsewhere (14% vs 37%, $p < 0.01$) brain failure. Of note, although this study is sometimes criticized for failing to demonstrate a survival benefit with WBRT, it was not powered to do so; however, patients receiving WBRT had over a 10% nonsignificant increase in median survival (48 weeks vs 43 weeks, $p = 0.39$). Also, WBRT did result in a lower rate of neurological deaths (14% vs 44%, $p = 0.003$). This sole randomized trial examining the role of adjuvant WBRT after surgical resection is summarized in **Table 26.1**.

Recently, consideration has been given to SRS to the resection cavity in patients who have had tumor resection. Given that the trial by Patchell et al demonstrated a 44% local recurrence rate when radiation therapy was withheld, it is felt that surgical resection alone of single brain metastases is inadequate. In an attempt to improve local control yet spare the patient the potential neurotoxicity attributed to WBRT, some have used SRS to the resection cavity alone. Although no randomized data are available to validate such an approach, several institutional experiences have been published that suggest reasonable local control with SRS to the resection cavity. To our knowledge, the largest such experience, from Stanford, examined 120 resection cavities in 112 patients (Level III evidence).[9] Over all, they found a 12-month incidence of local failure of 9.5%, although the distant failure was 54%. Interestingly, they noted improved local control with no difference in toxicity with use of a 2 mm margin on the resection cavity. Whether or not adjuvant SRS results in equivalent local control as WBRT in patients with resected brain metastases, a concern with use of this strategy is that it will lead to increased brain failures elsewhere. The NCCTG is currently evaluating this approach by enrolling patients in the N107C trial, which is randomizing patients with one to four brain metastases, at least one of which has been resected, to SRS to the resection cavity/residual brain metastases versus WBRT.

WBRT ± SRS in Patients with Limited (1–3) Brain Metastases

Although no randomized trials have been performed comparing surgery to SRS, they are generally felt to result in comparable local control rates of 80 to 90% when used in conjunction with WBRT.[2] They are complementary modalities, where the decision to use one or the other is influenced by the number of metastases, the need for pathological tissue sampling or relieving mass effect, the volume of the metastatic lesion(s), and the timing of planned systemic therapies.

The ease of delivery of SRS with its low complication rates, combined with its excellent local control (when combined with WBRT), inspired investigators to further examine its use in patients with brain metastases. The initial randomized trial utilizing SRS in addition to WBRT was performed at the University of

Table 26.1 Summary of Level I evidence for postoperative WBRT in patients with a single brain metastasis

			Local failure		Distant failure		Median survival	
Study	**Study arms**	**N**	**Obs.**	**WBRT**	**Obs.**	**WBRT**	**Obs.**	**WBRT**
Patchell et al	Sx ± WBRT	95	46%	10%	37%	14%	43 wk	48 wk

Abbreviations: Obs., observation; Sx, surgery; WBRT, whole-brain radiation therapy.

Pittsburgh, where 27 patients with two to four brain metastases were randomized to 30 Gy WBRT with or without 16 Gy SRS (Level I evidence).[10] The authors noted a considerable improvement in 1-year local control with SRS (100% vs 8%, $p = 0.0016$); however, the resultant difference in survival did not reach statistical significance. The benefits of SRS following WBRT were further evaluated in the multi-institutional Radiotherapy Oncology Group (RTOG) 9508 trial (Level I evidence).[11] This study enrolled 333 patients with one to three intracranial metastases who were randomized to 37.5 Gy WBRT with or without 15 to 24 Gy SRS. When analyzing the entire cohort, there was no difference in the primary end point of survival, although there was a local recurrence benefit favoring the addition of SRS (18% vs 29%, $p = 0.01$). It should be noted, however, that nearly 20% of patients randomized to the combined modality arm failed to receive the SRS portion of their treatment, which may partially obscure the true benefit of SRS following WBRT. In a planned subgroup analysis, patients with a single brain metastasis had an improvement in median survival (6.5 vs 4.9 months, $p = 0.0390$). Also, several unplanned subgroup analyses demonstrated improved survival with SRS among patients with recursive partitioning analysis (RPA) class 1, squamous non-small-cell lung cancer, or tumors > 2 cm. Similar to the quality of life benefits seen with the addition of surgery to WBRT, patients receiving SRS were more likely to have an improved or stable KPS at 6 months as well as a decreased steroid requirement. The latter finding challenges previous conventional wisdom that when combining SRS with WBRT, WBRT should be first so as to allow for tumor shrinkage and SRS treatment of a potentially smaller volume. Given the fundamental goal of "palliation" in many of these patients, patients requiring steroids due to associated tumor edema may be considered for SRS prior to WBRT. Given the findings of RTOG 9508, this approach may more quickly relieve patients of the need for steroids (thus sooner palliating symptoms and minimizing steroidal side effects). The randomized evidence for the addition of WBRT to SRS is summarized in **Table 26.2**.

SRS ± WBRT in Patients with Limited (One to Three) Brain Metastases

Favorable local control with SRS combined with concerns about neurotoxicity related to WBRT have led some investigators to treat brain metastases with SRS alone, delaying WBRT until time of progression. In perhaps the most well known of such experiences, a multi-institutional retrospective study of 569 patients demonstrated no difference in survival between patients receiving SRS alone or SRS + WBRT (8.6 months vs 8.2 months, $p = 0.93$) (Level III evidence).[12] This paradigm has since been tested in three important randomized trials, which are summarized in **Table 26.3**.

The Japanese were the first to report a randomized study examining the benefit of WBRT after SRS (Level I evidence).[13] In this study, 160 patients with one to four brain metastases were randomized to 30 Gy WBRT or observation following 18 to 25 Gy SRS. This study demonstrated no difference in survival with WBRT, which was not surprising because it was underpowered to evaluate this end point (the enrollment numbers were similar to the aforementioned study by Patchell et al, whose primary end point was intracranial recurrence[8]). There was, however, a brain tumor control benefit with the addition of WBRT (76% vs 47%, $p < 0.001$), including benefits to local control (89% vs 73%, $p = 0.002$) as well as to brain tumor recurrence elsewhere (42% vs 64%, $p = 0.003$). Interestingly, among patients with a normal Mini–Mental State Examination (MMSE) at baseline, WBRT resulted in an increased average duration until deterioration (17 vs 8 months, $p = 0.05$). This led the authors to conclude that "for most brain metastatic patients, control of the brain tumor is the most important factor for stabilizing neurocognitive function."[14]

A recently published study performed by the European Organization for Research and Treatment of Cancer also examined WBRT after local therapy (including both SRS and surgery) (Level I evidence).[15] The authors randomized 353 patients with brain metastases to SRS ($n = 199$) or surgery ($n = 160$) with

Table 26.2 Summary of Level I evidence for WBRT ± SRS in patients with limited (one to three) brain metastases

			Local failure		Median survival	
Study	**Study arms**	**N**	**WBRT**	**WBRT + SRS**	**WBRT**	**WBRT + SRS**
Kondziolka et al 1999[10]	WBRT ± SRS	27	100%	8%	7.5 mo	11 mo
Andrews et al 2004[11]	WBRT ± SRS	333	29%	18%	5.7 mo	6.5 mo

Abbreviations: SRS, stereotactic radiosurgery; WBRT, whole-brain radiation therapy.

Table 26.3 Summary of Level I evidence for SRS ± WBRT in patients with limited (1–3) brain metastases

			Local failure		Distant failure		Median survival	
Study	**Study arms**	**N**	**Obs.**	**WBRT**	**Obs.**	**WBRT**	**Obs.**	**WBRT**
Aoyama et al[13]	SRS ± WBRT	132	27%	11%	64%	42%	8 mo	8 mo
Chang et al 2009[16]	SRS ± WBRT	58	33%	0%	55%	27%	15 mo	6 mo
Kocher et al 2011[15]	Sx/SRS ± WBRT	353	59/31%	27/19%	42/48%	23/33%	11 mo	11 mo

Abbreviations: Obs., observation; SRS, stereotactic radiosurgery; Sx, surgery; WBRT, whole-brain radiation therapy.

or without 30 Gy WBRT. Although the study did not meet its primary end point of increased duration of functional independence (a subjective measure affected by factors other than control of brain metastases including extracranial disease status), WBRT did increase median progression-free survival (4.6 vs 3.9 months, $p = 0.020$) and decrease intracranial progression (48% vs 78%;, $p < 0.001$), including local and elsewhere failure, as well as the rate of neurological death (28% vs 44%, $p < 0.002$).

A third study evaluating the role of WBRT following SRS for patients with one to three brain metastases was reported by Chang et al from MD Anderson Cancer Center (Level II evidence).[16] Patients in this study were randomized to 15 to 24 Gy SRS with or without 30 Gy WBRT in 12 fractions. The primary end point was a decline in Hopkins Verbal Learning Treatment–Revised (HVLT-R) at 4 months. The trial closed early after accrual of only 58 patients based on concern for significantly worse neurocognitive outcomes secondary to the addition of WBRT. WBRT patients were found to have a 52% decline in HVLT-R at 4 months, whereas patients in the SRS-alone arm had only a 24% decline. Once again, the addition of WBRT resulted in decreased 1-year intracranial recurrence (27% vs 73%, $p = 0.0003$), including both improved local (100% vs 67%, $p = 0.012$) and elsewhere (73% vs 45%, $p = 0.02$) brain tumor control. Paradoxically, and unprecedented in similar randomized trials, patients in the WBRT arm had a significantly compromised median survival (5.7 vs 15.2 months, $p = 0.003$).

The trial, while commendable for its effort to prospectively study neurocognitive function following central nervous system (CNS)-directed WBRT, has several shortcomings that make its findings difficult to generalize.[17] For one, the study used patient stratification variables not prognostic of the study's primary neurocognitive end point. In this study, patients were stratified by RPA class, number of brain metastases, and histology, which are factors linked to survival rather than to neurocognitive function. The authors did not stratify by baseline neurocognitive function, examination of which suggests at least a trend toward increased neurocognitive dysfunction in the WBRT group. Also important is the fact that the authors failed to account/stratify for many medications commonly prescribed to cancer patients—including opioids, sedatives, anticonvulsants, and steroids—that are known to cause neurocognitive dysfunction. Second, the authors chose an end point with questionable clinical relevance. The primary end point of their study was an assessment of neurocognitive function using only the HVLT-R at a single time point of 4 months; however, given the complexity of cognitive function, a battery of tests over time is required to accurately depict the neurocognitive effects of radiotherapy (RT).[18] In addition, this primary end point inadvertently biased the trial against WBRT because previous work had already shown that RT has a transient effect on memory, as measured by verbal learning tests. In serial neuropsychological studies, Armstrong and colleagues[19] assessed patients with low-grade glioma who received RT, and found a transient decline in verbal memory, with the nadir after RT corresponding exactly to the 4-month time interval used by Chang and colleagues.[16] Finally, as already mentioned, patients receiving WBRT inexplicably had a significantly shorter median survival than patients who received SRS alone, on the order of a threefold difference (5.7 vs 15.2 months). This is particularly perplexing given the improved CNS disease control with WBRT (27% vs 73% at 1 year). Moreover, three previous randomized studies reported equivalent survival with the addition of WBRT to local therapy.[8,13,15] It is unclear what specifically led to such a survival difference, although close inspection of the baseline patient characteristics suggests at least a trend toward more favorable factors (RPA class I, female gender, and lower median tumor volume) in the SRS-alone group. The authors suggest that the survival difference might be due in part to more frequent surgical salvage in patients who received SRS alone; however, the greater use of surgical salvage is more likely to be the result of increased CNS disease recurrence rather than a disproportionate rationing of salvage treatments. Also, although patients receiving WBRT had a higher proportion of systemic deaths, this is due to a delay in neurological mortality rather than an increased systemic disease burden, a finding originally reported by Patchell et al.[8] Perhaps, then, the survival difference was simply the result of statistical anomaly due to small patient numbers. Regardless, this survival difference could in itself explain the neurocognitive dysfunction found in patients receiving WBRT. The primary end point of this study was an assessment of neurocognitive function at 4 months (~ 1 month prior to the median date of death of patients in the WBRT group). Many studies suggest that patients with terminal cancer experience profound neurocognitive dysfunction.[20,21] For example, Pereira and colleagues followed 348 cancer patients with serial MMSEs and found that patients who died had a trend toward decreased scores, with 68% of patients having abnormal MMSE scores before death.[20] The decline in MMSE score was most profound 1 month before death. As such, the higher neurocognitive dysfunction noted in the WBRT group cannot be confidently ascribed to radiation given the large survival difference noted between treatment groups along with the timing of death in the WBRT group in relation to the single 4-month study end point (~ 1 month prior to median survival in the WBRT group).

To shed more light on this area of controversy and potentially elucidate the effect of WBRT on neurocognition, the NCCTG is currently enrolling a large number of patients in the N0574 trial, which is randomizing patients to SRS with or without WBRT, with the primary end point looking at neurocognitive function.

WBRT in Patients with Multiple (More Than Three) Brain Metastases

Whereas there is some controversy regarding the optimal management of patients with limited (one to three) brain metastases, WBRT is the cornerstone of management of patients with more than three brain metastases. SRS is only selectively employed in this setting, given the concern for irradiating large volumes of intracranial disease to high doses. In this setting, WBRT can, however, provide palliative as well as survival benefits. Responses to radiation can be seen early in the treatment course, with 50% of patients experiencing an improvement in neurological symptoms by the second week of treatment.[22] Over all, the clinical and radiographic response to brain radiation ranges from 50 to 75%.[2] The addition of WBRT to steroids is also generally felt to improve the survival for patients with multiple brain metastases from 2 to 4 months.[23] To our knowledge, only one randomized trial (performed prior to the advent of computed tomography) has evaluated the addition of WBRT to supportive care (Level II evidence).[24] In this trial, 48 patients with presumed brain metastases were randomized to steroids with or without 40 Gy WBRT. Although *p*-values were not given, the addition of WBRT led to improved duration of remission as well as median survival (14 vs 10 weeks).

Unfortunately, despite multiple randomized trials, we have been unable to improve upon standard fractionated WBRT for such patients. Multiple randomized trials evaluating altered fractionation of WBRT have been attempted without any difference in survival.[2] Similarly, multiple randomized trials have failed to identify a benefit with the addition of radiosensitizers or chemotherapy to WBRT.[2] Investigators, nonetheless, continue to search for drugs that will improve the therapeutic ratio between normal brain tissue and tumor cells.

Discussion Regarding WBRT and Neurocognitive Toxicity

The debate about the risks and benefits of WBRT in patients with brain metastases must keep in mind the original goals of therapy. The primary intent of WBRT is to effectively palliate symptoms associated with brain metastases, to improve quality of life, and, perhaps to a lesser degree, to improve overall survival. We feel that the toxicities of WBRT—specifically the risk of neurocognitive dysfunction—are overstated and, for the majority of patients with brain metastases, WBRT provides an overall benefit in terms of palliation and improved quality of life.

When discussing neurotoxicity, it is important to note that nearly all patients with brain metastases present with neurocognitive deficits prior to beginning WBRT.[25] Meyers et al reported the most extensive study evaluating neurocognitive function in patients with brain metastases. This detailed work examined neurocognitive function in patients with brain metastases randomized to WBRT with or without the radiation sensitizer motexafin gadolinium.[25] The study enrolled 401 patients and each patient underwent a battery of eight neurocognitive function tests at baseline and following treatment. At baseline, 91% of patients had a deficit, and 42% had deficits seen in four or more tests. Lesion volume was predictive of initial neurocognitive deficit. These data are critical because most studies do not describe baseline neurocognitive deficits.

When considering withholding WBRT, one must be mindful that patients not receiving WBRT are more likely to have tumor progression at local and distant brain sites. Withholding WBRT results in a significantly increased risk of failure locally and elsewhere in the brain. Such progression is often accompanied by irreversible neurological symptoms requiring invasive salvage treatments. In the study by Chang et al, for instance, patients who received SRS alone had a 33% rate of requiring salvage craniotomy, with most patients being symptomatic at the time of recurrence.[16] Similar findings were noted in a University of Kentucky study detailing their experience with 36 consecutive patients treated with SRS alone.[26] In this study, patients were followed with serial magnetic resonance imaging (MRI) ~ 3 months apart, despite which nearly half of patients (17/36, 47%) had brain tumor recurrence; of these, 12 (71%) presented with symptoms and 10 (59%) presented with neurological deficits. This study demonstrated a 1-year neurological-deficit-free survival of only ~ 50% with this approach.

Not only does recurrence of intracranial disease result in significant symptoms, it is also one of the most important predictors of neurocognitive dysfunction. In a reanalysis of the study by Meyers et al, Li et al noted a correlation between tumor progression and worsening neurocognitive function.[27] Following treatment, patients with tumor shrinkage at 2 months greater than the population median had improved survival as well as a longer time to neurocognitive dysfunction. Patients with a partial response also had an improvement in executive function and visual motor scanning from baseline. In comparison, patients with progressive disease had a significant worsening of neurocognitive symptoms. Similar results were seen in the RTOG 9104 study.[28] This trial randomized patients to two different radiation schedules and examined changes related to MMSE scores. The study demonstrated that, at 3 months, the average change in MMSE for patients with brain metastases that were controlled was –0.5, whereas it was –6.3 for patients with uncontrolled metastases, again suggesting that control of metastases plays a large role in the maintenance of neurocognitive function. These data suggest that the most significant threat to neurocognitive function is the recurrence/progression of brain metastases, and, much less likely, radiation-related toxicity. In addition, patients who respond to therapy can in fact have neurocognitive improvement.

Perhaps the most cited work regarding the risks of neurotoxicity in patients receiving WBRT is the retrospective series from Memorial Sloan Kettering published by DeAngelis et al.[29] This study evaluated 47 long-term survivors (≥ 1 year following the diagnosis of brain metastases) and noted that five patients (11%) developed severe dementia associated with ataxia and urinary incontinence. It should remembered, however, that these patients represented a select subgroup of patients who were long-term survivors and, therefore, the 11% severe dementia rate does not apply to those newly diagnosed with brain metastasis. Moreover, on closer examination, each of these five patients was treated using a nonstandard treatment regimen, placing them at higher risk of neurotoxicity. Four of the five patients received high dose per fraction radiation therapy (5 to 6 Gy/fraction), which is concerning given that fraction size is one of the most important predictors of late toxicity. The fifth patient received a standard dose per fraction of 3 Gy; however, this patient was treated with concurrent chemotherapy. Importantly, and not often discussed, is that no patient treated with 3 Gy or less per fraction without concurrent chemotherapy developed dementia. Perhaps, then, the most valuable finding from this study is to be wary of both the use of large fraction sizes and concurrent chemotherapy when delivering WBRT.

It is not to say that WBRT is not associated with some risk of neurotoxicity. The RTOG recently published the results of a randomized trial, 0214, in which patients with stage III non-small-cell lung cancer were randomized to prophylactic cranial RT (30 Gy) versus observation.[30] Although the trial failed to meet accrual goals, the authors noted that WBRT resulted in a decreased incidence of 1-year brain metastases (8% vs 18%), although overall survival was not different. Relevant to our discussion regarding neurocognitive dysfunction, patients receiving prophylactic cranial RT did have a slightly worse immediate and delayed recall, albeit without an effect on global quality of life; however, this required sensitive neurocognitive testing to detect (and again did not stratify for all factors known to affect neurocognitive dysfunction). As such, the question is not whether WBRT alone results in any neurotoxicity but rather whether its overstated risks are outweighed by the benefits of reduced intracranial failure with associated neurocognitive dysfunction. In our view, it generally is. When discussing the pros and cons of WBRT with patients, it is important that the physician maintain an appropriate perspective regarding the toxicities associated with WBRT. For instance, recently, there have been accumulating data suggesting that many systemic chemotherapies are associated with long-term neurotoxicities.[31,32] This is not to say that all chemotherapy need be abandoned, but rather, whenever prescribing treatment, one must make sure that the benefits outweigh the risks.

Researchers are exploring many avenues for potentially decreasing the neurotoxicity associated with WBRT for the treatment of brain metastases. Recently, the RTOG completed accrual on a phase 3 trial randomizing patients to WBRT with or without memantine, an *N*-methyl-D-aspartate (NMDA) receptor antagonist that has proven to be effective in the treatment of vascular and Alzheimer dementia.[33] The drug has minimal side effects, and if proven successful it would represent an important step forward in reducing radiation-induced neurotoxicity. Other groups are taking a different approach by limiting the dose to regions of the brain thought to be central to RT-induced neurocognitive toxicity. A retrospective analysis from Tata Memorial Hospital of patients with low-grade gliomas demonstrated that, following RT, one third of patients had a greater than 10% decrease in IQ.[34] Dosimetric analysis demonstrated that dose to the left temporal lobe was correlated with the decline in IQ. A separate analysis from MD Anderson Cancer Center of patients with low-grade or anaplastic brain tumors demonstrated a dose response, with hippocampal dose correlated with decline in learning and delayed recall.[35] These studies, along with preclinical data, have brought the hippocampus forward as the prime target of current investigations. This has led the RTOG to develop a trial, 0933, which will test a hippocampal-sparing WBRT technique for brain metastases patients. The primary outcome will be delayed recall using the HVLT at 4 months posttreatment, which is an unfortunate limitation as previously critiqued in our earlier discussion regarding the trial by Chang et al. Although specifically avoiding dose to regions of the brain does raise concern for potentially resulting in high failure rates at these sites, retrospective analyses have shown that ~ 8% of metastases occur near the hippocampus.[36] Were the trial to be successful in reducing neurocognitive dysfunction compared with a planned cohort of historical controls, the trade-off of a slightly higher failure rate in return for decreased neurotoxicity would likely be acceptable to most practitioners. Unfortunately, there are several reasons to be skeptical of such an approach, namely, hippocampal-sparing WBRT requires time-intensive contouring, planning, QA, and increased cost; sparing of the hippocampus by currently available techniques may not lead to a clinically significant benefit; and hippocampal-sparing WBRT downplays the importance of other parts of the brain (i.e., remainder of limbic circuit and cerebral cortex) in memory function.

■ Summary and Conclusions

Brain metastases remain a common problem in cancer patients, and as systemic therapies improve, leading patients to live longer, the brain's role as a "sanctuary" site will make this an even more frequent occurrence. The management of brain metastases remains a complex challenge, and the field remains filled with more questions than answers. Still, treatments have progressed considerably from the era of steroids as the sole treatment. Subsets of patients can be long-term survivors despite brain metastases. Attempting to discern who these patients are, based on established prognostic systems, or an individual patient's disease history, allows for an appropriate level of care. Although WBRT remains the standard of care for most patients, its judicious use in patients who are at high risk for toxicity should be a consideration. Aggressive local treatments with surgery and SRS can improve outcomes, including survival in select groups of patients. Future developments, including radiosensitizers, radioprotectors, alternative fractionation schemes, and techniques to reduce dose to sensitive brain tissues, may lead to improved results in the future.

Expert Recommendations

1. WBRT should be considered postoperatively in patients with resected brain metastases as a means to improve local and distant brain control of brain metastases. SRS to the resection cavity warrants further investigation and may be considered in those patients felt to be at high risk for neurotoxicity (e.g., elderly patients with evidence of cerebrovascular disease or risk factors); however, it comes with the risk of increased intracranial disease progression (Grade 1B Recommendation, Level I–III Evidence).
2. SRS should be considered in addition to WBRT in patients with one to three brain metastases to improve local control of brain metastases. Its use should be particularly considered in those patients in whom it has been found to improve survival (patients with a single lesion, RPA level 1, or squamous non-small-cell lung cancer histology) (Grade 1A Recommendation, Level I Evidence).
3. WBRT should be considered in addition to SRS/surgery in patients with one to three brain metastases to improve local and distant control of brain metastases. Withholding WBRT may be considered in those patients felt to be at high risk for neurotoxicity (e.g., elderly patients with evidence of cerebrovascular disease or risk factors); however, it comes with the risk of increased intracranial disease progression (Grade 1A Recommendation, Level I Evidence).
4. WBRT is the mainstay of treatment for patients with multiple (more than three) brain metastases. SRS/surgery should be used selectively in this setting (particularly, when the predominant symptom requiring palliation is related to significant mass effect) (Grade 1B Recommendation, Level II Evidence).

References

1. Sperduto PW, Chao ST, Sneed PK, et al. Diagnosis-specific prognostic factors, indexes, and treatment outcomes for patients with newly diagnosed brain metastases: a multi-institutional analysis of 4,259 patients. Int J Radiat Oncol Biol Phys 2010;77:655–661
2. Kwok Y, Pathchell RA, Regine WF. Management of overt central nervous system metastases: brain and spinal cord. In: Pass HI, ed. Principles and Practice of Lung Cancer, 4th ed. Philadelphia, PA: Lippincott Williams & Wilkins; 2010:911–926
3. Wen PY, Loeffler JS. Overview of the clinical manifestations, diagnosis, and management of patients with brain metastases. UpToDate. Posner JB, ed. 2011. http://www.uptodate.com. Accessed May 29, 2012
4. Flannery TW, Suntharalingam M, Regine WF, et al. Long-term survival in patients with synchronous, solitary brain metastasis from non-small-cell lung cancer treated with radiosurgery. Int J Radiat Oncol Biol Phys 2008;72:19–23
5. Gaspar L, Scott C, Rotman M, et al. Recursive partitioning analysis (RPA) of prognostic factors in three Radiation Therapy Oncology Group (RTOG) brain metastases trials. Int J Radiat Oncol Biol Phys 1997;37:745–751
6. Sperduto PW, Berkey B, Gaspar LE, Mehta M, Curran W. A new prognostic index and comparison to three other indices for patients with brain metastases: an analysis of 1,960 patients in the RTOG database. Int J Radiat Oncol Biol Phys 2008;70:510–514
7. Patchell RA, Tibbs PA, Walsh JW, et al. A randomized trial of surgery in the treatment of single metastases to the brain. N Engl J Med 1990;322:494–500
8. Patchell RA, Tibbs PA, Regine WF, et al. Postoperative radiotherapy in the treatment of single metastases to the brain: a randomized trial. JAMA 1998;280:1485–1489
9. Choi CY, Chang SD, Gibbs IC, et al. Stereotactic radiosurgery of the postoperative resection cavity for brain metastases: Prospective evaluation of target margin on tumor control. Int J Radiat Oncol Biol Phys 2012; Epub ahead of print
10. Kondziolka D, Patel A, Lunsford LD, et al. Stereotactic radiosurgery plus whole brain radiotherapy versus radiotherapy alone for patients with multiple brain metastases. Int J Radiat Oncol Biol Phys 1999;45:427–434
11. Andrews DW, Scott CB, Sperduto PW, et al. Whole brain radiation therapy with or without stereotactic radiosurgery boost for patients with one to three brain metastases: phase III results of the RTOG 9508 randomised trial. Lancet 2004;363:1665–1672
12. Sneed PK, Suh JH, Goetsch SJ, et al. A multi-institutional review of radiosurgery alone vs. radiosurgery with whole brain radiotherapy as the initial management of brain metastases. Int J Radiat Oncol Biol Phys 2002;53:519–526
13. Aoyama H, Shirato H, Tago M, et al. Stereotactic radiosurgery plus whole-brain radiation therapy vs stereotactic radiosurgery alone for treatment of brain metastases: a randomized controlled trial. JAMA 2006;295:2483–2491
14. Aoyama H, Tago M, Kato N, et al. Neurocognitive function of patients with brain metastasis who received either whole brain radiotherapy plus stereotactic radiosurgery or radiosurgery alone. Int J Radiat Oncol Biol Phys 2007;68:1388–1395
15. Kocher M, Soffietti R, Abacioglu U, et al. Adjuvant whole-brain radiotherapy versus observation after radiosurgery or surgical resection of one to three cerebral metastases: results of the EORTC 22952–26001 study. J Clin Oncol 2011;29:134–141
16. Chang EL, Wefel JS, Hess KR, et al. Neurocognition in patients with brain metastases treated with radiosurgery or radiosurgery plus whole-brain irradiation: a randomised controlled trial. Lancet Oncol 2009;10:1037–1044
17. Mahmood U, Kwok Y, Regine WF, Patchell RA. Whole-brain irradiation for patients with brain metastases: still the standard of care. Lancet Oncol 2010;11:221–222
18. Regine WF, Schmitt FA, Scott CB, et al. Feasibility of neurocognitive outcome evaluations in patients with brain metastases in a multi-institutional cooperative group setting: results of Radiation Therapy Oncology Group trial BR-0018. Int J Radiat Oncol Biol Phys 2004;58:1346–1352
19. Armstrong CL, Corn BW, Ruffer JE, et al. Radiotherapeutic effects on brain function: double dissociation of memory systems. Neuropsychiatry Neuropsychol Behav Neurol 2000;13:101–111
20. Pereira J, Hanson J, Bruera E. The frequency and clinical course of cognitive impairment in patients with terminal cancer. Cancer 1997;79:835–842
21. Lawlor PG, Gagnon B, Mancini IL, et al. Occurrence, causes, and outcome of delirium in patients with advanced cancer: a prospective study. Arch Intern Med 2000;160:786–794
22. Borgelt B, Gelber R, Kramer S, et al. The palliation of brain metastases: final results of the first two studies by the Radiation Therapy Oncology Group. Int J Radiat Oncol Biol Phys 1980;6:1–9
23. Sneed PK, Larson DA, Wara WM. Radiotherapy for cerebral metastases. Neurosurg Clin N Am 1996;7:505–515
24. Horton J, Baxter DH, Olson KB. The management of metastases to the brain by irradiation and corticosteroids. Am J Roentgenol Radium Ther Nucl Med 1971;111:334–336
25. Meyers CA, Smith JA, Bezjak A, et al. Neurocognitive function and progression in patients with brain metastases treated with whole-brain radiation and motexafin gadolinium: results of a randomized phase III trial. J Clin Oncol 2004;22:157–165
26. Regine WF, Huhn JL, Patchell RA, et al. Risk of symptomatic brain tumor recurrence and neurologic deficit after radiosurgery alone in patients with newly diagnosed brain metastases: results and implications. Int J Radiat Oncol Biol Phys 2002;52:333–338
27. Li J, Bentzen SM, Renschler M, et al. Regression after whole-brain radiation therapy for brain metastases correlates with survival and improved neurocognitive function. J Clin Oncol 2007;25:1260–1266
28. Regine WF, Scott C, Murray K, Curran W. Neurocognitive outcome in brain metastases patients treated with accelerated-fractionation vs. accelerated-hyperfractionated radiotherapy: an analysis from Radiation Therapy Oncology Group Study 91–04. Int J Radiat Oncol Biol Phys 2001;51:711–717
29. DeAngelis LM, Mandell LR, Thaler HT, et al. The role of postoperative radiotherapy after resection of single brain metastases. Neurosurgery 1989;24:798–805
30. Sun A, Bae K, Gore EM, et al. Phase III trial of prophylactic cranial irradiation compared with observation in patients with locally advanced non-small-cell lung cancer: neurocognitive and quality-of-life analysis. J Clin Oncol 2011;29:279–286
31. Koppelmans V, Breteler MM, Boogerd W, et al. Neuropsychological performance in survivors of breast cancer more than 20 years after adjuvant chemotherapy. J Clin Oncol 2012;30:1080–1086
32. Deprez S, Amant F, Smeets A, et al. Longitudinal assessment of chemotherapy-induced structural changes in cerebral white matter and its correlation with impaired cognitive functioning. J Clin Oncol 2012;30:274–281
33. Orgogozo J, Rigaud A, Stöffler A, et al. Efficacy and safety of memantine in patients with mild to moderate vascular dementia: a randomized, placebo-controlled trial (MMM 300). Stroke 2002;33:1834–1839
34. Jalali R, Mallick I, Dutta D, et al. Factors influencing neurocognitive outcomes in young patients with benign and low-grade brain tumors treated with stereotactic conformal radiotherapy. Int J Radiat Oncol Biol Phys 2010;77:974–979
35. Mahajan A, Dong L, Prabhu S, et al. Application of deformable image registration to hippocampal doses and neurocognitive outcomes. Soc Neuro Oncol 2007:538
36. Gondi V, Tome WA, Marsh J, et al. Estimated risk of perihippocampal disease progression after hippocampal avoidance during whole-brain radiotherapy: safety profile for RTOG 0933. Radiother Oncol 2010;95:327–331

27

Evidence-Based Management of Leptomeningeal Metastasis from Solid Tumors

Jennie W. Taylor and Andrew Norden

Introduction

Leptomeningeal metastasis (LM), also known as carcinomatous meningitis when related to primary solid tumors, or lymphomatous/leukemic meningitis when related to hematologic malignancies, is a dreaded complication of systemic cancer in which tumor cells invade the cerebrospinal fluid (CSF) and leptomeninges. With an overall prevalence of 5 to 10%,[1] LM is most commonly associated with adenocarcinoma (> 70%),[2] but the prevalence varies depending on the primary tumor type (**Table 27.1**), though breast and lung are the most common primary histology (**Table 27.2**). Approximately 1 to 7% of all cases arise from unknown primary sites.[3] Usually a complication of advanced malignancy, LM is associated with progressive disseminated disease in > 70% of cases, as the primary site of progressive disease in 20%, and as the initial manifestation of cancer in 5 to 10%.[3] However, it is likely underdiagnosed given a 20% incidence at autopsy in patients with known malignancies and neurological complaints.[4]

Prognosis is poor, with a dismal median survival for untreated patients of 4 to 16 weeks.[5,6] Poor performance status, advanced age, and presence of bulky disease have been identified as adverse prognostic factors in several studies.[7–10] Other prognostic factors may include duration of clinical signs at presentation, protein levels in the CSF, and treatment with intrathecal chemotherapy.[11]

Table 27.1 Prevalence of leptomeningeal metastasis among solid tumor types[1,24]

Breast	5 to 35%
Lung	10 to 26%
Melanoma	5 to 25%
Gastrointestinal	4 to 14%
Cancers of unknown primary	1 to 7%
Primary brain tumors	1 to 2%

Pathophysiology and Clinical Presentation

Upon entering the CSF space, malignant cells quickly disperse, which often results in multifocal seeding. The most common sites of tumor infiltration are the basilar cisterns at the skull base and the dorsal aspect of the spinal cord, particularly at the cauda equina[12,13]; these sites explain the high frequency of cranial nerve dysfunction and lumbosacral radiculopathy. The routes of central nervous system (CNS) invasion are similar to those taken by parenchymal metastases: hematogenous spread, particularly

Table 27.2 Distribution (%) of leptomeningeal metastasis from solid tumors

	Bruna et al 2009[2]	Waki et al 2009[10]	Clarke et al 2010[23]	Range
Breast	43	39	43	39 to 43
Lung	39	42	31	31 to 42
Gastointenstinal	6	11	7	6 to 11
Skin (melanoma)	4	2	6	2 to 6
Other	8	4	9	4 to 9

through the choroid plexus or the valveless vertebral venous system; direct tumor invasion; or migration along perivascular or perineural spaces.[12,13] The cancer stem cell hypothesis may also apply to LM in that clonal expansion within the CSF is a potential mechanism of entry and a therapeutic target.[14]

Iatrogenic spread after resection of an intraparenchymal metastasis, especially in the posterior fossa, may be an important mechanism of tumor cell dispersion.[15] Large retrospective data show that piecemeal resection, as compared with en bloc resection, is associated with an increased incidence of leptomeningeal dissemination, irrespective of primary tumor type. In one study, 9% of patients who had a piecemeal resection developed leptomeningeal dissemination, versus 3% of those treated with gross total resection or 1% of those treated with stereotactic radiosurgery (SRS).[15] The incidence is even higher if the lesion is in the posterior fossa, with 14% of patients developing LM after piecemeal resection, as compared with 6% treated with en bloc resection or SRS.[16] This difference may be explained by the lower CSF flow rate in the infratentorial compartment, allowing for easier deposition of circulating tumor cells, especially after a piecemeal resection.[15] There may also be a shorter time to development of LM after surgery (3.4 months) versus after SRS (4.2 months).[15] However, the overall survival is 2.8 months regardless of treatment[15] (Level III).

Classically, LM manifests as a triad of cerebral dysfunction (e.g., headache, altered mental status, confusion, memory impairment, and seizures), cranial neuropathies, and radiculopathies. Multifocal signs are present in 70% of patients, and 50% have evidence of spinal or radicular symptoms.[17] Cranial nerve (CN) VI is the most commonly affected cranial nerve, leading to diplopia, though CN III or IV palsies may also cause double vision. Facial weakness, numbness, vertigo, tinnitus, and blurry vision are other common symptoms that implicate involvement of nerves VII, V, VIII, and II, respectively. Spinoradicular symptoms most commonly affect the legs and manifest as weakness, numbness, pain, and bowel or bladder dysfunction.[11] Symptoms vary depending on the primary tumor, with solid tumors more likely to affect nerves II, III, IV, and VI and hematologic malignancies more likely to affect CN VII. Headaches may be the result of increased intracranial pressure (ICP) or leptomeningeal irritation.[18] CSF flow abnormalities are also noted in 50% of patients when flow studies are performed.[11] Synchronous intraparenchymal brain metastases are evident in 30 to 60% of patients presenting with leptomeningeal disease,[10] as are synchronous intramedullary spinal metastases.[6]

■ Diagnosis

Computed tomography (CT) has a low sensitivity of 30% for detecting LM. Magnetic resonance imaging (MRI) of the entire neuroaxis, ideally prior to lumbar puncture to eliminate artifact related to intracranial hypotension,[19] should be performed when there is a clinical suspicion for LM. Typical MRI findings include focal areas of contrast enhancement of the leptomeninges that are nodular deposits along the subependymal lining or subarachnoid space. Diffuse dural enhancement is rare. The cerebellar folia and cauda equina are areas where leptomeningeal enhancement may be more easily seen (**Fig. 27.1**). Cranial and spinal nerves may be thickened and enhancing. When contrast-enhanced sequences are unrevealing, T2-weighted or fluid-attenuated axial inversion recovery (FLAIR) imaging may be useful.[20] MRI has a sensitivity of 85% in solid tumors versus 20% in leukemia and 37.5% in lymphoma.[21] Despite its superior sensitivity, MRI reveals abnormal enhancement in only ~50% of cases (Level II).

In patients with an underlying malignancy, diffuse dural enhancement on CT or MRI is usually associated with skull metastases causing underlying dural inflammation rather than LM. The presenting symptoms of headache and cranial neuropathies may be similar to those seen in LM, and CSF studies may also show elevated protein and hypoglycorrhachia. However, it is critical to distinguish these two groups of patients because calvarial metastases usually re-

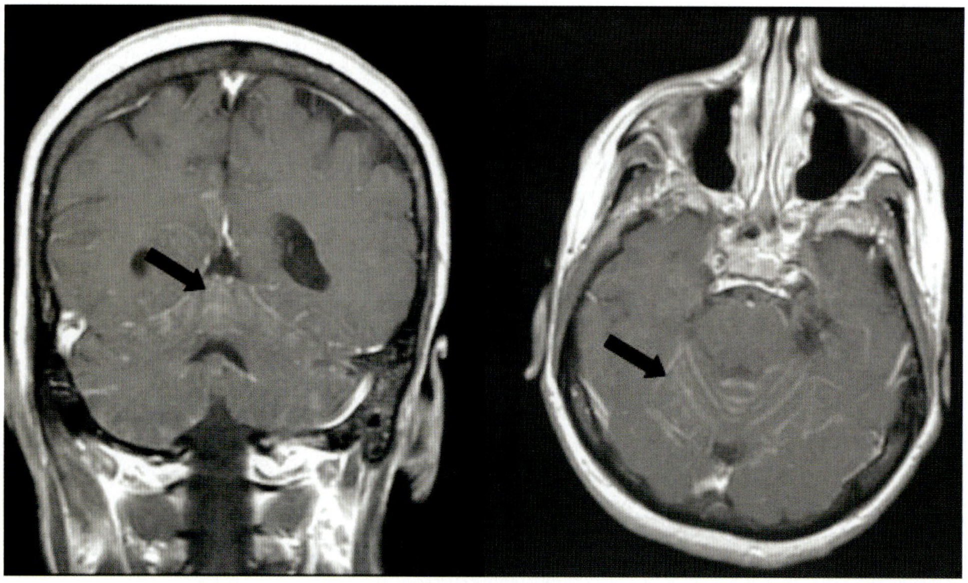

Fig. 27.1 Coronal and axial T1-contrast-enhancing magnetic resonance imaging scan of a patient with leptomeningeal metastasis from breast cancer with leptomeningeal enhancement in the folia of the cerebellum.

spond to systemic treatment, which is rarely effective in LM.[22]

When clinical or imaging findings raise suspicion for LM, CSF examination is usually required to confirm the diagnosis. The classic CSF abnormalities seen in LM are elevated opening pressure, elevated protein, low glucose, and lymphocytic pleocytosis. In a large study of 150 patients with LM from solid tumors, 56% had an elevated opening pressure (> 20 cm H_2O), 57% with a leukocytosis (> 5/mm^2), 62% had elevated protein (> 50 mg/dL), and 38% had low glucose (<40 mg/dL). Only 5% of patients had completely normal CSF.[23] Cytology has a sensitivity of ~ 85% for solid tumors versus 94 to 100% for meningitis secondary to lymphoproliferative disorders (Level II).[21] Patients with solid tumor LM who have definitive clinical and imaging findings may in some circumstances avoid CSF evaluation.[21] Even after repeated CSF examinations, 10 to 20% of patients will have false-negative cytology.[24] Cytology is positive in 96% of LM patients with neurological dysfunction and in 84% of those with a CSF pleocytosis.[25] For malignant cells to be detected by cytology they must make up at least 5% of the cell sample[26]; for this reason a minimum of 10 mL of CSF should be processed.[27] Samples should be processed as quickly as possible, with the addition of fixative, ethylenediaminetetraacetic acid (EDTA), prolonging cellular degradation for up to several days.[5,26] Some groups recommend that cytology not be sent at night, over the weekend, or in other circumstances when processing will be delayed (Level II).[27] Up to 45% of samples will be falsely negative on the first CSF cytology evaluation, with an improved yield of 80% on the second sample[24] (**Table 27.3**).

Abnormal CSF circulation is evident in 30 to 70% of patients with LM and is associated with a poor prognosis.[7,28] Intrathecal treatment for these patients leads to poor drug distribution and increases risk of toxicity. Blockage of flow can be diagnosed with a radionuclide study using either ^{111}indium-diethylenetriaminepentaacetic acid or ^{99}Tc macroaggregated albumin that is injected intrathecally. Radiotherapy restores flow in 30% of patients with spinal CSF blockage and 50% of those with intracranial blockage. However, patients with improved CSF flow seem to accrue greater benefits from intrathecal chemotherapy[7,28] (Level III).

Unfortunately, biomarkers and immunohistochemical analysis of CSF have not significantly in-

Table 27.3 Maximizing cerebrospinal fluid cytology results[27]

Obtain cerebrospinal fluid from a symptomatic or radiographically involved site (e.g., cisternal tap if cranial nerves are involved)
Collect > 10.5 mL of cerebrospinal fluid
Process the sample within 48 hours
Collect > 2 samples if first cytology was negative but clinical suspicion is high

creased the yield of cytology.[3] The exception is with antibody-specific markers and cytogenetic analysis that may help distinguish pathological from reactive cells in the case of lymphomatous or leukemic meningitis.[3] The differential diagnosis for leptomeningeal disease in patients with suspicious symptoms includes infectious etiologies, such as tickborne illnesses, varicella zoster virus, human herpesvirus-6, toxoplasmosis, legionellosis, listeriosis, bacterial meningitis, and tuberculous meningitis.[21]

Recommendations for Evaluation of Leptomeningeal Metastases[29]

1. All patients without contraindications (e.g., pacemaker placement) should undergo a contrasted MRI scan of the entire neuroaxis to evaluate extent of disease and direct appropriate therapy (Grade 2A Recommendation, Level II Evidence).
2. All patients without contraindications (e.g., severe thrombocytopenia or mass effect from intracranial lesion) should have a lumbar puncture for detection of malignant cells by cytology. To optimize results, a minimum of 10 mL of CSF should be collected and processed immediately in EDTA to prevent degradation. The opening pressure should be measured and CSF sent for glucose, protein, cell count, cytology, and flow cytometry and gene rearrangement studies when hematologic malignancies are suspected. If CSF is suspicious, but malignant cells are not detected by cytology, a repeat LP should be performed[24] (Grade 2A Recommendation, Level II Evidence).
3. Patients with good performance status and prognosis should undergo a radionucleotide CSF flow study to detect fluid obstruction[7,28] (Grade 2B Recommendation, Level II Evidence).
4. If LM is the initial manifestation of malignancy, then a thorough workup with whole-body scanning and a medical oncology consult should be obtained (Grade 2A Recommendation, Level II Evidence).

■ Literature Review

Treatment

Clinical studies of treatment for LM are challenging, and the published results can be difficult to interpret. In most studies, diagnosis is defined by positive cytology or enhancement on imaging. Treatment response is typically determined by clearing of CSF. Because cytology has low sensitivity, and often patients are not subjected to repeated LP, it is an imperfect measure of response. Clinical improvement alone as a primary end point is infrequently used. Another complicating factor is that patients who are treated with one modality over another often differ in terms of important prognostic factors.

Treatment of LM is palliative; long-term survival is rare, and neurological dysfunction is usually irreversible. Therefore the intent of treatment is to stabilize current deficits and prevent progression.[30] Three treatment modalities are available: intrathecal (IT) chemotherapy, systemic chemotherapy that penetrates the blood–brain barrier, and radiation therapy. For patients with a good performance status and positive cytology, normal CSF flow and no bulky disease, IT chemotherapy should be considered, though penetration is only 1 to 2 mm and fails to address disease outside the CNS.[31] For those with a good performance status with bulky disease or CSF flow blockage, and good systemic treatment options, a combination of modalities may be beneficial. Patients with poor performance status, fixed neurological deficits, and bulky CNS disease may be best treated with focused radiation to symptomatic areas or whole brain radiation (National Comprehensive Cancer Network [NCCN] 2012).[29] The likelihood of treatment response also depends on tumor histology, though this has been rigorously evaluated only in patients with LM secondary to lymphoproliferative disorders and breast cancer, both of which are associated with a better overall prognosis.

Unfortunately, no large prospective, randomized trials exist for the treatment of LM; therefore recommendations and guidelines are based on several small phase 2 and 3 studies, case series, and expert opinion. The most recent NCCN guidelines from July 2012 provide an algorithm for treatment of LM.[29]

Level II to Level III Evidence

Overall survival and time to neurological progression are comparable between IT chemotherapy and radiotherapy. A review of the current literature on LM from solid tumors reports a response rate for IT chemotherapy of 27% and median survival of 14 weeks, compared with radiation, which has a 20% response rate and median survival of 11 weeks. Although the combination of the two methods improves response rates to 34%, overall survival is still only 13 weeks. More intensified treatment, combining IT and systemic chemotherapy along with radiation, further improves response rates to 67%, but again no overall survival benefit is seen (Level II).[20]

Patients with a poor functional status are less likely to tolerate systemic or IT chemotherapy, and radiation should be considered in these cases. Radiotherapy does not improve overall survival in patients with LM but is very useful as a palliative treatment. Whole-brain radiation, 30 Gy over 10 fractions, is often used to treat synchronous intraparenchymal lesions or bulky leptomeningeal disease that would preclude IT chemotherapy administration. If infratentorial lesions are present, the field should include the spinal cord down to the caudal margin of the second vertebral body.[20] A recently published retrospective study of 27 patients with solid tumors, treated with whole-brain radiation as monotherapy, reported a median overall survival of 8 weeks, with 26% alive at 6 months and 15% alive at 1 year. On multivariate analysis, the only significant prognostic marker was fixed cranial nerve deficit, which carried a poor prognosis—19 versus 4 weeks[32] (Level III). Radiation is also used focally throughout the neuroaxis to treat symptomatic lesions and bulky disease causing CSF flow block[7,8,10] (Level II). Craniospinal radiation, however, is not generally recommended because of its toxicity in this heavily pretreated population.

Long-term whole brain radiation therapy survivors (longer than 4 months) often develop leukoencephalopathy with diffuse confluent white matter changes seen on imaging, or communicating hydrocephalus. The overall incidence is probably underreported but is estimated to be roughly 20%. Clinical symptoms include variable degrees of cognitive impairment, and neuroimaging reveals white matter T2/FLAIR changes[33] (**Fig. 27.2**). Systemic methotrexate and any IT chemotherapies during or after radiation increase the risk of leukoencephalopathy.[20,33,34] Clinically, patients and their families note impaired cognitive function with decreased memory, gait disturbance, and urinary incontinence, and these patients may benefit from ventriculoperitoneal shunting.[20]

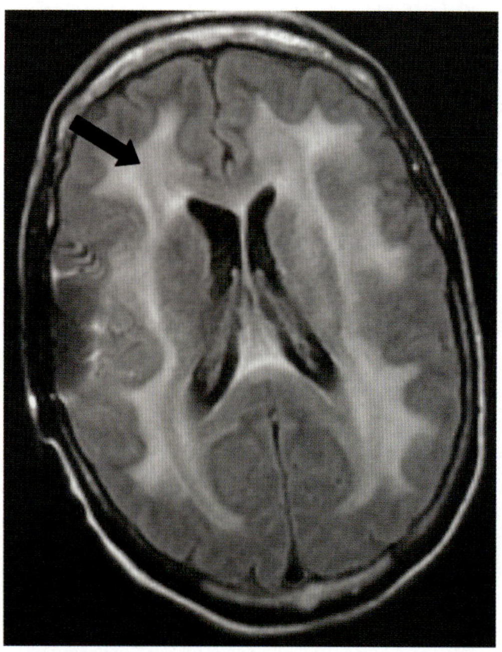

Fig. 27.2 Axial T2/fluid-attenuated inversion recovery magnetic resonance imaging scan of a patient with leptomeningeal metastasis from breast cancer with diffuse white matter changes consistent with leukoencephalopathy from radiation and systemic chemotherapy.

The most commonly used IT medications are methotrexate, cytarabine, or its longer-acting liposomal derivative liposomal cytarabine (DepoCyt, Sigma-Tau Pharmaceuticals, Gaithersburg, MD), and less often thiotepa and topotecan (**Table 27.4**). Their widespread use and approval are based on a few randomized trials and several smaller phase 2 studies.

Methotrexate, a folate antimetabolite with a CSF half-life of 4.5 to 8.0 hours, is dosed IT at 10 to 15 mg twice a week for 4 weeks as induction, followed by 10 to 15 mg weekly for 4 weeks, and then monthly thereafter. It is generally used to treat LM from breast cancer or lymphoproliferative disorders. Cytarabine is a pyrimidine nucleoside analogue. IT dosing is 25 to 100 mg twice a week for 4 weeks, followed by weekly injections for 4 weeks, and then monthly thereafter.[3] DepoCyt, a long-acting liposomal derivative of cytarabine, produces cytotoxic cytarabine levels throughout the CSF at a dose of 50 mg (irrespective of site of delivery) for more than 14 days.[35] Induction treatment is given every 2 weeks for 8 weeks, followed by monthly doses until disease progression or toxicity develops.[5] The most common acute toxicity related to IT DepoCyt administration is aseptic meningitis, which occurs in up to 20 to 40% of patients and can last up to 72 hours after drug administration. Symptoms include fever, headache, photophobia, nausea, vomiting, and lethargy. Treatment consists of oral steroids, antipyretics, and antiemetics[3] and can be prevented when dexamethasone 4 mg twice a day is administered on days 1 through 5 of each cycle.[30]

A phase 3 randomized trial of 61 patients with LM from solid tumors (all with positive cytology) comparing IT DepoCyt (50 mg every 2 weeks) to IT methotrexate (10 mg twice a week) was published in 1999. Response was defined as negative cytology and stable or improved neurological exam. DepoCyt had a response rate of 26% with a median survival of 105 days, compared with methotrexate with a 20% response rate and median survival of 78 days. Those treated with DepoCyt had a statistically significant prolonged median time to neurological progression (58 vs 30 days), with an easier dosing schedule and similar toxicity profile (Level II).[36] These findings were later validated in a large, open-label trial of 110 patients with a response rate of 27% with a median overall survival of 95 days and time to neurological progression of 55 days (Level II).[30] DepoCyt showed a similar response rate of 28% when evaluated in 58 patients with breast cancer, with median time to neurological progression of 49 days, overall survival of 88 days, and 1-year survival of 19% (Level II).[37]

Table 27.4 Commonly used intrathecal chemotherapies

Drug	Dose	Induction	Consolidation/maintenance
Methotrexate[33,36,38]	10 to 12 mg	Twice weekly for 4 weeks	Weekly for 4 to 8 weeks; monthly
DepoCyt[a] (liposomal cytarabine)[36]	50 mg	Every 2 weeks for 8 weeks	Monthly
Thiotepa[38]	10 mg	Twice weekly for 4 weeks	Weekly for 4–8 weeks; monthly
Topotecan[39]	0.4 mg	Twice weekly for 6 weeks	Twice weekly for 6 weeks/every 2 weeks for 4 months

[a]Sigma-Tau Pharmaceuticals, Gaithersburg, MD.

IT methotrexate (10 mg twice a week) was compared with IT thiotepa (10 mg twice a week) in a prospective randomized study of 52 patients with LM from solid and hematologic malignancies. No patients demonstrated a response, and no significant difference in overall survival (15.9 weeks vs 14.1 weeks) or toxicity profiles was seen (Level II).[38] Preliminary small studies with IT topotecan were promising. However, a phase 2 study of IT topotecan (400 µg twice a week) in 62 patients with predominantly solid tumors revealed a cytologic response rate of 21% and clinical response of 16%. Median overall survival was 105 days and 32% experienced chemical meningitis (Level II).[39] A small phase 2 trial of 22 patients with LM from solid tumors and lymphoproliferative disorders were treated with IT interferon-α with a 45% cytologic response but a 60% rate of transient chemical arachnoiditis (Level II).[40]

Because LM is often a late complication of malignancies, patients are usually heavily pretreated and have poor performance status, making them more susceptible to toxicities from systemic chemotherapy. Though the blood–brain barrier is likely compromised in LM, concentrations of systemic chemotherapy are often inadequate to be cytotoxic. Although this accounts for the historical use of IT chemotherapy over systemic therapy, IT chemotherapy fails to address disease outside the CNS.[31] One study prospectively compared two groups of patients with LM from solid tumors. The groups were well matched by age and primary tumor histology. Of 104 patients treated with systemic chemotherapy and radiation, 54 received concurrent IT methotrexate. There was no difference in the duration of response (4 to 5 months), overall survival (4 months), or percentage of long-term survivors (~ 20%). However, the group who received IT methotrexate had a statistically significant higher rate of CNS-related toxicity (Level II).[41]

A small prospective trial of 35 patients with LM from breast cancer randomized patients to receive IT methotrexate as part of their treatment versus not, with both groups receiving radiation and systemic chemotherapy as clinically indicated. The median survival in the IT group was 18 weeks compared with 30 weeks in the non-IT group. Moreover, 53% of patients treated with IT chemotherapy developed cognitive impairment compared with 22% in the non-IT group (Level II).[34] A case-control study of high-dose intravenous methotrexate (8 g/m^2) looked at 16 patients with LM from solid tumors and lymphoproliferative disorders who were not candidates for IT treatment and compared them to 15 matched controls who received standard IT methotrexate. Median survival in the systemic methotrexate group was 13.8 months with a longer cytotoxic CSF concentration, compared with 2.3 months in the IT methotrexate group (Level III).[33]

Small phase 2 trials have evaluated other cytotoxic systemic agents. Etoposide (0.5 mg orally or intravenously for 5 days every other week for 8 weeks) was also studied in a phase 2 trial of 27 patients with LM from hematologic and solid tumors. There was a 27% response rate, median survival of 70 days, and 13% toxicity rate, and 30% of patients were unable to complete the 8 weeks of therapy (Level II).[42]

Development of communicating hydrocephalus is an important complication of LM when the kinetics of CSF flow and reabsorption are impaired. It may also be a delayed complication from whole-brain radiation. Symptoms of increased ICP, with headache, gait disturbance, nausea/vomiting, and cognitive impairment, can be debilitating for patients. Symptoms may be out of proportion to the degree of ventricular enlargement, and papilledema is rarely noted. However, the opening pressure is usually elevated on lumbar puncture, and there is often a transient improvement in symptoms following the procedure. Symptoms may be quickly reversible with ventriculoperitoneal shunting, which is both palliative and therapeutic by improving functional status. In one study of 37 patients treated at Memorial Sloan-Kettering Cancer Center, 77% had improvement in symptoms after shunting, with complication rates of < 10% and median overall survival of 2 months (Level III).[43] However, administering IT chemotherapy to patients with functioning ventriculoperitoneal shunts can be counterproductive and can lead to diversion of drug out of the CSF space.[44] Introducing a reservoir with an on-off valve in conjunction with a ventriculoperitoneal shunt (RO-VPS) was shown in one case-controlled retrospective trial to be safe and efficacious (Level III).[44] However, no prospective data have been published to address this issue. Nonetheless, RO-VPS can be considered in patients with good functional status, favorable histology, and symptoms related to increased ICP.

Level IV Evidence

Several newer cytotoxic and molecularly targeted agents are being evaluated for their response rates in treatment of LM. Case reports of capecitabine (an oral fluoropyrimidine) in patients with LM from breast and esophageal cancer[45,46] are promising in combination with temozolomide (an oral alkyating agent) in breast cancer (Level IV).[46] Trastuzumab, a monoclonal antibody to the HER2 receptor, has significantly improved the overall survival of patients with HER2+ breast cancer but is too large a molecule to penetrate the CNS, leaving it a sanctuary for relapse. An estimated 40% of HER2+ patients relapse in the CNS, though the incidence of isolated leptomeningeal disease without parenchymal involvement is only 2 to 3%.[24,46] IT administration of trastuzumab is controversial, with some case reports demonstrating safety and efficacy (Level IV).[46] Bevacizumab, another monoclonal antibody, which targets vascular endothelial growth factor (VEGF) receptor, has been evaluated for safety in animal models with promising results.[47]

Tyrosine kinase inhibitors (TKIs), another molecularly targeted therapy, are being widely used in several malignancies and contribute to improved survival. Epidermal growth factor receptor (EGFR) somatic mutations are present in up to 25% of patients with non-small-cell lung cancer (NSCLC) and are very sensitive to EGFR TKIs, such as gefitinib (Iressa, AstraZeneca, Wilmington, DE) and erlotinib (Tarceva, Genentech, South San Francisco, CA). Typical mutations are either a deletion in exon 19 or a missense mutation at the L858R position on exon 21. However, there is also a high rate of acquired resistance to TKIs, with T790M substitution in exon 20 occurring in up to 50% of cases at progression. When patients treated with TKIs relapse in the CNS (in either the leptomeninges or the parenchyma), the acquired resistance mutation is often absent, suggesting persistent sensitivity to TKIs. Evidence suggests that pulsatile dosing of erlotinib (1,500 to 2,000 mg weekly) has superior CNS penetration and efficacy over chronic daily dosing (150 to 200 mg daily) (Level IV).[48,49] There are also several case reports of improved efficacy with high-dose erlotinib despite exposure to daily erlotinib or gefitinib (Level IV).[48,50] Lapatinib, a dual EGFR/HER TKI, in combination with capecitabine has been studied in parenchymal metastasis from breast cancer, but its efficacy is unknown in LM (Level IV).[46]

Expert Recommendations[29]

1. Focal radiation should be considered in the following patients:
   a. A poor performance status or prognosis, or those with significant bulky leptomeningeal or parenchymal disease, for symptomatic relief with a focus on comfort and best supportive care (Grade 2A Recommendation, Level II/III Evidence)
   b. A good performance status or prognosis and evidence of CSF flow obstruction on radionucleotide study or focal bulky disease on MRI (Grade 2A Recommendation, Level III Evidence)
   c. For symptomatic treatment at any point during the course of the disease (Grade 2A Recommendation, Level II Evidence)
2. IT chemotherapy (either DepoCyt [Sigma-Tau Pharmaceuticals] or methotrexate) via an Ommaya reservoir, should be considered in the following patients, all with good performance status and prognosis:
   a. Without bulky leptomeningeal disease or concern for increased ICP (as detected by elevated opening pressure on LP and subsequent improvement in symptoms) (Grade 2A Recommendation, Level II/III Evidence).
   b. With LM from hematologic or breast malignancies without bulky leptomeningeal disease or increased ICP (Grade 2A Recommendation, Level II Evidence)
   c. Who are not receiving concurrent radiation, and synchronous treatment with systemic chemotherapy should be used with caution and close monitoring for neurotoxicities[34,41] (Grade 2A Recommendation, Level II/III Evidence)
3. Systemic chemotherapy with high-dose methotrexate should be considered in breast cancer or lymphoma patients with a good performance status and prognosis[33] (Grade 2A Recommendation, Level II Evidence).
4. Ventriculoperitoneal shunting should be considered in patients with evidence of communicating hydrocephalus for symptomatic relief of increased ICP. RO-VPS can also be considered in patients with good performance status and prognosis who may need IT chemotherapy in the future[44] (Grade 2B Recommendation, Level III Evidence).

■ Summary and Conclusions

In summary, LM from solid tumors is a devastating, usually late, complication of several malignancies and is likely to increase in incidence as systemic control improves and cancer patients live longer. Presenting signs and symptoms are often multifocal, and diagnosis is best made by CSF cytology or leptomeningeal enhancement on MRI. Treatment is palliative and should be tailored based on the patient's performance status and projected survival. Radiation, intrathecal and systemic chemotherapy, and ventriculoperitoneal shunt placement all have a role in the treatment of LM, though outcomes are still poor. Notable ongoing trials for treatment of LM from solid tumors include a phase 1/2 study evaluating the safety and efficacy of IT bevacizumab in LM that will correlate VEGF levels with treatment response (NCT00924820), and two phase 1/2 studies assessing the safety and efficacy of IT trastuzumab in LM from breast cancer (NCT01373710) and HER2+ breast cancer (NCT01325207). GRN1005, an intravenous novel peptide-drug conjugate of paclitaxel that penetrates the blood–brain barrier, is being studied in patients with brain metastases from breast cancer and may warrant evaluation in treatment of patients with LM.

■ References

1. Posner J, Neurologic Complications of Cancer. Philadelphia, PA: FA Davis; 1995
2. Bruna J, González L, Miró J, Velasco R, Gil M, Tortosa A; Neuro-Oncology Unit of the Institute of Biomedical Investigation of Bellvitge. Leptomeningeal carcinomatosis: prognostic implications of clinical and cerebrospinal fluid features. Cancer 2009;115(2):381–389
3. Chamberlain MC. Neoplastic meningitis. Semin Neurol 2004;24(4):363–374
4. Pavlidis N. The diagnostic and therapeutic management of leptomeningeal carcinomatosis. Ann Oncol 2004;15(Suppl 4): iv285–iv291
5. Pace A, Fabi A. Chemotherapy in neoplastic meningitis. Crit Rev Oncol Hematol 2006;60(3):194–200
6. Groves MD. The pathogenesis of neoplastic meningitis. Curr Oncol Rep 2003;5(1):15–23
7. Glantz MJ, Hall WA, Cole BF, et al. Diagnosis, management, and survival of patients with leptomeningeal cancer based on cerebrospinal fluid-flow status. Cancer 1995;75(12): 2919–2931
8. Herrlinger U, Förschler H, Küker W, et al. Leptomeningeal metastasis: survival and prognostic factors in 155 patients. J Neurol Sci 2004;223(2):167–178
9. Boogerd W, Hart AA, van der Sande JJ, Engelsman E. Meningeal carcinomatosis in breast cancer. Prognostic factors and influence of treatment. Cancer 1991;67(6):1685–1695
10. Waki F, Ando M, Takashima A, et al. Prognostic factors and clinical outcomes in patients with leptomeningeal metastasis from solid tumors. J Neurooncol 2009;93(2):205–212
11. Balm M, Hammack J. Leptomeningeal carcinomatosis. Presenting features and prognostic factors. Arch Neurol 1996; 53(7):626–632
12. Gonzalez-Vitale JC, Garcia-Bunuel R. Meningeal carcinomatosis. Cancer 1976;37(6):2906–2911
13. Grossman SA, Krabak MJ. Leptomeningeal carcinomatosis. Cancer Treat Rev 1999;25(2):103–119
14. Grewal J, Saria MG, Kesari S. Novel approaches to treating leptomeningeal metastases. J Neurooncol 2012;106(2): 225–234
15. Suki D, Hatiboglu MA, Patel AJ, et al. Comparative risk of leptomeningeal dissemination of cancer after surgery or stereotactic radiosurgery for a single supratentorial solid tumor metastasis. Neurosurgery 2009;64(4):664–674
16. Suki D, Abouassi H, Patel AJ, Sawaya R, Weinberg JS, Groves MD. Comparative risk of leptomeningeal disease after resection or stereotactic radiosurgery for solid tumor metastasis to the posterior fossa. J Neurosurg 2008;108(2):248–257
17. Chowdhary S, Chamberlain M. Leptomeningeal metastases: current concepts and management guidelines. J Natl Compr Canc Netw 2005;3(5):693–703
18. Wolfgang G, Marcus D, Ulrike S. LC: clinical syndrome in different primaries. J Neurooncol 1998;38(2-3):103–110
19. Mokri B. Low cerebrospinal fluid pressure syndromes. Neurol Clin 2004;22(1):55–74, vi.
20. Gleissner B, Chamberlain MC. Neoplastic meningitis. Lancet Neurol 2006;5(5):443–452
21. Pauls S, Fischer AC, Brambs HJ, Fetscher S, Höche W, Bommer M. Use of magnetic resonance imaging to detect neoplastic meningitis: limited use in leukemia and lymphoma but convincing results in solid tumors. Eur J Radiol 2012;81(5): 974–978
22. River Y, Schwartz A, Gomori JM, Soffer D, Siegal T. Clinical significance of diffuse dural enhancement detected by magnetic resonance imaging. J Neurosurg 1996;85(5):777–783
23. Clarke JL, Perez HR, Jacks LM, Panageas KS, Deangelis LM. Leptomeningeal metastases in the MRI era. Neurology 2010;74(18):1449–1454
24. Wasserstrom WR, Glass JP, Posner JB. Diagnosis and treatment of leptomeningeal metastases from solid tumors: experience with 90 patients. Cancer 1982;49(4):759–772
25. Bromberg JE, Breems DA, Kraan J, et al. CSF flow cytometry greatly improves diagnostic accuracy in CNS hematologic malignancies. Neurology 2007;68(20):1674–1679
26. Quijano S, López A, Manuel Sancho J, et al; Spanish Group for the Study of CNS Disease in NHL. Identification of leptomeningeal disease in aggressive B-cell non-Hodgkin's lymphoma: improved sensitivity of flow cytometry. J Clin Oncol 2009;27(9):1462–1469
27. Glantz MJ, Cole BF, Glantz LK, et al. Cerebrospinal fluid cytology in patients with cancer: minimizing false-negative results. Cancer 1998;82(4):733–739
28. Chamberlain MC, Kormanik PA. Prognostic significance of ^{111}indium-DTPA CSF flow studies in leptomeningeal metastases. Neurology 1996;46(6):1674–1677
29. National Comprehensive Cancer Network. NCCN clinical practice guidelines in oncology. Central nervous system cancers. Version 2.2012. Leptomeningeal metastases. 2012 7/6/2012 10/25/2012. http://www.nccn.org.
30. Chamberlain MC, Kormanik P, Howell SB, Kim S. Pharmacokinetics of intralumbar DTC-101 for the treatment of leptomeningeal metastases. Arch Neurol 1995;52(9):912–917
31. Kim L, Glantz MJ. Neoplastic meningitis. Curr Treat Options Oncol 2001;2(6):517–527
32. Gani C, Müller AC, Eckert F, et al. Outcome after whole brain radiotherapy alone in intracranial leptomeningeal carcinomatosis from solid tumors. Strahlenther Onkol 2012;188(2): 148–153
33. Glantz MJ, Cole BF, Recht L, et al. High-dose intravenous methotrexate for patients with nonleukemic leptomeningeal cancer: is intrathecal chemotherapy necessary? J Clin Oncol 1998;16(4):1561–1567
34. Boogerd W, van den Bent MJ, Koehler PJ, et al. The relevance of intraventricular chemotherapy for leptomeningeal metas-

tasis in breast cancer: a randomised study. Eur J Cancer 2004; 40(18):2726–2733
35. Kim S, Chatelut E, Kim JC, et al. Extended CSF cytarabine exposure following intrathecal administration of DTC 101. J Clin Oncol 1993;11(11):2186–2193
36. Glantz MJ, Jaeckle KA, Chamberlain MC, et al. A randomized controlled trial comparing intrathecal sustained-release cytarabine (DepoCyt) to intrathecal methotrexate in patients with neoplastic meningitis from solid tumors. Clin Cancer Res 1999;5(11):3394–3402
37. Jaeckle KA, Phuphanich S, Bent MJ, et al. Intrathecal treatment of neoplastic meningitis due to breast cancer with a slow-release formulation of cytarabine. Br J Cancer 2001;84(2): 157–163
38. Grossman SA, Finkelstein DM, Ruckdeschel JC, Trump DL, Moynihan T, Ettinger DS; Eastern Cooperative Oncology Group. Randomized prospective comparison of intraventricular methotrexate and thiotepa in patients with previously untreated neoplastic meningitis. J Clin Oncol 1993;11(3): 561–569
39. Groves MD, Glantz MJ, Chamberlain MC, et al. A multicenter phase II trial of intrathecal topotecan in patients with meningeal malignancies. Neuro-oncol 2008;10(2):208–215
40. Chamberlain MC. A phase II trial of intra-cerebrospinal fluid alpha interferon in the treatment of neoplastic meningitis. Cancer 2002;94(10):2675–2680
41. Bokstein F, Lossos A, Siegal T. Leptomeningeal metastases from solid tumors: a comparison of two prospective series treated with and without intra-cerebrospinal fluid chemotherapy. Cancer 1998;82(9):1756–1763
42. Chamberlain MC, Tsao-Wei DD, Groshen S. Phase II trial of intracerebrospinal fluid etoposide in the treatment of neoplastic meningitis. Cancer 2006;106(9):2021–2027
43. Omuro AM, Lallana EC, Bilsky MH, DeAngelis LM. Ventriculoperitoneal shunt in patients with leptomeningeal metastasis. Neurology 2005;64(9):1625–1627
44. Lin N, Dunn IF, Glantz M, et al. Benefit of ventriculoperitoneal cerebrospinal fluid shunting and intrathecal chemotherapy in neoplastic meningitis: a retrospective, case-controlled study. J Neurosurg 2011;115(4):730–736
45. Giglio P, Tremont-Lukats IW, Groves MD. Response of neoplastic meningitis from solid tumors to oral capecitabine. J Neurooncol 2003;65(2):167–172
46. Lin NU. Concordance of HER2 in primary tumor and leptomeningeal metastases: now what? Breast Cancer Res Treat 2010;123(1):129–131
47. Brastianos PK, Brastianos HC, Hsu W, et al. The toxicity of intrathecal bevacizumab in a rabbit model of leptomeningeal carcinomatosis. J Neurooncol 2012;106(1):81–88
48. Grommes C, Oxnard GR, Kris MG, et al. "Pulsatile" high-dose weekly erlotinib for CNS metastases from EGFR mutant non-small cell lung cancer. Neuro-oncol 2011;13(12):1364–1369
49. Clarke JL, Pao W, Wu N, Miller VA, Lassman AB. High dose weekly erlotinib achieves therapeutic concentrations in CSF and is effective in leptomeningeal metastases from epidermal growth factor receptor mutant lung cancer. J Neurooncol 2010;99(2):283–286
50. Masuda T, Hattori N, Hamada A, et al. Erlotinib efficacy and cerebrospinal fluid concentration in patients with lung adenocarcinoma developing leptomeningeal metastases during gefitinib therapy. Cancer Chemother Pharmacol 2011; 67(6):1465–1469

▪ SECTION VII ▪

Extra-Axial Tumors and Skull Base Tumors

28

The Role of Radiosurgery in Newly Diagnosed Meningiomas

Douglas Kondziolka, Neal Luther, Hideyuki Kano, Ajay Niranjan, John C. Flickinger, and L. Dade Lunsford

Meningiomas are generally slow-growing, intracranial or intraspinal extra-axial tumors that develop from the arachnoid cap cells of the dura mater.[1-3] Most meningiomas are histologically benign (World Health Organization [WHO] grade I). Others can have atypical features with a faster growth rate (WHO grade II), or features of anaplasia (malignant meningioma, WHO grade III). Meningiomas can occur sporadically or in the setting of neurofibromatosis.

Meningiomas can be found incidentally with neuroimaging or due to the symptoms of headache, seizures, or neurological deficits depending on location. In years past it was uncommon to diagnose a meningioma when it was small, but over the last 20 years most tumors are found earlier due to an awareness by both patients and physicians who obtain neuroimaging, particularly magnetic resonance imaging (MRI) for less specific complaints, such as headache. Under observation, three separate growth patterns may eventually emerge: (1) no or very slow growth, (2) slow growth (i.e., 2 mm/y linear growth on imaging studies), and (3) fast growth (i.e., > 8 mm/y). More rapid growth patterns increase the level of concern that the tumor may have atypical features. Although not common, some tumors double in volume within 6 months to a year. Stereotactic radiosurgery (SRS) has expanded the management options for meningiomas because patients no longer have to choose simply between craniotomy and resection and observation. To date, Level I prospective randomized trials that compare radiosurgery to resection or observation have not been performed. Similarly, there are no randomized comparisons between resection and observation. However, there are numerous large case series with large numbers of patients that include follow-up evaluations beyond 5 years. There is also one cohort comparison. These are discussed in this chapter. The criteria for inclusion of articles are listed in **Table 28.1**.

Table 28.1 Inclusion criteria for literature review: gamma knife radiosurgery for meningiomas

Inclusion Criteria
– Maximum tumor diameter < 3.5 cm
– Data collected prospectively
– Minimum number of subjects =100
– Median follow-up > 4 years
– Treating centers experienced in meningioma management
– Gamma knife radiosurgery patients managed since 1987 (magnetic resonance imaging era)
– Data available on outcomes of tumor response, clinical function, and presenting symptoms

■ Gamma Knife Radiosurgery versus Surgical Resection for Intracranial Meningiomas

Resection is indicated for larger tumors with clinically symptomatic brain or cranial nerve compression, hydrocephalus, intractable headache, or trigeminal neuralgia. Many patients have smaller-volume tumors with no or minimal associated symptoms. Symptoms in turn correlate with the tumor location. A convexity meningioma in the anterior fossa may lead to cognitive or personality dysfunction. A convexity tumor over the motor cortex may produce seizures or motor weakness. A tumor arising in the cavernous sinus typically presents with diplopia.[4]

Surgical resection can be performed via many different cranial, cranial base, and endoscopic approaches. Although the outcomes of surgical removal at centers of excellence have improved markedly over the last 2 decades, patients increasingly seek less invasive options. It is important to understand the different goals of microsurgery and SRS. During resection, removal of both the tumor and its neoplastic dural base provides the best chance for cure (Simpson grade 1 resection).[1] A grade 1 resection is still associated with a 9% recurrence rate, with a mean time to recurrence of 62 months. A grade 2 resection (19% recurrence at mean 59 months) includes tumor removal and cauterization of the adjacent dura. A grade 3 resection (29% recurrence rate) reflects tumor removal only (lumpectomy). A grade 4 resection (40% recurrence rate) reflects subtotal tumor removal. Simpson did not report average follow-up times to progression for grade 3 and grade 4 resections.[1] Because many meningiomas are found at critical locations in the skull base or attached to venous sinuses, grade 2, 3, and 4 resections are common.[2] These surgical recurrence rates can be compared with those observed after gamma knife radiosurgery (GKRS), which is performed to inactivate tumor growth while preserving existing neurological function.

Meningioma SRS using the Gamma Knife (Elekta, Atlanta, GA) was first performed in Stockholm in the mid-1970s. The first comprehensive analysis of 50 patients was provided by the University of Pittsburgh group in 1991 but included only short-term outcomes.[5] During the past 2 decades, radiosurgery has emerged as an effective alternative to surgical removal of small to moderate-sized meningiomas. The long-term results have established radiosurgery as an important minimally invasive alternative to resection. Advanced dose-planning software, high-resolution magnetic resonance imaging (MRI) for targeting, dose optimization, and robotic delivery reflect the evolution of this technology. The goals of meningioma radiosurgery are to prevent further tumor growth, preserve neurological function where possible, avoid the risks associated with open resection, and, in selected patients, improve preexisting symptoms.

Gamma Knife Radiosurgery Technique for Meningiomas

Patients with meningiomas are evaluated with high-resolution MRI (computed tomography [CT] may be substituted in patients who cannot undergo MRI scans) and other tests depending on location (e.g., audiometry for cerebellopontine angle tumors, visual field testing for parasellar tumors). In GKRS, the procedure begins with rigid fixation of an MRI-compatible Leksell stereotactic frame (model G, Elekta Instruments, Atlanta, GA) to the patient's head. Local anesthetic scalp infiltration (5% marcaine and 1% xylocaine) is used, supplemented by mild intravenous sedation as needed. High-resolution images are acquired with a fiducial system attached to the stereotactic frame. For meningioma radiosurgery, a three-dimensional (3-D) volume-acquisition MRI using a gradient pulse sequence (divided into 28 to 36 axial slices, 1 or 1.5 mm thick) is performed to cover the entire lesion and surrounding critical structures. A T2-weighted 3-D volume sequence is performed to visualize the brain parenchyma, any edema, and cranial nerves if appropriate. Planning is performed on narrow-slice-thickness axial MRI scans with coronal and sagittal reconstructions.[6,7]

Radiosurgical Dose Planning

Dose planning is a critical aspect of radiosurgery, and GammaPlan software (Elekta) provides the platform for reliable tumor irradiation when gamma knife technique is used. Complete coverage of the tumor and preservation of brain and cranial nerve function are given priority during dose planning. Conformality (confining the tumor marginal dose to the 3-D geometry of the tumor) and selectivity (rapid fall-off of the dose beyond the tumor margin) are necessary for neurological function preservation.[8] Specific GKRS techniques include accurate definition of the tumor volume, use of multiple isocenters, beam weighting, and selective use of plug patterns to reduce dose to adjacent critical structures. This degree of conformality can be achieved through complex multi-isocenter planning (**Fig. 28.1**). Meningioma planning is usually performed using a combination of small beam diameter (4 and 8 mm) collimators. For larger tumors, 14-, 16-, or 18-mm collimators (depending on which gamma knife technology is available) are used. The selective use of 4-mm isocenters near critical structures like the optic nerves and chiasm are used to reduce risk.

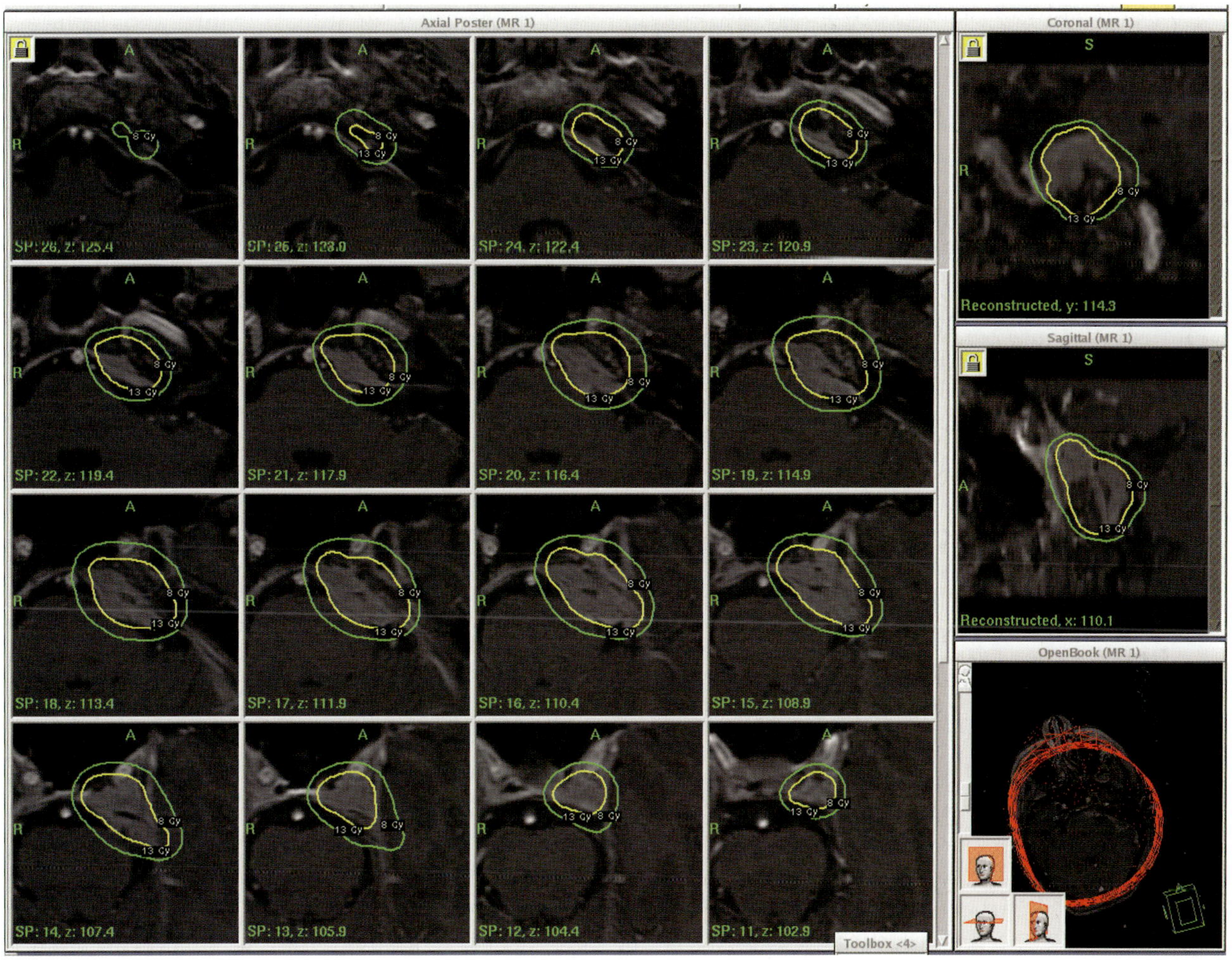

Fig. 28.1 Gamma knife radiosurgery dose plan for a left petrous apex meningioma of the skull base.

After optimizing the plan, a maximum dose inside the target is determined as well as the dose to the tumor margin. The treatment isodose, maximum dose, and dose to the margin (edge) are jointly decided by a neurosurgeon, radiation oncologist, and medical physicist. In GKRS, a dose of 11 to 16 Gy is typically prescribed to the 50% (or other) isodose line that conforms to the tumor margin. The commonest doses are 12 or 13 Gy, which are associated with long-term tumor growth control in more than 90% of grade I tumors. For histologically confirmed grade II or III tumors residual or recurrent after prior surgery, higher doses may improve long-term tumor response, although an optimum dose has not yet been defined.

Dose prescription for meningiomas changed significantly during the first 10 years of experience at our center. Current margin dose ranges as already described are associated with a low complication rate and yet maintain a high rate of tumor control (**Fig. 28.2**). This gradual dose de-escalation has now been stable for more than 10 years and maintains the long-term tumor control rates previously reported. Further dose reduction, except when critical structures are at risk, is likely to impact tumor control rates negatively. For example, we try to limit the maximum optic nerve dose to 8 to 10 Gy, but the volume of the optic apparatus receiving a certain dose is more important.[4,9,10] Using SRS, the tumor margin is receiving a radiobiological dose equivalent to the maximum dose that can be delivered by fractionated radiation therapy. Therefore, the majority of the tumor volume is receiving a radiobiological dose two to four times the radiobiological dose delivered by fractionated radiation therapy even using intensity-modulated radiation therapy techniques. A maximum radiosurgical dose of 25 Gy may be radiobiologically equivalent to 100 Gy of fractionated radiation.

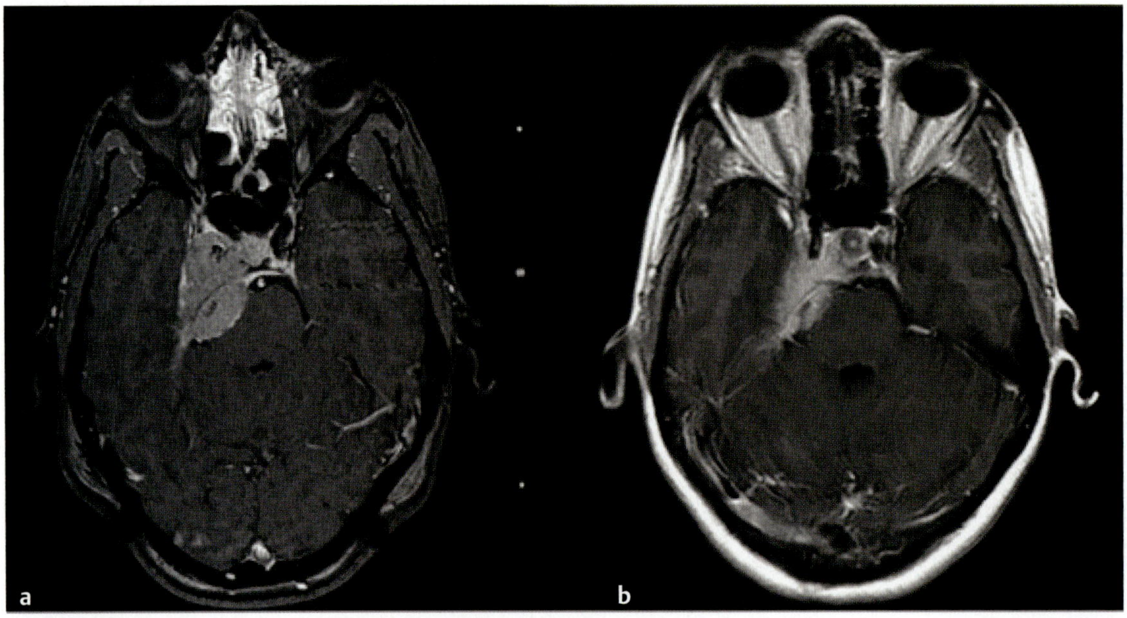

Fig. 28.2 A 37-year-old female with a right cavernous sinus meningioma. Axial T1 with contrast magnetic resonance imaging shown at the time of radiosurgery **(a)** and 6 years following the procedure **(b)**. Preexisting cranial nerve V and VI palsies improved within 2 years following treatment with gamma knife radiosurgery.

After radiosurgery, patients are followed up with serial gadolinium-enhanced MRI scans, which are generally requested at 6 months, 12 months, and 2, 4, 8, 12, 16, and 20 years. Clinical tests are obtained at regular intervals depending on initial symptoms and tumor location.

■ Literature Search

We performed a literature search from 1990 to 2011 (www.pubmed.org). The following literature sources were used to identify data: PubMed from the U.S. National Library of Medicine and the World Science Network software (www.world-sci.com).

Gamma Knife Radiosurgery: Clinical Results

The long-term results of GKRS for meningiomas have been documented,[8,9,11-20] all of which were determined to be Level III series (**Table 28.2**). These reports suggest a postradiosurgery tumor control rate greater than 90% for grade I tumors. Kondziolka et al studied 5- to 10-year outcomes in meningioma patients who had radiosurgery at the University of Pittsburgh. In that 1999 report, the authors evaluated 99 consecutive patients who underwent radiosurgery for meningioma between 1987 and 1992.[20] Evaluation was performed using serial imaging tests, clinical assessments, and a patient survey that was administered between 5 and 10 years after radiosurgery. The average tumor margin dose was 16 Gy, and the median tumor volume was 4.7 mL (range 0.24 to 24.0 mL). Fifty-seven patients (57%) had under-

Table 28.2 Summary of tumor control outcomes following gamma knife radiosurgery in select major contemporary series

Study	*N*	WHO grades	Long-term PFS
Kondziolka et al 2008[8]	1,045	I, II, III	91% (WHO I 10-year)
Santacroce et al 2012[6]	5,300	I, II, III	88.6% (all grades 10-year)
Kreil et al 2005[16]	200	I	97.2% (WHO I 10-year)
Zada et al 2010[13]	137	I	84% (WHO I 10-year)
Stafford et al 2001[19]	206	I, II, III	93% (WHO I 5-year)

Abbreviations: N, number of meningiomas treated; PFS, progression-free survival; WHO, World Health Organization.

gone prior resection, of which 12 procedures were considered total. Five patients received fractionated radiation therapy before radiosurgery. Eighty-nine patients (89%) had skull base tumors. The clinical tumor control rate (no resection required) was 93%. Sixty-one (63%) of 97 tumors became smaller, 31 (32%) remained unchanged in size, and five (5%) were enlarged. Resection was performed in seven patients (7%), six of whom had undergone prior resection. New neurological deficits developed in five patients (5%) 3 to 31 months after radiosurgery.

Patients also were surveyed about their clinical status and satisfaction. Twenty-seven (42%) of 65 responding patients were employed at the time of radiosurgery and 20 (74%) of them remained so. Radiosurgery was believed to have been "successful" by 67 of 70 patients who completed an outcomes questionnaire 5 to 10 years later. At least one complication was described by nine patients (14%), and in four patients the complications resolved. Thus, 5 to 10 years after radiosurgery, 96% of surveyed patients believed that radiosurgery provided a satisfactory outcome for their meningioma. Over all, 93% of patients required no other tumor surgery. Radiosurgery provided long-term tumor control associated with high rates of neurological function preservation and patient satisfaction.

In 2001, Stafford et al reported the Mayo Clinic experience.[19] One hundred ninety consecutive patients with 206 meningiomas underwent radiosurgery between 1990 and 1998, including 147 tumors (77%) at the cranial base. The median age at the time of radiosurgery was 58 years (range, 20 to 90 years). Prior surgery had been performed in 59%. Twenty-two patients (12%) had either atypical (n = 13) or malignant (n = 9) tumors. The median prescription isodose volume was 8.2 cm^3 (range, 0.5 to 50.5 mL^3), and the median tumor margin dose was 16 Gy (range, 12 to 36 Gy). The median clinical follow-up was 4 years. The cause-specific survival rates at 5 years for patients with benign, atypical, and malignant tumors were 100, 76, and 0%, respectively ($p < 0.0001$). The 5-year local control rate for benign tumors was 93%, compared with 68% and 0% for patients with atypical or malignant meningiomas, respectively. No correlation was observed between radiation dose and local control rate. Twenty-four patients (13%) experienced treatment-related complications, including cranial nerve deficits (8%), symptomatic parenchymal changes (3%), internal carotid artery stenosis (1%), and symptomatic cyst formation (1%). Only six patients (3%) exhibited decreases in functional status that were directly related to radiosurgery. Tumor volume, tumor margin dose, or previous radiotherapy was not associated with the development of radiation-related complications.

In 2005, Kreil et al reported results in 200 patients treated at Graz, Austria.[16] Ninety-nine patients were treated with a combination of resection and GKRS. In 101 patients, GKRS was performed as the sole treatment. Tumor volumes varied from 0.38 to 89.8 mL^3 (median 6.5 mL^3), and doses of 7 to 25 Gy (median 12 Gy) were given to the tumor margin. The actuarial progression-free survival rate was 98.5% at 5 years and 97.2% at 10 years. Radiation-induced edema occurred in two patients (1%). The neurological status improved in 83 cases (41.5%), remained unaltered in 108 (54%), and worsened in 9 (4.5%). Repeat surgical resection was performed in five patients following GKRS (2.5%).

In a subsequent 2008 report, the University of Pittsburgh group provided further data.[8] This larger patient cohort consisted of 972 patients with 1,045 intracranial meningiomas managed during an 18-year period. The series included 70% women, 49% of whom had undergone a previous resection and 5% of whom had received previous fractionated radiation therapy. Tumor locations included middle fossa (n = 351), posterior fossa (n = 307), convexity (n = 126), anterior fossa (n = 88), parasagittal region (n = 113), or other (n = 115). The overall control rate for patients with benign meningiomas (WHO grade I) was 93%. In those without previous histological confirmation (n = 482), the tumor control was 97%. However, for patients with WHO grade II and III tumors, tumor control was 50 and 17%, respectively. Delayed resection after radiosurgery was necessary in 51 patients (5%) at a mean of 35 months. After 10 years, grade I tumors were controlled in 91% (n = 53); in those without histology, 95% (n = 22) were controlled. None of the patients developed a radiation-induced tumor. The overall morbidity rate was 7.7%. Symptomatic peritumoral imaging changes developed in 4% of the patients at a mean of 8 months.

Zada et al provided data from the University of Southern California.[13] Data were retrospectively reviewed in 116 patients who underwent 136 gamma knife procedures for benign intracranial meningiomas between 1996 and 2004. Patients with atypical or malignant meningiomas were excluded. Surgical resection preceded SRS in 72 patients (62%). The median tumor volume was 3.4 mL, and the median prescription dose to the 50% isodose line was 16 Gy. The median follow-up time was 75 months (range, 4 to 146 months). Overall tumor control was achieved in 128 of 136 lesions (94%), of which tumor size was stable in 68% and decreased in 26%. Seven patients experienced disease progression in 8 tumors, occurring at a mean time of 90 months. The overall 5-year and 10-year actuarial tumor control rates were 98.9% and 84%, respectively. Characteristics corresponding to tumor progression included insufficient tumor coverage (98% vs 93%, p = 0.007), cavernous sinus lesions, and meningiomatosis. Complications after GKRS developed in 8% of patients, in whom the mean tumor volume was nearly double that in patients with no adverse effects (11.0 vs 5.7 cm^3, $p = 0.003$). The findings of this series are consistent with results reported earlier in the chapter from the University of Pittsburgh.

Recently, Santacroce et al provided results from a large European multicenter retrospective study.[6] Using data from 15 participating centers, they reported an observational analysis of 4,565 consecutive patients who had 5,300 benign meningiomas. All patients underwent gamma knife radiosurgery at least 5 years before assessment. The median tumor volume was 4.8 cm^3, and the median dose to the tumor margin was 14 Gy. Detailed results from 3,768 meningiomas (71%) were analyzed. Median imaging follow-up was 63 months. The volume of treated tumors decreased in 2,187 lesions (58%), remained unchanged in 1,300 lesions (34.5%), and increased in 281 lesions (7.5%), giving a control rate of 92.5%. Only 84 (2.2%) enlarging tumors required further treatment. Five- and 10-year progression-free survival (PFS) rates were 95.2% and 88.6%, respectively. Tumor control was higher for imaging-defined tumors versus grade I meningiomas ($p < 0.001$), for female versus male patients ($p < 0.001$), for sporadic versus multiple meningiomas ($p < 0.001$), and for skull base versus convexity tumors ($p < 0.001$). Permanent morbidity rate was 6.6% at the last follow-up. Again, this large series shows results consistent with other reports.

Linear Accelerator–Based Radiosurgery for Meningioma

Although gamma knife series make up the vast majority of the radiosurgery literature on meningioma (and the results serve as the primary basis for performing radiosurgery in appropriately selected patients), a growing experience in linear accelerator (LINAC)-based techniques also confirms favorable outcomes. The University of Florida group initially published their results in 1999, performing LINAC radiosurgery in a series of 70 patients harboring a total of 76 skull base and convexity tumors with a mean follow-up of 23 months. The mean marginal dose was 12.7 Gy delivered most commonly to the 80% isodose line. Forty-eight tumors had radiographic follow-up of more than 1 year, and all tumors were found to be stable or decreased in size. One patient required craniotomy for resection as a result of postradiosurgical edema.[21] In 2010, Korah et al reported a 94% PFS of 41 convexity and skull base meningiomas treated with LINAC SRS.[22] More recently, El Majdoub et al reported stable or decreased tumor size in 100% of 70 grade I convexity and skull base meningiomas treated at a median 12 Gy marginal dose with median follow-up of 79.7 months (range 24 to 109 months). Two patients in this series developed permanent trigeminal neuralgia; otherwise, all morbidities were transient.[23]

Other LINAC series have described similarly favorable results for patients with skull base meningiomas. The Stanford University group published their initial radiosurgical experience using the Cyberknife (Accuray, Sunnyvale, CA) with skull base and cavernous sinus meningiomas that had had initial management between 1997 and 1998.[24,25] They noted tumor control or shrinkage in 98% and 100% of 55 skull base and 24 cavernous sinus meningiomas, respectively. The mean follow-up was 48.4 months in skull base meningiomas overall and 45.6 months in cavernous sinus tumors (and > 1 year in all patients). Chuang et al in 2004 reported 43 skull base meningiomas treated with LINAC radiosurgery and found a 90% PFS at 5 years.[26] Spiegelmann et al in 2002 presented a 97.5% 5-year PFS following LINAC radiosurgery for cavernous sinus meningiomas.[27] In cases of WHO grade II and III meningiomas, outcomes were less satisfactory. El-Khatib et al in 2011 described PFSs of 74%, 67%, and 58% at 3, 5, and 10 years, respectively, in a series of 28 patients with atypical and anaplastic tumors.[28]

Initial patient management costs as well as initial potential morbidity are significantly reduced when SRS is used compared with microsurgical resection.[29] Larger tumor volumes, higher marginal doses, and a parasagittal tumor location confer a higher risk of postradiosurgical reactive changes or edema.[30] Cranial nerve and neurological deficits are seen more often following treatment of skull base meningiomas (5 to 20% in the previously discussed reported series), but most such symptoms are transient and respond to a short course of corticosteroids. Although studies to date have not defined the clear superiority of one radiosurgical modality in the management of meningiomas, it is important to realize that high-definition intraoperative MRI performed in stereotactic frame–based conditions, precise volumetric dose planning, and accurate dose delivery are critical to achieving tumor control and reducing potential risks of SRS.

Comparison of Radiosurgery and Surgical Resection

Level II Evidence

It is unlikely that a randomized clinical trial will emerge to compare surgical resection with radiosurgery for meningioma patients eligible for either option. A single Level II matched cohort study compared outcomes for patients with tumors < 3.5 cm in diameter. Pollock et al reported the Mayo Clinic experience between 1990 and 1997.[31] Adult meningioma patients (n = 198) underwent either surgical resection (n = 136) or GKRS (n = 62) as primary management for a benign meningioma. Tumor recurrence or progression rates were calculated by the Kaplan-Meier method according to an independent imaging review. The mean follow-up was 64 months. The tumor resections were Simpson grade 1 in 57 (42%), grade 2 in 57 (42%), and grade 3 to 4 in 22 (16%). The mean margin and maximal radiation dose at radiosurgery was 17.7 Gy and 34.9 Gy, respectively. Tumor recurrence or progression was more frequent in the surgical resection group (12%) than in the radiosurgical group (2%; p = 0.04). No statistically significant difference was detected in the 3- and 7-year actuarial PFS rate between patients with Simpson grade 1 resections (100% and 96%, respectively) and patients who underwent radiosurgery (100% and 95%, respectively; p = 0.94). Radiosurgery provided a higher PFS rate compared with patients with Simpson grade 2 (3- and 7-year PFS rate, 91% and 82%, respectively; $p < 0.05$) and grade 3 to 4 (3- and 7-year PFS rate, 68% and 34%, respectively; $p < 0.001$) resections. Subsequent tumor treatments were more common after surgical resection (15% vs 3%, p = 0.02). Complications occurred in 10% of patients after radiosurgery compared with 22% of patients after surgical resection (p = 0.06). The authors found that the control rate after radiosurgery was equivalent to that after resection of a Simpson grade 1 tumor and was superior to grade 2 and 3 to 4 resections. They concluded that, after additional long-term follow-up, these initial results continue to confirm the high tumor control rate and low morbidity of radiosurgery. They suggested that radiosurgery would become the preferred initial management for patients with small- to moderate-size meningiomas not associated with symptomatic mass effect

Summary and Conclusions

SRS has become a well-documented and successful management option for patients with intracranial meningiomas. Data are most available for the results in patients with known or presumed grade 1 tumors. Outcomes in excess of 10 years of follow-up are now published, and systematic, serially collected outcomes data are available on large numbers of patients. Radiosurgery is now a frequent management for patients with newly diagnosed, recurrent, and progressive meningiomas. Worldwide by 2010, more than 91,000 patients had undergone GKRS for meningiomas (Leksell Gamma Knife Society, 2013).

References

1. Simpson D. The recurrence of intracranial meningiomas after surgical treatment. J Neurol Neurosurg Psychiatry 1957;20(1):22–39
2. Mahmood A, Qureshi NH, Malik GM. Intracranial meningiomas: analysis of recurrence after surgical treatment. Acta Neurochir (Wien) 1994;126(2-4):53–58
3. Borovich B, Doron Y. Recurrence of intracranial meningiomas: the role played by regional multicentricity. J Neurosurg 1986;64(1):58–63
4. Lee JY, Niranjan A, McInerney J, Kondziolka D, Flickinger JC, Lunsford LD. Stereotactic radiosurgery providing long-term tumor control of cavernous sinus meningiomas. J Neurosurg 2002;97(1):65–72
5. Kondziolka D, Lunsford LD, Coffey RJ, Flickinger JC. Stereotactic radiosurgery of meningiomas. J Neurosurg 1991;74(4):552–559
6. Santacroce A, Walier M, Régis J, et al. Long-term tumor control of benign intracranial meningiomas after radiosurgery in a series of 4565 patients. Neurosurgery 2012;70(1):32–39
7. Kondziolka D, Nathoo N, Flickinger JC, Niranjan A, Maitz AH, Lunsford LD. Long-term results after radiosurgery for benign intracranial tumors. Neurosurgery 2003;53(4):815–821
8. Kondziolka D, Mathieu D, Lunsford LD, et al. Radiosurgery as definitive management of intracranial meningiomas. Neurosurgery 2008;62(1):53–58
9. Nicolato A, Foroni R, Alessandrini F, Bricolo A, Gerosa M. Radiosurgical treatment of cavernous sinus meningiomas: experience with 122 treated patients. Neurosurgery 2002;51(5):1153–1159
10. Tishler RB, Loeffler JS, Lunsford LD, et al. Tolerance of cranial nerves of the cavernous sinus to radiosurgery. Int J Radiat Oncol Biol Phys 1993;27(2):215–221
11. Starke RM, Nguyen JH, Rainey J, et al. Gamma knife surgery of meningiomas located in the posterior fossa: factors predictive of outcome and remission. J Neurosurg 2011;114(5):1399–1409
12. Skeie BS, Enger PO, Skeie GO, Thorsen F, Pedersen PH. Gamma knife surgery of meningiomas involving the cavernous sinus: long-term follow-up of 100 patients. Neurosurgery 2010;66(4):661–668
13. Zada G, Pagnini PG, Yu C, et al. Long-term outcomes and patterns of tumor progression after gamma knife radiosurgery for benign meningiomas. Neurosurgery 2010;67(2):322–328
14. Iwai Y, Yamanaka K, Ikeda H. Gamma knife radiosurgery for skull base meningioma: long-term results of low-dose treatment. J Neurosurg 2008;109(5):804–810
15. Zachenhofer I, Wolfsberger S, Aichholzer M, et al. Gamma-knife radiosurgery for cranial base meningiomas: experience of tumor control, clinical course, and morbidity in a follow-up of more than 8 years. Neurosurgery 2006;58(1):28–36
16. Kreil W, Luggin J, Fuchs I, Weigl V, Eustacchio S, Papaefthymiou G. Long term experience of gamma knife radiosurgery for benign skull base meningiomas. J Neurol Neurosurg Psychiatry 2005;76(10):1425–1430
17. Pollock BE, Stafford SL. Results of stereotactic radiosurgery for patients with imaging defined cavernous sinus meningiomas. Int J Radiat Oncol Biol Phys 2005;62(5):1427–1431
18. Flickinger JC, Kondziolka D, Maitz AH, Lunsford LD. Gamma knife radiosurgery of imaging-diagnosed intracranial meningioma. Int J Radiat Oncol Biol Phys 2003;56(3):801–806
19. Stafford SL, Pollock BE, Foote RL, et al. Meningioma radiosurgery: tumor control, outcomes, and complications among 190 consecutive patients. Neurosurgery 2001;49(5):1029–1037

20. Kondziolka D, Levy EI, Niranjan A, Flickinger JC, Lunsford LD. Long-term outcomes after meningioma radiosurgery: physician and patient perspectives. J Neurosurg 1999;91(1):44–50
21. Shafron DH, Friedman WA, Buatti JM, Bova FJ, Mendenhall WM. Linac radiosurgery for benign meningiomas. Int J Radiat Oncol Biol Phys 1999;43(2):321–327
22. Korah MP, Nowlan AW, Johnstone PA, Crocker IR. Radiation therapy alone for imaging-defined meningiomas. Int J Radiat Oncol Biol Phys 2010;76(1):181–186
23. El Majdoub F, Elawady M, Bührle C, et al. mMLC-LINAC radiosurgery for intracranial meningiomas of complex shape. Acta Neurochir (Wien) 2012;154(4):599–604
24. Chang SD, Adler JR Jr, Martin DP. LINAC radiosurgery for cavernous sinus meningiomas. Stereotact Funct Neurosurg 1998;71(1):43–50
25. Chang SD, Adler JR Jr. Treatment of cranial base meningiomas with linear accelerator radiosurgery. Neurosurgery 1997;41(5):1019–1025
26. Chuang CC, Chang CN, Tsang NM, et al. Linear accelerator-based radiosurgery in the management of skull base meningiomas. J Neurooncol 2004;66(1-2):241–249
27. Spiegelmann R, Nissim O, Menhel J, Alezra D, Pfeffer MR. Linear accelerator radiosurgery for meningiomas in and around the cavernous sinus. Neurosurgery 2002;51(6):1373–1379
28. El-Khatib M, El Majdoub F, Hoevels M, et al. Stereotactic LINAC radiosurgery for incompletely resected or recurrent atypical and anaplastic meningiomas. Acta Neurochir (Wien) 2011;153(9):1761–1767
29. Tan SS, van Putten E, Nijdam WM, et al. A microcosting study of microsurgery, LINAC radiosurgery, and gamma knife radiosurgery in meningioma patients. J Neurooncol 2011; 101(2):237–245
30. Patil CG, Hoang S, Borchers DJ III, et al. Predictors of peritumoral edema after stereotactic radiosurgery of supratentorial meningiomas. Neurosurgery 2008;63(3):435–440
31. Pollock BE, Stafford SL, Utter A, Giannini C, Schreiner SA. Stereotactic radiosurgery provides equivalent tumor control to Simpson Grade 1 resection for patients with small- to medium-size meningiomas. Int J Radiat Oncol Biol Phys 2003; 55(4):1000–1005

29

The Role of Preoperative Embolization for Meningiomas (Skull Base and Non–Skull Base)

Alex M. Witek, Geoffrey P. Colby, Li-Mei Lin, and Alexander L. Coon

Meningiomas are the most common primary intracranial tumors.[1] Their standard treatment is surgical resection, and complete excision, including the dural tail, offers the highest likelihood of cure.[2] The ease of resection depends on various factors, including location, size, blood supply, and involvement of critical structures. Although most meningiomas are treated with resection alone, preoperative endovascular embolization has emerged as an attractive adjunct option for highly vascular and large tumors. The invention of cerebral angiography by Egas Moniz in 1927[3] paved the way for the field of endovascular procedures, ultimately including tumor embolization. Transfemoral meningioma embolization was first reported in 1972 by Djindjian and colleagues, who embolized an anterior fossa meningioma via the internal maxillary artery (IMA).[4] This was soon followed by other case reports and eventually by large series. Preoperative endovascular embolization has been employed by many neurosurgical centers with the goal of facilitating resection, and at some it has become a standard component of treatment for these common tumors. Despite its widespread use, meningioma embolization is a controversial practice, and its indications and usefulness continue to be defined.

■ Vascular Supply

The blood supply to a meningioma generally parallels that of the adjacent dura and can include branches of both the external carotid artery (ECA) and the internal carotid artery (ICA). Tumors of the cerebral convexity and superior falcine region tend to be supplied by the middle meningeal artery (MMA) (**Fig. 29.1**). Anterior skull base meningiomas can be supplied by various branches, including the ethmoidal arteries, artery of the falx, or branches of the ICA or IMA. Tumors of the middle fossa can derive their vascular supply from both ICA and ECA branches. The vascular supply to posterior fossa meningiomas is highly variable and often includes multiple feeding vessels that may be branches of the ICA, ECA, or posterior circulation. In addition to these dural-based feeders, which supply the bulk of the tumor, large tumors may recruit adjacent pial vessels to supply their periphery.[5]

■ Patient Selection

Each patient and tumor must be considered on an individual basis, specifically with respect to the arterial access available to perform the embolization

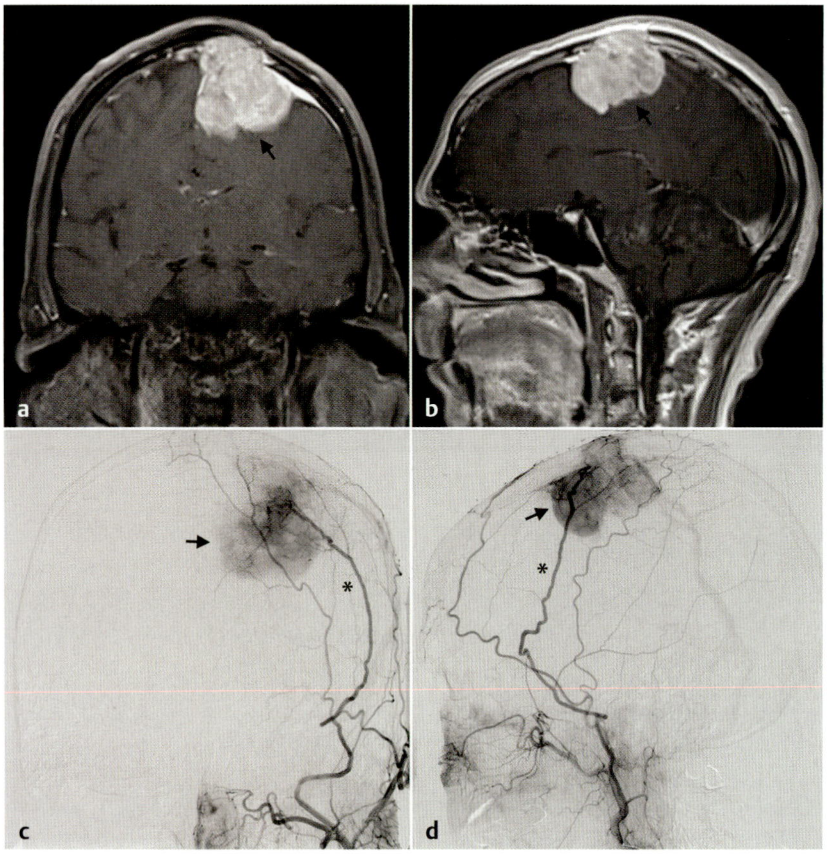

Fig. 29.1 Arterial supply to a parasagittal/convexity meningioma. Coronal **(a)** and sagittal **(b)** views of a T1-weighted magnetic resonance imaging scan of the brain with contrast demonstrating a 4 cm left-sided parafalcine meningioma (*arrow*). Left external carotid artery DSA in anteroposterior **(c)** and lateral **(d)** views demonstrates a prominent vascular blush (*arrow*) corresponding to the meningioma that receives arterial supply predominantly from a hypertrophied middle meningeal artery (*asterisk*).

procedure and to the vascular supply of the tumor. Preoperative embolization is commonly thought to be most beneficial for patients with large, hypervascular tumors and tumors located at the skull base. Skull base tumors tend to have feeding arteries that are located deep to the tumor during the surgical approach, meaning they are encountered late in the surgery after significant tumor debulking has been performed. Preoperative occlusion of these vessels may therefore permit earlier devascularization of the tumor. In contrast, convexity and parasagittal meningiomas tend to derive their blood supply from the overlying dura, so the major feeding arteries are encountered early during the approach and can be ligated prior to tumor debulking.[6] Although there has been an evolution in cranial base approaches that facilitate early access to any skull base feeders (i.e., extended bifrontal for anterior cranial fossa meningiomas), lesions such as petroclival meningiomas and certain posterior fossa meningiomas still pose great difficulty with regard to early intraoperative devascularization.

Catheter angiography, including selective ECA and ICA injections, is the optimal imaging modality for characterizing the tumor vascular blush and can identify feeding arteries that are suitable for embolization. Angiography is also useful for identifying nearby vessels supplying the cerebrum or cranial nerves, dangerous extracranial–intracranial anastomoses, vessel encasement by tumor, venous drainage pathways, and patency of the dural sinuses.[5] The relative contributions from ECA and ICA feeders should also be considered. Embolization via the ICA is often avoided because reflux of embolic material may result in a neurological deficit. Furthermore, embolization of ECA branches may be less beneficial if significant ICA supply remains. A more detailed discussion of the evidence available to select patients for preoperative embolization takes place in the following sections.

■ Embolization Technique

Embolization is most commonly performed following superselective catheterization of feeding vessels. Although subselective embolization has also been employed,[7,8] a retrospective comparison found the superselective technique to be more effective.[9] A variety of guide catheter and microcatheter systems are commercially available for intracranial embolization procedures, but a discussion of these details is beyond the scope of this chapter.

Distal embolization of the tumor microcirculation is considered preferable to more proximal occlusion of feeding arteries because there is less risk of collateral perfusion to the tumor bed.[10] The depth of penetration depends on microcatheter position, type of embolic material, and flow in the embolized vessel. A more distal microcatheter position facilitates penetration of the embolic material into the tumor and reduces the risk of unwanted reflux. Once a microcatheter position is established, superselective angiography is performed to assess the safety of the position. As an additional safety measure, provocative testing can be performed to identify any small anastomotic channels or vasa nervorum that may not be angiographically evident. Methods of provocative testing employing both lidocaine and amobarbital have been described.[11] If no neurological changes are noted on provocative testing, embolization can be performed from the current microcatheter position.

A variety of embolic agents are available for clinical use. **Table 29.1** lists those most commonly employed for intracranial meningiomas, including particulate agents (the most common), liquid embolics, and coils. Compared with larger particles, liquids and small particles provide deeper penetration into the tumor vascular bed. One study concluded that 50 to 150 µm polyvinyl alcohol (PVA) particles induce more tumor necrosis and lead to decreased blood loss compared with 150 to 300 µm particles without added complications,[12] but the smaller particles were associated with increased rates of postembolization hemorrhage in a different study.[13] Small particles may also increase the risk of occluding dangerous anastomoses or vasa nervorum. One study found microspheres to be more effective than PVA,[14] and another reported no difference in operative blood loss following chemoembolization with mannitol as compared with particulate embolization with PVA.[15] No other direct comparisons have been made between the various materials, and few data are available on some of the newer agents. The choice of embolic material for meningiomas is therefore primarily governed by operator preference.

The desired end point of embolization is decreased tumor blush and stasis of flow in the embolized artery. Overly aggressive injection of embolisate should be avoided because it may lead to unwanted reflux into other vessels. Postembolization angiography is performed to estimate the degree of devascularization. Caution is advised when performing postembolization angiography because there is a risk of neurological deficits from retained embolic particles in the microcatheter.[16] Following the procedure, a thorough neurological examination should

Table 29.1 Embolic agents

	Agent[a]	Characteristics
Particles	Polyvinyl alcohol[7,12–14,24,26,31]	The most commonly reported material for tumor embolization Available in multiple sizes Easy to deliver, though particles have a tendency to aggregate Rapidly absorbed
	Trisacryl gelatin microspheres (Embospheres[b])[14,23,30]	Hydrophilic spheres Precisely calibrated with multiple sizes Less aggregation and catheter occlusion Nonabsorbable
	Gelatin powder (Gelfoam[c])[7,18,24,25]	Rapidly absorbed No longer frequently used
Liquids	*N*-butyl-2-cyanoacrylate	Polymerizes rapidly Nonabsorbable
	Ethylene vinyl alcohol copolymer (Onyx[d])	Newer agent Precise control and deep penetration Nonabsorbable
	Metallic coils	Produce proximal vessel occlusion Precise positioning without danger of reflux

[a] References are provided for notable studies that have used a given agent. This is not all-inclusive and includes only comparative studies and large series ($n \geq 30$). Some less commonly used embolic materials include fibrin glue, cellulose porous beads, microfibrillar collagen, lyophilized dura, silastic spheres, ethanol, and mannitol.
[b] BioSphere Medical, Rockland, MA.
[c] Baxter, Deerfield, IL.
[d] Covidien, Mansfield, MA.

be performed, with special attention to the cranial nerve function following embolization of skull base tumors. The patient should then be monitored closely in a neurological intensive care unit given the risk of intracranial hemorrhage and severe edema.

Examples of meningioma embolizations are shown in **Fig. 29.2** and **Fig. 29.3**. **Fig. 29.2** demonstrates successful embolization of occipital artery and MMA pedicles to a tentorial meningioma using *N*-butyl-2-cyanoacrylate (NBCA). **Fig. 29.3** demonstrates successful embolization of MMA feeders to a sphenoid wing meningioma using NBCA and then coils to close the main arterial branch.

Recommendations for Embolization Technique

1. Superselective embolization is preferable to a subselective technique (Grade 1C Recommendation, Level III Evidence).
2. There is insufficient evidence to recommend a particular embolic agent.

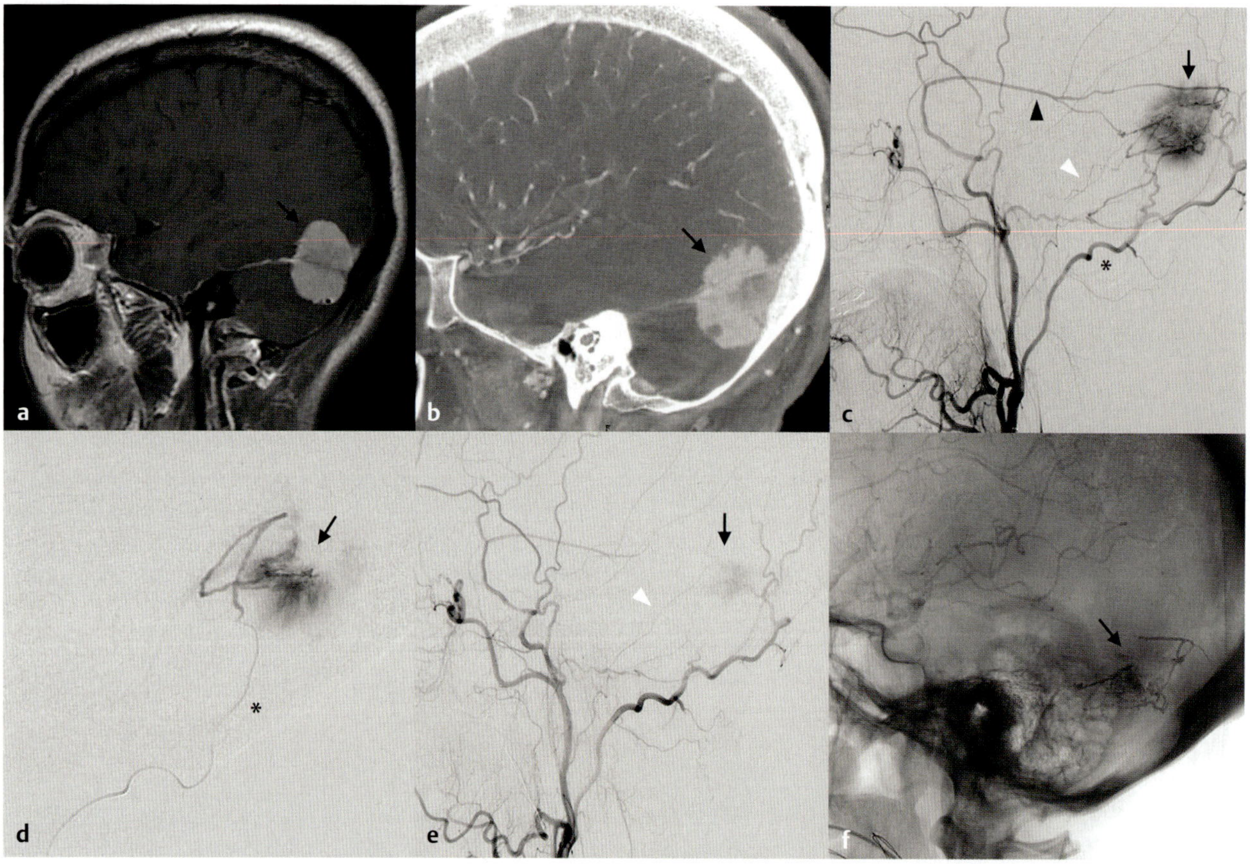

Fig. 29.2 *N*-butyl-2-cyanoacrylate (NBCA) embolization of a tentorial meningioma. **(a)** T1-weighted magnetic resonance imaging scan of the brain with contrast, sagittal view, demonstrating a 3.5 cm right-sided tentorial-based meningioma (*arrow*). **(b)** Right common carotid artery DynaCTA, sagittal reconstruction, demonstrating the vascular blush of the meningioma (*arrow*). **(c)** Right external carotid artery digital subtraction angiography (DSA), lateral view, demonstrates a prominent vascular blush (*arrow*) corresponding to the meningioma. This tumor receives arterial supply from the right middle meningeal artery posterior division (*black arrowhead*), the right occipital artery (*asterisk*), and the right ascending pharyngeal artery (*white arrowhead*). Minor arterial supply is also from the right posterior meningeal artery and temporal branches of the right posterior cerebral artery (not shown). **(d)** Superselective microcatheter DSA, lateral view, of an occipital artery feeder to the tumor. The microcatheter is marked with an asterisk and the tumor blush is marked with an arrow. **(e)** Right external carotid artery DSA, lateral view, post-NBCA embolization of a right occipital artery feeder and the posterior division of the middle meningeal artery. There is marked reduction in the vascularity of the tumor, and only a faint blush (*arrow*) is visualized with residual supply from the ascending pharyngeal artery (*white arrowhead*). **(f)** Native lateral view demonstrating the final NBCA cast (*arrow*).

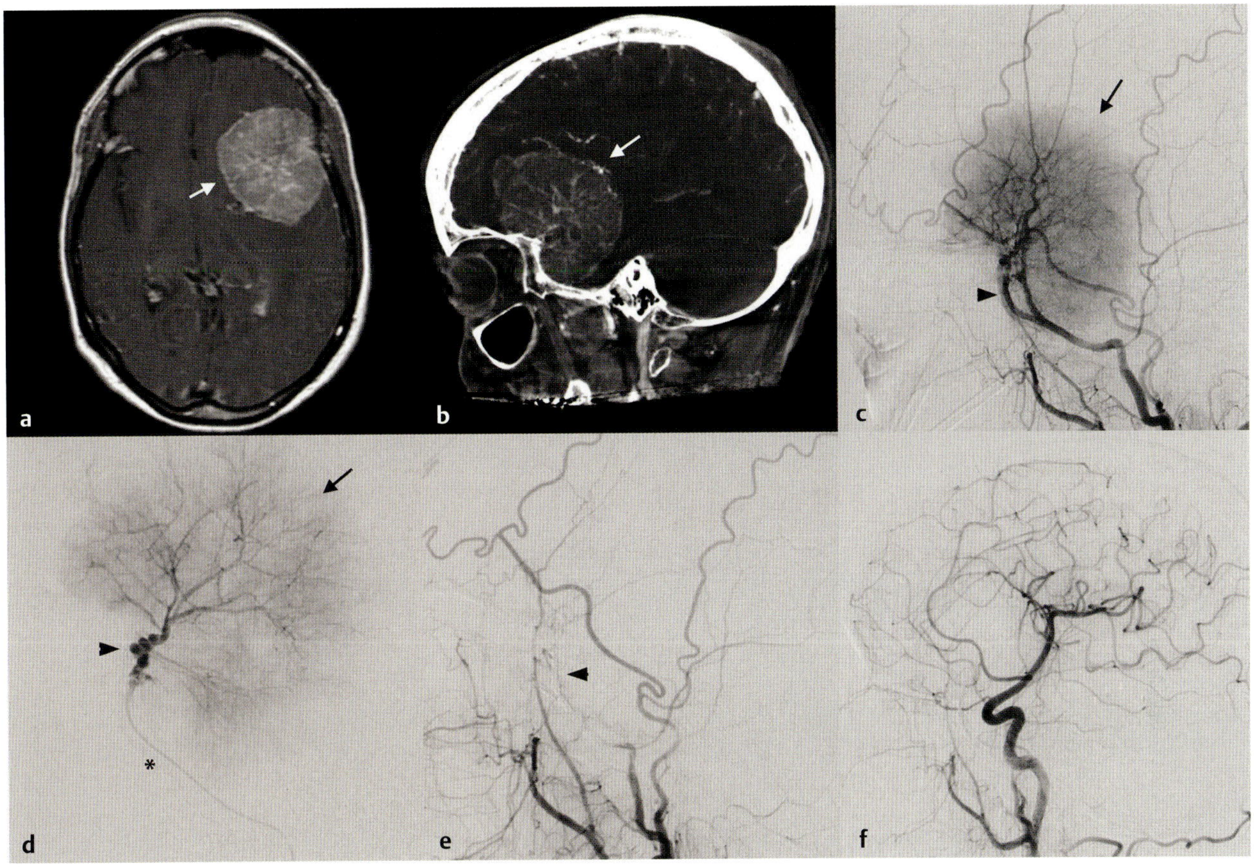

Fig. 29.3 *N*-butyl-2-cyanoacrylate (NBCA) and coil embolization of a sphenoid wing meningioma. **(a)** T1-weighted magnetic resonance imaging scan of the brain with contrast, axial view, demonstrating a 5 cm left-sided meningioma (*arrow*) arising from the lesser wing of the sphenoid bone. **(b)** Left common carotid artery DynaCTA, sagittal reconstruction, demonstrating the vascular blush of the meningioma (*arrow*). **(c)** Left external carotid artery DSA, lateral view, demonstrates a prominent vascular blush (*arrow*) corresponding to the meningioma. This tumor receives arterial supply primarily from two pedicles off the hypertrophied left middle meningeal artery (*black arrowhead*). **(d)** Superselective microcatheter digital subtraction angiography (DSA), lateral view, of a middle meningeal arterial pedicle (*black arrowhead*). The microcatheter is marked with an asterisk, and the tumor blush is marked with an arrow. **(e)** Right external carotid artery DSA, lateral view, post-NBCA embolization of both middle meningeal pedicles and coil embolization of the distal middle meningeal artery. The coil pack is marked with a black arrowhead. No residual tumor blush is visualized. **(f)** Left common carotid final control DSA, lateral view, demonstrating no tumor blush. Note the displacement of the left middle cerebral artery secondary to mass effect from the tumor.

Interval between Embolization and Surgery

No consensus exists on the ideal time interval between embolization and surgical resection. The interval should be long enough to allow adequate devascularization and necrosis of the tumor. However, an interval that is too long can allow for absorption of nonpermanent embolisate, development of collateral circulation, hemorrhage into a necrotic tumor bed, or fibrosis, which makes resection more difficult.[17] A wide range of intervals has been reported in published series, and experts have recommended intervals of 3 to 5 days,[5] 2 to 5 days,[6] and less than 1 week.[17,18]

Two retrospective studies examined the relationship between the time until resection and surgical outcomes. Kai and colleagues reported that tumor softening was maximal from days 7 through 9 after embolization, and those undergoing resection after more than 7 days had shorter operative times and better Simpson grades, whereas there was no difference in operative blood loss, length of hospital stay, or complication rates.[19] Chun and colleagues found that patients undergoing resection within 24 hours of embolization had greater blood loss compared with those who underwent resection at a later time, and there was no difference in duration of surgery or length of hospital stay.[20] In conclusion, a wide range of intervals has been used, and an ideal length has not been precisely identified. Most published studies have reported intervals between 1 and 10 days, and any interval within this range may be reasonable, but waiting at least 1 to several days may allow for tumor softening and easier resection.

Recommendation for Interval between Embolization and Surgery

The interval should be at least 24 hours, and the ideal interval may be several days (Grade 2C Recommendation, Level III Evidence).

Evidence to Support the Benefits of Embolization

The rationale behind performing preoperative embolization of meningiomas is to facilitate surgical resection by softening the tumor and reducing its vascularity. A possible benefit of decreasing the risk of recurrence has also been proposed,[21,22] but this idea has not been fully explored. There are five studies comparing embolization to resection alone, and their level of evidence regarding the efficacy of embolization is summarized in **Table 29.2**.

The end points used to measure efficacy deserve attention. Some studies have used radiographic or histological criteria to measure efficacy, and although such nonclinical parameters can be valuable for demonstrating the effects of embolization, they should not be considered desirable end points to inform clinical decision making and will not be discussed in this chapter. The optimal end points to use would be those most closely tied to quality of life, such as mortality, neurological outcome, symptomatic tumor recurrence, or reoperation rates. However, these outcomes are difficult to measure without large sample sizes and long-term follow-up. Most of the studies discussed in this section have therefore relied on operative time and blood loss to assess efficacy.

Level I Evidence

There is no Level I evidence comparing embolization versus no embolization for intracranial meningiomas.

Table 29.2 Comparative studies—embolization versus no embolization

Evidence level	Study	Design	Embolic agent	Results[a]
Level I	No studies			
Level II	Macpherson 1991[7]	Prospective cohort (n = 52)	Gelatin powder PVA	Fewer operative complications Lower transfusion requirement Higher likelihood of good outcome Resection subjectively less bloody
Level III	Bendszus et al 2000[23]	Prospective cohort (n = 60)	Trisacryl gelatin microspheres	Longer operative times in embolized group[b] No difference in blood loss (unless > 90% devascularized), transfused blood units, extent of resection, Barthel index, or length of hospital stay
	Dean et al 1994[24]	Retrospective cohort (n = 36)	Gelatin powder PVA	Less blood loss[b] Lower transfusion requirement[b] No difference in operative time, length of hospital stay, or cost
	Alberione et al 2009[25]	Retrospective cohort (n = 33)	Gelatin sponge	Less blood loss[b] Shorter operative time[b] No difference in transfusion requirement
Level IV	Oka et al 1998[26]	Retrospective cohort (n = 20)	PVA Microfibrillar collagen	Lower transfusion requirement (for tumors < 6 cm)[b] Trend toward better Glasgow Outcome Score No difference in operative time

Abbreviation: PVA, polyvinyl alcohol.
[a] Outcome in embolized group compared with nonembolized group.
[b] $p < 0.05$.

Level II Evidence

There is one Level II study comparing preoperative embolization to surgery alone. Macpherson prospectively compared outcomes in 52 patients considered for embolization with gelatin powder or PVA, which included 22 tumors of the convexity, 16 parasagittal/falx, 6 sphenoid, 5 subfrontal, 2 occipital, and 1 posterior fossa. Patients who underwent embolization had fewer surgical complications (21% vs 54%), a lower transfusion requirement, and a higher likelihood of a good outcome (79% vs 58%) than those who did not. Based on analysis of the surgeons' opinions regarding the ease of hemostasis, resection was less likely to be bloody following preoperative embolization (25% vs 62%).[7] The ability to draw conclusions from this and other observational studies is limited by selection bias. In this study, the nonembolized group was selected because embolization was considered technically infeasible or unlikely to be beneficial. It is also important to note that they performed subselective catheterization (with embolisate injected into the distal ECA), whereas superselective catheterization is the predominant method used in most published studies and in current practice.

Level III Evidence

There are three Level III studies. Bendszus and colleagues prospectively studied 60 patients, with tumors consisting of 44 convexity/falx, 13 skull base, and 3 posterior fossa. Half of the patients underwent embolization with trisacryl gelatin microspheres. Contrary to the belief that embolization decreases operative time, surgery was longer in the embolized group (310 min vs 234 min; $p < 0.05$), which the authors attribute to their use of intraoperative ultrasonography only in the embolized patients. They found no difference in blood loss, transfusion requirement, Simpson grade, 6-month Barthel index, length of hospital stay, or the surgeon's subjective evaluation of tumor consistency, extent of necrosis, and ease of hemostasis. However, a subgroup analysis showed that there was less blood loss for embolized tumors with greater than 90% devascularization compared with nonembolized tumors (335 mL vs 646 mL; $p < 0.05$). The two groups of patients in this study were treated at different institutions, and although a prestudy comparison showed no difference in operative times or blood loss between the two centers, this limits our ability to draw conclusions from their surgical outcomes.[23]

Dean and colleagues retrospectively compared 18 pairs of patients who were matched based on tumor size, location (although the location of the tumors is not specified), and histological subtype. Patients who underwent embolization with either gelatin powder or PVA had less blood loss (533 mL vs 836 mL; $p = 0.048$) and received fewer units of blood (0.39 units vs 1.56 units; $p = 0.041$). There was no difference in operating time (306 min vs 338 min; $p = 0.171$), length of hospital stay (10.6 d vs 15.0 d; $p = 0.192$), or cost ($29,605 vs $38,449; $p = 0.246$).[24]

Alberione et al retrospectively compared outcomes in 33 patients undergoing angiography and surgical resection for meningiomas > 4 cm, with tumor locations including 16 convexity/falx, 11 sphenoid, 3 anterior fossa, and 3 petroclival. They observed less blood loss (614 mL vs 988 mL; $p \le 0.001$) and shorter operating times (218 min vs 292 min; $p \le 0.002$) in those patients who underwent embolization, but no difference in units of red cells transfused.[25]

Level IV Evidence

Oka and colleagues compared outcomes in 20 patients with meningiomas of at least 4 cm, of which 12 underwent embolization with a combination of PVA and microfibrillar collagen. All of the tumors were located at the skull base, with 12 being classified as sphenoid, 6 temporal, 1 parasellar, and 1 clivus. There was a lower transfusion requirement following preoperative embolization only for those tumors between 4 and 6 cm in size (1.1 units vs 12.8 units; $p < 0.001$) but not for those > 6 cm, and there was no difference in operative time. Embolization was associated with a trend toward a higher proportion of "good recovery" outcomes as measured by the Glasgow Outcome Scale (83% vs 38%; $p = 0.052$). Although this is a comparative study, it does not qualify as a Level III study because it used a historical control group; the nonembolized patients were treated during a period before the standard of care at the authors' institution included preoperative embolization.[26]

Quiñones-Hinojosa and colleagues performed multivariate logistic regression on a series of 67 patients with giant (> 5 cm) intracranial meningiomas to identify positive and negative predictors of attaining gross total resection. Their series included 34 convexity/parasagittal/falx tumors, 11 sphenoid wing, 7 suprasellar, 6 olfactory groove, 5 clivus/foramen magnum, 2 cerebellopontine angle, and 2 cerebellar hemisphere. Performing preoperative embolization was the only factor that was associated with increased odds of gross total resection (odds ratio [95% confidence interval] = 8.087 [1.719 to 38.044]; $p = 0.008$).[27]

Some of the earlier case series of preoperative meningioma embolization subjectively reported that resection was easier or less bloody than it would have been without embolization.[8,10,17,18,28] However, given that several higher-quality, controlled studies are available, it is not necessary to discuss these findings in detail.

Conclusion

The existing data derived from several low-quality studies suggests that embolization decreases blood loss. There is not enough evidence to support decreased operating times. There may be a decrease in surgical complications, as evidenced by one Level II study. There have been no randomized trials, and the existing observational studies are subject to selection bias. Presumably, the meningiomas selected for embolization are those judged to be more likely to benefit (e.g., more vascular or more difficult to resect), which would create a bias against observing a difference in surgical outcomes. Although expert opinion has suggested that embolization is most beneficial for skull base meningiomas,[6,18,29] the available studies have not stratified outcomes based on tumor location, so an evidence-based statement regarding the relative benefit of embolization for tumors of various locations cannot be made.

Evidence Assessing the Safety of Embolization

In addition to determining the efficacy of preoperative embolization, it is important to assess the risks of the procedure in order to define the risk:benefit ratio. A list of some of the complications associated with preoperative meningioma embolization is provided in **Table 29.3**.

Level I Evidence

There is no Level I evidence comparing preoperative embolization versus resection alone for intracranial meningiomas.

Table 29.3 Complications of meningioma embolization

Minor	Major
Headache Face/scalp pain Nausea/vomiting Groin hematoma Transient neurological deficit	Persistent neurologic deficit – Monocular blindness – Hemiparesis – Aphasia – Neglect – Cranial nerve deficit Scalp necrosis Urgent craniotomy for edema or hemorrhage Death

Level II Evidence

Three comparative studies have reported complications of embolization as well as surgical complications in both embolized and nonembolized patients (**Table 29.4**). Macpherson reported five complications attributed to embolization in the 28 patients who underwent the procedure (18%), which included one patient each with lip numbness, scalp cyanosis, scalp necrosis, temporary paresis, and ischemia requiring embolectomy. Although surgical complications were lower in those who underwent preoperative embolization (21%) than in those who did not (54%), this difference is offset by the complications of the embolization procedure.[7]

Level III Evidence

Bendszus and colleagues reported a single complication attributed to embolization (monocular blindness) out of 30 patients (3%). Surgical complications resulting in permanent neurological deficits were experienced by five patients in the embolized group

Table 29.4 Complication rates from comparative studies

			Embolized group		
Evidence level	Study	Embolic agent	Complications of embolization	Surgical complications	Nonembolized group
Level I	No studies				
Level II	Macpherson 1991[7] (*n* = 52)	Gelatin powder PVA	5/28 (18%)	6/28 (21%)	13/24 (54%)
Level III	Bendszus et al 2000[23] (*n* = 60)	Trisacryl gelatin microspheres	1/30 (3%)	5/30 (17%)	6/30 (20%)
	Dean et al 1994[24] (*n* = 36)	Gelatin powder PVA	3/18 (17%)	6/18 (33%)	10/18 (56%)

Abbreviation: PVA, polyvinyl alcohol.

(17%) and six patients in the nonembolized group (20%).[23] Dean and colleagues reported four complications attributed to embolization in 18 patients who underwent the procedure. These embolized patients experienced zero major and six minor complications related to surgery, whereas the 18 nonembolized patients experienced three major and nine minor complications.[24]

Level IV Evidence

Three large case series have been published with the aim of characterizing the risks associated with embolization of meningiomas (**Table 29.5**). Carli and colleagues reported 11 total complications out of 198 embolized meningiomas (5.6%), of which 10 were hemorrhagic and one ischemic. A multivariate analysis of potential risk factors found that the use of smaller (50 to 150 µm) particles was associated with an increased complication rate. Tumor location and arterial supply were not found to be significant risk factors.[13] Bendszus and colleagues published a series of 185 patients, of which 12 (6.5%) experienced complications related to embolization (6 hemorrhagic and 6 ischemic).[30] In a series of 167 embolized skull base meningiomas, Rosen and colleagues noted that 22% of patients experienced a neurological complication, with 9% having permanent deficits.[31]

Some of the other large case series have reported complication rates of 2.5% (5 complications out of 203 embolized patients),[32] 2.5% (5 of 199),[33] 2.5% (2 of 80),[17] 13% (8 of 62),[34] 4.8% (3 out of 63),[29] and 2% (1 of 50).[20]

Effect of Tumor Location and Arterial Supply

To improve patient selection, it would be helpful to know the risk of embolization based on tumor location, but such a difference has not been demonstrated. As mentioned earlier, Carli and colleagues did not find an association between tumor location and complications.[13] Two studies of complications have dealt specifically with skull base tumors. In the first, Rosen and colleagues performed embolization on all of their skull base tumors, which included a substantial number with ICA feeders. Although the risk associated with embolization via the MHT or ophthalmic arteries was similar to that of the ECA branches, the overall rates of total (22%) and permanent (9%) neurological disability in the series were high.[31] More recently, Waldron and colleagues used a conservative strategy favoring complication avoidance over aggressive devascularization. By considering only select ICA feeding arteries for embolization (mainly the MHT and the anterior temporal artery), they observed no complications in 64 patients with skull base tumors, but this resulted in only 18% of feeding arteries from the ICA circulation being embolized.[33] The marked difference in complication rates between these two studies, which employed different strategies for skull base tumors, suggests that the arterial supply may be more important than the location of the tumor, although technical improvements may also play a role.

Although embolization of ICA branches is commonly avoided, the question of whether this can be accomplished safely is important given that some tumors receive a majority of their blood supply from these branches. Whereas one study reported a high rate of complications when embolizing branches of the cavernous carotid,[28] others have performed this with no complications,[29,33,35,36] so embolization of cavernous carotid branches may be reasonable provided that judicious patient selection and safe technique are employed. In this situation, temporary balloon occlusion may be helpful for preventing unwanted ICA emboli.[28,37] Successful embolization of a small number of ophthalmic[16,29,38,39] and pial[29,40,41] vessels has been reported with few complications, but little experience exists with these techniques and they are not recommended.

Table 29.5 Embolization complication rates from large series

Study	N	Embolic agent	Complications	Notes
Carli et al 2010[13]	198	PVA	11 (5.6%)	10 hemorrhagic complications 1 ischemic complication Smaller particles (45 to 150 µm) were associated with a higher complication rate
Bendszus et al 2005[30]	185	Trisacryl gelatin microspheres, Acrylamido PVA microspheres	12 (6.5%)	6 hemorrhagic complications 6 ischemic complications (1 fatality)
Rosen et al 2002[31]	167	PVA	36 (22%)	9% suffered permanent neurological deficit Included only skull base tumors

Abbreviation: PVA, polyvinyl alcohol.

Recommendations for Embolization of Internal Carotid Artery Branches

1. Embolization of ICA branches carries higher risk than that of ECA branches, and its routine use should be avoided (Grade 1C Recommendation, Level IV Evidence).
2. Embolization of ICA branches can be accomplished safely with sound technique in carefully selected cases (Grade 2C Recommendation, Level IV Evidence).

■ Summary and Conclusions

Several large case series have published data on complications related to embolization of meningiomas. Although these series provide the best estimate of the nature and frequency of complications, the risk associated with embolization remains difficult to quantify, given that reported complication rates vary greatly. This variation is likely due to differences in factors such as patient selection, embolization technique, type of embolic material, the definition used to define a complication, and the skill of the interventionalist. Perhaps more important than the total complication rate is the rate of major complications, which also varies between studies but is consistently less than 10%.

Putting It All Together: The Risk:Benefit Ratio

To make a clinical decision regarding embolization, all factors must be weighed together, including the anticipated benefits, added risks, and effect on cost. Unfortunately, the question of whether to perform preoperative embolization of meningiomas cannot be easily answered using the available evidence. The evidence does support decreased operative blood loss, but the clinical significance of this is not clear. Meanwhile, the extensive experience of neurosurgeons in dealing with meningiomas has shown that gross total resection can be safely achieved in the majority of cases without preoperative embolization, suggesting that the marginal benefit of embolization may be small for most tumors. Additionally, embolization is associated with certain complications, some serious, although these may be offset by decreased complications of the ensuing resection.

Patients with meningiomas are a highly heterogeneous group. Because factors such as tumor size, location, and origin of the feeding arteries may affect the risks and benefits of embolization, it is necessary to consider how these variables are represented in the literature. The comparative studies and large case series mentioned in the preceding sections were limited to large tumors, with the average size being ~ 5 cm, and with some studies including only tumors at least 4 cm in diameter.[25,26,32] Tumor location was limited to the skull base in some studies,[26,31,33] whereas the rest presented combined data from both skull base and more superficial locations. With regard to the vascular supply, most of the studies have included only tumors deriving the majority of their blood supply from ECA branches or performed embolization only in the ECA or its branches.[7,13,25,26,30,32] Variations in technique may also limit generalizability.

In light of the limitations in the existing data combined with the subjective opinion that embolization is beneficial for certain cases, it is reasonable to assume that preoperative embolization has a net benefit for some patients. However, it is not possible to identify these patients based on the existing literature, and the decision to perform the procedure must rely on clinical judgment.

Expert Recommendations

1. Preoperative embolization is reasonable to perform in select cases based on the clinician's judgment that it will be beneficial, which is most likely to be true for large, hypervascular tumors (Grade 2C Recommendation, Level II–IV Evidence).
2. There is insufficient evidence to make a statement regarding the relative benefit of embolization for tumors of different locations (i.e., skull base and non–skull base).

Considerations for Future Studies

Several large case series have reported data on complications of the embolization procedure, but complications have not been a primary focus of studies comparing preoperative embolization to surgery alone. Because embolization has the potential to decrease surgical complications, future comparative studies should include a carefully defined group of complications as a primary end point.

Additional data on clinical outcomes would be extremely valuable in determining the benefit of embolization. The existing literature has focused heavily on blood loss and operative times as measures of efficacy, but data on outcomes such as reoperation rates and neurological function would be more useful.

Further defining the risks and benefits of embolization for specific subgroups of patients, especially with regard to tumor location, may allow for a more evidence-based approach to patient selection. However, this will be challenging given the multitude of variables that may affect outcomes, the relatively small number of patients who undergo preoperative embolization, and the inherent weakness of subgroup analyses. Preoperative embolization of meningiomas remains a controversial practice, but centers that perform a significant number of embolizations can help us work toward answers through publication of their results, and a well-designed randomized, controlled trial would be invaluable.

■ References

1. Central Brain Tumor Registry of the United States. CBTRUS statistical report: primary brain and central nervous system tumors diagnosed in the United States in 2004–2007. 2011. Central Brain Tumor Registry of the United States, Hinsdale, IL. www.cbtrus.org
2. Simpson D. The recurrence of intracranial meningiomas after surgical treatment. J Neurol Neurosurg Psychiatry 1957; 20(1):22–39
3. Moniz E. L'encéphalographie artérielle, son importance dans la localisation des tumeurs cérébrales. Rev Neurol (Paris) 1927;2:72–90
4. Djindjian R, Cophignon J, Théron J, Merland JJ, Houdard R. L'embolisation en neuro-radiologie vasculaire. Technique et indications à propos de 30 cas. Nouv Presse Med 1972; 1(33):2153–2158
5. Nelson PK, Setton A, Choi IS, Ransohoff J, Berenstein A. Current status of interventional neuroradiology in the management of meningiomas. Neurosurg Clin N Am 1994;5(2):235–259
6. Manelfe C, Lasjaunias P, Ruscalleda J. Preoperative embolization of intracranial meningiomas. AJNR Am J Neuroradiol 1986;7(5):963–972
7. Macpherson P. The value of pre-operative embolisation of meningioma estimated subjectively and objectively. Neuroradiology 1991;33(4):334–337
8. Teasdale E, Patterson J, McLellan D, Macpherson P. Subselective preoperative embolization for meningiomas: a radiological and pathological assessment. J Neurosurg 1984;60(3): 506–511
9. Ng SH, Wan YL, Wong HF, et al. Preoperative embolization of meningiomas: comparison of superselective and subselective techniques. J Formos Med Assoc 1998;97(3):153–158
10. Hieshima GB, Everhart FR, Mehringer CM, et al. Preoperative embolization of meningiomas. Surg Neurol 1980;14(2): 119–127
11. Deveikis JP. Sequential injections of amobarbital sodium and lidocaine for provocative neurologic testing in the external carotid circulation. AJNR Am J Neuroradiol 1996;17(6): 1143–1147
12. Wakhloo AK, Juengling FD, Van Velthoven V, Schumacher M, Hennig J, Schwechheimer K. Extended preoperative polyvinyl alcohol microembolization of intracranial meningiomas: assessment of two embolization techniques. AJNR Am J Neuroradiol 1993;14(3):571–582
13. Carli DF, Sluzewski M, Beute GN, van Rooij WJ. Complications of particle embolization of meningiomas: frequency, risk factors, and outcome. AJNR Am J Neuroradiol 2010;31(1): 152–154
14. Bendszus M, Klein R, Burger R, Warmuth-Metz M, Hofmann E, Solymosi L. Efficacy of trisacryl gelatin microspheres versus polyvinyl alcohol particles in the preoperative embolization of meningiomas. AJNR Am J Neuroradiol 2000;21(2):255–261
15. Feng L, Kienitz BA, Matsumoto C, et al. Feasibility of using hyperosmolar mannitol as a liquid tumor embolization agent. AJNR Am J Neuroradiol 2005;26(6):1405–1412
16. Terada T, Kinoshita Y, Yokote H, et al. Preoperative embolization of meningiomas fed by ophthalmic branch arteries. Surg Neurol 1996;45(2):161–166
17. Probst EN, Grzyska U, Westphal M, Zeumer H. Preoperative embolization of intracranial meningiomas with a fibrin glue preparation. AJNR Am J Neuroradiol 1999;20(9):1695–1702
18. Richter HP, Schachenmayr W. Preoperative embolization of intracranial meningiomas. Neurosurgery 1983;13(3): 261–268
19. Kai Y, Hamada J, Morioka M, Yano S, Todaka T, Ushio Y. Appropriate interval between embolization and surgery in patients with meningioma. AJNR Am J Neuroradiol 2002;23(1): 139–142
20. Chun JY, McDermott MW, Lamborn KR, Wilson CB, Higashida R, Berger MS. Delayed surgical resection reduces intraoperative blood loss for embolized meningiomas. Neurosurgery 2002;50(6):1231–1235
21. Berenstein A, Kricheff II. Microembolization techniques of vascular occlusion: radiologic, pathologic, and clinical correlation. AJNR Am J Neuroradiol 1981;2(3):261–267
22. Sughrue ME, Kane AJ, Shangari G, et al. The relevance of Simpson Grade I and II resection in modern neurosurgical treatment of World Health Organization Grade I meningiomas. J Neurosurg 2010;113(5):1029–1035
23. Bendszus M, Rao G, Burger R, et al. Is there a benefit of preoperative meningioma embolization? Neurosurgery 2000;47(6):1306–1311
24. Dean BL, Flom RA, Wallace RC, et al. Efficacy of endovascular treatment of meningiomas: evaluation with matched samples. AJNR Am J Neuroradiol 1994;15(9):1675–1680
25. Alberione F, Iturrieta P, Schulz J, et al. Embolización preoperatoria con esponja de gelatina absorbente en meningiomas intracraneales. Rev Neurol 2009;49(1):13–17
26. Oka H, Kurata A, Kawano N, et al. Preoperative superselective embolization of skull-base meningiomas: indications and limitations. J Neurooncol 1998;40(1):67–71
27. Quiñones-Hinojosa A, Kaprealian T, Chaichana KL, et al. Preoperative factors affecting resectability of giant intracranial meningiomas. Can J Neurol Sci 2009;36(5):623–630
28. Jungreis CA. Skull-base tumors: ethanol embolization of the cavernous carotid artery. Radiology 1991;181(3):741–743
29. Gruber A, Killer M, Mazal P, Bavinzski G, Richling B. Preoperative embolization of intracranial meningiomas: a 17-years single center experience. Minim Invasive Neurosurg 2000; 43(1):18–29
30. Bendszus M, Monoranu CM, Schütz A, Nölte I, Vince GH, Solymosi L. Neurologic complications after particle embolization of intracranial meningiomas. AJNR Am J Neuroradiol 2005;26(6):1413–1419
31. Rosen CL, Ammerman JM, Sekhar LN, Bank WO. Outcome analysis of preoperative embolization in cranial base surgery. Acta Neurochir (Wien) 2002;144(11):1157–1164
32. Kai Y, Hamada JI, Morioka M, et al. Clinical evaluation of cellulose porous beads for the therapeutic embolization of meningiomas. AJNR Am J Neuroradiol 2006;27(5):1146–1150
33. Waldron JS, Sughrue ME, Hetts SW, et al. Embolization of skull base meningiomas and feeding vessels arising from the internal carotid circulation. Neurosurgery 2011;68(1): 162–169
34. Perry A, Chicoine MR, Filiput E, Miller JP, Cross DT. Clinicopathologic assessment and grading of embolized meningiomas: a correlative study of 64 patients. Cancer 2001;92(3):701–711

35. Robinson DH, Song JK, Eskridge JM. Embolization of meningohypophyseal and inferolateral branches of the cavernous internal carotid artery. AJNR Am J Neuroradiol 1999; 20(6):1061–1067
36. Hirohata M, Abe T, Morimitsu H, Fujimura N, Shigemori M, Norbash AM. Preoperative selective internal carotid artery dural branch embolisation for petroclival meningiomas. Neuroradiology 2003;45(9):656–660
37. Théron J, Cosgrove R, Melanson D, Ethier R. Embolization with temporary balloon occlusion of the internal carotid or vertebral arteries. Neuroradiology 1986;28(3):246–253
38. Lefkowitz M, Giannotta SL, Hieshima G, et al. Embolization of neurosurgical lesions involving the ophthalmic artery. Neurosurgery 1998;43(6):1298–1303
39. Trivelatto F, Nakiri GS, Manisor M, et al. Preoperative onyx embolization of meningiomas fed by the ophthalmic artery: a case series. AJNR Am J Neuroradiol 2011;32(9):1762–1766
40. Yoon YS, Ahn JY, Chang JH, et al. Pre-operative embolisation of internal carotid artery branches and pial vessels in hypervascular brain tumours. Acta Neurochir (Wien) 2008;150(5):447–452
41. Kaji T, Hama Y, Iwasaki Y, Kyoto Y, Kusano S. Preoperative embolization of meningiomas with pial supply: successful treatment of two cases. Surg Neurol 1999;52(3):270–273

30

Adjuvant Therapies (Chemotherapy and Radiation Therapy) for Atypical and Anaplastic Meningiomas

Manmeet S. Ahluwalia, Rohan Garje, Patrick Y. Wen, and Minesh Mehta

The treatment of atypical and anaplastic meningiomas includes resection, radiotherapy, systemic therapy, or a combination of these modalities. The chemotherapy and radiation therapy recommendations for atypical and anaplastic meningiomas are usually based on data from retrospective series or small phase 2 studies because there are no randomized clinical studies comparing various treatment options.

Tumor Grade and Prognosis

Meningiomas are classified histologically by the World Health Organizaation as grade I (benign tumors without atypia or mitosis); grade II or atypical meningioma (rare mitosis and some cellular atypia), and grade III or atypical or malignant meningioma (abundant vascularization, numerous mitoses, and presence of cell atypia).[1–4] Atypical meningiomas (AMs) account for 5 to 20%[1–4] of the cases and anaplastic or malignant meningiomas (MMs) account for 1 to 5% of cases of meningiomas.[1–3,5] The goal of treatment for meningiomas is to achieve better survival and local control with the least possible morbidity. After definitive resection, AM carries a seven- to eightfold increased risk of recurrence in the initial 3 to 5 years, compared with grade I meningioma, with only 40 to 60% of patients disease free after 10 years.[2,3,5–8] MMs are even more aggressive tumors, with a 5-year recurrence rate of 72 to 78% and median recurrence-free survival < 2 years,[2,3,5] making a case for testing adjuvant therapies such as radiation therapy and chemotherapy.

Management of Atypical and Anaplastic Meningiomas

Radiotherapy

Fractionated external beam radiotherapy (EBRT) may have an important role in the management of AM and MM. In multiple retrospective studies, postoperative EBRT has shown improved progression-free survival (PFS) following subtotal resection and a reduction in long-term failures following an apparent gross total resection, in comparison with unirradiated patients from historical control data. The use of EBRT has grown in recent years as improved neuroimaging techniques enable better identification and treatment of skull-base lesions, which are not easily resectable. Optic nerve sheath meningiomas represent an example of the use of definitive EBRT, given the frequent visual sequelae of surgery or observation. EBRT planning is individualized and involves tumor grade, adjacent radiosensitive structures, such as the anterior optic apparatus, and radiographic characteristics of the tumor, such as hyperostosis.

Treatment Planning and Dose

Exact classification of these tumors is of importance because histology not only influences the decision to add radiotherapy (RT) to the treatment recommendation but also impacts the target volume definition as well as the RT dose.

Level I and Level II Evidence

There are no studies providing Level I or II evidence regarding the role of RT in patients with AM or MM.

Level III and IV Evidence

Target Volume

Gross target volume (GTV) is representative of the measurable disease and is contoured using magnetic resonance imaging (MRI), with computed tomography (CT) as an adjunct to visualize bony involvement or infiltration. Inclusion of the dural tail in the GTV is controversial. Pathophysiologically, the dural tail is representative of the hypervascular dura where a meningioma attaches or, to varying degrees, invades.[9,10] Radiographically, this appears as a linear enhancement of dura that usually trails off within a few millimeters to centimeters.[11] Pathologically, occasional microscopic clusters of meningioma cells have been reported in these regions.[9] Ahmadi and colleagues reported two patterns of dural enhancement: continuous and discontinuous. Dural tumor invasion was observed in every case of discontinuous enhancement; however, it was not present with continuous enhancement.[12] At the current time, it is unclear whether a tumor's dural tail (as defined by the linear enhancement radiographically) should be included in GTV.

Published reports have varied considerably on the optimal margin to be applied to the GTV in calculating the clinical target volume (CTV), which by definition would include subclinical disease, and the subsequent expansion of this CTV to the planning target volume (PTV) that accounts for all the geometric uncertainties in daily treatment delivery. Recommendations for margin expansion have ranged from as small as 1 to 2 mm in recent stereotactic fractionated series[13,14] to 1 cm,[15] 2 cm,[7,16] and even as large as 4 cm.[17] Milker-Zabel et al have recommended the use of margins of 1 to 2 mm along normal brain parenchyma, 3 mm along osseous structures, and 5 mm along dura.[18] Intriguingly, with the tight conformity of 2 mm, achieved with stereotactic techniques, margin failures have actually been uncommon, with Debus and colleagues reporting no marginal failures in 189 patients with 3 years of median follow-up, calling into question whether larger margins are really necessary.[13]

Grade 1 Simpson resection requires removal of abnormal bone.[19] However, the question of inclusion of hyperostotic bone within the radiotherapy target volume remains unanswered. In reported series, complete resection of the tumor but not of the hyperostotic bone has been associated with low recurrence rates. Similar observations have been made in radiosurgery or fractionated EBRT series. Most radiation oncologists individualize the decision to include or exclude hyperostotic bone from the RT field, based on the known histopathological involvement of it or not, and the extent of resection.

Dose

A firm dose–response relationship for meningiomas has not been established. A retrospective series of 140 patients with meningioma (all grades) treated at the University of California, San Francisco (1967 to 1990) included 23 patients with subtotal resection of MM treated with adjuvant RT (a median dose = 54 Gy).[20] The PFS and the overall survival (OS) rate at 5 years were 48 and 58%, respectively, for the MM group.[20] In another retrospective study, 15 patients with AM and 16 patients with MM were treated with fractionated RT.[8] RT was delivered using megavoltage photons in 15 patients and combined photons and 160 MeV protons in 16 patients. Total target doses for AM and MM ranged from 50 to 68 Gy (mean dose of 62 Gy) and 40 to 72 Gy (mean dose of 58 Gy) or D cobalt-gray-equivalent (CGE), respectively. Actuarial local control rates were similar for both groups at 5 and 8 years (38 and 19% for AM and 52 and 17% for MM). Significantly improved local control was seen for proton, compared with photon RT (80 vs 17% at 5 years) at target doses ≥ 60 Gy for both AM ($p = 0.025$) and MM ($p = 0.0006$) groups. The study suggested that conformal, high-dose RT resulted in significant improvement of local control for AM and MM, and increased local control resulted in improved survival in MM.

In a multicenter retrospective study, 119 patients (82 with AM and 37 with MM) were treated with RT with a mean dose of 54.6 ± 5.1 Gy (range, 40 to 66 Gy) after surgery or for recurrence.[21] The 5- and 10- year disease-free survival was 58 and 48%, respectively, for the whole group. The actuarial OS was 65 and 51% at 5 and 10 years, respectively.[21] On multivariate analysis, age > 60 years ($p = 0.001$) and high mitotic rate ($p = 0.02$) were significant adverse prognostic factors for survival, but dose was not. In a retrospective study of 59 patients with AM and MM treated with RT (average dose = 50 Gy), the 5-year actuarial OS was 28% and cause-specific survival was 34%.[22] Twenty of 59 patients were disease-free after RT. In this retrospective analysis, RT dose > 50 Gy, age < 58 years, and treatment planning (in favor of MR-based volume definitions) were prognostically significant.

In an effort to evaluate whether a more aggressive course of RT resulted in improved outcomes, 36 patients with AM (n = 27) or MM (n = 9) were treated with 60 Gy, 1.5 Gy per fraction twice daily with or without radiosurgery boost.[23] The overall 5-year local control was 45%, and cause-specific survival and absolute survival rates were 39 and 36%, respectively, in this study. Accelerated hyperfractionated RT resulted in a local control rate of 45% compared with 50% for patients treated with less aggressive schedules (p = 0.99). Radiosurgery boost in this study did not improve tumor control. The complication rate was dramatically higher in those treated with accelerated hyperfractionated RT (grade 3 through 5: 55% vs 0%, grade 4 and 5: 27% vs 0%; both $p < 0.05$). The authors suggested that a dose of 50 to 60 Gy delivered with conventional, once-daily fractionation is optimal for AM and MM, and more aggressive therapy added toxicity without improvement in efficacy.

In a retrospective analysis to assess the efficacy of conformal fractionated RT combining proton (mean dose 34.05 CGE) and photon beam (mean dose 30.96 CGE), a total mean dose of 65.01 CGE was utilized as postoperative management of 24 patients with AM (n = 19) and MM (n = 5).[24] The overall mean local relapse-free interval was 28.3 (10 to 50) and 23 (13 to 33) months for the AM and MM groups, respectively. The 5- and 8-year OS for the whole group was 53.2% ± 11.6% and 42.6% ± 13%, respectively. One patient developed radiation necrosis 16 months after treatment. Overall the high-dose RT was well tolerated and not associated with acute radiation-related morbidity. The study concluded that postoperative combination of conformal RT with protons and photons for AM and MM is a well-tolerated treatment producing long-term tumor stabilization. Increase of the total dose to > 60 Gy resulted in better cause-specific survival, and OS with increase of the total dose to > 65 Gy demonstrating a trend for a possible additional benefit of OS.

In a recently published retrospective study of 85 patients with AM (n = 62) or MM (n = 23), 60% underwent RT after surgical resection, 19% received RT at disease progression, and 8.3% as a primary treatment.[25] The median dose of RT was 57.6 Gy, and different methods used to deliver RT included fractionated stereotactic RT (FSRT), intensity-modulated RT (IMRT), and carbon ions. PFS at 5 years for AM and MM was 50 and 13%, respectively, resulting in an OS of 81 and 53% at 5 years, respectively.

Despite the need for randomized trials and for larger studies with longer median follow-up, RT is highly effective for the management of AM and MM with an acceptable incidence of complications. Increased EBRT doses appear to be associated with superior local control for AM and PFS, cause-specific survival, and even OS for MM.[8,22,26] Standard RT techniques use accelerated photons to deliver the radiation dose to the PTV. Proton therapy has a possible advantage over standard photon therapy because of the possibility of substantially reducing the exit dose delivered to normal tissue. Thus proton irradiation can achieve better target dose conformality than is attainable with conventional EBRT and IMRT, and the advantage becomes more apparent for large volumes. However, currently there are no randomized trials showing how effective proton irradiation alone or in combination with photons is for treatment of AM and MM. The Radiotherapy Oncology Group study (RTOG 0539), "Observation or Radiation Therapy in Treating Patients with Grade I, Grade II, or Grade III Meningioma," is an ongoing trial that will help answer questions regarding the natural history of meningioma and utility of RT in AM and MM further. There is an urgent need for the brain tumor community to come together to conduct trials like RTOG 0539 to further address the role of RT in patients with AM and MM (**Table 30.1**).

Table 30.1 Trials with radiotherapy for atypical and anaplastic meningiomas

Study	No. patients	Radiation technique	Dose	Local control
Milosevic et al 1996[22]	59	Photons	50 Gy	34% local control at median 40 months
Hug et al 2000[8]	31	Photons and protons	40 to 72 Gy E	AM: 38% at 5 years MM: 52% at 5 years
Katz et al 2005[23]	36	Hyperfractionated photons, radiosurgery boost		45% at 5 years
Pasquier.et al 2008[21]	119	Photons	40 to 66 Gy E	58% at 5 years
Boskos et al 2009[24]	24	Photons and protons	65 Gy E	61.3% at 5 years
Adeberg et al 2012[25]	85	Photon, photon + carbon ion		AM: 81% at 5 years MM: 53% at 5 years

Abbreviations: AM, atypical meningioma; MM, malignant or anaplastic meningioma.

Recommendations for Radiotherapy in AM and MM

1. AM and MM have a significant probability of recurrence even after gross total resection.
2. Use of RT is generally recommended at a dose of 54 to 60 Gy postoperatively in patients with AM to improve local control (Grade 1C Recommendation, Level III/IV Evidence).
3. Higher EBRT (60 to 64 Gy) doses have been associated with superior progression-free survival, cause-specific survival, and even OS for MM (Grade 1C Recommendation, Level III/IV Evidence).

Chemotherapy

Medical therapy (hormonal therapy, chemotherapy, or targeted therapy) is usually limited to treatment of meningiomas that recur after surgical and RT options have been exhausted. Evidence from small clinical trials and retrospective case series suggest only minimal activity of chemotherapy against AM and MM.[27] One of the challenges in evaluation of these therapies is the limited number of patients, the heterogeneous group (benign meningiomas are often combined with AM and MM), and the lack of data regarding the natural history of untreated meningiomas (**Table 30.2**).

Table 30.2 Trials with chemotherapy and target agents in patients with meningioma

Study	Drug	No. patients	WHO histology grade	Prior surgery	Prior RT	Outcomes in AM and MM
Rosenthal (2002)	Hydroxyurea	15	AM = 5	All	1/15	Not reported separately for AM or MM
Mason et al 2002[31]	Hydroxyurea	20	AM = 3 MM = 1	All	All	Median TTP in AM = 19 weeks MM = 24 weeks
Loven et al 2004[30]	Hydroxyurea	12	AM = 4	All	No	SD: 25%
Newton et al 2004[32]	Hydroxyurea	21	AM = 1	Yes	No	Median TTP in AM = 176 weeks
Chamberlain 2011[29]	Hydroxyurea	35	AM = 22 MM = 13	Yes	Yes	Median PFS = 2 months PFS-6 = 3%
Wen et al 2009[36]	Imatinib mesylate	23	AM = 5 MM = 5	yes	20/23	Median PFS = 2 months PFS-6 = 0%
Horak et al 2012[35]	Imatinib mesylate	18	AM = 2 MM = 6	NA	NA	PFS in AM = 16, 32 months Median PFS in MM = 15 months
Reardon et al 2012[37]	Imatinib + hydroxyurea	21	AM = 9 MM = 4	Yes	Yes	OS=6 months for AM + MM = 76.9% PFS-6 = 46.2%
Johnson et al 2011[42]	Subcutaneous octreotide	12	AM = 2 MM = 5	7/7	6/7	TTP in AM = 118 and 6,700 days Median TTP in MM = 33 days
Chamberlain et al 2007[43]	Sustained-release somatostatin	16	AM = 3 MM = 5	Yes	yes	PR in AM = 33% PR in MM = 20%
Norden (2011)	Pasireotide	26	AM + MM = 17	Yes	Yes	Median PFS = 16 weeks PFS-6 = 20%
Lou et al 2012[45]	Bevacizumab	14	AM = 5 MM = 3	Yes	Yes	Median PFS = 15.8 months PFS-6 = 87.5%
Nayak et al 2012[46]	Bevacizumab	15	AM = 6 MM = 9	Yes	Yes	Median PFS = 26 weeks PFS-6 = 43.8% Median OS = 15 months
Kaley and Schiff 2010[48]	Sunitinib	36	MM = 30	Yes	Yes	Median PFS = 5.1 months PFS-6 = = 36%
Raizer and Grimm 2010[47]	Vatalinib	25	AM = 14 MM = 8	Yes	Yes	PFS-6 = 57.2% Median TTP = 7.5 months Median OS = 26.9 months
Norden et al 2010[50]	Erlotinib or gefitinib	25	AM = 9 MM = 8	Yes	Yes	Median PFS = 16 weeks Median OS = 33 months.

Abbreviations: AM, atypical meningioma; MM, malignant or anaplastic meningioma; OS, overall survival; PFS, progression-free survival; PFS-6, progression-free survival at 6 months; RT, radiotherapy; SD, stable disease; TTP, time to progression; WHO, World Health Organization.

Level I and Level II Evidence

There are no Level I or II evidence studies evaluating the role of chemotherapy in patients with AM or MM.

Level III and Level IV Evidence

Hydroxyurea

Schrell and colleagues showed that oral hydroxyurea (HU), a ribonucleotide reductase inhibitor, inhibits primary human melanoma cells in the S phase of the cell cycle, and induces apoptosis in both cell culture and meningioma transplants.[28] This preclinical efficacy led to several retrospective and phase 2 clinical trials evaluating the efficacy of hydroxyurea in medical management of meningiomas. In a retrospective case series analysis of 35 patients with progressive AM (n = 22) and MM (n = 13) who underwent prior surgery and RT, patients were treated with oral hydroxyurea (1000 mg/m^2/single daily dose) every 4 weeks.[29] In this study, no patient achieved complete response (CR) or partial response (PR), 15 patients (43%) had stable disease (SD) as best response, and 20 patients (57%) progressed after two cycles of HU. The median PFS was 2 months (95% confidence interval [CI] 1.6 to 2.4), PFS-6 months was 3% and PFS-12 months was zero. This study concluded that efficacy of HU in AM and MM was limited.

In a prospective study, 12 patients (benign = 8 and AM = 4) with nonresectable meningioma were treated by HU.[30] All four patients with AM had undergone surgical resection; however, they did not receive any prior RT. One patient achieved SD both clinically and by imaging after 3 months of HU but discontinued therapy due to hematological toxicity. The remaining three patients progressed after 9 to 13 months of therapy. In a prospective study of 20 patients with recurrent or unresectable meningioma, three patients with AM and one patient with MM (all had prior surgery and RT) were treated with HU.[31] Median time to progression in AM patients was 19 weeks (range: 12 to 45 weeks), and the patient with MM progressed after 24 weeks of therapy. In a prospective cohort study, 21 patients (one patient had AM) with unresectable or residual meningioma were treated with HU alone.[32] Median time to progression for all the patients was 176 weeks, and the only patient with AM progressed after 286 weeks. These studies demonstrate that HU has minimal, if any, activity in meningiomas.

Imatinib

In vitro studies showed increased expression of platelet-derived growth factor (PDGF) ligands AA and BB, PDGF-β receptors, and a possible autocrine signaling loop promoting meningioma cell growth and maintenance.[33,34] In a retrospective study of 18 patients with recurrent meningiomas that included nine patients with at least one PGDF receptor positive were treated with a daily dose of 400 mg of imatinib mesylate.[35] This included two patients with AM and six patients with MM. No objective response was seen in this study, and overall median PFS was 16 months. The PFS for two patients with AM was 16 and 32 months, respectively. The median PFS for patients with grade III meningioma was 15 months (R, 1 to 26 months). In a phase 2 study done by the North American Brain Tumor Consortium (NABTC), 23 patients with recurrent meningiomas (five with AM and five with MM) were treated with 400 to 800 mg daily dose of imatinib.[36] The median PFS was 2 months (0.7 to 3.7 months), and 6 month PFS was 0%. Although well tolerated, imatinib demonstrated minimal activity as a single agent in recurrent meningiomas.

Imatinib plus Hydroxyurea

A prospective study of 21 patients with recurrent meningiomas (9 AM, 4 MM) were treated with a combination of imatinib and HU.[37] These patients had previously undergone surgery, RT, and/or stereotactic radiosurgery (SRS). The PFS and OS at 6 months for AM and MM patients were 46.2% (95% CI 19.2 to 69.6) and 76.9% (95% CI 44.2 to 91.9), respectively. The combination showed only modest antitumor activity in this patient population.

Somatostatin Analogues

In vitro studies have shown that meningiomas express somatostatin receptors, especially sstr2a receptor.[38,39] Somatostatin analogues have been shown to inhibit meningioma cell growth in previous case reports and series.[40,41] In a phase 2 study, 12 patients with recurrent meningioma (two AM and five MM, two of whom had previous chemotherapy) were treated with subcutaneous octreotide.[42] Time to progression (TTP) was 118 and 6,700 days for the two patients with AM and median TTP of 33 days (range 22 to 939) for the patients with MM. However, no clinical improvement was seen in any of the patients. In another prospective pilot trial of 16 patients with recurrent meningioma (three with AM and five with MM), patients were treated with sustained-release somatostatin once every 28 days.[43] One out of five patients (20%) with MM achieved PR, one patient (20%) achieved SD, and one out of three patients (33%) with AM achieved a PR, and one had SD as best response.[43] Over all, this regimen was well tolerated, with minimal toxicity of grade II diarrhea in 3/16 patients.

In a phase 2 study of 26 patients with recurrent or progressive meningioma (17 patients with AM or MM) were treated with monthly pasireotide LAR (SOM230C). The median PFS was 16 weeks and a PFS-6 of 20% was seen for the whole cohort. The therapy was relatively well tolerated, with grade 3 hyperglycemia in five patients and grade 4 hyperglycemia in one patient. Aforementioned studies confirm that somatostatin analogues are well tolerated; however, they have minimal efficacy in AM and MM.

Vascular Endothelial Growth Factor Inhibition

Bevacizumab Multiple in vitro studies have shown evidence for increased VEGF and VEGF receptor (VEGFR) expression in high-grade meningiomas.[44] Bevacizumab is a monoclonal antibody directed against VEGF that is approved for the pretreatment of recurrent glioblastoma multiforme (GBM). In a retrospective case series study, 14 patients with recurrent/progressive meningioma (WHO grade I = 5, AM = 5, MM = 3) were treated with bevacizumab either as a single agent or combined with chemotherapy.[45] The patients in this series were heavily pretreated, with multiple surgical resections, RT, SRS, and other previous chemotherapy/target therapy. Median PFS and median PFS-6 were 15.8 months (95% CI 5.5 to 17.9) and 87.5% (38.7 to 98.1), respectively, for patients with AM and MM. In a multicenter retrospective case series of 15 patients with AM (n = 6) and MM (n = 9) who had undergone prior surgery, RT and 7/15 had received prior chemotherapy/targeted therapy, were treated with bevacizumab.[46] None of the patients achieved any objective response, and stable disease was the best response seen in this report. The median PFS was 26 weeks (95% CI, 10 to 29 weeks), PFS-6 was 43.8% (95% CI 15.7 to 69.1%), median OS was 15 months (range, 10 to 22 months). Three patients had intratumoral hemorrhage (2: grade I, 1: grade II), and one patient had grade II fatigue. These studies show very modest efficacy for bevacizumab but suggest that bevacizumab may be considered in patients who have exhausted radiation and surgical options, especially if there is significant peritumoral edema.

Vatalinib In a phase 2 trial, 25 patients with recurrent or progressive meningiomas (14 AM and 8 MM) were treated with PTK787 (vatalanib), a tyrosine kinase inhibitor that targets VEGF and PDGF.[47] Of the 21 evaluable patients, partial response (PR) was seen in one patient, SD was seen in 15 patients, and progressive disease (PD) was reported in five patients. Over all, PFS-6 was 57.2% and median TTP was 7.5 months in the intent-to-treat analysis. Median OS was 26.9 months. The study suggested that combination VEGF/PDGF inhibition in patients with recurrent or progressive meningiomas can lead to disease stabilization in some patients.

Sunitinib In a phase 2 trial of sunitinib, a small-molecule multiple tyrosine kinase inhibitor that targets VEGF and PDGF receptors, in 36 heavily pretreated patients (30 AM and 6 MM), the median PFS was 5.1 months, and the PFS-6 was 36%, suggesting modest activity, although at the cost of fairly significant toxicity.[48]

Epidermal Growth Factor Receptor Inhibitors

In vitro studies have shown expression of epidermal growth factor receptor (EGFR) in most meningiomas. Preclinical evidence indicates meningiomas express EGF and tumor growth factor (TGF)-α messenger RNA (mRNA), which activate EGFRs (autocrine or paracrine mechanism) and result in proliferation of meningioma cells.[49] A phase 2 pilot study of erlotinib and gefitinib, tyrosine kinase inhibitors (TKIs) that inhibit EGFR, was conducted by NABTC.[50] Twenty-five patients with meningiomas that included nine with AM, received erlotinib 150 mg daily (nine patients) or gefitinib 500 to 1,000 mg daily (16 patients) as part of the study. A median PFS of 16 weeks (95% CI 8 to 23), PFS-6 of 29%, and PFS-12 of 18% were seen in patients with AM or MM. The median OS was 33 months. Six patients reported grade 3 rashes. This study suggests that both of these drugs have minimal activity in the management of recurrent meningioma.

Expert Recommendation

There is no demonstrated benefit of adjuvant chemotherapy in AM and MM, and it is generally reserved as a salvage therapy for recurrent tumor or failed response to radiation-based adjuncts (Grade 2C Recommendation, Level III/IV Evidence).

■ Summary and Conclusions

In summary, further exploration of the molecular biology of meningioma will hopefully provide new insights that will guide future treatments. Genomic studies will likely help to identify growth factors and their cognate receptors, intracellular signaling pathways, and hormonal influences that will represent novel targets for therapy. Angiogenesis is important for higher-grade meningiomas and can be targeted with a variety of approved and investigational drugs. There is some hint for activity with bevacizumab and some VEGFR inhibitors, although the level of evidence is low. In future, these novel therapies will complement the traditional approaches like RT and lead to more effective treatments for patients with AM or MM.

■ References

1. Willis J, Smith C, Ironside JW, Erridge S, Whittle IR, Everington D. The accuracy of meningioma grading: a 10-year retrospective audit. Neuropathol Appl Neurobiol 2005;31(2): 141–149
2. Perry A, Scheithauer BW, Stafford SL, Lohse CM, Wollan PC. "Malignancy" in meningiomas: a clinicopathologic study of 116 patients, with grading implications. Cancer 1999; 85(9):2046–2056
3. Perry A, Stafford SL, Scheithauer BW, Suman VJ, Lohse CM. Meningioma grading: an analysis of histologic parameters. Am J Surg Pathol 1997;21(12):1455–1465
4. Claus EB, Bondy ML, Schildkraut JM, Wiemels JL, Wrensch M, Black PM. Epidemiology of intracranial meningioma. Neurosurgery 2005;57(6):1088–1095
5. Jääskeläinen J, Haltia M, Servo A. Atypical and anaplastic meningiomas: radiology, surgery, radiotherapy, and outcome. Surg Neurol 1986;25(3):233–242
6. Perry A. Unmasking the secrets of meningioma: a slow but rewarding journey. Surg Neurol 2004;61(2):171–173
7. Condra KS, Buatti JM, Mendenhall WM, Friedman WA, Marcus RB Jr, Rhoton AL. Benign meningiomas: primary treatment selection affects survival. Int J Radiat Oncol Biol Phys 1997;39(2):427–436
8. Hug EB, Devries A, Thornton AF, et al. Management of atypical and malignant meningiomas: role of high-dose, 3D-conformal radiation therapy. J Neurooncol 2000;48(2):151–160
9. Borovich B, Doron Y. Recurrence of intracranial meningiomas: the role played by regional multicentricity. J Neurosurg 1986;64(1):58–63
10. Nägele T, Petersen D, Klose U, Grodd W, Opitz H, Voigt K. The "dural tail" adjacent to meningiomas studied by dynamic contrast-enhanced MRI: a comparison with histopathology. Neuroradiology 1994;36(4):303–307
11. Kawahara Y, Niiro M, Yokoyama S, Kuratsu J. Dural congestion accompanying meningioma invasion into vessels: the dural tail sign. Neuroradiology 2001;43(6):462–465
12. Ahmadi J, Hinton DR, Segall HD, Couldwell WT. Surgical implications of magnetic resonance-enhanced dura. Neurosurgery 1994;35(3):370–377
13. Debus J, Wuendrich M, Pirzkall A, et al. High efficacy of fractionated stereotactic radiotherapy of large base-of-skull meningiomas: long-term results. J Clin Oncol 2001;19(15): 3547–3553
14. Henzel M, Gross MW, Hamm K, et al. Stereotactic radiotherapy of meningiomas: symptomatology, acute and late toxicity. Strahlenther Onkol 2006;182(7):382–388
15. Goldsmith B. Meningioma. In: Leibel SA, Phillips TS, eds. Textbook of Radiation Oncology. Philadelphia, PA: WB Saunders; 1998:324–340
16. Sibtain A, Plowman PN. Stereotactic radiosurgery, VII: Radiosurgery versus conventionally-fractionated radiotherapy in the treatment of cavernous sinus meningiomas. Br J Neurosurg 1999;13(2):158–166
17. Glaholm J, Bloom HJ, Crow JH. The role of radiotherapy in the management of intracranial meningiomas: the Royal Marsden Hospital experience with 186 patients. Int J Radiat Oncol Biol Phys 1990;18(4):755–761
18. Milker-Zabel S, Zabel-du Bois A, Huber P, Schlegel W, Debus J. Intensity-modulated radiotherapy for complex-shaped meningioma of the skull base: long-term experience of a single institution. Int J Radiat Oncol Biol Phys 2007;68(3):858–863
19. Simpson D. The recurrence of intracranial meningiomas after surgical treatment. J Neurol Neurosurg Psychiatry 1957; 20(1):22–39
20. Goldsmith BJ, Wara WM, Wilson CB, Larson DA. Postoperative irradiation for subtotally resected meningiomas: a retrospective analysis of 140 patients treated from 1967 to 1990. J Neurosurg 1994;80(2):195–201
21. Pasquier D, Bijmolt S, Veninga T, et al; Rare Cancer Network. Atypical and malignant meningioma: outcome and prognostic factors in 119 irradiated patients: a multicenter, retrospective study of the Rare Cancer Network. Int J Radiat Oncol Biol Phys 2008;71(5):1388–1393
22. Milosevic MF, Frost PJ, Laperriere NJ, Wong CS, Simpson WJ. Radiotherapy for atypical or malignant intracranial meningioma. Int J Radiat Oncol Biol Phys 1996;34(4):817–822
23. Katz TS, Amdur RJ, Yachnis AT, Mendenhall WM, Morris CG. Pushing the limits of radiotherapy for atypical and malignant meningioma. Am J Clin Oncol 2005;28(1):70–74
24. Boskos C, Feuvret L, Noel G, et al. Combined proton and photon conformal radiotherapy for intracranial atypical and malignant meningioma. Int J Radiat Oncol Biol Phys 2009; 75(2):399–406
25. Adeberg S, Hartmann C, Welzel T, et al. Long-term outcome after radiotherapy in patients with atypical and malignant meningiomas—clinical results in 85 patients treated in a single institution leading to optimized guidelines for early radiation therapy. Int J Radiat Oncol Biol Phys 2012;83(3):859–864
26. Goldsmith BJ, Wara WM, Wilson CB, Larson DA. Postoperative irradiation for subtotally resected meningiomas. A retrospective analysis of 140 patients treated from 1967 to 1990. J Neurosurg 1994;80(2):195–201
27. Wen PY, Quant E, Drappatz J, Beroukhim R, Norden AD. Medical therapies for meningiomas. J Neurooncol 2010;99(3): 365–378
28. Schrell UM, Rittig MG, Anders M, et al. Hydroxyurea for treatment of unresectable and recurrent meningiomas, I: Inhibition of primary human meningioma cells in culture and in meningioma transplants by induction of the apoptotic pathway. J Neurosurg 1997;86(5):845–852
29. Chamberlain MC. Hydroxyurea for recurrent surgery and radiation refractory high-grade meningioma. J Neurooncol 2012;107(2):315–321
30. Loven D, Hardoff R, Sever ZB, et al. Non-resectable slow-growing meningiomas treated by hydroxyurea. J Neurooncol 2004;67(1-2):221–226
31. Mason WP, Gentili F, Macdonald DR, Hariharan S, Cruz CR, Abrey LE. Stabilization of disease progression by hydroxyurea in patients with recurrent or unresectable meningioma. J Neurosurg 2002;97(2):341–346
32. Newton HB, Scott SR, Volpi C. Hydroxyurea chemotherapy for meningiomas: enlarged cohort with extended follow-up. Br J Neurosurg 2004;18(5):495–499
33. Shamah SM, Alberta JA, Giannobile WV, et al. Detection of activated platelet-derived growth factor receptors in human meningioma. Cancer Res 1997;57(18):4141–4147
34. Yang SY, Xu GM. Expression of PDGF and its receptor as well as their relationship to proliferating activity and apoptosis of meningiomas in human meningiomas. J Clin Neurosci 2001;8(Suppl 1):49–53
35. Horak P, Wöhrer A, Hassler M, Hainfellner J, Preusser M, Marosi C. Imatinib mesylate treatment of recurrent meningiomas in preselected patients: a retrospective analysis. J Neurooncol 2012;109(2):323–330
36. Wen PY, Yung WK, Lamborn KR, et al. Phase II study of imatinib mesylate for recurrent meningiomas (North American Brain Tumor Consortium study 01-08). Neuro-oncol 2009; 11(6):853–860
37. Reardon DA, Norden AD, Desjardins A, et al. Phase II study of Gleevec® plus hydroxyurea (HU) in adults with progressive or recurrent meningioma. J Neurooncol 2012;106(2): 409–415
38. Arena S, Barbieri F, Thellung S, et al. Expression of somatostatin receptor mRNA in human meningiomas and their implication in in vitro antiproliferative activity. J Neurooncol 2004;66(1-2):155–166
39. Reubi JC, Maurer R, Klijn JG, et al. High incidence of somatostatin receptors in human meningiomas: biochemical characterization. J Clin Endocrinol Metab 1986;63(2):433–438

40. Rünzi MW, Jaspers C, Windeck R, et al. Successful treatment of meningioma with octreotide. Lancet 1989;1(8646):1074
41. García-Luna PP, Relimpio F, Pumar A, et al. Clinical use of octreotide in unresectable meningiomas. A report of three cases. J Neurosurg Sci 1993;37(4):237–241
42. Johnson DR, Kimmel DW, Burch PA, et al. Phase II study of subcutaneous octreotide in adults with recurrent or progressive meningioma and meningeal hemangiopericytoma. Neurooncol 2011;13(5):530–535
43. Chamberlain MC, Glantz MJ, Fadul CE. Recurrent meningioma: salvage therapy with long-acting somatostatin analogue. Neurology 2007;69(10):969–973
44. Pistolesi S, Boldrini L, Gisfredi S, et al. Angiogenesis in intracranial meningiomas: immunohistochemical and molecular study. Neuropathol Appl Neurobiol 2004;30(2):118–125
45. Lou E, Sumrall AL, Turner S, et al. Bevacizumab therapy for adults with recurrent/progressive meningioma: a retrospective series. J Neurooncol 2012;109(1):63–70
46. Nayak L, Iwamoto FM, Rudnick JD, et al. Atypical and anaplastic meningiomas treated with bevacizumab. J Neurooncol 2012;109(1):187–193
47. Raizer JJ, Grimm S. J C. A phase II trial of PTK787/ZK 222584 (PTK787) in recurrent or progressive meningiomas. Neurooncol 2010;12:iv36–iv57
48. Kaley TJ, Schiff D. S K. Phase II trial of sunitinib (SU011248) for recurrent meningioma. Neuro-oncol 2010;12:iv69–iv78
49. Carroll RS, Black PM, Zhang J, et al. Expression and activation of epidermal growth factor receptors in meningiomas. J Neurosurg 1997;87(2):315–323
50. Norden AD, Raizer JJ, Abrey LE, et al. Phase II trials of erlotinib or gefitinib in patients with recurrent meningioma. J Neurooncol 2010;96(2):211–217

31

Extent of Resection and Selection of Operative Approaches in the Surgical Management of Petroclival Meningiomas

David S. Xu, Nader Sanai, and Robert F. Spetzler

Petroclival meningiomas remain one of the most formidable intracranial pathologies for surgical management. These lesions are typically large at presentation, and their removal is fraught with challenges like deep locations, extension into multiple cranial fossae, and eloquent adjoining neurovascular structures. Even in the modern microsurgical era, cumulative outcomes data from the late 1980s show that, on average, a third of patients will experience a new cranial nerve deficit and 14% will incur motor deficits after surgery.[1] As a result, multiple controversies still exist regarding selection of the appropriate surgical approach as well as how aggressively one should pursue gross total resection given the perilous nature of surgery. This chapter explores contemporary evidence concerning extent of resection of petroclival meningiomas as well as prevailing data concerning common operative approaches employed in resection of these tumors.

Classification and Anatomy

Posterior fossa meningiomas were first classified into five groups by the work of Castellano and Ruggiero in 1953.[2] Their system was based on the site of dural attachment, which included (1) cerebellar convexity, (2) tentorium, (3) posterior surface of the petrous bone, (4) clivus, and (5) foramen magnum. Beginning in the early 1980s with the advent of computed tomography (CT) and the use of the operative microscope, numerous studies called for the classification system to change based on observations that many tumors of the basal posterior fossa exhibited transitional dural attachments that could no longer be assigned solely to the clivus or cerebellopontine angle.[3,4] As summarized by Bricolo et al, the term *petroclival meningioma* best refers to a group of lesions arising along the clivus, but most importantly medial and anterior to the trigeminal nerve and acoustic canal.[5] The dural attachment is frequently not limited to the clivus proper and can involve the tentorium, petrous apex, and cavernous sinus, making tumoral expansion into multiple cranial fossae and the extradural space common. As these lesions grow, they typically wedge into the brainstem and can encase or compress the basilar artery and neighboring cranial nerves.[6]

Natural History and Presentation

The natural history of petroclival meningiomas is no different than that of all meningiomas—unremitting growth with eventual compression of critical adjacent structures. In a natural history study by Van Havenbergh et al, 21 patients harboring petroclival meningiomas were followed without therapy for a minimum of 4 years.[7] Tumor growth was seen in 76% of patients and clinical deterioration was seen in 63%

of patients, with the majority of those patients having been initially asymptomatic. Presenting clinical symptoms correspond closely with compromise of the neighboring cranial nerves, brainstem, and critical vasculature, with the most frequent presenting symptoms being cranial nerve deficits, gait and balance disturbances, and headaches.

■ Literature Review

Role of Surgery

Multiple historical datasets have shown that the extent of meningioma resection significantly determines subsequent progression and long-term follow-up progression or recurrence of meningiomas.[8,9] The most contemporary data regarding long-term follow-up of cranial base meningiomas after surgical resection demonstrate that even 10 to 15% of tumors that undergo complete resection (Simpson grade 1 or 2) still recur after 10 years of follow-up, and 100% of subtotally resected tumors will recur or progress 15 years after surgery.[10] However, given the intimidating challenges associated with removal of petroclival meningiomas, a more aggressive surgical philosophy may incur higher rates of up-front neurological deficits and decreased long-term patient quality of life.[11] Conversely, less aggressive pursuit of total tumor resection may reduce the incidence of operative complications, but at the cost of leaving more residual tumor that may lead to earlier recurrences or need for repeat surgery. The level of evidence in literature examining the effect of extent of surgical resection on immediate and long-term outcomes with follow-up data past 24 months is summarized in **Table 31.1**.

Level I and Level II Evidence

There is no Level I or Level II evidence comparing extent of resection with patient outcomes or tumor recurrence.

Level III Evidence

Natarajan et al published the largest case series of petroclival meningiomas, consisting of 150 patients with a mean follow-up of 102 months.[12] They defined extent of resection as being gross total if no residual tumor was present, subtotal if more than 90% of the tumor was removed, and partial if less than 90% of the tumor was resected. Using those definitions, 48 patients (32%) received gross total resection, 65 patients (43%) received subtotal resection, and 37 patients (25%) received partial resection. At the end of follow-up, two of 48 patients (4%) who received gross total resection developed tumor recurrence and five of the 102 patients (5%) who had an incomplete resection showed evidence of progression. One of the patients with a recurrence eventually died of tumor progression, whereas the other six remain stable

Table 31.1 Evidence table for extent of resection impact on operative complications and tumor recurrence/progression

Level of evidence	Study	Findings
Level I and II	None	None
Level III	Natarajan et al 2007[12]	Extent of resection was not associated with tumor recurrence in 150 patients after a mean follow-up of 102 months.
	Little et al 2005[13]	Uniformly pursuing gross total resection was associated with increased operative complications. Leaving more than 1 mL of residual tumor was associated with increased rate of recurrence. Among 15 patients with recurrence/progression, only 4 were symptomatic after 29.8 months of follow-up.
	Park et al 2006[14]	Aggressive surgical planning resulted in high rates of gross total resection but increased cranial nerve complications and lower Karnofsky performance scale scores.
Level IV	Couldwell et al 1996[15]	Cavernous sinus invasion is associated with higher rates of progression/recurrence of tumor, likely due to the difficulty of surgical management.
	Jung et al 2000[16]	This retrospective study found high rates of tumor progression in 16 of 38 patients with subtotally resected tumors after a mean of 47.5 months.
	Bricolo et al 1992[5]	This retrospective case series presented a high rate of gross total resection irrespective of tumor size, and all patients experienced a new or worsened cranial nerve deficit postoperatively.

with an average Karnofsky performance scale (KPS) score higher than 85. Kaplan-Meier analysis did not show a statistically significant difference in progression-/recurrence-free survival between patients receiving gross total resection or incomplete resection.

Little et al conducted a retrospective cohort study of 137 patients harboring petroclival meningiomas at their institution from 1993 to 2002 with a mean follow-up of 29.8 months.[13] Their experience was fractioned into two parts, an "early" group from 1993 to 1996 where gross total resection was pursued uniformly in all patients, and a "late" group from 1996 to 2002 where the degree of resection was guided by intraoperatively defined tumor characteristics. Specifically, remnant tumor was left in the latter group with fibrous tumors that had portions embedded in vascular perforators and with tumor portions adherent to vital neurovascular structures. Over all, there was a higher (although not statistically significant) rate of gross total resection of tumor in the early group (45.2% vs 38.7%). There was a statistically significant difference in the rates of postoperative cranial nerve deficits (38.7% vs 17.9%) as well as an almost statistically significant increase in the incidence of paresis/ataxis (19.4% vs 7.5%, $p = 0.056$) between the early and late groups.

Their study also found that the extent of resection correlated negatively with recurrence and progression. As defined in the study, *gross total resection* referred to no intraoperative or subsequent radiological evidence of tumor, *near total resection* referred to evidence of intraoperative tumor but radiologically measured to be < 1 mL, and *subtotal resection* referred to > 1 mL of tumor remaining after surgery. Specifically, after gross total resection, one of 31 patients (3.6%) had a tumor recur, whereas after near total or subtotal resection, five of 31 patients (16.1%) and nine of 26 patients (34.6%) had a tumor recurrence, respectively. Only four of the 15 patients who had recurrences were symptomatic from them. These differences were only statistically significant when patients who underwent a gross total or near total resection were compared with those who underwent a subtotal resection.

Park et al reviewed all patients with petroclival meningiomas who were cared for at their institution from 1986 to 2000.[14] Of 75 patients identified, 49 received surgical treatment (median follow-up 86 months). At the end of follow-up, 11 patients (28%) of 39 who underwent subtotal resection experienced tumor progression, and none of the 10 patients who underwent gross total resection had evidence of tumor recurrence compared with patients undergoing gross total resection. They also found that patients who underwent a subtotal resection had outcomes that were statistically more favorable in terms of cranial neuropathies as well as improved or stable postoperative long-term KPS scores. Specifically, 12 of 39 patients (30.8%) in the subtotal resection group and eight of 10 patients (80%) in the complete resection group developed new cranial nerve deficits after surgery. Similarly, nine of 39 patients (23.1%) in the subtotal resection group and seven of 10 patients (70%) in the gross total resection group had a lower KPS score at the end of follow-up.

Level IV Evidence

Couldwell et al reported 109 consecutive cases of petroclival meningiomas with a mean follow-up of 73.2 months.[15] Among 75 patients who underwent gross total resection, two patients (2.6%) developed a recurrence 18 months and 24 months after resection, respectively. Among 34 patients with more than 90% of the tumor resected, 12 patients (35.2%) developed progression, all of which involved extension into the cavernous sinus.

Jung et al published data on 38 cases of petroclival meningioma that were subtotally resected, with a mean follow-up of 47.5 months.[16] At the end of their follow-up, tumor had progressed in 16 (42%) patients and the 5-year progression-free survival rate was 60%. A criticism of this study is that the authors defined subtotal resection as remaining tumor (i.e., 1 to 50% of the original size), which is too insensitive. Furthermore, they did not specify the patients' causes of death and whether they were associated with tumor progression.

Bricolo et al followed 33 patients for a mean length of 51.6 months after tumor resection.[5] They achieved gross total resection in 26 patients (79%), which was a high rate, but noted that all patients awoke with new or worsened neurological deficits. Ten years after the initial procedure, there was a recurrence in one patient who underwent gross total resection and died soon after a second procedure. Progression occurred in two patients 3 and 4 years after their initial partial resection after less than 50% of their original tumor had been removed.

Conclusion

Surgical resection of petroclival meningiomas remains the most reliable route to obtain durable remission of tumor progression as well as to provide patients with a permanent cure. However, an overly aggressive operative philosophy can incur higher rates of neurological complications. For follow-up times shorter than 5 years, rates of tumor progression or recurrence did not appear to vary significantly between patients who underwent gross total resection and those who underwent partial resection in which more than 90% of the tumor was removed. This finding may reflect inherently slow growth rates of these tumors, but it cannot be generalized to longer follow-up periods. Therefore, the surgical philosophy used to dictate how aggressively to pursue gross total resection must consider the patient's expected life span and must balance potential gains in progression-free survival with the short-term risks of perioperative complications resulting from a more aggressive operative plan.

Key Points for Surgical Therapy

1. Gross total resection should not be a universal goal, especially for tumors densely adherent to or encasing critical neurovascular structures.
2. Greater extent of surgical resection may not affect patient survival or tumor progression during short follow-up. For patients with a life expectancy greater than 10 years, gross or near-total resection offers the best possibility of a durable cure.
3. Cavernous sinus invasion has been associated with a high risk of future recurrence or progression of petroclival meningiomas.

Surgical Approaches

Various surgical approaches have been used in the resection of petroclival meningiomas (**Fig. 31.1**), but controversy remains regarding the optimal approach that will allow the greatest extent of tumor resection while also minimizing operative morbidity. Options include classic "workhorse" approaches, such as the orbitozygomatic, retrosigmoid, and subtemporal approaches. These approaches have been utilized with success but may necessitate staged usage with additional approaches for large tumors that encompass multiple cranial fossae. Other options involve lateral transmastoid skull base approaches that can be combined with a supratentorial transpetrous approach to offer a single procedure that can expose the length of lower clivus to the parasellar area.

Enthusiasm for skull base approaches has been garnered by the principle that a lateral trajectory reduces the operative distance and, when combined with extradural dissection, allows wider exposure with decreased need for brain retraction and better visualization of critical neurovascular structures.[17] Disadvantages of the approach are historical case series that document a high rate of new-onset cranial nerve palsies, most notably of the seventh and eighth cranial nerves, the demanding technical expertise required in the approach and dissection, as well as a potential intraoperative bias for overaggressive resection of the tumor.[11,18,19]

Currently, no studies offer a direct comparative analysis of approach-specific outcomes in the operative management of petroclival meningiomas. Most case series or institutional experiences report data for patients who underwent a mixture of different

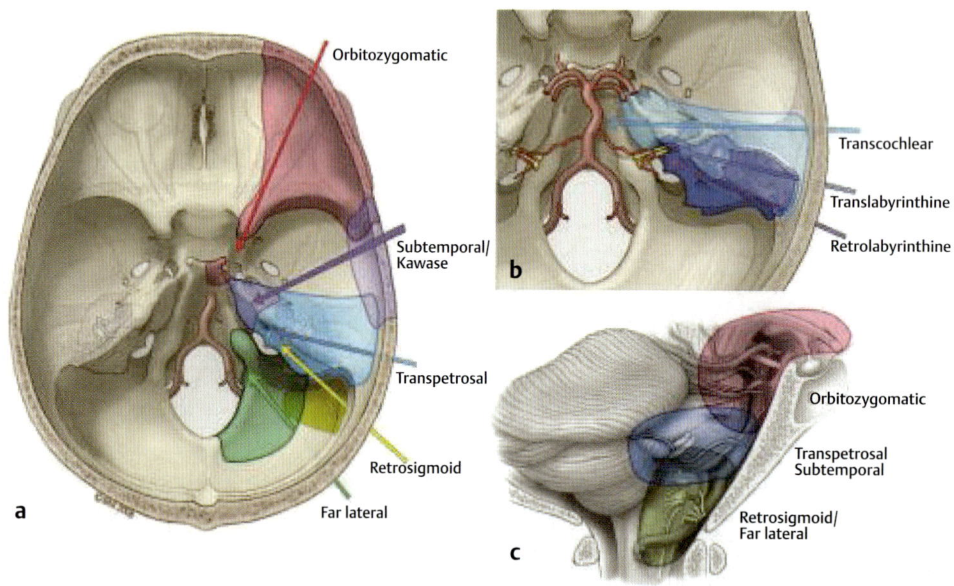

Fig. 31.1 Approaches to the cranial base and clival region. **(a)** Multiple surgical approaches to petroclival meningiomas are available depending on the anatomical features of the tumor. **(b)** The three transpetrosal approaches to the cranial base include the transcochlear approach, the translabyrinthine approach, and the retrolabyrinthine approach. **(c)** Sagittal view of the clivus shows that it can be divided into thirds. The top third is accessed most easily via the orbitozygomatic approach, the middle third via the various transpetrosal approaches, such as the subtemporal approach with an anterior petrosectomy, and the posterior third via the retrosigmoid and far-lateral approaches. (Used with permission from Barrow Neurological Institute.)

approaches depending on the historical time period, individual surgeon preference, or anatomical features of the tumor. The clearest evidence that can be drawn from the literature is a handful of studies that offer historical comparisons between their cases as well as studies where patients underwent a uniform operative plan. A summary of these studies is presented in **Table 31.2**.

Level I Evidence

There are no Level I evidence studies comparing outcomes between single-stage combined approaches and two-stage surgical approaches for the resection of petroclival meningiomas.

Level II Evidence

Siwanuwatn et al compared the quantitative working areas exposed by the retrosigmoid, combined petrosal, and transcochlear approaches to the petroclival region in cadaveric heads utilizing stereotactic imaging.[20] They found that the transcochlear approach had a statistically significant greater working area for the ventral brainstem and petroclival surface than the retrosigmoid and combined petrosal approaches. In comparing the retrosigmoid with the combined petrosal approaches, there was no difference in working area for the petroclivus, but the combined petrosal approach afforded greater exposure of the ventral brainstem.

Little et al obtained quantitative measurements of the working area offered by a combined retrosigmoid and orbitozygomatic approach in six cadaveric heads utilizing stereotactic imaging.[21] The two approaches were complementary and had little overlap, while providing extensive exposure of the ventral brainstem and clivus up to the parasellar area.

Level III Evidence

Bambakidis et al documented their institution's experience with petroclival meningioma resection across two historical periods.[19] Their first "early" group consisted of seven patients, all of whom un-

Table 31.2 Evidence table for selection of operative approach

Evidence	Study	Findings
Level I	None	None
Level II	Siwanuwatn et al 2006[20]	The retrosigmoid and combined petrosal approaches offer statistically similar exposure of the petroclival surface. The transcochlear approach offers greater exposure than both.
	Little et al 2008[21]	A staged retrosigmoid and orbitozygomatic exposure allows extensive exposure of the clivus and ventral brain stem up to the parasellar region with minimal redundancy.
Level III	Bambakidis et al 2007[19]	Lower rates of cranial nerve injuries occurred after authors changed their preferred approach from lateral skull base to traditional retrosigmoid with or without an additional staged orbitozygomatic approach. Rates of gross total resection did not change.
	Spallone et al 1999[22]	No differences in average extent of resection or long-term neurological deficits from surgery between patients operated on via a presigmoid approach versus a retrosigmoid approach with or without a subtemporal staged procedure.
Level IV	Mathiesen et al 2008[23]	Outcomes of combined petrosal approach in 29 patients (mean follow-up 66 months). Gross total resection rate 41%, 18% incidence of facial palsy, and 26% incidence of diminished hearing.
	Sekhar et al 1999[24]	Utilization of presigmoid partial labyrinthectomy associated with a 19% incidence of loss of hearing. Rates of cerebrospinal fluid leaks were initially as high as 33%. Authors stated this issue resolved after they began packing the eustachian tube.
	Watanabe et al 2011[25]	Modified retrosigmoid approach performed in 26 patients, with gross total resection rate of 46%. After 6 months, persistent facial palsy present in 4% of patients, and hearing decline persisted in 12%.
	Samii et al 1999[26]	Traditional retrosigmoid approach used in 24 patients, with gross total resection rate of 58%. Facial palsy and worsening hearing each occurred in 25% of the patients and persisted 3 weeks after surgery.

derwent a lateral skull base approach. Their second group consisted of 39 patients, all of whom underwent a retrosigmoid approach with or without an additional orbitozygomatic approach. Rates of gross total resection were similar between the two groups (43% vs 53%, respectively). However, the operative complication rate was significantly higher in group 1, with an incidence of 85% versus 33%. The most common complication was a new cranial nerve deficit, which occurred in 71% of patients in group 1 versus 23% of patients in group 2. Among those deficits, facial nerve weakness occurred in 71% of the patients in group 1 and in 23% of the patients in group 2.

Criticisms of the study include absence of long-term clinical or quality-of-life functional data between the two groups outside the immediate postoperative period. In addition, data for group 1 patients were collected when lateral skull base approaches were still newly adopted at the institution, and the average tumor size in group 1 was much larger than that in group 2, although this difference did not reach statistical significance.

Spallone et al reviewed all petroclival meningioma resections over a 4-year period and divided their cohort into group A, consisting of 13 cases operated on using a combination of the retrosigmoid and subtemporal approaches, and group B, comprising 18 cases operated on with a presigmoid transmastoid approach.[22] Rates of gross total resection were similar between the two groups (77% vs 83%, respectively), but the skull base approach group had higher initial rates of immediate postoperative cranial nerve V and VIII palsies compared with group A (40% and 60% vs 23% and 23%, respectively). Seven patients in group A also had cerebellar ataxia after surgery, likely related to cerebellar retraction during the procedure, compared with none of the patients in group B. At the end of an average of 3.2 years of follow-up, rates of residual cranial nerve deficits were not significantly different between the two groups.

Level IV Evidence

Mathiesen et al reported 29 consecutive petroclival meningiomas operated on via a combined supra- and infratentorial transpetrosal approach (mean follow-up 66 months).[23] They obtained gross total resection in 41% of their patients but incurred new or worsening postoperative cranial nerve VII deficits in five patients (17%). These deficits persisted at the end of follow-up, and new or exacerbated auditory deficits were present in six of 23 patients (26%) who underwent an auditory sparing approach. At the end of follow-up, 16 patients were able to take the 36-item Short Form Health Survey (SF-36). A majority scored under the age-adjusted population mean for psychosocial functioning, irrespective of the patient's neurological outcome.

Sekhar et al presented their group's utilization of a presigmoid partial labyrinthectomy and petrous apicectomy approach to 33 petroclival neoplasms.[24] Although isolated surgical outcomes for petroclival meningiomas were unavailable, the authors reported that hearing was lost in seven patients (19%) with serviceable preoperative hearing. They also reported that 12 patients (33%) developed cerebrospinal fluid (CSF) leaks, five of which required reexploration. The last nine patients in their series had no CSF leaks after the authors began performing reversible packing of the eustachian tube with Surgicel (Ethicon, Somerville, NJ) during wound closure.

A modified retrosigmoid approach was utilized by Watanabe et al to treat 26 patients with a petroclival meningioma located predominantly in the posterior fossa.[25] The authors achieved gross total resection in 11 patients (42%) and subtotal resection in 10 patients (38%). Immediate postoperative cranial nerve deficits were found in six patients (23%), predominantly involving cranial nerves VII and VIII. At the end of 6 months of follow-up, three patients (12%) had persistent diminished hearing and one patient (4%) still had deficits of cranial nerve VII.

Samii et al utilized the retrosigmoid approach in 24 cases of petroclival meningioma and obtained gross total resection in 14 cases (58%).[26] Facial palsy occurred in six patients (25%). After 2 to 3 weeks of follow-up, five patients partially improved. An additional six patients (25%) with preoperative hearing deficits experienced further decline of their hearing loss.

Expert Recommendations

1. Both traditional and skull base approaches can be used effectively to resect petroclival meningiomas, and outcomes in contemporary literature do not significantly differ between them.
2. It is currently unclear whether there are approach-specific impacts on long-term patient outcomes.
3. For large tumors, a two-stage approach and a combined skull base approach are both viable surgical plans, but the risks and economic impact of repeat rounds of anesthesia and longer operative times have not been examined. Surgeons should select what is anatomically appropriate and most familiar to their training.

Summary and Conclusions

Since the late 1990s, contemporary studies have not shown definitive differences in the rate of cranial nerve palsies or gross total resection between traditional approaches and skull base approaches for resection of petroclival meningiomas. Direct comparison among these case series cannot reliably isolate approach-specific operative risks, given differences in patient baseline function and tumor characteristics. For the most challenging large tumors with extensive expansion into the middle cranial fossa, a staged procedure continues to be a valid option, although the risks and economic factors associated with two rounds of anesthesia as well as prolonged operative time have yet to be fully studied. Ultimately, operative planning of these challenging lesions depends predominantly on the anatomical characteristics of the tumor as well as on the surgeon's fluency with the proposed operative plan. Given the already intimidating nature of these lesions, it may be prudent for less-experienced surgeons to allow familiarity and refinement of their existing skill sets to dictate surgical planning, rather than preconceived notions of a particular approach.

References

1. Diluna ML, Bulsara KR. Surgery for petroclival meningiomas: a comprehensive review of outcomes in the skull base surgery era. Skull Base 2010;20(5):337–342
2. Castellano F, Ruggiero G. Meningiomas of the posterior fossa. Acta Radiol Suppl 1953;104:1–177
3. Sekhar LN, Jannetta PJ. Cerebellopontine angle meningiomas: microsurgical excision and follow-up results. J Neurosurg 1984;60(3):500–505
4. Mayberg MR, Symon L. Meningiomas of the clivus and apical petrous bone: report of 35 cases. J Neurosurg 1986;65(2):160–167
5. Bricolo AP, Turazzi S, Talacchi A, Cristofori L. Microsurgical removal of petroclival meningiomas: a report of 33 patients. Neurosurgery 1992;31(5):813–828
6. Ramina R, Tatagiba M, Fernandes YB, Neto MC. Petroclival meningiomas: diagnosis, treatment, and results. In: Ramina R, Aquiar PHP, Tatagiba M, eds. Samii's Essentials in Neurosurgery. Berlin: Springer; 2008;121–134
7. Van Havenbergh T, Carvalho G, Tatagiba M, Plets C, Samii M. Natural history of petroclival meningiomas. Neurosurgery 2003;52(1):55–62
8. Adegbite AB, Khan MI, Paine KW, Tan LK. The recurrence of intracranial meningiomas after surgical treatment. J Neurosurg 1983;58(1):51–56
9. Simpson D. The recurrence of intracranial meningiomas after surgical treatment. J Neurol Neurosurg Psychiatry 1957;20(1):22–39
10. Mathiesen T, Lindquist C, Kihlström L, Karlsson B. Recurrence of cranial base meningiomas. Neurosurgery 1996;39(1):2–7
11. Seifert V. Clinical management of petroclival meningiomas and the eternal quest for preservation of quality of life: personal experiences over a period of 20 years. Acta Neurochir (Wien) 2010;152(7):1099–1116
12. Natarajan SK, Sekhar LN, Schessel D, Morita A. Petroclival meningiomas: multimodality treatment and outcomes at long-term follow-up. Neurosurgery 2007;60(6):965–979
13. Little KM, Friedman AH, Sampson JH, Wanibuchi M, Fukushima T. Surgical management of petroclival meningiomas: defining resection goals based on risk of neurological morbidity and tumor recurrence rates in 137 patients. Neurosurgery 2005;56(3):546–559
14. Park CK, Jung HW, Kim JE, Paek SH, Kim DG. The selection of the optimal therapeutic strategy for petroclival meningiomas. Surg Neurol 2006;66(2):160–165
15. Couldwell WT, Fukushima T, Giannotta SL, Weiss MH. Petroclival meningiomas: surgical experience in 109 cases. J Neurosurg 1996;84(1):20–28
16. Jung HW, Yoo H, Paek SH, Choi KS. Long-term outcome and growth rate of subtotally resected petroclival meningiomas: experience with 38 cases. Neurosurgery 2000;46(3):567–574
17. Al-Mefty O, Fox JL, Smith RR. Petrosal approach for petroclival meningiomas. Neurosurgery 1988;22(3):510–517
18. Samii M, Gerganov V, Giordano M, Samii A. Two step approach for surgical removal of petroclival meningiomas with large supratentorial extension. Neurosurg Rev 2010;34(2):173–179
19. Bambakidis NC, Kakarla UK, Kim LJ, et al. Evolution of surgical approaches in the treatment of petroclival meningiomas: a retrospective review. Neurosurgery 2007;61(5, Suppl 2):202–209
20. Siwanuwatn R, Deshmukh P, Figueiredo EG, Crawford NR, Spetzler RF, Preul MC. Quantitative analysis of the working area and angle of attack for the retrosigmoid, combined petrosal, and transcochlear approaches to the petroclival region. J Neurosurg 2006;104(1):137–142
21. Little AS, Jittapiromsak P, Crawford NR, et al. Quantitative analysis of exposure of staged orbitozygomatic and retrosigmoid craniotomies for lesions of the clivus with supratentorial extension. Neurosurgery 2008;62(5, Suppl 2):ONS318–ONS323
22. Spallone A, Makhmudov UB, Mukhamedjanov DJ, Tcherekajev VA. Petroclival meningioma. An attempt to define the role of skull base approaches in their surgical management. Surg Neurol 1999;51(4):412–419
23. Mathiesen T, Gerlich A, Kihlström L, Svensson M, Bagger-Sjöbäck D. Effects of using combined transpetrosal surgical approaches to treat petroclival meningiomas. Neurosurgery 2008;62(6, Suppl 3):1213–1223
24. Sekhar LN, Schessel DA, Bucur SD, Raso JL, Wright DC. Partial labyrinthectomy petrous apicectomy approach to neoplastic and vascular lesions of the petroclival area. Neurosurgery 1999;44(3):537–550
25. Watanabe T, Katayama Y, Fukushima T, Kawamata T. Lateral supracerebellar transtentorial approach for petroclival meningiomas: operative technique and outcome. J Neurosurg 2011;115(1):49–54
26. Samii M, Tatagiba M, Carvalho GA. Resection of large petroclival meningiomas by the simple retrosigmoid route. J Clin Neurosci 1999;6(1):27–30

32

Need for Gross Total Resection of Cranial Base Meningiomas

Gustavo Pradilla and Jacques Morcos

Skull base meningiomas represent a multitude of lesions located along the anatomical compartments of the cranial base, with varying degrees of biological activity. Despite multiple advances in microsurgical techniques, surgical approaches, diagnostic modalities, and intraoperative neurophysiological monitoring, their propensity to involve neurovascular structures, invade dural sinuses, and extend to multiple cranial fossae can significantly complicate surgical resection and may result in considerable morbidity. Although surgical resection remains the primary treatment modality, the role of gross total resection in these complex lesions remains unclear. This chapter clarifies the mixed nomenclature of skull base meningiomas, discusses particular anatomical considerations, defines the impact of pathological grading on intraoperative decision making and postoperative adjuvant therapies, reviews available evidence for gross total and subtotal resection, and mentions nonoperative therapeutic alternatives for these lesions.

Definition of Skull Base Meningiomas

Skull base meningiomas are defined as those arising from the dura mater overlying the cranial base. Although other lesions not arising from the skull base dura may require a surgical approach through the skull base for resection, they are not discussed in this chapter. In other words, the "skull base" connotation is applied to location of the tumor, and not to the surgical approach.

■ Anatomical Considerations of Skull Base Meningiomas

The traditional categorization into three cranial fossae will be followed.

Anterior Fossa

The anterior cranial fossa is structurally composed of the orbital plates of the frontal bone, the cribriform plate of the ethmoid bone, the lesser wing of the sphenoid bone, and the anterior aspect of the body of the sphenoid bone. The junction of these plates gives rise to the frontoethmoidal, sphenoethmoidal, and sphenofrontal sutures. Relevant neurovascular structures include the olfactory bulb, the nasociliary nerve, and the anterior and posterior ethmoidal vessels. Meningiomas arising in this compartment are typically located in the cribriform plate, along the olfactory groove, over the planum sphenoidale, or at the tuberculum sellae.

Middle Fossa

The middle cranial fossa is limited anteriorly by the posterior border of the lesser wings of the sphenoid bone, the anterior clinoid processes, and the anterior margin of the chiasmatic groove; posteriorly by the petrous ridge and the dorsum sella; and laterally by the temporal squamae, sphenoidal angles of the parietal bone, and the greater wings of the sphenoid bones. The squamosal, sphenosquamosal, sphenopetrosal, and sphenoparietal sutures traverse the middle fossa.

Medially, the middle fossa includes the chiasmatic groove, optic foramen, tuberculum sella, clinoid processes (anterior, middle, and posterior), foraminal opening of the Dorello canal, and carotid groove. Laterally, it includes the foramen spinosum; temporal squama; superior orbital fissure; orbital plate of the frontal bone, foramen rotundum, ovale, and lacerum; proximal portion of the pterygoid canal; petrous ridge with the arcuate eminence; facial hiatus; and gasserian depression of the Meckel cave.

Meningiomas in this compartment are most commonly located in the sellar region, the sphenoid wing, and the cavernous sinus.

Posterior Fossa

The posterior fossa extends anteriorly to the petrous apex and is bounded posteriorly by the basioccipital bone to the level of the occipital condyles. Laterally it includes the inferior portion of the temporal squama and the mastoid segment of the temporal bone. Meningiomas in this compartment are most commonly located in the cerebellopontine angle (CPA), the petrous segment of the temporal bone, the clivus, and the foramen magnum. Neural structures commonly involved by tumors in this location include the cerebellar tonsils, cerebellar hemispheres and vermis, fourth ventricle, caudal medulla, cranial nerves III through XII, rostral aspect of the spinal cord, and upper cervical roots (C1 and C2). Arteries of the vertebrobasilar system, the petrosal contributors of the venous system, the transverse and sigmoid sinuses, and the jugular bulb surround these structures.

■ Skull Base Meningiomas by Location

Skull base meningiomas can occur in a variety of intracranial locations. In a study of 262 patients treated for meningiomas at the University of Florida between 1964 and 1992, Condra et al[1] reported that the most common location of meningiomas was the sphenoid ridge (16%), followed by convexity meningiomas (14%), cerebellopontine angle (13%), parasellar (12%), parasagittal (11%), posterior fossa (8%), olfactory groove (8%), falx (7%), foramen magnum (3%), orbital (3%), and other (6%) meningiomas.

Olfactory Groove Meningiomas

Between 9 and 18% of all meningiomas occur along the olfactory groove, between the crista galli and the planum sphenoidale.[2,3] Most meningiomas in this region are classified by the World Health Organization as Grade I lesions with meningothelial and fibrous characteristics[4] and appear to arise from the frontosphenoidal suture. Although lesions in this location are in close proximity to the tuberculum sella, the mass effect exerted on the optic chiasm separates them into different clinical entities. Whereas olfactory groove meningiomas (OGMs) depress the optic chiasm posteriorly, tuberculum sella meningiomas (TSMs) elevate it superiorly. OGMs are typically associated with significant hyperostosis of the anterior cranial fossa floor, and in up to 20% of cases may erode into the ethmoid sinus.[3,5] Vascular supply to these lesions most commonly arises from the anterior and posterior ethmoidal arteries, with occasional contributions from sphenoidal branches of the middle meningeal artery. The anterior cerebral arteries (ACAs) are often displaced posteriorly and superiorly, but unlike the orbitofrontal and frontopolar branches, they are rarely embedded inside the tumor capsule. Similarly, the olfactory nerves and tracts are laterally displaced over the orbital roof and are infrequently encased by tumor. Due to meningiomas' slow and indolent growth pattern, patients can present with large tumors and nonspecific, slowly evolving cognitive deficits and personality changes.

Given their accessibility and favorable anatomical features, surgical resection of OGMs is favored, with the goals of treatment being complete tumor resection, including removal of tumor extending into the ethmoid sinuses, with resection of all infiltrated hyperostotic bone. Multiple surgical approaches have been described, including subfrontal with unilateral or bifrontal craniotomies, unilateral pterional, interhemispheric, lateral supraorbital, and endoscopic. Most reported series demonstrate a high percentage of tumor resection, irrespective of size. Solero et al presented their results in 153 patients, 98 of whom had OGMs, in 1983.[3] All patients underwent resection via a unilateral frontal craniotomy, often accompanied by partial frontal lobe resection. Gross total resection was achieved in 93.8% of patients. Mortality was 17.3%, all related to vascular injury or occlusion.

Procedure-related morbidity was also significant and included CSF leak (2%), infection (3%), seizures (6%), and hematoma (1%). Since then, reported morbidity and mortality rates have steadily declined.

In 2005 Spektor et al[6] reported their 13-year institutional experience in 81 patients with OGMs treated surgically using multiple open approaches (unilateral subfrontal 11.1%, pterional 22.2%, fronto-orbital craniotomy 8.6%, and subcranial 14.8%). Gross-total resection was achieved in 90% of patients. Follow-up ranged from 6 to 164 months (mean, 70.8 months). No operative mortality was reported, and although anosmia was the only new permanent focal neurological deficit, 25 patients (31.3%) experienced surgery-related complications. These included cerebrospinal fluid (CSF) leaks (12.5%), meningitis (5%, one fatal 6 months after surgery), intracranial hematoma requiring surgical evacuation (5%), postoperative seizures (3.8%), deep vein thrombosis (DVT) (6.3%), and pulmonary embolism (PE) (2.5%). Recurrence occurred in two patients who had subtotal tumor resections.

Over all, oncological results in modern series are excellent, with high rates of gross total resection, small percentages of recurrent disease, and minimal mortality. Recurrence is clearly determined by the extent of tumor resection and the removal of all affected bony and dural surfaces.[6–9] Significant morbidity, however, still exists, and more recent series have favored lateral-based approaches over bifrontal craniotomies to minimize complications.[10,11]

Tuberculum Sellae Meningiomas

Meningiomas in the tuberculum sellae represent a small percentage of all meningiomas. Lesions in this region most often present with unilateral or bilateral vision loss (frequently with bitemporal hemianopsia) related to compression of the optic apparatus, and surgical resection is the treatment of choice in all cases. Proximity of the optic apparatus and inability to rapidly relieve tumor compression render nonoperative therapies (i.e., stereotactic radiosurgery, three-dimensional conformal therapy, or intensity-modulated radiotherapy) ineffective in most cases. Although the optic nerves tend to be displaced superiorly and laterally, the optic chiasm is usually found superiorly or posteriorly. Extension of the tumor into the medial aspect of the optic canals is often encountered, and direct visualization following decompression of the optic canal is recommended. Posterior ethmoidal branches, meningeal branches of the cavernous internal carotid artery (ICA), and small pial branches often provide vascular supply to these lesions. The pattern of invasion of the optic canal can help determine the preferred surgical approach. Lesions with involvement of the medial aspect of the optic canal could be explored via endonasal approaches; however, dural reconstruction poses significant challenges and CSF leak rates can be significant. Therefore, most authors recommend a transcranial approach in these cases. Similarly, bilateral compromise of the optic canals is often best approached via bifrontal or anterolateral approaches (pterional/orbitofrontal, etc.). Involvement of the lateral aspect of the optic canal precludes an endonasal approach because the optic nerve gets in the way of adequate and complete resection. The position of the optic chiasm in relation to the tumor and the area of the interoptic space can also influence the choice of approach. Lesions with large infrachiasmatic tumor burden and a small anterior interoptic space resulting from a pre-fixed optic chiasm might be more favorably approached via an endonasal route. Multiple surgical series of tuberculum sellae meningiomas (TSMs) have been reported, and recent advances in endonasal endoscopic technique have expanded the existing literature. Goel and Muzumdar[12] published their results with 70 patients treated surgically for TSMs in 2002. In this series, gross total resection was achieved in 59 patients (84.2%). In all patients with subtotal resection, a pathological diagnosis of atypical or malignant meningioma was reported. Mortality occurred in two patients (2.9%), one secondary to CSF leak-related meningitis, and one from complications of postoperative stroke. Mean follow-up was 46 months (range, 6 to 108 months). Surgical approaches included unilateral frontal approach in 63 patients, bifrontal craniotomies in four patients, pterional craniotomies with orbitozygomatic osteotomies in two patients, and transsphenoidal resection in one patient. Of note, no special attempt was made to remove bony hyperostosis unless it compromised the surgical exposure. Vascular injury occurred in four patients. The overall visual outcomes after surgery showed improvement in 44 of the 63 patients with visual deficits (70%), no change in 10 patients (16%), and worsening vision in seven patients (10%). Only one recurrence of a subtotally resected grade II lesion was reported at last follow-up.

De Divitiis and colleagues[13] in 2007 presented their results with fully endoscopic extended transsphenoidal resections in 6 patients with TSMs. In five patients gross total resection and visual improvement were achieved. One patient, however, had a postoperative CSF leak that required three additional operations for repair of the cranial base defect, rapidly deteriorated secondary to a delayed intraventricular hemorrhage, and died 6 days later. Postoperative permanent diabetes insipidus developed in another patient. Since this report, improvement of reconstructive techniques and increased operator experience have minimized CSF leaks and complication rates. In 2011, Ceylan and colleagues[14] reported their experience with the endoscopic transsphenoidal approach in nine patients with TSMs. In this series, gross total resection and visual improvement were achieved in six of nine patients, no mortality was encountered, and no CSF leaks were seen.

A recent review of the literature encompassing 25 contemporary surgical series conducted by Sughrue and colleagues[15] showed an estimated pooled gross total resection of 88 to 92% in patients treated with a transcranial approach. In this group, postoperative visual improvement was achieved in 57 to 63% of patients, but visual decline occurred in 12 to 17% of patients. For patients treated via endonasal approaches, gross total resection rates ranged from 55 to 78%, and stable or improved vision was reported in 91 to 100% of patients. The authors concluded that endonasal approaches achieved slightly better visual outcomes at the expense of conservative resection rates with significant residual tumor, but they limited their interpretation of these findings in light of the relatively limited reports of long-term outcomes for patients treated with endonasal approaches, as well as the inherent selection bias that would expectedly assign larger tumors to the "open" group and "smaller" tumors to the "endoscopy" group. In addition, technical difficulties leading to CSF leaks and meningitis were commonly seen in earlier series of patients treated with endonasal approaches, although their frequency continues to decrease in recent reports.

Lateral and Middle Sphenoid Wing Meningiomas

The sphenoid wing is the site of origin of 11 to 18% of all meningiomas reported in large surgical series.[16,17] The clinical presentation and surgical management of lateral and small middle third sphenoid wing meningiomas presenting with a "globular" pattern of growth, without significant hyperostosis, are similar to those of convexity meningiomas because the neurovascular involvement seen in these tumors is significantly less than that in medial and large middle sphenoid wings meningiomas, in which involvement of the carotid artery and its early branches as well as the optic apparatus is frequently seen.

Lateral and middle sphenoid wing meningiomas can also present with significant hyperostosis, which frequently involves the bony structures that constitute the orbit. These lesions are commonly referred to as hyperostosing or *en plaque* meningiomas, and patients frequently present with exophthalmos and diplopia, which result from either mass effect of intraorbital tumor, from intraosseus tumor growth, or from venous stasis due to decreased orbital venous drainage. Diplopia is generally secondary to restriction or compression of the extraocular muscles rather than to cranial neuropathies. Symptoms of optic nerve compression tend to develop in later stages with larger tumors. These lesions can also invade the surrounding soft tissues and compromise the integrity of the skin.

Patients with large globular or *en plaque* lesions can develop significant edema and present with associated motor deficits, seizures, or symptoms of frontal lobe compression (cognitive or memory difficulties, flat affect, personality changes, etc.). Although some lesions can encase or compress ACA and middle cerebral artery (MCA) branches, they tend to remain silent.

The goals of surgical treatment vary according to the extent of tumor involvement and the biology of the lesion, but overall gross total resection is the main objective. As discussed for meningiomas in other locations, local control and recurrence rates are directly affected by the extent of resection, which includes removal of all tissues involved, including bone and periorbita among others. Blood supply to these lesions is primarily derived from the superficial temporal and middle meningeal arteries, with lesser contributions from the anterior meningeal and other branches of the ethmoidal arteries. Although major branches of the MCAs are often encased by tumor, true invasion of the arterial wall is rare.[18] Middle sphenoid wing tumors may invade the anterior clinoid process and the optic canal. Early extradural clinoidectomy and decompression of the optic canal have been advocated to minimize the risk of additional compression of the optic nerve by manipulation during the microdissection.[19] Clinoidal meningiomas, however, are different clinical entities and are discussed separately. Similarly, although extension of middle sphenoid wing tumors into the cavernous sinus is common, these are discussed under cavernous sinus meningiomas.

Rates of postoperative residual disease, recurrence, and complications vary widely among reported series, reflecting the multiplicity of presentations and the various philosophies on extent of resection and use of up-front adjuvant radiosurgery or radiotherapy. Most series report extent of resection as determined by contrast-enhanced magnetic resonance imaging; however, Simpson grades are reported based on the surgeon's intraoperative observations. Together these make comparison among surgical series more challenging. In general, all meningiomas located in the lateral sphenoid wing and most of those located in the middle third of the sphenoid can be resected fully, including their dural origin, if the hyperostotic changes in the surrounding bone are accessible for removal, which occurs in a large proportion of patients. In these patients, reported recurrence rates range between 5 and 10% and are comparable to those of convexity-located lesions.[16] These rates increase to 9 to 23% for hyperostosing meningiomas extending to the medial wing[20] and to 8 to 31% for spheno-orbital tumors.[21–24]

Radiotherapy for lateral and middle sphenoid wing meningiomas, to our knowledge, has not been selectively studied. Reported series include either sphenoid wing meningiomas irrespective of their mediolateral location or lesions defined as skull base meningiomas, which included cavernous sinus and clinoidal meningiomas. In general, progression-free survival for patients with benign skull base meningiomas treated with fractionated radiotherapy is ~ 90% at 5 years and 80 to 90% at 10 years.[16] Nutting and colleagues reported their experience with conservative subtotal resection of sphenoid wing meningiomas followed by fractionated radiotherapy and showed substantially lower progression-free survival rates of ~ 69% at 10 years.[25] Lateral and middle sphenoid wing meningiomas with orbital extension that are partially resected have been shown to benefit significantly from radiotherapy.[24]

Medial Sphenoid Wing and Clinoidal Meningiomas

Although true medial sphenoid wing meningiomas without involvement of the clinoidal region constitute a separate entity from clinoidal meningiomas, medial sphenoid wing meningiomas often progress to involve the clinoidal region and the cavernous sinus and are discussed together in this section. These lesions often involve the optic nerve, optic chiasm, and/or the ICA; may expand and compress the mesial inferior frontal and temporal lobes, resulting in cerebral edema and seizures; and may extend into the cavernous sinus, further involving the cavernous cranial nerves. Clinoidal meningiomas in particular can be further classified according to the site of origin along the anterior clinoid process (ACP) into three different types, as described by Al-Mefty.[18] Type I arise from the subclinoidal dura just before the ICA enters the arachnoidal cisternal space; therefore, these lesions are "extra-arachnoidal" and are more frequently adherent to the wall of the ICA, which makes resection more challenging and increases the subtotal resection and recurrence rates. Type II lesions originate from the superior and lateral aspect of the ACP and are commonly surrounded by an arachnoidal layer from the carotid cisterns that separates the ICA from the tumor, which facilitates dissection. Because type I and II lesions originate distal to the optic nerve, the arachnoidal layers of the chiasmatic cisterns can envelope the optic nerve and isolate it from the tumor capsule.[26] Type III originate from the optic foramen region, extend into the optic canal, and, due to early symptomatic presentation, tend to be diagnosed earlier.

Surgical resection remains the most effective therapeutic option for patients with medial sphenoid wing and clinoidal meningiomas. The involvement of the optic nerve and optic apparatus limits the use of radiosurgery or radiation therapy in many cases. Surgical resection can be performed through multiple approaches, including pterional, orbitofrontal or extended pterional, cranio-orbitozygomatic approaches. Several authors advocate extradural resection of the anterior clinoid because it facilitates early visualization of the proximal ICA and contributes to tumor devascularization from orbitomeningeal and middle meningeal feeders. Decompression of the optic canal with removal of the optic strut is also recommended by most authors, along with resection of all tissues involved along the anterior skull base. Intradural exploration of the optic canal following bony decompression can reveal additional tumor components not clearly apparent on radiological studies and may prevent recurrence at this site with resultant visual compromise. Although gross total resection is the goal in all cases, type I lesions can be significantly adherent to the adventitial wall of the ICA, and intraoperative judgment often calls for conservative resection. Reconstruction of the skull base with auto- or allografts prevents CSF leaks that may manifest in a delayed fashion.

In contemporary series, the rates of gross total resection range between 43 and 91%.[18–20,26–33] Mortality in these series ranged from 0 to 15%, and major morbidity ranged from 0 to 18.6%. Recurrence rates were closely associated with extent of resection. While series with higher resection rates, such as Al-Mefty's[18] (83% GTR), resulted in lower recurrence rates (4% overall), series with lower resection rates, such as Puzzilli's (54.5% GTR), resulted in higher recurrence rates (26% overall) at comparable follow-up intervals (57 vs 53.7 mean follow-up months, respectively. The most common postoperative deficits involve visual deterioration secondary to manipulation of the optic nerve, ischemic neuropathy due to devascularization of small optic capillaries involved in the tumor capsule, and thermal injury from the drill during decompression of the optic canal.

Cavernous Sinus Meningiomas

Among skull base meningiomas, cavernous sinus lesions remain one of the most controversial. Although evolving techniques in skull base approaches to the cavernous sinus have significantly decreased the morbidity and mortality of surgical resection, the increasing efficacy of radiosurgery and radiotherapy has modified the goals of treatment and the surgical indications for these tumors. Cavernous sinus meningiomas can be grossly divided into two categories depending on their origin: some lesions arise from the dura of the cavernous sinus proper, whereas others constitute extension of lesions originating primarily from the medial sphenoid wing, clinoidal, or petroclival regions. Surgical resection is limited by the anatomical constraints of the cavernous sinus, the degree of neurovascular and dural sinus involvement, and the involvement of the underlying bony structures. Limited data on the natural history of cavernous sinus meningiomas followed for 5 to 7 years after diagnosis suggests that 25 to 27% of patients will show tumor progression with neurological decline.[34,35] In a recent review of the available data on growth rates as well as radiographic and clinical progression, Dunn and Al-Mefty[36] concluded that ~ 60% of cavernous sinus meningiomas remain quiescent, and that factors such as older age, T2 hypointensity, and calcification are associated with a more benign course. Based on the scarce evidence available, the authors suggest that conservative management can be recommended for patients with asymptomatic or minimally symptomatic lesions as long as close radiographic and clinical follow-up can be guaranteed. In patients with symptomatic lesions and those exhibiting significant progression, treatment options include surgical resection with the goal of gross total resection, radiotherapy to achieve growth control without cytoreduction, or a combined strategy of maximally safe resection with adjuvant radiosurgery of the residual disease. As discussed for meningiomas in other locations, gross total resection includes removal of all affected dural and bony structures. Multiple surgical approaches to the cavernous sinus have been described, including pterional transsylvian, cranio-orbitozygomatic, subtemporal, and transzygomatic, among others, with recent isolated reports of transnasal endoscopic resection in selected cases. Approach selection is based on the extent of tumor involvement, the goals of resection, the experience and preference of the surgeon, and the extent of postoperative reconstruction required, following the basic principles of minimal brain retraction, maximal exposure, and adequate neurovascular control through targeted bone removal. Rates of gross total resection in contemporary series vary widely, from 12 to 92%.[37–45] Although greater extent of resection is associated with decreased recurrence rates, series with higher gross total resection also report higher rates of new cranial neuropathies and increased mortality.

Knosp et al[40] treated 29 patients for meningiomas primarily arising in the cavernous sinus. Complete resection was achieved in five patients (17%); the long-term local control rate was not stated. There was no operative mortality. Procedure-related complications included injuries to the oculomotor (14%), trochlear (7%), ophthalmic (3%), maxillary (10%), mandibular (17%), and abducens nerves (3%). Two patients required a second operation, one for a pseudoaneurysm of the internal carotid artery and one for a CSF leak.

DeMonte et al[39] reported 41 patients who underwent resection by Al-Mefty and colleagues for benign meningiomas involving the cavernous sinus between 1982 and 1992. Follow-up information was available for 38 patients (mean follow-up, 45 months; range, 2 months to 10 years). Complete resection was achieved in 31 patients (76%). Improved function was observed in 14% of affected cranial nerves. After complete resection, local control was obtained in 25 of 28 patients (89%) for whom follow-up was available and in eight of 10 patients (80%) with a subtotal resection. However, the follow-up in eight patients who remained progression free after subtotal resection was very short. Three patients (7%) died postoperatively. New cranial neuropathies occurred in seven patients (18%, mostly involving the oculomotor and trigeminal nerves). Other complications included stroke with a permanent deficit of the dominant hemisphere (two patients) and CSF leak (two patients).

O'Sullivan et al[41] reported their results on 39 patients surgically treated for meningiomas involving the cavernous sinus between 1985 and 1994. There were no postoperative deaths. Complete resection was achieved in 20%. At 6 months postsurgery, permanent deficits included new optic neuropathy (one patient) and new oculomotor nerve deficits (seven patients, 18%).

Sindou and colleagues[45] reported their experience with cavernous sinus meningiomas treated with surgical resection alone and showed that, in cases in which aggressive gross total resection was achieved (92%), the recurrence rate at 8.3 years of mean follow-up was 12.5%, compared with a recurrence rate of 26% in patients in which a subtotal resection was achieved. A recent retrospective series reported by Pichierri and colleagues[44] of 147 patients treated with either extensive resection by "open cavernous sinus surgery" (24 patients, with a gross total resection of 91.7%) or conservative resection (removing only the extracavernous component, 123 patients, 83.7%) showed a recurrence rate of 12.5% for the first group compared with a 26.2% recurrence rate in the second group. Worsening of the preoperative neurological status occurred in 62.5% of patients in the first group versus 31.7% in the second group. Although perioperative mortality was 8.3% in the first group, no deaths were reported for the second group. Mean follow-up in this series was 8.3 years. Cranial nerve injury remains the most frequent surgical morbidity. In general, preoperative deficits rarely improve, and new or worsening deficits occur in 3 to 29% of patients, with the oculomotor nerve being most commonly affected (14 to 29%).[36] Although radiosurgical treatment for these lesions has been shown to be effective in achieving local tumor control with minimal procedure-related morbidity in some series (as will be discussed) and may be used in lesions with adequate margins for optic nerve protection, considerable rates of delayed complications have also been reported. Delayed progression after failed radiosurgery is of significant concern, as reported by Couldwell and colleagues.[46] This report reviewed 13 patients with benign skull base meningiomas with radiographic progression following radiosurgical treatment as a primary or adjuvant treatment. Rate of progression varied widely, with some patients showing progression 14 years after the initial treatment. Recurrences in these series were seen within as well as outside the radiation field. Most authors therefore recommend up-front postoperative radiosurgery only for patients with grade II or III residual disease and delayed radiosurgery in patients with postoperative symptomatic progression of benign lesions. Long-term results of combined strategies of maximal safe resection with adjuvant postoperative radiation are yet to be reported.

Cerebellopontine Angle Meningiomas

Lesions considered as cerebellopontine angle (CPA) meningiomas are those arising from the posterior petrous dura lateral to the trigeminal nerve, although for practical purposes lesions arising in adjacent areas but extending to the CPA and that encase most of the tumor burden in this region are also considered CPA meningiomas. The location of these lesions along the internal acoustic meatus (IAM) has been traditionally used to classify them into premeatal and postmeatal tumors.[47] Whereas premeatal tumors tend to manifest early with trigeminal symptoms as well as facial and cochlear signs, postmeatal tumors tend to be diagnosed later, when mass effect generates cerebellar signs and symptoms. These classifications have been expanded further by Samii and colleagues into premeatal, postmeatal, suprameatal, inframeatal, and centered at the IAM,[22] with the majority of cases presenting as premeatal tumors (33%). Early detection of CPA meningiomas continues to increase as MRI use expands and presents clinicians with the challenge of recommending conservative management of asymptomatic patients versus proactive surgical resection in light of the well-documented improved outcomes in neurologically intact patients with smaller lesions. Although gross total resection is the treatment of choice for CPA meningiomas, most centers advocate for conservative management of smaller tumors in elderly patients and in those with significant comorbidities, as long as continued follow-up confirms clinical and radiographic stability. Multiple surgical techniques have been described in the treatment of CPA meningiomas, including retrosigmoid with or without suprameatal extension, far-lateral, presigmoid (translabyrinthine, transcochlear, transpetrosal), middle fossa, and combination approaches.[22,47,48] The choice of approach is influenced by the extension of the lesion along the posterior fossa, the possibility of hearing preservation, the functional state of the cranial nerves involved, and the experience of the surgical team. In contrast to vestibular schwannomas, hearing preservation remains a reasonable goal even in large CPA meningiomas because hearing loss occurs from external compression of the cochlear nerve. Postoperative hearing loss in some cases is more related to interruption of vascular supply to cochlear structures than to manipulation of the cisternal or meatal cochlear nerve. Hearing preservation is, as expected, more frequently achieved in postmeatal tumors.[49]

Tumor location and consistency appear to play a more determinant role in the surgical outcomes than the overall size of the lesion. Other contributing factors include extent of skull base involvement and the adherence of the capsule to the pial surface of the brainstem and to the surrounding neurovascular structures. In general, facial nerve and hearing preservation are decreased in premeatal tumors. Most contemporary series report gross total resection rates > 80%, with low mortality rates and variable degrees of perioperative morbidity.[48,50–53] In a series of 421 patients reported by Nakamura and colleagues,[22] gross total resection (Simpson 1 and 2) was achieved in 86% of tumors. Tumors classified as supra- and postmeatal exhibited the highest rates of gross total resection (90 and 89%, respectively). Tumors classified as pre- and inframeatal had the lowest rate of gross total resection (83 and 78%, respectively). Facial nerve preservation in this series (House-Brackmann 1 or 2) was accomplished in 89% of patients, and hearing was preserved in 91%. Recurrence rates in some series range from 0 to 9.5%[48,50,52]; therefore, postoperative radiographic follow-up is strongly recommended. Patients exhibiting symptomatic recurrence can be treated by reoperation, radiosurgery, or radiotherapy. In patients with subtotally resected meningiomas, adjuvant postoperative radiation therapy has been shown to increase time-to-recurrence rates and prolong overall survival.

Clival and Petroclival Meningiomas

Whereas the dural attachment of clival meningiomas is typically located at the upper two thirds of the clivus near the midline, the dural attachment of petroclival meningiomas is centered on the petroclival junction, posterior to the gasserian ganglion and medial to the IAM. The pattern of growth progresses accordingly, with clival meningiomas causing posterior displacement of the brainstem and petroclival meningiomas causing posterolateral displacement to the opposite side. Extension into the posterior cavernous sinus, parasellar region, tentorium, or foramen magnum is frequently encountered.[54] Due to their insidious nature, most clival and petroclival meningiomas are diagnosed later, once cranial nerve compression has become symptomatic or when hydrocephalus or balance/gait abnormalities become more pronounced.[54]

As in all skull base meningiomas, surgical approaches have been developed to minimize brain retraction and to facilitate visualization of neurovascular structures, while limiting approach-related morbidity. Traditional approaches, including pterional, subtemporal, and suboccipital, were used initially,[12,55–57] followed by targeted skull base approaches that included suboccipital or subtemporal corridors with anterior or posterior petrosectomies, supplemented in some cases by presigmoid or lateral transcondylar exposures.[58–60] Natural history studies are scarce and have shown wide variability in growth rates of unresected or residual lesions. One observational study of 21 patients reported a growth rate of 0.81 mm/year,[61] whereas another of 38 patients reported a rate of 0.37 cm/year.[62] Radiological progression, however, does appear to correlate with clinical deterioration, as shown by Van Havenbergh and colleagues,[61] who reported radiological progression in 76% of the 21 patients studied at 4 years, with functional decline in 63% of these. In addition, Jung and colleagues[62] also showed radiological progression in 42% of subtotally resected meningiomas at 4 years, with an increase in the growth pattern (doubling time was 8 years). In Van Havenbergh et al's study,[61] 24% of untreated patients showed no radiological progression at 4 years. Similarly, in Jung et al's study, 58% of subtotally resected lesions remained radiologically stable at 4 years. These findings suggest that conservative management with close radiographic follow-up can be entertained in asymptomatic patients with smaller lesions who are elderly or not ideal surgical candidates.

Although modern skull base techniques have significantly decreased the morbidity and mortality associated with resection of these lesions, CSF leaks, hearing loss, and facial paralysis remain significant in recent series from specialized high-volume centers.[59,63] Rates of gross total resection vary among contemporary series from 20 to 79%, with a mortality ranging from 0 to 7%,[12,55,56,58,59,62,64–67] but the overall goal is maximal safe resection to achieve optimal brainstem decompression. Preoperative cranial neuropathies, fibrous or adherent consistency, previous resection, and radiological evidence of brainstem edema have been associated with the worst outcomes.[54] Worsening of preexisting cranial neuropathies and new cranial nerve deficits occur in up to 76% of cases, with the fourth cranial nerve being the most frequently injured.[68] Some cranial neuropathies are transient, and delayed improvement has been reported.[66] Recurrence rates vary widely in the literature, ranging from 0 to 42%[12,55,56,58,59,62,64–67] and are increased in lesions that are subtotally resected, higher grade, or extending into the cavernous sinus.

Of 33 patients treated by Bricolo et al,[55] 26 (79%) underwent complete and seven (21%) underwent subtotal resection of a petroclival meningioma. Three patients died postoperatively. The mean follow-up for the remaining 30 patients was 4.3 years. Three patients (10%) died from tumor progression. Karnofsky performance 1 month after surgery and at last follow-up, respectively, was as follows: unchanged, 60% and 70%; improved, 17% and 30%; and worse, 23% and 0%. Three patients (9%) died perioperatively. Worsening of a preexisting deficit occurred in 12 patients (36%), and at least one new cranial nerve deficit was present in 25 (76%). Cranial nerve deficits per patient averaged 2.2 preoperatively, 3.6 perioperatively, and 2.7 at last follow-up.

Couldwell et al[64] surgically treated 109 patients with petroclival meningiomas. Seventy-five patients (69%) underwent gross total resection. Follow-up ranged from 25.2 to 168 months (mean, 73.2 months). One hundred and five patients had benign tumors, and 10% experienced local recurrence or progression. Procedure-related postoperative mortality was 4%, and permanent cranial neuropathies were observed in 36 patients (33%).

More recently, a combination of subtotal resection followed by postoperative stereotactic radiosurgery has been proposed, with recurrence or progression rates ranging from 4.5 to 22% at 6 to 8 years of mean follow-up.[64,66,67] Whereas progression of subtotally resected tumors can be as high as 42% at 4 years,[62] progression rates of patients treated with radiosurgery following subtotal resection range from 0 to 13% at 3 years.[69]

Foramen Magnum Meningiomas

Anatomically, the region of the foramen magnum (FM) extends anteriorly from the lower third of the clivus to the superior border of the body of C2, laterally from the jugular tubercle superiorly to the superior border of the lamina of C2 inferiorly, and posteriorly from the anterior border of the squamous portion of the occipital bone to the spinous process of C2. FM meningiomas frequently have an intradural origin, although transdural and extradural tumors can also develop. Although FM meningiomas are rare (1.8 to 3.2% of all meningiomas), they represent three quarters of all benign tumors found in this location.[70–72] Analogous to petroclival meningiomas, FM meningiomas have an indolent course, with vague complaints of headache or neck pain resulting in a delayed diagnosis when long tract signs become manifest, causing the classic FM presentation with unilateral upper extremity sensory and motor deficits that progress to the ipsilateral lower extremity, followed by the contralateral lower extremity, and finally up to the contralateral upper extremity. Surgical resection remains the treatment of choice, with the primary goal of maximal safe tumor resection, decompression of the cervicomedullary junction, and protection of the lower cranial nerves and the posterior circulation.

Although most FM meningiomas arise anterolaterally (68 to 98%), classification according to their site of origin and their relationship with the vertebral artery (VA) has valuable surgical implications.[71,72] Tumors arising primarily from the rostral cervical spine, also referred to as spinocranial, tend to displace the VA superiorly, almost always originate below the FM, and also displace the lower cranial nerves superiorly. Tumors originating at the point of dural entry of the distal V3 segment of the VA tend to encase the artery, displacing the VA away from the petrous surface and separating it from the medulla. Tumors with a cranial, anterolateral, or anterior origin arise ventral to the VA and medial to the hypoglossal and jugular foramen and displace the VA and the medulla away from the petrous surface, also displacing the lower cranial nerves posterolaterally. Careful analysis of the preoperative neurovascular imaging guides the choice of surgical approach, based on the natural corridor created by the lesion, and allows the surgeon to anticipate potential complications due to anatomical variability, such as an extradural posteroinferior cerebellar artery (PICA) origin (occurring in 5 to 20% of patients). The presence of T2 changes suggestive of brainstem or spinal cord edema secondary to pial infiltration by the tumor has been used by some authors as a determinant factor for a conservative subtotal resection aimed primarily at function preservation.[73] Similarly, evidence of narrowing or encasement of the VA should prompt consideration of a more conservative resection because the adventitial wall may be compromised and emphasizes the need for early vascular control of the proximal VA. In these cases, formal angiographic evaluation can be helpful in elucidating potential collaterals and the exact point of origin of PICA in case emergent VA sacrifice is required. Most contemporary series report high rates of gross total resection with minimal morbidity and mortality regardless of the approach selected. Cusimano and colleagues reported their results in 20 patients with FM meningiomas treated between 1992 and 2009.[72] Gross total resection was achieved in 15/20 patients with a suboccipital approach without condylar resection with no evidence of recurrence on last follow-up (mean follow-up 33.1 months). Surgery-related morbidity included CSF leaks in three patients and hydrocephalus requiring shunting in two patients. Although no deaths were reported, one patient developed lateral medullary ischemia and another developed a mild Brown-Séquard syndrome. Functional status at last follow-up was improved in 15 patients, unchanged in two patients, and worse than preop in three patients. Other complications reported in the literature include intracranial hematomas, meningitis, lower cranial neuropathies, hemiparesis, quadriparesis, and aspiration pneumonia.[51,71,74–89] Factors related to worse outcomes include anterior location, smaller size, pial invasion, extradural extension, and recurrence after prior resection. The addition of condylar resection has not been correlated with superior outcomes, although prospective comparative analysis has not been conducted. In patients with surgical contraindications, those electing nonoperative treatment, and those with residual tumors after microsurgical resection, radiosurgical options should be considered, as potential growth within the confined space of the FM can result in significant irreversible deficits.

Table 32.1 summarizes some larger select surgical series, stratified by skull base location, including key indicators of outcome, morbidity, and follow-up.

■ Management of Skull Base Meningiomas

Gross Total Resection versus Subtotal Resection

Level I and Level II Evidence

There are no published studies on the topic.

Level III and Level IV Evidence

In 1996, Mathiesen et al[7] reported a large series of skull base meningiomas treated almost exclusively with surgery between 1947 and 1982. In this series, 338 patients were followed for a minimum of 10 years until tumor recurrence or death. The majority of their lesions were classified as benign (98%). Extent of resection was graded according to the Simpson criteria.[90] The 10-year survival rate for 315 patients treated surgically with and without postoperative radiation was ~ 79%. Of these, 46 had tumors located in the central skull base, with 13 of the 46 central tumors requiring postoperative radiotherapy. The 10-year survival rate for those treated with surgery alone was 42%, compared with 72% for those treated with surgery and radiotherapy. Similarly, at 20 years, survival rates after treatment for those treated with surgery alone compared with surgery and radiotherapy were as follows: 10 years, 14 of 33 (42%) versus 10 of 13 (77%) ($p < 0.05$); and 20 years, 6 of 33 (18%) versus 5 of 13 (38%) (not statistically significant).

All patients with a Simpson grade 4 or 5 resection and follow-up longer than 20 years showed disease progression. Local recurrences occurred more frequently in patients with central skull base tumors.

Table 32.1 Partial listing of some key published clinical series on skull base meningiomas categorized by location and treatment

Study	Study type	Class	Reference	N	Location in skull base
Mathiesen et al 1996[7]	RCS	4	Neurosurgery 1996;39: 2–9	338	All
Condra et al 1997[1]	RCS	4	Int J Radiat Oncol Biol Physiol 1997;39:427–436	262	All
Olfactory groove					
Spektor et al 2005[6]	RCS	4	Neurosurgery. 2005 Oct;57(4 Suppl):268–80	80	Olfactory groove
Tuberculum sellae					
Goel[12]	RCS	4	Neurosurgery 51:1358–1364, 2002	70	Tuberculum sellae
Clinoidal					
Al-Mefty 1990[18]	RCS	4	J Neurosurg. 1990 Dec;73[50]:840–9	24	Clinoidal
Lee et al 2001[19]	RCS	4	Neurosurgery 2001;48[27]:1012–1019	15	Clinoidal
Bassiouni et al 2009[27]	RCS	4	J Neurosurg 2009;111[27]:1078–1090	106	Clinoidal
Goel et al 2000[29]	RCS	4	Neurol Med Chir (Tokyo) 2000;40[55]:610–616	60	Clinoidal
Nakamura et al 2006[30]	RCS	4	Neurosurgery 2006;58[71]:626–639	39	Medial sphenoid wing
Pamir et al 2008[31]	RCS	4	Acta Neurochir (Wien) 2008;150[74]:625–635	43	Clinoidal
Tobias et al 2003[33]	RCS	4	Neurosurg Focus 2003;14[50]:e5	26	Clinoidal
Cavernous Sinus					
Knosp et al 1996[40]	RCS	4	Neurosurgery 1996;38:434–444	29	Cavernous sinus
De Monte et al 1994[39]	RCS	4	J Neurosurg 1994;81:245–251	41	Cavernous sinus
O'Sullivan et al 1997[41]	RCS	4	Neurosurgery 1997;40:238–247	39	Cavernous sinus
Cusimano	RCS	4	Neurosurgery 1995;37[58]:1–9	89	Cavernous sinus
Sindou et al 2007[45]	RCS	4	J Neurosurg 2007;107[27]:937–944	100	Cavernous sinus
Pichierri et al 2009[44]	RCS	4	Neurosurgery 2009;64[50]:1090–1099	147	Cavernous sinus
De Jesús et al 1996[38]	RCS	4	Neurosurgery 1996;39:915–920	119	Cavernous sinus
Petroclival					
Couldwell et al 1996[64]	RCS	4	J Neurosurg 1996;84:20–28	109	Petroclival
Bricolo et al 1992[55]	RCS	4	Neurosurgery 1992;31:813–828	33	Petroclival
Goel and Muzumdar 2004[12]	RCS	4	Surg Neurol 2004;62[71]:332–338	28	Petroclival
Spallone et al 1999[57]	RCS	4	Surg Neurol 1999;51[71]:412–419	31	Petroclival
Mathiesen et al 2007[60]	RCS	4	Neurosurgery 2007;60[50]:982–991	29	Petroclival
Abdel Aziz et al 2000[58]	RCS	4	Neurosurgery 2000;47[58]:139–150	35	Clival and petroclival
Natarajan et al 2007[66]	RR of PACS	4	Neurosurgery 2007;60[50]:965–979	150	Petroclival
Park et al 2006[67]	RCS	4	Surg Neurol 2006;66[70]:160–165	75	Petroclival
Cerebellopontine angle					
Voss et al 2000[52]	RCS	4	Surg Neurol 2000;53[27]:439–446	40	CPA
Thomas and King 1996[48]	RCS	4	Br J Neurosurg 1996;10[1]:59–68	41	CPA
Wu et al 2005[53]	RCS	4	J Neurosurg 2005;102[70]:284–289	82	Posterior petrosal

(Continued on page 308)

Table 32.1 *(Continued)* Partial listing of some key published clinical series on skull base meningiomas categorized by location and treatment

Study	Study type	Class	Reference	*N*	Location in skull base
Foramen magnum					
Kandenwein et al 2009[79]	RCS	4	Br J Neurosurg 2009;23[58]:33–39	16	Foramen magnum
Wu et al 2009[87]	RCS	4	Surg Neurol 2009;72[71]:376–382	114	Foramen magnum
Borba et al 2009[76]	RCS	4	Neurosurg Rev 2009;32[58]:49–58	15	Foramen magnum
Bassiouni et al 2006[74]	RCS	4	Neurosurgery 2006;59[50]:1177–1185	25	Foramen magnum
Pamir et al 2004[84]	RCS	4	J Clin Neurosci 2004;11[75]:863–867	22	Foramen magnum
George et al 1997[78]	RCS	4	Surg Neurol 1997;47[71]:371–379	40	Foramen magnum
Samii[89]	RCS	4	Neurosurgery 1996;39[50]:1086–1094	38	Foramen magnum
Gamma knife radiosurgery					
Stafford et al 2001[90]	RR of PACS	4	Neurosurgery 2001;49:1029–1038	147	All
Subach et al 1998[69]	RCS	4	Neurosurgery 1998;42:437–445	62	Petroclival
Lee et al 2002[91]	RCS	4	J Neurosurg 2002;97:65–72	176	Cavernous sinus
Linear accelerator					
Hakim et al 1998[93]	RCS	4	Neurosurgery 1998;42:446–454	127	All (53% skull base)
Shafron et al 1999[94]	RR of PACS	4	Int J Radiat Oncol Biol Physiol 1999;43:321–327	70	All (45% skull base)
Fractionated radiotherapy					
Debus et al 2001[95]	RCS	4	J Clin Oncol 2001;19:3547–3553	189	All (82% skull base)
Nutting et al 1999[25]	RCS	4	J Neurosurg 1999;90:823–827	82	Skull base
Dufour et al 2001[96]	RCS	4	Neurosurgery 2001;48:285–294	31	Cavernous sinus
Maguire et al 1999[97]	RCS	4	Int J Radiat Oncol Biol Physiol 1999;44:75–79	28	Cavernous sinus
Proton beam					
Wenkel et al 2000[98]	RCS	4	Int J Radiat Oncol Biol Physiol 2000;48:1363–1370	46	96% skull base
Intensity-modulated radiotherapy					
Uy et al 2002[99]	RCS	4	Int J Radiat Oncol Biol Physiol 2002;48:1363–1370	40	80% skull base

Abbreviations: CPA, cerebellopontine angle; RCS, retrospective case series; PACS, prospectively acquired case series; RR, retrospective review.

Although this series comprises a 35-year experience in which surgical techniques, surgical adjuncts, and perioperative care have drastically evolved, the principles of resection-dependent recurrence are still applicable today.

In Condra et al's series[1] of 262 patients, 229 (87.4%) were treated with surgery alone, 21 (8%) were treated with surgery and postoperative radiation, seven (2.7%) were treated with radiation alone, and five (1.9%) were treated with radiosurgery alone. The 15-year cause-specific survival rate for patients in which a gross total resection was achieved was 88%, which was similar to that of patients with subtotal resection and radiotherapy (86%), but the rates decreased significantly in patients who underwent subtotal resection alone (51%). In this series, 60% of tumors involved the skull base, and 18% were atypical.

De Jesús et al[38] described 119 patients with skull base meningiomas treated surgically by Sekhar and colleagues at the University of Pittsburgh between 1983 and 1993. Twenty-nine percent had confined tumors (< 3 cm and involving the cavernous sinus and immediately adjacent areas), and 71% had extensive tumors (≥ 3 cm and involving multiple areas of the skull base). Forty-four percent of the patients had undergone prior surgery, and 7% had received prior radiotherapy. The mean follow-up was 34 months. Gross total resection was achieved in 73 (61%) patients (confined, 72%; extensive, 58%). There was no relationship between the likelihood of gross total resection and whether the patient had received prior treatment. Local recurrence, progression, or both were observed in seven (10%) of the 73 patients after gross total resection compared with seven (15%) of the 46 patients after subtotal resection. The 5-year local control rate was 81% after complete resection, compared with 62% after subtotal resection. Of the 46 patients who underwent incomplete resection, 17 (37%) subsequently received radiotherapy. Complications included CSF leak (21%), pituitary dysfunction (14%), stroke (5%), infection (4%), and brain hematoma or contusion (3%).

Recommendations for the Role of Gross Total Resection

1. When feasible, gross total resection (GTR) correlates well with recurrence-free survival and is recommended (Grade 1C Recommendation, Level III/IV Evidence).
2. When GTR is not feasible, subtotal resection (STR) supplemented with adjuvant radiotherapy (RT) achieves equivalent long-term survival rates (Grade 1C Recommendation, Level III/IV Evidence).
3. STR alone results in more long-term recurrences/progression compared with GTR and/or STR + RT. Upfront or delayed RT for residual disease, after maximal safe resection, is recommended in the younger patient (Grade 2C Recommendation, Level III/IV Evidence).

Stereotactic Radiosurgery and Other Nonoperative Options

Level I and Level II Evidence

There are no published studies on the topic.

Level III and Level IV Evidence

Studies specifically analyzing local control rates for skull base meningiomas treated with radiotherapy or stereotactic radiosurgery are scarce, with reported control rates for meningiomas of all grades ranging from 0 to 100%.

Stafford et al[91] reported their experience with gamma knife radiosurgery (GKRS) (Gamma Knife, Elekta, Atlanta, GA) at the Mayo Clinic for 206 meningiomas in 190 patients, of which 147 (77%) involved the skull base. This series included 168 patients with benign meningiomas and 22 patients (12%) with atypical or malignant lesions, with a 5-year local control rate of 93% for benign tumors, 68% for atypical tumors, and 0% for malignant tumors. The 5-year cause-specific survival rate in this series was 100%. Procedure-related complications occurred in 24 patients (13%), new cranial nerve deficits occurred in 8%, symptomatic parenchymal changes occurred in 3%, internal carotid artery stenosis developed in 1%, and symptomatic cyst formation was seen in 1%. Decreased functional status was attributed to radiosurgery in 3% of patients.

Subach et al[69] reported the University of Pittsburgh Medical Center experience with GKRS for residual or recurrent petroclival meningiomas in 62 patients treated between 1987 and 1995. Previous resections were performed in 39 patients (63%), and prior external-beam radiotherapy had been delivered to seven patients (11%). Overall local control was obtained in 92% of patients until last follow-up (follow-up ranged from 12 to 101 months, mean, 42 months). Neurological status improved in 21%, remained stable in 66%, but worsened in 13%. Patients with benign tumors who had not received prior radiotherapy had a local control rate of 92% at 96 months. New, persistent cranial nerve deficits occurred in three patients (5%), without evidence of disease progression.

Lee et al[92] reported the results of 176 patients treated with GKRS for cavernous sinus meningiomas at the University of Pittsburgh Medical Center (UPMC) between 1987 and 2000. Mean follow-up was 35 months (range 2 to 138 months). Prior radiotherapy was delivered to two patients, and only four patients had atypical or malignant meningiomas. Although resection was performed in 76 patients (48%) prior to radiation, radiosurgery alone was given to 83 patients (52%). Neurological status improved in 29%, remained stable in 62%, and worsened in 9%. The 10-year local control rate was 93% for patients with benign meningiomas but only 25% at 5 years for malignant and atypical lesions. Significant complications resulting in permanent deficits occurred in 11 patients (7%) and included visual deterioration,[18] trigeminal nerve dysfunction,[27] partial complex seizures responsive to medical management,[70] and cognitive deterioration.[58]

The latest reported series to date, by Starke et al,[93] presents a retrospective review of a prospectively acquired database of 255 patients with skull base meningiomas treated at the University of Virginia between 1989 and 2006. Although surgical resection followed by GKRS was chosen in 146 patients, 109 were treated with radiosurgery alone. Patients were assessed clinically and radiographically at routine intervals following GKRS. Tumors involved the cerebellopontine angle in 17% of patients, the clivus in 16%, the petroclival region in 11%, the petrous region in 2%, and the parasellar region in 54%. Median follow-up was 6.5 years (range 2 to 18 years).

Treatment with linear accelerated–based radiosurgery has been more scarcely reported. Hakim et al[94] reported their results in 127 patients with 155 meningiomas (half of which involved the skull base) treated with linear accelerator–based radiosurgery with a follow-up of 1.2 to 79.8 months. Grade I lesions were found in 106 tumors (68%). The 5-year local control rate for benign tumors was 89%. Two patients died of procedure-related complications. Other severe permanent complications occurred in six patients (5%) and included unilateral blindness,[58] unilateral deafness,[58] monoparesis,[58] and hemiparesis.[58] Similarly, Shafron et al[95] reported linear accelerator–based results in 70 patients with 76 benign meningiomas treated at the University of Florida between 1989 and 1997. Mean follow-up was 23 months (range 2 to 88 months). Thirty-four tumors (45%) involved the skull base. The local control rate was 100%.

Fractionated stereotactic radiotherapy has also been used in the treatment of skull base meningiomas. Debus et al[96] reported the results of 189 patients with meningiomas treated at the University of Heidelberg with conformal fractionated radiotherapy between 1985 and 1998. In 155 patients (82%) the skull base was involved. Median follow-up was 35 months (range 3 months to 12 years). The average dose delivered was 56.8 Gy, with a median fraction size of 1.8 Gy. Local control was achieved in 177 (98%) patients with WHO grade I meningiomas. Forty-five percent of patients experienced neurological improvement after treatment. Overall survival for grade I meningiomas (180 patients) at 5 and 10 years was 97% and 96%, respectively.

Significant late toxicity was observed in four patients (2%) but no fatal complications were reported. Nutting et al[25] reported the results of 82 patients with benign skull base meningiomas treated with fractionated external beam radiation showing a 10-year progression-free survival rate of 83% with a 71% overall survival rate. Treatment-associated complications included visual decline in six patients (7%, five due to cataracts and one due to retinopathy), decreased short-term memory,[71] and hypopituitarism.[18] Dufour et al[97] reviewed their experience with 31 patients with benign meningiomas involving the cavernous sinus treated with radiotherapy, with and without previous resection. In this study, 17 patients underwent surgery and radiotherapy, and 14 were treated with radiation alone; median follow-up was 73.2 months (range, 24 to 192 months). The 10-year overall progression-free survival rate was 93%, and a 100% 10-year cause-specific survival rate was also reported. One patient experienced short-term memory loss. Maguire et al[98] described the results of 28 patients with cavernous sinus meningiomas treated with fractionated radiotherapy at Duke University Medical Center between 1985 and 1998. Delayed toxicity occurred in two patients (7%) and consisted of decreased cognitive function[58] and orbital fibrosis.[58]

Proton beam therapy has also been used in the treatment of skull base meningiomas. Wenkel et al[99] reported the results of 46 patients with partially resected, unresectable, or recurrent grade I meningiomas treated with combined proton and photon radiotherapy at Harvard Medical School between 1981 and 1996. Median follow-up was 53 months (range, 12 to 207 months). The majority of tumors involved the skull base except for two orbital lesions. Recurrence-free survival at 10 years was 88%.

Intensity-modulated radiotherapy was used in 40 patients with benign meningiomas treated at Baylor College of Medicine between 1994 and 1999 by Uy and colleagues.[100] Median follow-up was 30 months (range 6 to 71 months). Eighty percent of these tumors involved the skull base. The 5-year local control rate was 93%. Significant toxicity occurred in three patients (8%) and included memory loss and personality changes in two patients and fatal brainstem necrosis in one patient.

Expert Recommendations

1. It is reasonable to treat selected meningiomas with radiosurgery alone, such as holocavernous meningiomas, when risks of surgery (cranial neuropathies) are deemed too high (Grade 1C Recommendation, Level III/IV Evidence).
2. The role of up-front postoperative radiosurgery for residual disease, as opposed to delayed radiosurgery based on time of regrowth/recurrence of symptoms, is not clear (Grade 2C Recommendation, Level III/IV Evidence).
3. It is reasonable to treat larger selected meningiomas with fractionated radiotherapy instead of surgery in patients with systemic comorbidities (Grade 1C Recommendation, Level III/IV Evidence).
4. It is reasonable to treat selected meningiomas with fractionated radiotherapy instead of radiosurgery if there are contiguous critically radiosensitive structures (optic apparatus, brainstem) (Grade 1C Recommendation, Level III/IV Evidence).
5. In the case of WHO grade II and III meningiomas, recurrence rates are higher than those for grade I, and postoperative adjuvant radiation therapy or radiosurgery for residual tumor is recommended (Grade 2C Recommendation, Level III/IV Evidence).
6. In the case of WHO grade II meningiomas, where gross total resection was achieved, it is unclear whether up-front postoperative adjuvant radiation therapy or radiosurgery is beneficial or not.

■ Summary and Conclusions

Skull base meningiomas represent formidable surgical and therapeutic challenges. Although local tumor control after surgery or radiotherapy can be achieved in a significant number of patients with benign tumors, the likelihood of progression-free survival decreases with time. Benign lesions exhibit comparable rates of long-term survival and local control following complete resection, radiosurgery, or radiotherapy. The risk of complications is, therefore, the main factor in determining the treatment of choice. The location and extent of the tumor as well as its biological idiosyncrasies largely determine the extent of resection. Gross total resection of large lesions, or partial resection of lesions in eloquent areas, can lead to significant permanent neurological deficits. Nonoperative therapies, such as radiosurgery and radiotherapy, are, however, not free of risk, with subsets of patients experiencing radiotherapy-related complications. General consensus exists on attempting gross total resection in patients with well-circumscribed tumors in which the long-term morbidity associated with resection is limited. Subtotal resection of extensive lesions may be attempted if decompression can improve existing neuropathies and decrease the severity of mass-effect-related symptoms. Improvement of preexisting cranial neuropathies is unlikely in most cases after subtotal resection. In subtotally resected lesions exhibiting persistent growth on follow-up and in higher-grade lesions, radiosurgery may be indicated if the lesion can be adequately encompassed within the treatment fields. Up-front radiosurgery without surgical decompression can be beneficial in patients who are not surgical candidates and in large multifocal lesions. In benign lesions treated with radiosurgery, no difference in outcomes has been found between GKRS-treated patients and those treated with linear accelerator–based systems. Radiotherapy can be used instead of radiosurgery in patients with irregularly shaped tumors, or in lesions too large to be treated with radiosurgery. Radiotherapy can also be recommended for patients with tumors located in close proximity to highly radiosensitive structures, such as the optic apparatus. Decreasing the volume of normal tissue included in the radiotherapy fields can reduce the risk of long-term complications.

■ References

1. Condra KS, Buatti JM, Mendenhall WM, Friedman WA, Marcus RB Jr, Rhoton AL. Benign meningiomas: primary treatment selection affects survival. Int J Radiat Oncol Biol Phys 1997;39(2):427–436
2. Chan RC, Thompson GB. Morbidity, mortality, and quality of life following surgery for intracranial meningiomas. A retrospective study in 257 cases. J Neurosurg 1984;60(1):52–60
3. Solero CL, Giombini S, Morello G. Suprasellar and olfactory meningiomas. Report on a series of 153 personal cases. Acta Neurochir (Wien) 1983;67(3-4):181–194
4. Hentschel SJ, DeMonte F. Olfactory groove meningiomas. In: DeMonte F, Mcdermott MW, al-Mefty O, eds. Al-Mefty's Meningiomas. New York, NY: Thieme; 2011:196–205
5. Maiuri F, Salzano FA, Motta S, Colella G, Sardo L. Olfactory groove meningioma with paranasal sinus and nasal cavity extension: removal by combined subfrontal and nasal approach. J Craniomaxillofac Surg 1998;26(5):314–317
6. Spektor S, Valarezo J, Fliss DM, et al. Olfactory groove meningiomas from neurosurgical and ear, nose, and throat perspectives: approaches, techniques, and outcomes. Neurosurgery 2005;57(4, Suppl):268–280
7. Mathiesen T, Lindquist C, Kihlström L, Karlsson B. Recurrence of cranial base meningiomas. Neurosurgery 1996;39(1):2–7
8. Obeid F, Al-Mefty O. Recurrence of olfactory groove meningiomas. Neurosurgery 2003;53(3):534–542
9. Snyder WE, Shah MV, Weisberger EC, Campbell RL. Presentation and patterns of late recurrence of olfactory groove meningiomas. Skull Base Surg 2000;10(3):131–139
10. Nakamura M, Struck M, Roser F, Vorkapic P, Samii M. Olfactory groove meningiomas: clinical outcome and recurrence rates after tumor removal through the frontolateral and bifrontal approach. Neurosurgery 2007;60(5):844–852
11. Romani R, Lehecka M, Gaal E, et al. Lateral supraorbital approach applied to olfactory groove meningiomas: experience with 66 consecutive patients. Neurosurgery 2009;65(1):39–52
12. Goel A, Muzumdar D. Conventional posterior fossa approach for surgery on petroclival meningiomas: a report on an experience with 28 cases. Neurosurg 2002;51(6):1358–1363
13. de Divitiis E, Cavallo LM, Esposito F, Stella L, Messina A. Extended endoscopic transsphenoidal approach for tuberculum sellae meningiomas. Neurosurgery 2007;61(5, Suppl 2):229–237
14. Ceylan S, Koc K, Anık I. Extended endoscopic transphenoidal approach for tuberculum sellae meningiomas. Acta Neurochir (Wien) 2011;153(1):1–9
15. Sughrue ME, Sanai N, Mcdermott MW. Tuberculum sellae meningiomas. In: DeMonte F, Mcdermott MW, al-Mefty O, eds. Al-Mefty's Meningiomas. New York, NY: Thieme; 2011:206–213
16. Simon M, Schramm J. Lateral and middle sphenoid wing meningiomas. In: DeMonte F, Mcdermott MW, al-Mefty O, eds. Al-Mefty's Meningiomas. New York, NY: Thieme; 2011:214–227
17. Stafford SL, Perry A, Suman VJ, et al. Primarily resected meningiomas: outcome and prognostic factors in 581 Mayo Clinic patients, 1978 through 1988. Mayo Clin Proc 1998;73(10):936–942
18. Al-Mefty O. Clinoidal meningiomas. J Neurosurg 1990;73(6):840–849
19. Lee JH, Jeun SS, Evans J, Kosmorsky G. Surgical management of clinoidal meningiomas. Neurosurgery 2001;48(5):1012–1019
20. Russell SM, Benjamin V. Medial sphenoid ridge meningiomas: classification, microsurgical anatomy, operative nuances, and long-term surgical outcome in 35 consecutive patients. Neurosurgery 2008;62(3, Suppl 1):38–50
21. Mirone G, Chibbaro S, Schiabello L, Tola S, George B. En plaque sphenoid wing meningiomas: recurrence factors and surgical strategy in a series of 71 patients. Neurosurgery 2009;65(6, Suppl):100–108
22. Nakamura M, Roser F, Dormiani M, Matthies C, Vorkapic P, Samii M. Facial and cochlear nerve function after surgery of cerebellopontine angle meningiomas. Neurosurgery 2005;57(1):77–90

23. Ringel F, Cedzich C, Schramm J. Microsurgical technique and results of a series of 63 spheno-orbital meningiomas. Neurosurgery 2007;60(4, Suppl 2):214–221
24. Schick U, Bleyen J, Bani A, Hassler W. Management of meningiomas en plaque of the sphenoid wing. J Neurosurg 2006; 104(2):208–214
25. Nutting C, Brada M, Brazil L, et al. Radiotherapy in the treatment of benign meningioma of the skull base. J Neurosurg 1999;90(5):823–827
26. Krisht AF. Clinoidal meningiomas. In: DeMonte F, Mcdermott MW, Al-Mefty O, eds. Al-Mefty's Meningiomas. New York, NY: Thieme: 2011:229–236
27. Bassiouni H, Asgari S, Sandalcioglu IE, Seifert V, Stolke D, Marquardt G. Anterior clinoidal meningiomas: functional outcome after microsurgical resection in a consecutive series of 106 patients. Clinical article. J Neurosurg 2009;111(5): 1078–1090
28. Day JD. Cranial base surgical techniques for large sphenocavernous meningiomas: technical note. Neurosurgery 2000;46(3):754–759
29. Goel A, Gupta S, Desai K. New grading system to predict resectability of anterior clinoid meningiomas. Neurol Med Chir (Tokyo) 2000;40(12):610–616
30. Nakamura M, Roser F, Jacobs C, Vorkapic P, Samii M. Medial sphenoid wing meningiomas: clinical outcome and recurrence rate. Neurosurgery 2006;58(4):626–639
31. Pamir MN, Belirgen M, Ozduman K, Kiliç T, Ozek M. Anterior clinoidal meningiomas: analysis of 43 consecutive surgically treated cases. Acta Neurochir (Wien) 2008;150(7):625–635
32. Puzzilli F, Ruggeri A, Mastronardi L, Agrillo A, Ferrante L. Anterior clinoidal meningiomas: report of a series of 33 patients operated on through the pterional approach. Neuro-oncol 1999;1(3):188–195
33. Tobias S, Kim CH, Kosmorsky G, Lee JH. Management of surgical clinoidal meningiomas. Neurosurg Focus 2003;14(6): e5
34. Bindal R, Goodman JM, Kawasaki A, Purvin V, Kuzma B. The natural history of untreated skull base meningiomas. Surg Neurol 2003;59(2):87–92
35. Golnik KC, Miller NR, Long DM. Rate of progression and severity of neuro-ophthalmologic manifestations of cavernous sinus meningiomas. Skull Base Surg 1992;2(3):129–133
36. Dunn IF, al-Mefty O. Cavernous sinus meningiomas. In: DeMonte F, Mcdermott MW, al-Mefty O, eds. Al-Mefty's Meningiomas. New York, NY: Thieme; 2011:237–247
37. Cusimano MD, Sekhar LN, Sen CN, et al. The results of surgery for benign tumors of the cavernous sinus. Neurosurgery 1995;37(1):1–9
38. De Jesús O, Sekhar LN, Parikh HK, Wright DC, Wagner DP. Long-term follow-up of patients with meningiomas involving the cavernous sinus: recurrence, progression, and quality of life. Neurosurgery 1996;39(5):915–919
39. DeMonte F, Smith HK, al-Mefty O. Outcome of aggressive removal of cavernous sinus meningiomas. J Neurosurg 1994; 81(2):245–251
40. Knosp E, Perneczky A, Koos WT, Fries G, Matula C. Meningiomas of the space of the cavernous sinus. Neurosurgery 1996;38(3):434–442
41. O'Sullivan MG, van Loveren HR, Tew JM Jr. The surgical resectability of meningiomas of the cavernous sinus. Neurosurgery 1997;40(2):238–244
42. Sekhar LN, Patel S, Cusimano M, Wright DC, Sen CN, Bank WO. Surgical treatment of meningiomas involving the cavernous sinus: evolving ideas based on a ten year experience. Acta Neurochir Suppl (Wien) 1996;65:58–62
43. Heth JA, Al-Mefty O. Cavernous sinus meningiomas. Neurosurg Focus 2003;14(6):e3
44. Pichierri A, Santoro A, Raco A, Paolini S, Cantore G, Delfini R. Cavernous sinus meningiomas: retrospective analysis and proposal of a treatment algorithm. Neurosurgery 2009;64(6): 1090–1099
45. Sindou M, Wydh E, Jouanneau E, Nebbal M, Lieutaud T. Long-term follow-up of meningiomas of the cavernous sinus after surgical treatment alone. J Neurosurg 2007;107(5):937–944
46. Couldwell WT, Cole CD, Al-Mefty O. Patterns of skull base meningioma progression after failed radiosurgery. J Neurosurg 2007;106(1):30–35
47. Samii M, Gerganov VM. Cerebellopontine angle meningiomas. In: DeMonte F, Mcdermott MW, Al-Mefty O, eds. Al-Mefty's Meningiomas. New York, NY: Thieme; 2011:262–269
48. Thomas NW, King TT. Meningiomas of the cerebellopontine angle. A report of 41 cases. Br J Neurosurg 1996;10(1): 59–68
49. Schaller B, Heilbronner R, Pfaltz CR, Probst RR, Gratzl O. Preoperative and postoperative auditory and facial nerve function in cerebellopontine angle meningiomas. Otolaryngol Head Neck Surg 1995;112(2):228–234
50. Bassiouni H, Hunold A, Asgari S, Stolke D. Meningiomas of the posterior petrous bone: functional outcome after microsurgery. J Neurosurg 2004;100(6):1014–1024
51. Matthies C, Carvalho G, Tatagiba M, Lima M, Samii M. Meningiomas of the cerebellopontine angle. Acta Neurochir Suppl (Wien) 1996;65:86–91
52. Voss NF, Vrionis FD, Heilman CB, Robertson JH. Meningiomas of the cerebellopontine angle. Surg Neurol 2000;53(5): 439–446
53. Wu ZB, Yu CJ, Guan SS. Posterior petrous meningiomas: 82 cases. J Neurosurg 2005;102(2):284–289
54. Coppens JR, Couldwell WT. Clival and petroclival meningiomas. In: DeMonte F, Mcdermott MW, al-Mefty O, eds. Al-Mefty's Meningiomas. New York, NY: Thieme; 2011:270–282
55. Bricolo AP, Turazzi S, Talacchi A, Cristofori L. Microsurgical removal of petroclival meningiomas: a report of 33 patients. Neurosurgery 1992;31(5):813–828
56. Goel A. Extended lateral subtemporal approach for petroclival meningiomas: report of experience with 24 cases. Br J Neurosurg 1999;13(3):270–275
57. Spallone A, Makhmudov UB, Mukhamedjanov DJ, Tcherekajev VA. Petroclival meningioma. An attempt to define the role of skull base approaches in their surgical management. Surg Neurol 1999;51(4):412–419
58. Abdel Aziz KM, Sanan A, van Loveren HR, Tew JM Jr, Keller JT, Pensak ML. Petroclival meningiomas: predictive parameters for transpetrosal approaches. Neurosurgery 2000;47(1): 139–150
59. Erkmen K, Pravdenkova S, Al-Mefty O. Surgical management of petroclival meningiomas: factors determining the choice of approach. Neurosurg Focus 2005;19(2):E7
60. Mathiesen T, Gerlich A, Kihlström L, Svensson M, Bagger-Sjöbäck D. Effects of using combined transpetrosal surgical approaches to treat petroclival meningiomas. Neurosurgery 2007;60(6):982–991
61. Van Havenbergh T, Carvalho G, Tatagiba M, Plets C, Samii M. Natural history of petroclival meningiomas. Neurosurgery 2003;52(1):55–62
62. Jung HW, Yoo H, Paek SH, Choi KS. Long-term outcome and growth rate of subtotally resected petroclival meningiomas: experience with 38 cases. Neurosurgery 2000;46(3):567–574
63. Sekhar LN, Schessel DA, Bucur SD, Raso JL, Wright DC. Partial labyrinthectomy petrous apicectomy approach to neoplastic and vascular lesions of the petroclival area. Neurosurgery 1999;44(3):537–550
64. Couldwell WT, Fukushima T, Giannotta SL, Weiss MH. Petroclival meningiomas: surgical experience in 109 cases. J Neurosurg 1996;84(1):20–28
65. Kawase T, Shiobara R, Toya S. Middle fossa transpetrosal-transtentorial approaches for petroclival meningiomas. Selective pyramid resection and radicality. Acta Neurochir (Wien) 1994;129(3-4):113–120
66. Natarajan SK, Sekhar LN, Schessel D, Morita A. Petroclival meningiomas: multimodality treatment and outcomes at long-term follow-up. Neurosurgery 2007;60(6):965–979

67. Park CK, Jung HW, Kim JE, Paek SH, Kim DG. The selection of the optimal therapeutic strategy for petroclival meningiomas. Surg Neurol 2006;66(2):160–165
68. Carvalho GA, Matthies C, Tatagiba M, Eghbal R, Samii M. Impact of computed tomographic and magnetic resonance imaging findings on surgical outcome in petroclival meningiomas. Neurosurgery 2000;47(6):1287–1294
69. Subach BR, Lunsford LD, Kondziolka D, Maitz AH, Flickinger JC. Management of petroclival meningiomas by stereotactic radiosurgery. Neurosurgery 1998;42(3):437–443
70. Akalan N, Seçkin H, Kiliç C, Ozgen T. Benign extramedullary tumors in the foramen magnum region. Clin Neurol Neurosurg 1994;96(4):284–289
71. Arnautović KI, Al-Mefty O, Husain M. Ventral foramen magnum meningiomas. J Neurosurg 2000;92(1, Suppl):71–80
72. Cusimano MD, Faress A, Chang Y, Luong W. Foramen magnum meningiomas. In: DeMonte F, Mcdermott MW, al-Mefty O, eds. Al-Mefty's Meningiomas. New York, NY: Thieme; 2011: 297–307
73. Sekhar LN, Swamy NK, Jaiswal V, Rubinstein E, Hirsch WE Jr, Wright DC. Surgical excision of meningiomas involving the clivus: preoperative and intraoperative features as predictors of postoperative functional deterioration. J Neurosurg 1994;81(6):860–868
74. Bassiouni H, Ntoukas V, Asgari S, Sandalcioglu EI, Stolke D, Seifert V. Foramen magnum meningiomas: clinical outcome after microsurgical resection via a posterolateral suboccipital retrocondylar approach. Neurosurgery 2006;59(6): 1177–1185
75. Bertalanffy H, Gilsbach JM, Mayfrank L, Klein HM, Kawase T, Seeger W. Microsurgical management of ventral and ventrolateral foramen magnum meningiomas. Acta Neurochir Suppl (Wien) 1996;65:82–85
76. Borba LA, de Oliveira JG, Giudicissi-Filho M, Colli BO. Surgical management of foramen magnum meningiomas. Neurosurg Rev 2009;32(1):49–58
77. Boulton MR, Cusimano MD. Foramen magnum meningiomas: concepts, classifications, and nuances. Neurosurg Focus 2003;14(6):e10
78. George B, Lot G, Boissonnet H. Meningioma of the foramen magnum: a series of 40 cases. Surg Neurol 1997;47(4): 371–379
79. Kandenwein JA, Richter HP, Antoniadis G. Foramen magnum meningiomas—experience with the posterior suboccipital approach. Br J Neurosurg 2009;23(1):33–39
80. Kratimenos GP, Crockard HA. The far lateral approach for ventrally placed foramen magnum and upper cervical spine tumours. Br J Neurosurg 1993;7(2):129–140
81. Margalit NS, Lesser JB, Singer M, Sen C. Lateral approach to anterolateral tumors at the foramen magnum: factors determining surgical procedure. Neurosurgery 2005;56(2, Suppl):324–336
82. Meyer FB, Ebersold MJ, Reese DF. Benign tumors of the foramen magnum. J Neurosurg 1984;61(1):136–142
83. Nanda A, Vincent DA, Vannemreddy PS, Baskaya MK, Chanda A. Far-lateral approach to intradural lesions of the foramen magnum without resection of the occipital condyle. J Neurosurg 2002;96(2):302–309
84. Pamir MN, Kiliç T, Ozduman K, Türe U. Experience of a single institution treating foramen magnum meningiomas. J Clin Neurosci 2004;11(8):863–867
85. Pirotte B, David P, Noterman J, Brotchi J. Lower clivus and foramen magnum anterolateral meningiomas: surgical strategy. Neurol Res 1998;20(7):577–584
86. Strang RD, al-Mefty O. Small skull base meningiomas. Surgical management. Clin Neurosurg 2001;48:320–339
87. Wu Z, Hao S, Zhang J, et al. Foramen magnum meningiomas: experiences in 114 patients at a single institute over 15 years. Surg Neurol 2009;72(4):376–382
88. Marin Sanabria EA, Ehara K, Tamaki N. Surgical experience with skull base approaches for foramen magnum meningioma. Neurol Med Chir (Tokyo) 2002;42(11):472–478
89. Samii M, Klekamp J, Carvalho G. Neurosurgery 1996; 39(6):1086–1094
90. Simpson D. The recurrence of intracranial meningiomas after surgical treatment. J Neurol Neurosurg Psychiatry 1957; 20(1):22–39
91. Stafford SL, Pollock BE, Foote RL, et al. Meningioma radiosurgery: tumor control, outcomes, and complications among 190 consecutive patients. Neurosurgery 2001;49(5):1029–1037
92. Lee JY, Niranjan A, McInerney J, Kondziolka D, Flickinger JC, Lunsford LD. Stereotactic radiosurgery providing long-term tumor control of cavernous sinus meningiomas. J Neurosurg 2002;97(1):65–72
93. Starke RM, Williams BJ, Hiles C, Nguyen JH, Elsharkawy MY, Sheehan JP. Gamma knife surgery for skull base meningiomas. J Neurosurg 2012;116(3):588–597
94. Hakim R, Alexander E III, Loeffler JS, et al. Results of linear accelerator-based radiosurgery for intracranial meningiomas. Neurosurgery 1998;42(3):446–453
95. Shafron DH, Friedman WA, Buatti JM, Bova FJ, Mendenhall WM. Linac radiosurgery for benign meningiomas. Int J Radiat Oncol Biol Phys 1999;43(2):321–327
96. Debus J, Wuendrich M, Pirzkall A, et al. High efficacy of fractionated stereotactic radiotherapy of large base-of-skull meningiomas: long-term results. J Clin Oncol 2001;19(15): 3547–3553
97. Dufour H, Muracciole X, Métellus P, Régis J, Chinot O, Grisoli F. Long-term tumor control and functional outcome in patients with cavernous sinus meningiomas treated by radiotherapy with or without previous surgery: is there an alternative to aggressive tumor removal? Neurosurgery 2001;48(2):285–294
98. Maguire PD, Clough R, Friedman AH, Halperin EC. Fractionated external-beam radiation therapy for meningiomas of the cavernous sinus. Int J Radiat Oncol Biol Phys 1999;44(1): 75–79
99. Wenkel E, Thornton AF, Finkelstein D, et al. Benign meningioma: partially resected, biopsied, and recurrent intracranial tumors treated with combined proton and photon radiotherapy. Int J Radiat Oncol Biol Phys 2000;48(5):1363–1370
100. Uy NW, Woo SY, Teh BS, et al. Intensity-modulated radiation therapy (IMRT) for meningioma. Int J Radiat Oncol Biol Phys 2002;53(5):1265–1270

▪ SECTION VIII ▪

Hemangiopericytomas

33

Is There a Need for Gross Total Resection in Management of Hemangiopericytomas in the Era of Radiosurgery?

Syed M. A. Karim, Anand Veeravagu, and Steven D. Chang

Hemangiopericytomas are a rare and aggressive subtype of meningeal tumors. Routine radiographic evaluation of patients with hemangiopericytoma does not easily differentiate this tumor type from the more common and more benign meningioma. The clinical course and treatment response for meningiomas and hemangiopericytomas, however, differ considerably. Hemangiopericytomas are known for their aggressiveness, high recurrence rates, and propensity for extracranial metastasis.[1] Intraoperative (frozen section) pathology of hemangiopericytoma is commonly mistaken for meningioma, thus potentially affecting clinical decision making for degree of resection at the time of surgery. Postoperative (permanent section) pathology may also be mistaken for meningiomas in centers with low tumor volume surgery, thus affecting postoperative decision making with respect to aggressive treatment of residual disease.

This chapter discusses the role of radiosurgery for residual and recurrent disease focusing on the Stanford experience with cyberknife (CK) radiosurgery (Cyberknife, Accuray, Sunnyvale, CA) treatment of patients with hemangiopericytoma. Radiosurgery experiences of other centers in treating residual or recurrent hemangiopericytomas with gamma knife radiosurgery (GKRS) (Gamma Knife, Elekta, Atlanta, GA) are also reviewed. Despite the noteworthy successes of radiosurgery in controlling disease progression in hemangiopericytoma, surgical resection remains by far the first-line treatment.

■ Clinical Presentation and Diagnosis

Hemangiopericytomas occur between the third and fifth decade of life with a slight predominance in males.[2–4] Hemangiopericytomas are most commonly located within the supratentorial compartment within the convexity or parasagittal region.[5] Posterior fossa[6–8] and Meckel cave[9] locations have also been reported. A rare case of hemangiopericytoma in a pediatric patient has also been reported by Arshad and Normala.[10] The majority of patients with hemangiopericytoma develop metastases years after the initial diagnosis,[11] with one reported case of metastasis developing 22 years after the initial intracranial resection.[12] Metastatic disease has been reported between 63 and 99 months after the initial diagnosis of hemangiopericytoma.[13,14] The incidence of distant metastasis increases with time and has been reported as 13, 33, and 64% at 5, 10, and 15 years, respectively.[15]

Common presenting symptoms in patients with hemangiopericytomas include headaches, seizures, and paresis, with symptoms consistent with the anatomical location of the tumor.[13] Patients with hemangiopericytomas demonstrate imaging findings on magnetic resonance imaging (MRI) and computed tomography (CT) similar to those of meningiomas. Tumor margins may often be lobulated and irregular, with dural attachments that are less prominent than those in meningiomas.[4] Calcifications and peritumoral edema are less likely in hemangiopericytoma than in meningiomas.[4] Furthermore, enhancement patterns are more heterogeneous in hemangiopericytoma, with adjacent bone erosion and little to no hyperostosis, in contradistinction to meningiomas, where homogeneous enhancement and hyperostosis are characteristic.[4] Despite these serially observed findings, it is difficult to differentiate meningioma from hemangiopericytoma with absolute certainty based on preoperative radiographic evaluation alone. Magnetic resonance spectroscopy findings in patients with hemangiopericytoma suggest that myoinositol to choline ratio higher than 0.9 may favor a diagnosis of hemangiopericytoma, with a 3.56 ppm shift attributable to myoinositol.[16,17] Furthermore, CT perfusion imaging may provide information differentiating the vascularity of hemangiopericytoma from meningioma.[18] Further advances in imaging are required for preoperative differentiation of these radiographically similar pathologies with divergent natural history and clinical course, particularly in the era of radiosurgery, where diagnostic tumor pathology is not a prerequisite for radiosurgical treatment.

■ World Health Organization Classification and Histopathology

Hemangiopericytomas were considered variants of meningiomas until 1993, when the World Health Organization (WHO) classified them as a distinct tumor type.[1,19] It is probable that the true incidence of hemangiopericytoma prior to 1993 was grossly underestimated due to the confusion with meningiomas and lack of a consistent classification scheme.

First described by Stout and Murray in 1942, hemangiopericytomas arise from Zimmerman pericytes associated with capillary walls[20] and classic staghorn vessels seen on hematoxylin and eosin (H&E) staining.[21] Central nervous system (CNS) hemangiopericytomas are rare and account for < 1% of primary CNS tumors.[15,22] There is no familial clustering, and karyotypic abnormalities are inconsistently found on chromosome 3 and chromosome 12.[2] Histopathologically, hemangiopericytomas are classified as differentiated (WHO grade II) or anaplastic (WHO grade III) tumors.[3] Whereas imaging-based differential diagnosis of hemangiopericytoma should always include meningioma, histopathologically based differential diagnosis should consider the possibility of solitary fibrous tumor.[23,24] Although meningioma and hemangiopericytoma can easily be differentiated on histopathology, the distinction between solitary fibrous tumor and hemangiopericytoma may be more difficult. Fibrous meningiomas consist of psammoma bodies not seen in solitary fibrous tumors. Furthermore, solitary fibrous tumor cells have rich reticulin fibers seen on silver staining.[25] Both solitary fibrous tumor and hemangiopericytoma express CD34 and Bcl-2 antigen and are negative for epithelial membrane antigen (EMA) and S-100 protein.[23,25] Solitary fibrous tumors stain reticulin fibers with coarse collagenous fibers with higher reactivities with CD34 and Bcl-2 than hemangiopericytomas.[23] Most hemangiopericytomas are uniformly cellular and composed of oval to round rather than spindle cells and are immunohistochemically weakly reactive with CD34 and Bcl-2.[24]

■ Surgical and Radiosurgical Treatment of Hemangiopericytomas

Given the current understanding of the natural history of hemangiopericytomas, a randomized study comparing outcomes of radiosurgery alone versus outcomes of surgical resection alone is not possible, since the benefits of surgical resection in prolonging median survival are evident.[1,14] All series published to date, therefore, evaluate outcomes from surgical resection of the primary lesion or outcomes with surgical resection followed by external beam radiation therapy or stereotactic radiosurgery. Chemotherapy may have a modest benefit in improving progression-free survival in hemangiopericytoma.[5]

The standard treatment of hemangiopericytomas consists of gross total resection combined with adjuvant radiotherapy.[26] Rutkowski et al[1] completed a thorough review of the literature focusing on the prognostic factors influencing the mortality rates from hemangiopericytoma.[1] Histories of 563 patients with hemangiopericytoma were reviewed, from which 277 patients could be evaluated. The median survival was 13 years, with 1-, 5-, 10-, and 20-year survival rates of 95%, 82%, 60%, and 23%, respectively. In 105 patients with gross total resection, the median survival was 13 years, whereas the 23 patients with subtotal resection had a median survival of 9.75 years. Patients with tumors of the posterior fossa had a median survival of 10.75 years, versus 15.6 years for those with tumors located elsewhere. Postoperative adjuvant radiation was not associated with a survival benefit. Radiosurgery was not the focus of this study because patients in this analysis had received external beam radiotherapy. However, the benefit of gross surgical resection in prolonging survival was clearly evident in Rutkowski's report. Interestingly, another report by Rutkowski et al[27] analyzing management of recurrent hemangiopericytoma with surgery combined with external beam radiotherapy extended the second-recurrence-free survival. Furthermore, patients undergoing GKRS without surgical resection of recurrence in this study had a decreased second-recurrence-free survival. Although these findings in Rutkowski's small series reiterate the role of surgical resection in hemangiopericytomas, they also suggest that further investigations are needed comparing outcomes of radiosurgery to external beam radiotherapy for hemangiopericytomas.[27]

Stereotactic radiosurgery combines the efficacy of resection with the more minimal rate of radiotherapy-induced morbidity because radiosurgery minimizes radiation to eloquent structures.[28] Given the proposed cellular origin, dural sinus invasion, anatomical inaccessibility, and high vascularity of hemangiopericytomas, gross total resection followed by radiotherapy conveys a mean survival of ~ 84 months from diagnosis.[8]

The role of CK and GKRS in the treatment of hemangiopericytomas has been previously described, with tumor control rates ranging from 46 to 100%.[13,26,28–33] The Stanford University experience using CK stereotactic radiosurgery to treat 14 patients with residual, metastatic, or recurrent CNS hemangiopericytomas has been previously published[7] and a summary of the findings are reviewed.

Stanford Cyberknife Series

Fourteen patients were treated with CK stereotactic radiosurgery between the years 2002 and 2009 at Stanford University Medical Center. All CNS hemangiopericytomas were documented as residual, metastatic, or recurrent, postresection lesions. Seven patients had undergone two or more surgical resections, and seven patients had undergone only one prior operation. Nine patients had received prior cranial irradiation. Presenting symptoms correlated with lesion location and included headache, seizures, visual dysfunction, motor weakness, and tandem gait. In total, the 14 patients harbored 24 hemangiopericytomas. Tumors were located in supra- and infratentorial sites as well as spinal locations (**Table 33.1**). All 14 patients and 24 tumors were treated with CK stereotactic radiosurgery. Patients underwent a stereotactic MRI scan (2.0 mm slice thickness) with gadolinium contrast, which was

Table 33.1 Summary of patient characteristics

Pt. no.	Age at onset/ gender	Clinical presentation	No. of surgeries before CK	Radiation therapy before CK	Site	Grade	Time to CK postsurgery	No. of CK treatments	Follow-up (months)
1	43M	HA, Vis	1	N	Torcular	3	2 years	1	73
2	39M	Vis	2	54 Gy	Parasellar	–	16 years	2	36, 64
3	58M	Leg weak	2	45 Gy	T6–8	3	6 years	1	37
4	47M	HA, ataxia, Vis	1	N	Parafalcine	1	1 month	1	37
5	42F	Leg weak, Sz	2	N	Parafalcine	–	10 years	1	39
6	29F	HA, hand weak	1	N	Tentorium	1	1 month	3	53, 30, 10
7	47F	Sen loss, Vis	1	GK	C- T- spine	–	10 years	1	26, 45
8	69F	Foot drop	1	N	Parafalcine	2	1 month	1	41
9	38M	HA, Sz	1	50.4 Gy	Left middle fossa	–	9 months	1	59
10	51F	Left buttock pain	4	Y	Lumbar spine	–	16 years	3	15
11	41F	HA, Vis	2	59.4 Gy	Rt inf. cerebellar	3	5 years	1	30
12	53F	Numbness, facial pain, diplopia	2	Y	Rt temporal, cav sinus	–	14 years	3	–
13	38F	Left facial palsy, tandem gait	2	54 Gy	Pineal space, left tentorium	–	15 years	2	–
14	35M	HA	1	Y	Posterior fossa	–	12 years	2	15

Abbreviations: GK, Gamma Knife, Elekta; HA, headache; N, none; Sen loss, sensory loss: Sz, seizure; Vis, visual deficits; Y, prior radiation but no dosage available.

Source: Veeravagu A, Jiang B, Patil CG, et al. CyberKnife stereotactic radiosurgery for recurrent, metastatic, and residual hemangiopericytomas. J Hematol Oncol 2011;4:26. Adapted with permission.

then fused to the stereotactic CT scan. Tumor volume was carefully contoured and inverse treatment planning was performed to achieve a conformal treatment plan that minimized dose to adjacent eloquent structures (**Fig. 33.1**). For spinal treatments prior to 2005, patients first underwent implantation of either straight gold fiducials or stainless steel screws for tracking of spinal bony landmarks. Following implantation, the patient returned for a treatment planning CT. The Xsight spine tracking system (Accuray, Sunnyvale, CA) has now eliminated the use of fiducial implantation.[34]

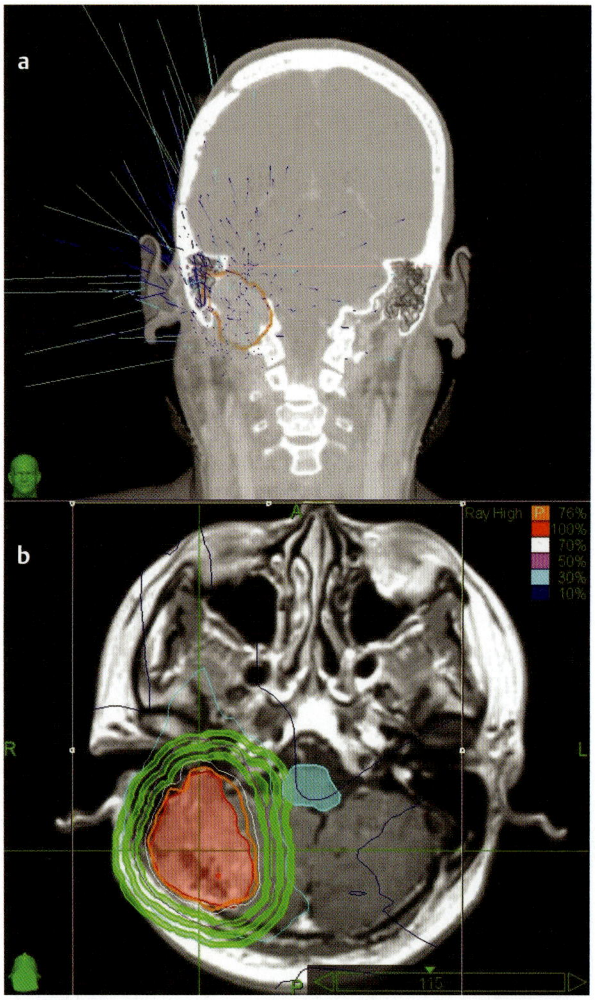

Fig. 33.1 CyberKnife (Accuray) contour for patient 14, a 47-year-old male who was treated for a 56.7 cm^3 in the posterior fossa. A single fraction at marginal dose of 21 Gy and maximum dose of 27.6 Gy was used. The isodose line was 76% and the conformity index was 1.19. At 15 months follow-up, the tumor was stable. (From Veeravagu A, Jiang B, Patil CG, et al. CyberKnife stereotactic radiosurgery for recurrent, metastatic, and residual hemangiopericytomas. J Hematol Oncol 2011;4:26. Used with permission.)

Of the 14 patients treated, follow-up data were available for 12 patients, accounting for a total of 22 tumors. Radiographic follow-up evaluation included gadolinium-enhanced MRI scans obtained every 4 months for the first year after treatment, every 6 months during the second year, and annually thereafter. Clinical follow-up examination was conducted at the same intervals. The median clinical and radiographic follow-up period was 37 months (range 10 to 73 months). In this series, all patients with brain hemangiopericytomas who were treated with more than one session had their hemangiopericytoma located next to the brainstem, cavernous sinus, or optic pathways. Of those 22 tumors, follow-up MRI showed 12 decreased in size (54.5%), 6 remained unchanged (27.3%), and 4 recurred or increased in size (18.2%) after CK therapy. The progression-free survival rate was 95%, 71.5%, and 71.5% at 1, 3, and 5 years, respectively, after multiple CK treatments. The 5-year survival rate after CK treatment in the Stanford series was 81%. There did not appear to be a correlation between treatment dose, tumor volume, and tumor response in the Stanford study.[7]

Gamma Knife Stereotactic Radiosurgery

Multiple series have reported the role of GKRS in the treatment of hemangiopericytomas.[14,26,28–33,35–38] In 1993, Coffey et al provided the first radiosurgical report for the treatment of hemangiopericytomas. GKRS treatment was delivered in five patients with 11 hemangiopericytomas after surgical resection of an initial intracranial lesion.[35] Galanis et al added five more patients to the Coffey series for a total of 20 hemangiopericytomas.[14] Of the radiosurgically treated lesions, 14 of the hemangiopericytomas decreased in size, four disappeared radiographically, and two were stable in size. However, lesions that decrease in size with radiosurgery may subsequently enlarge. Payne et al[31] reported on 10 patients with 12 lesions who had undergone treatment with GKRS.[31] Four of the nine tumors that decreased in size subsequently increased in size after a mean of 22 months postradiosurgery.

Olson et al reported 21 patients with 28 lesions who were treated with GKRS.[30] These patients had received a mean marginal dose of 17 Gy, and at last follow-up, the tumor control rate was 46.4%. Olson's series reported the lowest control rate, with the longest mean follow-up (69 months) of all the radiosurgery series. Iwai and Yamanaka[38] with the second-longest mean follow-up of 61 months in eight patients, had a tumor control rate of 100% on last follow-up. Thus, longer follow-up did not necessarily account for the lower tumor control rates seen by Olson et al.[30]

Kim et al published a series of 17 hemangiopericytomas in nine patients treated with surgery followed

Table 33.2 Published studies on stereotactic radiosurgery for hemangiopericytoma

Study	Institution	Study period	Treatment modality	No. patients/ lesions	Mean marginal dose (Gy)	Mean follow-up (months)	Tumor control at last follow-up (%)
Coffey 1993[35]	Mayo Clinic	1990–1992	Gamma Knife[c]	5/11	15.5	14.8	81.8
Galanis et al 1998[14]	Mayo Clinic	1976–1996	Gamma Knife	10/20	12 to 18	6 to 36	100[a]
Payne et al 2000[31]	U of Virginia	1991–1999	Gamma Knife	10/12	14	24.8	75
Sheehan et al 2002[26]	U of Pittsburgh	1987–2001	Gamma Knife	14/15	15	31.3	80
Chang and Sakamoto 2003[28]	Stanford	1992–2002	Linac, CyberKnife[d]	8/8	20.5	44	75
Ecker et al 2003[29]	Mayo Clinic	1980–2000	Gamma Knife	15/45	16	45.6	93[b]
Kano et al 2008[36]	U of Pittsburgh	1989–2006	Gamma Knife	20/29	15	37.9	72.4
Sun et al 2009[32]	Beijing Neu. Ins.	1994–2006	Gamma Knife	22/58	13.5	26	89.7
Iwai and Yamanaka 2009[38]	Osaka City Hosp	1994–2003	Gamma Knife	8/13	15.1	61	100
Olson et al 2010[30]	U of Virginia	1989–2008	Gamma Knife	21/28	17	69	46.4
Veeravagu et al 2011[7]	Stanford	2002–2009	CyberKnife	14/22	21.2	37	81.8
Kim et al 2010[33]	Seoul Nat'l Inst	1999–2008	Gamma Knife	9/17	18.1	33.8	82.4

Abbreviations: Linac, linear accelerator.

[a] Tumors responded to GKS with decrease or stability in volume, but effect lasted less than 1 year in majority of patients. Study also includes the five patients from Coffey et al. 1993 manuscript.

[b] Also includes five patients from Coffey et al. 1993 manuscript.

[c] Elekta, Atlanta, GA.

[d] Accuray, Sunnyvale, CA.

Source: From Veeravagu A, Jiang B, Patil CG, et al. CyberKnife stereotactic radiosurgery for recurrent, metastatic, and residual hemangiopericytomas. J Hematol Oncol 2011;4:26. Adapted with permission.

by GKRS.[33] The tumor control rate was noted to be 82.4%. Furthermore, statistical analysis in this series suggests that marginal doses > 17 Gy may be associated with better tumor control rates.

The 12 recently published studies on stereotactic radiosurgery for recurrent and residual hemangiopericytomas have been summarized in **Table 33.2.**[14,26,28–33,35–38]

Expert Recommendation

The clear benefits of surgery prohibit randomized trials of surgical resection versus radiosurgery alone, and thus baseline therapy often includes both modalities. Furthermore, the relatively low incidence of hemangiopericytomas prevents randomized, controlled trials. At this time, based on clinical case series from various institutions, the level of evidence remains IV for the treatment of intracranial hemangiopericytomas with radiosurgical therapy following surgical resection (Grade 2C Recommendation, Level IV Evidence).

■ Summary and Conclusions

Characteristic of hemangiopericytomas is their aggressive pathology, high recurrence rate, and propensity for distant metastasis.[1] Gross total resection remains the initial treatment of choice for those lesions that are surgically accessible[1,14,26]; however, postoperative stereotactic radiosurgery has been shown to be effective in increasing time to recurrence as well as survival. Due to the aggressive nature of hemangiopericytomas, initial decreases in tumor size or even disappearance may be followed by regrowth.[31] As suggested by the Stanford CK series and multiple published GKRS series, stereotactic radiosurgery results in effective tumor control (**Table 33.2**). Marginal doses > 17 Gy may be associated with better tumor control.[33] Despite surgical resection and subsequent radiosurgery, clinical and radiographic follow-up is necessary due to the high probability of local recurrence and distant metastases.

■ References

1. Rutkowski MJ, Sughrue ME, Kane AJ, et al. Predictors of mortality following treatment of intracranial hemangiopericytoma. J Neurosurg 2010;113(2):333–339
2. Lamar Z, Lesser GJ. Management of meningeal neoplasms: meningiomas and hemangiopericytomas. Curr Treat Options Oncol 2011;12(3):230–239
3. Zweckberger K, Jung CS, Mueller W, Unterberg AW, Schick U. Hemangiopericytomas grade II are not benign tumors. Acta Neurochir (Wien) 2011;153(2):385–394
4. Sibtain NA, Butt S, Connor SEJ. Imaging features of central nervous system haemangiopericytomas. Eur Radiol 2007; 17(7):1685–1693
5. Chamberlain MC, Glantz MJ. Sequential salvage chemotherapy for recurrent intracranial hemangiopericytoma. Neurosurgery 2008;63(4):720–726, author reply 726–727
6. Tashjian VS, Khanlou N, Vinters HV, Canalis RF, Becker DP. Hemangiopericytoma of the cerebellopontine angle: a case report and review of the literature. Surg Neurol 2009; 72(3):290–295
7. Veeravagu A, Jiang B, Patil CG, et al. CyberKnife stereotactic radiosurgery for recurrent, metastatic, and residual hemangiopericytomas. J Hematol Oncol 2011;4:26
8. Kumar R, Wani AA. Unusual tumors of the posterior fossa skull base. Skull Base 2006;16(2):75–84
9. Muto J, Kawase T, Yoshida K. Meckel's cave tumors: relation to the meninges and minimally invasive approaches for surgery: anatomic and clinical studies. Neurosurgery 2010;67(3, Suppl Operative):ons291–ons298
10. Arshad AR, Normala B. Infantile malignant hemangiopericytoma of the orbit. Ophthal Plast Reconstr Surg 2008;24(2): 147–148
11. van der Starre PJA, Sze DY, Guta C, Mitchell RS, Dake MD. Stent-graft repair of an aortic rupture caused by invasive hemangiopericytoma. Ann Thorac Surg 2006;81(6):2300–2302
12. Suzuki H, Haga Y, Oguro K, Shinoda S, Masuzawa T, Kanai N. Intracranial hemangiopericytoma with extracranial metastasis occurring after 22 years. Neurol Med Chir (Tokyo) 2002; 42(7):297–300
13. Dufour H, Métellus P, Fuentes S, et al. Meningeal hemangiopericytoma: a retrospective study of 21 patients with special review of postoperative external radiotherapy. Neurosurgery 2001;48(4):756–762
14. Galanis E, Buckner JC, Scheithauer BW, Kimmel DW, Schomberg PJ, Piepgras DG. Management of recurrent meningeal hemangiopericytoma. Cancer 1998;82(10):1915–1920
15. Guthrie BL, Ebersold MJ, Scheithauer BW, Shaw EG. Meningeal hemangiopericytoma: histopathological features, treatment, and long-term follow-up of 44 cases. Neurosurgery 1989;25(4):514–522
16. Fortuniak J, Jaskolski DJ, Stefanczyk L, Zawirski M, Gajewicz W. Magnetic resonance imaging of rare intracranial neoplasms—role of the in vivo ^{1}H spectroscopy in the radiological differential diagnostics. Cen Eur Neurosurg 2010;71:181–188
17. Barba I, Moreno A, Martinez-Pérez I, et al. Magnetic resonance spectroscopy of brain hemangiopericytomas: high myoinositol concentrations and discrimination from meningiomas. J Neurosurg 2001;94(1):55–60
18. Ren G, Chen S, Wang Y, Zhu RJ, Geng DY, Feng XY. Quantitative evaluation of benign meningioma and hemangiopericytoma with peritumoral brain edema by 64-slice CT perfusion imaging. Chin Med J (Engl) 2010;123(15):2038–2044
19. Spatola C, Privitera G. Recurrent intracranial hemangiopericytoma with extracranial and unusual multiple metastases: case report and review of the literature. Tumori 2004; 90(2):265–268
20. Stout AP, Murray MR. Hemangiopericytoma: a vascular tumor featuring Zimmerman's pericytes. Ann Surg 1942;116(1): 26–33
21. Burger PC, Scheithauer BW, Vogel FS. Surgical Pathology of the Nervous System and Its Coverings. 3rd ed. New York, NY: Churchill Livingstone; 1991
22. Akiyama M, Sakai H, Onoue H, Miyazaki Y, Abe T. Imaging intracranial haemangiopericytomas: study of seven cases. Neuroradiology 2004;46(3):194–197
23. Hori E, Kurimoto M, Fukuda O, et al. Recurrent intracranial solitary fibrous tumor initially diagnosed as hemangiopericytoma. Brain Tumor Pathol 2007;24(1):31–34
24. Bisceglia M, Dimitri L, Giannatempo G, et al. Solitary fibrous tumor of the central nervous system: report of an additional 5 cases with comprehensive literature review. Int J Surg Pathol 2011;19(4):476–486
25. Teranishi K, Yamamoto T, Nakao Y, Osada H, Wada R, Mori K. Recurrent solitary fibrous tumor of the falx cerebri with intraventricular extension: case report. Neurol Med Chir (Tokyo) 2007;47(6):269–272
26. Sheehan J, Kondziolka D, Flickinger J, Lunsford LD. Radiosurgery for treatment of recurrent intracranial hemangiopericytomas. Neurosurgery 2002;51(4):905–910
27. Rutkowski MJ, Bloch O, Jian BJ, et al. Management of recurrent intracranial hemangiopericytoma. J Clin Neurosci 2011;18(11):1500–1504
28. Chang SD, Sakamoto GT. The role of radiosurgery for hemangiopericytomas. Neurosurg Focus 2003;14(5):e14
29. Ecker RD, Marsh WR, Pollock BE, et al. Hemangiopericytoma in the central nervous system: treatment, pathological features, and long-term follow up in 38 patients. J Neurosurg 2003;98(6):1182–1187
30. Olson C, Yen CP, Schlesinger D, Sheehan J. Radiosurgery for intracranial hemangiopericytomas: outcomes after initial and repeat Gamma Knife surgery. J Neurosurg 2010;112(1): 133–139
31. Payne BR, Prasad D, Steiner M, Steiner L. Gamma surgery for hemangiopericytomas. Acta Neurochir (Wien) 2000; 142(5):527–536
32. Sun S, Liu A, Wang C. Gamma knife radiosurgery for recurrent and residual meningeal hemangiopericytomas. Stereotact Funct Neurosurg 2009;87(2):114–119
33. Kim JW, Kim DG, Chung HT, et al. Gamma Knife stereotactic radiosurgery for intracranial hemangiopericytomas. J Neurooncol 2010;99(1):115–122
34. Ho AK, Fu D, Cotrutz C, et al. A study of the accuracy of cyberknife spinal radiosurgery using skeletal structure tracking. Neurosurgery 2007;60(2, Suppl 1):ons147–ons156
35. Coffey RJ, Cascino TL, Shaw EG. Radiosurgical treatment of recurrent hemangiopericytomas of the meninges: preliminary results. J Neurosurg 1993;78(6):903–908
36. Kano H, Niranjan A, Kondziolka D, Flickinger JC, Lunsford LD. Adjuvant stereotactic radiosurgery after resection of intracranial hemangiopericytomas. Int J Radiat Oncol Biol Phys 2008;72(5):1333–1339
37. Glaholm J, Bloom HJ, Crow JH. The role of radiotherapy in the management of intracranial meningiomas: the Royal Marsden Hospital experience with 186 patients. Int J Radiat Oncol Biol Phys 1990;18(4):755–761
38. Iwai Y, Yamanaka K. Gamma knife radiosurgery for other primary intra-axial tumors. Prog Neurol Surg 2009;22: 129–141

SECTION IX

Meningeal Sarcoma

34

The Role of Surgery and Adjuvant Therapies for Meningeal Sarcoma with Brain Invasion

Edward W. Swanson and Chad R. Gordon

Primary sarcoma of the central nervous system (CNS) is rare, with the reported incidence varying from 0.1 to 3.0% of all CNS tumors.[1] Variation in incidence is due in part to its ill-defined nature. Historical reports grouped medulloblastoma, glioblastoma, gliosarcoma, oligodendroglioma, angioma, aneurysms, parasitic cysts, lymphoma, and granuloma as sarcoma.[2] Recent studies have included hemangiopericytoma, reticulum cell sarcoma, and diffuse sarcomatosis, resulting in falsely high rates. Furthermore, primary CNS sarcoma is often difficult to distinguish from other primary CNS tumors, and studies frequently include primaries of alternate origin with resultant sarcomatous differentiation. Although controversy remains, primary CNS sarcoma is thought to arise from pluripotent mesenchymal cells in the dura mater, the leptomeninges or their pial extensions, the stroma of the choroid plexus, the tela choroidea, and the vascular adventitia. The etiology of these tumors is unknown but can be associated with prior brain irradiation, immunocompromise with Epstein-Barr virus (EBV) infection, and possibly trauma, including surgical manipulation.[1,3–11] Primary CNS sarcoma can occur at any age, with more frequent reports in the pediatric population, including congenital primary CNS sarcoma. Both sexes are affected equally and there is no predilection for a certain site of origin.[12] There is a low propensity to spread, although there have been case reports of multifocal disease and metastasis. In general, prognosis is poor, and rapid growth and recurrence are common.

This chapter discusses the role of surgery and adjuvant therapy in the treatment of primary meningeal sarcoma with brain invasion. Only primary CNS sarcoma originating from the meninges is included, (1) aligning with the classification of Rubinstein as a tumor originating from the leptomeninges [and dura] invading the brain tissue and (2) after complete immunohistochemical analysis, carcinoma, lymphoma, glioma, and primitive neuroectodermal tumors (PNETs) are excluded.[13] The most recent World Health Organization (WHO) classification of CNS tumors includes fibrosarcoma, liposarcoma, leiomyosarcoma, rhabdomyosarcoma, chondrosarcoma, osteosarcoma, and angiosarcoma as mesenchymal tumors of the meninges (**Table 34.1**). In many cases, the sarcoma subtype cannot be identified, and the tumor is classified as undifferentiated sarcoma. Meningeal sarcomatosis is excluded here because it presents a different clinical picture and requires unique management strategies not applicable to localized primary meningeal sarcoma.

With sparse evidence in the literature, which is almost entirely populated by case reports, *no* standard treatment exists for primary meningeal sarcoma with brain invasion. The available evidence is reviewed and recommendations for future practice are provided, with emphasis on avoiding and managing surgical complications.

Table 34.1 2007 World Health Organization classification of tumors of the central nervous system: mesenchymal tumors of the meninges categorized as sarcoma

Fibrosarcoma
Liposarcoma
Leiomyosarcoma
Rhabdomyosarcoma
Chondrosarcoma
Osteosarcoma
Angiosarcoma

■ Diagnosis

Primary meningeal sarcoma presents with a similar clinical picture to meningioma, with new onset neurological signs and symptoms related to extrinsic compression. Neuroradiological features are nonspecific. Magnetic resonance (MR) signals are consistent with a vascular, edematous mass. Specifically, meningeal sarcoma displays iso-/hyperintense T1 signal, hyperintense T2 signal, with heterogeneous enhancement, irregular margins, and cystic and hemorrhagic areas. On computed tomographic (CT) examination, these tumors are iso-/hyperdense, with heterogeneous enhancement, irregular borders, and occasional calcifications.[14] Erosion of the calvaria and hyperostosis can be present (**Fig. 34.1**). The differential diagnosis based on radiological findings includes meningioma, metastasis from extracranial neoplasms, and intracranial extension from a cranial or parameningeal site. Moreover, radiological diagnosis is difficult.

Immunohistochemical analysis remains the gold standard for diagnosis of meningeal sarcoma. The tumor presents as a malignant mesenchymal neoplasm in which no meningothelial components are present. However, meningeal sarcoma can present with varying features and a wide range of subtypes, complicating the diagnosis. Furthermore, reports of meningeal sarcoma with meningothelial elements exist. Of note, the distinction between malignant meningioma and meningeal sarcoma can be difficult because sarcomatous progression of a preexisting meningioma occurs. Findings consistent with meningeal sarcoma include negative glial and neuronal markers with strong vimentin positivity. Electron microscopy aids in the diagnosis, with spindle-shaped cells, dilated rough endoplasmic reticulum, lack of well developed junctions, abundance of intermediate filaments, and the absence of neurosecretory granules and microvilli all pointing toward cells of mesenchymal origin. Special stains and electron microscopy can further define subtype. Grade of the tumor is based on cellularity, differentiation, pleomorphism, mitotic rate, and necrosis. Once diagnosis is confirmed, craniospinal axis imaging, bone scan, and chest/abdomen/pelvis CT and/or positron-emission tomographic (PET) scan should be performed to identify all sites of disease, allow for staging, and rule out extracranial primary with metastasis.[15] If not contradicted, lumbar puncture can additionally be performed to assess for leptomenogeal spread.

■ Management of Primary Meningeal Sarcoma

In general, the goal of treatment for primary meningeal sarcoma is complete eradication of the tumor. Moreover, management of meningeal sarcoma mirrors that of soft tissue sarcoma, relying heavily on radical operative resection with additional treatment regimens depending on subtype. Consequently, the use of adjuvant radiation and chemotherapy depends on tumor pathology, is inconsistent, and has evolved with improved technology and current chemotherapeutic regimens. With a paucity of long-term follow-up reported in the literature, the optimal treatment strategy in the presence of brain invasion is difficult to determine.

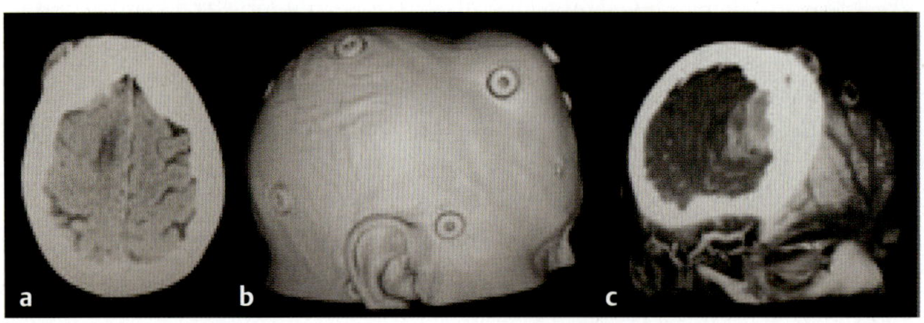

Fig. 34.1 Axial **(a)** and three-dimensional reconstruction **(b,c)** computed tomographic images of meningeal sarcoma with osseous invasion/degradation and extracranial extension.

Surgery

Radical operative resection is the mainstay of treatment for primary meningeal sarcoma with brain invasion. The goal is to achieve maximum feasible resection, with total extirpation providing the best outcomes while not risking neurological function. Subtotal and partial resection decrease chances for long-term disease-free survival.

Proper techniques with tension-free closures are essential for avoiding peri- and postoperative complications and providing the patient with the best results. Therefore, in certain cases a consultation with a craniofacial plastic surgeon may be of benefit. As with patients undergoing resection for meningioma, patients with meningeal sarcoma are often left with dural deficits, large bone flaps, and wide incisions. The initial soft tissue dissection can be performed in the subpericranial plane utilizing bone wax to control emissary vein bleeding, or in the suprapericranial plane, to minimize blood loss. However, suprapericranial dissection may result in compromise of vascularity when replacing the bone flap at closure, especially if the scalp has been irradiated. The incision should be performed in a segmental manner, using clips as the dissection proceeds. To avoid alopecia, bipolar electrocautery should be used prudently. Optimal closure includes strict adherence to sterile technique, complete dural integrity, rigid fixation of the bone flap, and layered closure of the scalp over closed suction drains (**Fig. 34.2**). Of note, drains should *not* be placed in any dissection areas located near invaded dura and/or sinus cavities (i.e., frontal sinus). Pericranial flaps and grafts are used to reinforce dural repairs and to cover defects, and can be further supported with fibrin glue. Larger dural defects may require fascial grafts or the use of a dural substitute. A final intraoperative examination must ensure complete hemostasis and the absence of cerebrospinal fluid (CSF) leaks.[16]

Level I and Level II Evidence

There are no Level I or II evidence studies comparing operative versus nonoperative management of primary meningeal sarcoma with brain invasion.

Level III Evidence

In general, all studies of meningeal sarcoma attempt maximum feasible resection as first-line therapy, making comparison of operative versus nonoperative therapy difficult. Furthermore, patients not undergoing operative resection are typically thought to have unresectable or systemic disease. However, case series exist documenting the extent of resection, and the need for total versus subtotal/partial resection is an important question to be addressed.

In a series of 16 pediatric patients with CNS sarcoma, Al-Gahtany et al reported their experience with various treatments of these rare tumors.[3] For patients who underwent total resection, survival ranged from 3 months to 16 years (mean, 6.2 years) versus survival in those who received subtotal resection ranging from 1 month to 14 years (mean, 3.4 years). In the subset of six patients with meningeal sarcoma, survival ranged from 10 months to 16 years for those who had total resection versus a survival of 22 months for the one patient who underwent subtotal resection. Over all, it is difficult to determine the effects of the extent of resection, but nevertheless, there appears to be a trend favoring total resection. However, those patients in whom only subtotal resection could be achieved may be presenting with more aggressive tumors, or tumors invading more critical areas, creating a bias in the data. In addition, patients received widely different combinations of adjuvant radiation and chemotherapy. Recurrence is common even in cases of total resection, implying that microscopic disease is often left behind, questioning the need for overly aggressive operations.

Level IV Evidence

Case reports govern the vast majority of literature pertaining to meningeal sarcoma, and maximum feasible resection is employed in nearly all. Therefore, deducing differences in outcomes based on the extent of resection is nearly impossible, and details of every case report would prove impractical. With the advent of improved radiation technology, it is possible that local control of residual disease may be better than overtly aggressive operations. Nonethe-

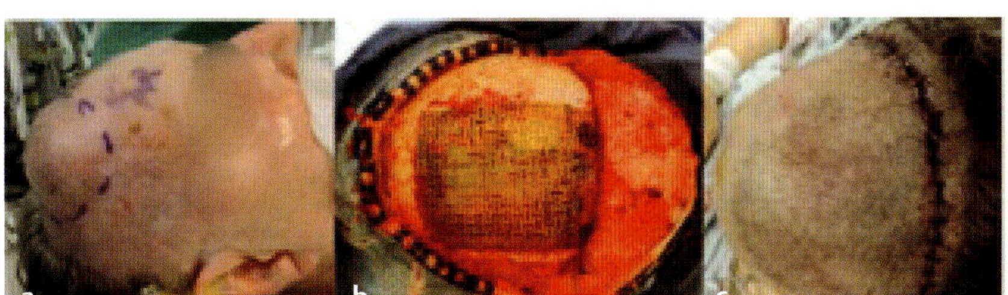

Fig. 34.2 Intraoperative photographs of a patient with meningeal sarcoma with extracranial extension demonstrating the planned incision **(a)**, titanium mesh cranioplasty **(b)**, and layered closure over closed suction drains **(c)**.

less, it is unlikely in such a rare disease that a conclusive study will be performed to elucidate the benefits of total versus subtotal resection. Moreover, the only true long-term survival has been seen in instances of total extirpation of well circumscribed tumors, such as the patient who achieved 21-year survival after two gross total resections by Christensen and Lara.[17]

Surgical Complications

In the immediate postoperative period, patients must be monitored closely. Hemorrhage requires emergent operative exploration. CSF leaks may present as rhinorrhea, otorrhea, or increased output from closed suction drains. High-output CSF leaks likely indicate significant dural compromise and require intraoperative repair.

Perioperative antibiotics should be utilized to minimize the risk of infection. Poor wound healing, incisional drainage, and purulence should raise suspicion of an infected bone flap. Irradiated scalp flaps require meticulous design with large base:width ratios and delicate preservation of underlying pericranium. Attempts to manage infected bone flaps with thorough irrigation and parenteral antibiotics often prove inadequate and typically, infected bone flaps require removal. In such cases, patients are left with large cranial defects and should be provided with a protective helmet. Definitive cranioplasty should be delayed 3 to 6 months to allow for resolution of the infection. Large cranial defects result in increased brain tissue compliance and consequently patients can develop herniation, even in the presence of normotensive intracranial pressure (ICP). Transcranial cerebral herniation presents a difficult problem, and patients desire definitive closure to return to their preoperative state. When conservative measures (such as head of bed elevation, hyperventilation, osmotic diuresis, durotomy with CSF evacuation, and manual compression) fail to reduce the herniation, *bipolar duraplasty* can be employed, as introduced by Gordon and colleagues in 2011.[18] In bipolar duraplasty, bipolar electrocautery is used to score the dura in a crosshatch pattern to safely and transiently reduce transcranial cerebral herniation and allow for definitive cranioplasty (**Fig. 34.3**). This technique has been used successfully to restore cranial integrity, providing an option for earlier closure, permanent protection, and a satisfying aesthetic result.[18]

In addition, from an aesthetic standpoint, following pterional craniotomies patients can develop unilateral or bilateral temporal hollowing. This may be related to the surgery itself, temporalis foreshortening/displacement, and/or postoperative irradiation. In either instance, the senior surgeon recommends subcutaneous temporal augmentation, which employs a methylmethacrylate implant attached to screws extending posterolaterally from the lateral orbit.[19]

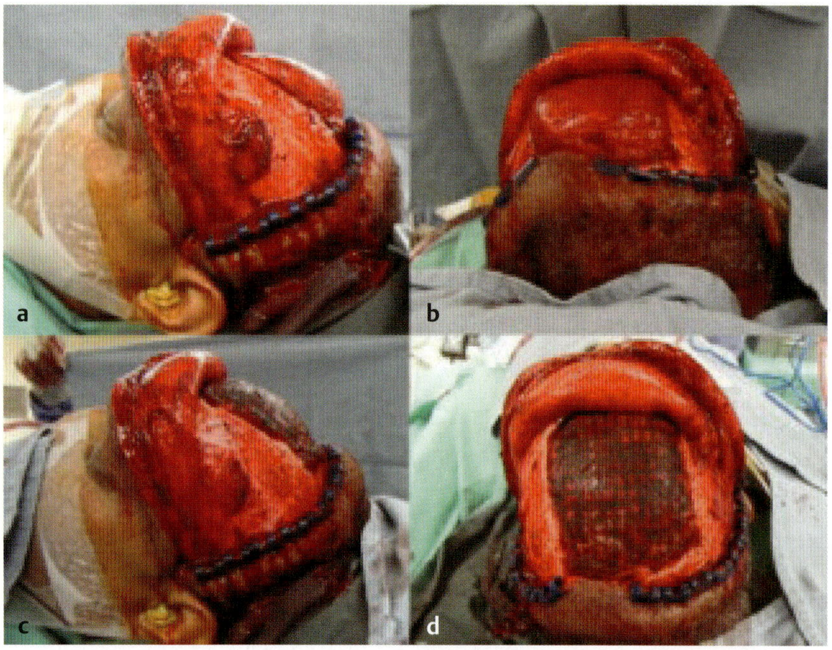

Fig. 34.3 Intraoperative images of external cerebral herniation **(a,b)** through a large bifrontal cranial defect with associated photographs **(c,d)** demonstrating immediate transient reduction following bipolar duraplasty. (With permission from Gordon CR, Swanson E, Westvik T, Yaremchuk MJ. Bipolar duraplasty: A new technique for transient correction of cerebral herniation during definitive cranioplasty. J Neurosurg. 2011;115(5):1026.)

Over all, patients must be observed continuously, and complications must be addressed promptly to provide patients with optimal outcomes. Although primary meningeal sarcoma carries a poor prognosis, long-term survival can be achieved, and proper peri- and postoperative management provides patients with the best chance to return to a normal quality of life.

Recommendations for Operative Management of Primary Meningeal Sarcoma

1. Maximum feasible resection is the mainstay of treatment for primary meningeal sarcoma with brain invasion (Grade 1C Recommendation, Level III/IV Evidence).
2. Definitive diagnosis is usually delayed until final microscopic analysis is complete, with the majority of meningeal sarcomas diagnosed radiologically as meningiomas preoperatively. Upon final diagnosis of meningeal sarcoma, investigation of the extent of disease should be undertaken, and the patient should be followed closely for signs of recurrence, and re-resection may be indicated.
3. With radical resection providing the best chance for long-term survival, steps must be taken to ensure peri- and postoperative morbidity and mortality are minimized. Complete aseptic technique, preserved dural integrity, and complex layered wound closure over closed suction drains remain at the heart of any craniofacial operation. In addition, it is important to avoid unnecessary cautery (i.e., alopecia), excessive temporal dissection (i.e., temporal fat pad atrophy), temporalis disinsertion, and high-tension scalp closures. For those difficult skin closures, careful galeal scoring with needle-point cautery parallel to the incision, in combination with contralateral subpericranial dissection, seems to improve wound edge approximation in most nonirradiated cases. Thorough perioperative care will give the patient the chance for maximum survival far exceeding any minimal gains that may be achieved with adjuvant therapies.

Adjuvant Radiation

Despite its aggressive nature and rapid growth, meningeal sarcoma is not particularly radiosensitive.[2] Nevertheless, adjuvant radiation is commonly employed to treat and control microscopic and gross residual disease (**Table 34.2**). However, this often adds complexity to scalp flap design and viability if and when secondary surgery may be indicated.

Level I and Level II Evidence

There are no Level I or II evidence studies comparing radiation versus no radiation in patients with primary meningeal sarcoma with brain invasion.

Level III Evidence

With no standard treatment regimen available, the use of adjuvant radiation is becoming typical for meningeal sarcoma because of its poor prognosis. Al-Gahtany and colleagues found clinically significant improved outcomes in patients with CNS sarcoma receiving radiation (4,500 to 5,900 cGy), with a mean survival of 7 years (range 10 months to 16 years) compared with only 6 months (range 3 to 22 months) in patients who did not receive radiation.[3] They concluded that maximal surgical resection followed by radiation provided the best treatment possible.

Level IV Evidence

The benefits of radiation in extracranial sarcoma have been repeatedly proven.[20,21] In their report of nine patients with primary cerebral sarcoma, Gaspar and coworkers quoted a required dose of 64 to 66 Gy to treat microscopic and residual extracranial fibrosarcoma.[22] However, these doses are at the upper limit of those tolerated by the normal brain, and the authors suggest using cone-down external beam techniques, with 3- to 4-cm margins for the first 60 Gy and 1- to 2-cm margins of 4 to 6 Gy thereafter. Furthermore, they advise against the use of craniospinal radiation because there is no evidence to suggest the dose of radiation tolerated by the neuraxis can control extracranial fibrosarcoma. In their own patients, for five that had meningeal fibrosarcoma, they employed adjuvant radiation at doses of 45 to 60 Gy in 2.0 to 2.7 Gy daily fractions, consisting of whole brain plus boost or local field. One patient was alive and well at 100 months, and the overall median survival was 9 months, with at least one local recurrence in every patient. Tomita and Gonzalez-Crussi also used adjuvant radiation in every patient in their series of CNS sarcoma, but they concluded that total resection afforded the best prognosis, whereas no conclusion could be drawn about the use of radiation or chemotherapy.[23]

Table 34.2 Evidence table for the role of adjuvant radiation in the treatment of meningeal sarcoma

Level of evidence	Study	Sarcoma subtype	Outcomes[a]
Level I and II	No Papers		
Level III	Al-Gahtany et al 2003[3]	Undifferentiated	Improved outcomes in patients receiving radiation
	Sugita et al 2009[31]	Sarcoma with leiomyoblastic differentiation	Series of two patients with one receiving 50 Gy and surviving 3 years
Level IV	Gaspar et al 1993[22]	Fibrosarcoma	Nine patients receiving 45 to 60 Gy whole brain plus boost or local field radiation
	Tomita and Gonzalez-Crussi 1984[23]	Undifferentiated	Eight patients receiving adjuvant radiation with no conclusions as to efficacy
	Romeo et al 2010[26]	Osteoblastic chondrosarcoma	60 Gy in 30 fractions with no relapse at 43 months
	Utsuki et al 2009[32]	Osteosarcoma with rhabdomyosarcoma component	Unspecified radiation used in a patient who developed osteosarcoma following radiation for previous astrocytoma who survived 5 years with eight recurrences
	Osipov et al 2002[10]	Osteosarcoma	54 Gy in 27 fractions given to patient with postradiation osteosarcoma who expired at 18 months
	Setzer et al 2002[33]	Osteosarcoma	Patient alive at 3 years following 60 Gy in 30 fractions
	Alleyne et al 2000[30]	Osteosarcoma	Patient died of thromboembolism following aggressive adjuvant radiation and chemotherapy
	Palta et al 2011[15]	Rhabdomyosarcoma	59.4 Gy plus radiosensitization employed safely without report of survival
	Lee et al 2010[25]	Rhabdomyosarcoma	Patient free of disease at 13 months following 45 Gy in 25 fractions
	Xu et al 2000[34]	Rhabdomyosarcoma	Patient alive at 1 month following biopsy plus radiation
	Zevallos-Giampietri et al 2004[5]	Leiomyosarcoma (Epstein-Barr virus+)	Lost to follow-up after 44 Gy in 30 fractions

[a] All patients underwent maximum feasible resection unless otherwise noted.

Recommendations for Adjuvant Radiation Treatment of Primary Meningeal Sarcoma

1. No definitive evidence exists supporting the use of adjuvant radiation specifically in meningeal sarcoma. Nonetheless, it is being used with increasing frequency in hopes of controlling and treating residual disease in this highly aggressive cancer. This practice is in large part due to its success in limb-sparing treatment of soft tissue sarcoma (Grade 2C Recommendation, Level III/IV Evidence).
2. Larger, multi-institutional studies are needed to compare treatment regimens in these exceedingly rare tumors.
3. Further advancements in radiotherapy may provide avenues to achieve localized doses high enough to treat residual disease without the detrimental effects of large-field brain radiation. Reduction of field will also aid in preserving skin perfusion via small vessels to the native, nonirradiated scalp. Adjuvant radiation may confer the greatest benefit in meningeal sarcoma subtypes with extracranial counterparts that are particularly radiosensitive.
4. Because there is inadequate evidence to support the use of adjuvant radiation, it must be considered carefully due to its known sequelae, especially in younger patients. In addition to potential functional deficits, radiation can predispose patients to neoplastic growth in the future because one risk factor for meningeal sarcoma is prior CNS radiation.

Adjuvant Chemotherapy

There is no standard chemotherapeutic regimen for meningeal sarcoma. Adjuvant therapy is targeted at histological subtype when employed. CNS-penetrating agents can be added to therapies utilized in soft tissue sarcoma. Due to the rarity of meningeal sarcoma, for which chemotherapy is based on even rarer subtypes, there is little proof of its overall utility. The level of evidence of comparative studies and case reports published in the literature is summarized in **Table 34.3**.

Level I and Level II Evidence

There are no Level I or II evidence studies comparing adjuvant chemotherapy versus no chemotherapy in patients with primary meningeal sarcoma with brain invasion.

Level III Evidence

Due to the scarcity of meningeal sarcomas, few case-control studies exist. Of the limited studies available to compare the use of adjuvant chemotherapy, sample size remains small, making interpretation difficult.

Gaspar et al published a series of nine patients with primary intracranial fibrosarcoma, five cases being meningeal fibrosarcoma. All patients with meningeal fibrosarcoma underwent operative resection with adjuvant radiation. Procarbazine, lomustine, and vincristine (PCV) was administered in one patient who died of disease at 7.5 months. The remaining four patients with meningeal fibrosarcoma had a median survival of 21 months (range 10 to 100 months). Conclusions cannot be drawn due to the small sample size and heterogeneity of disease.[22] Similarly, Tomita and Gonzalez-Crussi reported a series of eight patients with intracranial primary undifferentiated sarcoma; one patient received chemotherapy, but there is little information as to its efficacy.[23]

Level IV Evidence

The use of chemotherapy in meningeal sarcoma is largely documented through various case series and reports. In the series by Al-Gahtany et al, all patients surviving the initial months of presentation were

Table 34.3 Evidence table for the role of adjuvant chemotherapy in the treatment of meningeal sarcoma

Level of evidence	Study	Sarcoma subtype	Outcomes[a]
Level I and II	No Papers		
Level III	Gaspar et al 1993[22]	Fibrosarcoma	Case series of nine patients with intracranial fibrosarcoma; one patient received PCV therapy
	Tomita and Gonzalez-Crussi 1984[23]	Undifferentiated	Case series of eight patients with intracranial sarcoma; one patient received chemotherapy
Level IV	Al-Gahtany et al 2003[3]	Undifferentiated	Case series of six patients with meningeal sarcoma receiving VAC or ICE therapy; longer survival seen in those without brain invasion
	Celli et al 1998[24]	Rhabdomyosarcoma	Case reports of 38 RMs in review of literature of intraparenchymal tumors; 12 patients received varying chemotherapy regimens, with two thromboembolic deaths
	Palta et al 2011[15]	Rhabdomyosarcoma	Case report using VAC therapy in RMS without survival data
	Lee et al 2010[25]	Rhabdomyosarcoma	Case report of ICE therapy in RMS with no recurrence at 13 months
	Romeo et al 2010[26]	Osteoblastic chondrosarcoma	Case report using cisplatinum and doxorubicin with long-term survival at 43 months; similar results found upon review of four cases using chemotherapy in osteosarcoma (one died of thromboembolism)[27–30]
	Blumenthal et al 1999[6]	Leiomyosarcoma (Epstein-Barr virus+)	Case report of doxorubicin therapy alone (no operation or radiation) in leiomyosarcoma, with patient alive at 24 months

Abbreviations: ICE, isofosfamide, carboplatin, and etoposide; RMS, rhabdomyosarcoma; VAC, vincristine, actinomycin, and cyclophosphamide,

[a] All patients underwent maximum feasible resection unless otherwise noted.

treated with chemotherapy in addition to resection and radiation.[3] Of the six patients with meningeal sarcoma, three were found to have brain invasion, with survivals of 10 and 22 months (one patient was lost to follow-up at 7 months) following differing chemotherapeutic regimens consisting of vincristine, actinomycin, and cyclophosphamide (VAC) or isofosfamide, carboplatin, and etoposide (ICE), with the addition of various other agents including methotrexate and adriamycin. The three patients without brain invasion achieved long-term survivals, with two still alive at 12 and 16 years, following similar regimens.

Although their systematic review of the literature investigated intraparenchymal tumors as opposed to meningeal, Celli et al compiled 38 case reports of intracranial rhabdomyosarcoma (RMS), of which 12 received adjuvant chemotherapy. The median survival for the 12 patients receiving chemotherapy was 13.5 months, with four patients alive for more than 20 months. Two patients who underwent chemotherapy died from pulmonary embolism, which may have been related to the aggressive adjuvant therapy in addition to the cancer-related hypercoagulable state. However, patients received differing treatment regimens, and conclusions as to efficacy cannot be drawn.[24] Palta et al used VAC in treating meningeal rhabdomyosarcoma in one patient, who tolerated the regimen well, with no mention of survival status beyond the duration of therapy. In a five year-old boy with multifocal meningeal RMS extending into the right frontal lobe, Lee et al achieved near-total resection followed by bifrontal radiation (45 Gy in 25 fractions) and 13 cycles of ICE. At the time of report, their patient was alive at 13 months without recurrence.[25] The standard therapy for systemic RMS is VAC, and it is the regimen of choice when basing decisions on systemic counterparts. However, meningeal sarcoma may be an entirely different entity arising from neuroectodermal precursors, requiring further consideration.

Romeo and colleagues reported their experience treating a case of primary meningeal osteoblastic chondrosarcoma with total resection, radiation, and chemotherapy.[26] Chemotherapy consisted of six courses of cisplatinum (100 mg/m^2/d at day 1) and doxorubicin (20 mg/m^2/d from day 1 to 3) given every 3 weeks. The patient achieved long-term disease-free survival, and was alive at 43 months at the time of report. However, on microscopic examination, the tumor showed no intraparenchymal invasion. Upon review of the literature, they found 12 similar cases of primary meningeal osteosarcoma, with four patients undergoing adjuvant chemotherapy. In three of the cases, similar regimens consisting of cisplatinum and doxorubicin were used (with the addition of methotrexate in two), and disease-free survivals of 36, 24, and 12 months were achieved.[27-29] The fourth case employed adjuvant vincristine, bleomycin, methotrexate, and leucovorin, and the patient died 11 months postoperatively due to a hypercoagulable state likely related to aggressive chemoradiation therapy.[30] In the review by Romeo et al,[26] those patients not receiving chemotherapy with complete follow-up had a median survival of 8.5 months (range, perioperative death to 60 months); however, two patients with ongoing follow-up were alive at 24 and 33 months, complicating the comparison. Extracranial osteosarcoma is a chemosensitive tumor, with increased survival attained with the introduction of high-dose chemotherapy with methotrexate in the 1970s. Current treatment recommendations include complete surgical resection followed by methotrexate, cisplatin, and doxorubicin, as demonstrated in the majority of cases reviewed by Romeo et al.[26] However, the role of chemotherapy in craniofacial osteosarcoma continues to be controversial, and there is certainly no standard regimen with proven efficacy in meningeal osteosarcoma. As demonstrated in the studies presented, adjuvant chemotherapy is largely dictated by subtype.

Expert Recommendations

1. The role of adjuvant chemotherapy in the treatment of primary meningeal sarcoma remains to be defined. Each sarcoma subtype presents with different considerations, and when used, chemotherapy regimens in meningeal sarcoma mirror those utilized in extracranial counterparts. Certain subtypes known to be chemosensitive peripherally show promising results, such as meningeal osteosarcoma (Grade 2C Recommendation, Level IV Evidence).
2. Due to the highly aggressive nature of these tumors, the addition of chemotherapy is becoming more common as salvage therapy.
3. The potential benefit of chemotherapy must be weighed heavily against its potential harmful effects because case reports document deaths from venothromboembolism potentially related to aggressive regimens. Each patient should be evaluated on an individual basis, and adjuvant therapy should be reserved for those thought to be the most medically stable (Grade 2C Recommendation, Level IV Evidence).

■ Summary and Conclusions

Primary meningeal sarcoma is a rare disease with limited evidence as to the best treatment strategy. There is general consensus that the cornerstone of treatment revolves around maximum feasible resection. Meticulous care should be undertaken to avoid postoperative complications in order to afford the patient the best possible outcome. Controversy remains concerning the utilization of adjuvant radiation and chemotherapy. On the whole, treatment is dictated by the current standard of care for the extracranial sarcoma subtype. The use of radiation and chemotherapy should be weighed against potential detrimental effects, including poor wound healing and postoperative complications, increased risk of secondary malignancies (especially in younger patients), the development of venothromboembolism, and direct toxicities of the chemotherapeutic agents. Patients should be evaluated on an individual basis and receive appropriate adjuvant treatments for their level of stability.

■ References

1. Haddad GF, Al-Mefty O. Meningeal sarcomas. In: Kaye AH, Laws ER Jr, eds. Brain Tumors: An Encyclopedic Approach. London: Churchill Livingstone; 2001:759–770
2. Avgeropoulos NG, Henson JW. Meningeal sarcomas. In: Raghavan D, Brecher ML, Johnson DH, Meropol NJ, Moots PL, Rose PG, eds. Textbook of Uncommon Cancer. John Wiley & Sons; 2006:626–637
3. Al-Gahtany M, Shroff M, Bouffet E, et al. Primary central nervous system sarcomas in children: clinical, radiological, and pathological features. Childs Nerv Syst 2003;19(12):808–817
4. Cinalli G, Zerah M, Carteret M, et al. Subdural sarcoma associated with chronic subdural hematoma: report of two cases and review of the literature. J Neurosurg 1997;86(3):553–557
5. Zevallos-Giampietri EA, Yañes HH, Orrego Puelles J, Barrionuevo C. Primary meningeal Epstein-Barr virus-related leiomyosarcoma in a man infected with human immunodeficiency virus: review of literature, emphasizing the differential diagnosis and pathogenesis. Appl Immunohistochem Mol Morphol 2004;12(4):387–391
6. Blumenthal DT, Raizer JJ, Rosenblum MK, Bilsky MH, Hariharan S, Abrey LE. Primary intracranial neoplasms in patients with HIV. Neurology 1999;52(8):1648–1651
7. Brown HG, Burger PC, Olivi A, Sills AK, Barditch-Crovo PA, Lee RR. Intracranial leiomyosarcoma in a patient with AIDS. Neuroradiology 1999;41(1):35–39
8. Morgello S, Kotsianti A, Gumprecht JP, Moore F. Epstein-Barr virus-associated dural leiomyosarcoma in a man infected with human immunodeficiency virus. Case report. J Neurosurg 1997;86(5):883–887
9. Ritter AM, Amaker BH, Graham RS, Broaddus WC, Ward JD. Central nervous system leiomyosarcoma in patients with acquired immunodeficiency syndrome. Report of two cases. J Neurosurg 2000;92(4):688–692
10. Osipov V, Ho KC, Krouwer HG, Meyer G, Shidham VB. Post-radiation dedifferentiation of meningioma into osteosarcoma. BMC Cancer 2002;2:34
11. Ziewacz JE, Song JW, Blaivas M, Yang LJ. Radiation-induced meningeal osteosarcoma of tentorium cerebelli with intradural spinal metastases. Surg Neurol Int 2010;1:14
12. Galanis E. Malignant central nervous system neoplasms of mesenchymal origin. In: Baehring JM, Piepmeier JM, eds. Brain Tumors: Practical Guide to Diagnosis and Treatment. New York, NY: Informa Healthcare USA; 2007:325–340
13. McLendon RE, Enterline DS. Tumors of the meninges and related tissues. In: Bigner DD, McLendon RE, Bruner JM, eds. Russel and Rubinstein's Pathology of Tumors of the Nervous System. New York, NY: Oxford University Press; 1998:67–139
14. Büttner A, Pfluger T, Weis S. Primary meningeal sarcomas in two children. J Neurooncol 2001;52(2):181–188
15. Palta M, Riedel RF, Vredenburgh JJ, et al. Primary meningeal rhabdomyosarcoma. Sarcoma 2011;2011:312802
16. Jarrahy R, Lazareff J. Neurosurgical considerations in craniofacial surgery. In: Thaller SR, Bradley JP, Garri JI, eds. Craniofacial Surgery. New York, NY: Informa Healthcare USA; 2008:49–58
17. Christensen E, Lara DE. Intracranial sarcomas. J Neuropathol Exp Neurol 1953;12(1):41–56
18. Gordon CR, Swanson EW, Westvik T, Yaremchuk MJ. Bipolar duraplasty: a new technique for reducing transcranial cerebral herniation to allow for definitive cranioplasty. J Neurosurg 2011;115(5):1025–1028
19. Gordon CR, Yaremchuk MJ. Temporal augmentation with methyl methacrylate. Aesthet Surg J 2011;31(7):827–833
20. Tepper JE, Suit HD. Radiation therapy of soft tissue sarcomas. Cancer 1985;55(9, Suppl):2273–2277
21. Tepper JE, Suit HD. The role of radiation therapy in the treatment of sarcoma of soft tissue. Cancer Invest 1985;3(6):587–592
22. Gaspar LE, Mackenzie IR, Gilbert JJ, et al. Primary cerebral fibrosarcomas. Clinicopathologic study and review of the literature. Cancer 1993;72(11):3277–3281
23. Tomita T, Gonzalez-Crussi F. Intracranial primary nonlymphomatous sarcomas in children: experience with eight cases and review of the literature. Neurosurgery 1984;14(5):529–540
24. Celli P, Cervoni L, Maraglino C. Primary rhabdomyosarcoma of the brain: observations on a case with clinical and radiological evidence of cure. J Neurooncol 1998;36(3):259–267
25. Lee JY, Kim BS, Phi JH, et al. Primary meningeal rhabdomyosarcoma associated with chronic subdural effusion: case report. J Neurosurg Pediatr 2010;5(2):167–171
26. Romeo E, Gisserot O, de Jaureguiberry JP, et al. Meningeal chondroblastic osteosarcoma: case report and review of the literature. J Neurooncol 2010;100(2):305–309
27. Sanno N, Hayashi S, Shimura T, Maeda S, Teramoto A. Intracranial osteosarcoma after radiosurgery—case report. Neurol Med Chir (Tokyo) 2004;44(1):29–32
28. Bar-Sela G, Tzuk-Shina T, Zaaroor M, Vlodarsky Y, Tsalik M, Kuten A. Primary osteogenic sarcoma arising from the dura mater: case report. Am J Clin Oncol 2001;24(4):418–420
29. Bonilla F, Provencio M, Salas C, España P. Primary osteosarcoma of the meninges. Ann Oncol 1994;5(10):965–966
30. Alleyne CH Jr, Theodore N, Spetzler RF, Coons SW. Osteosarcoma of the temporal fossa with hemorrhagic presentation: case report. Neurosurgery 2000;47(2):447–450
31. Sugita Y, Shigemori M, Harada H, et al. Primary meningeal sarcomas with leiomyoblastic differentiation: a proposal for a new subtype of primary meningeal sarcomas. Am J Surg Pathol 2000;24(9):1273–1278
32. Utsuki S, Oka H, Sato K, Shimizu S, Suzuki S, Fujii K. Radiation-induced osteosarcoma with a rhabdomyosarcoma component arising from the dura mater: a case report. Clin Neuropathol 2009;28(2):96–100
33. Setzer M, Lang J, Turowski B, Marquardt G. Primary meningeal osteosarcoma: case report and review of the literature. Neurosurgery 2002;51(2):488–492
34. Xu F, De Las Casas LE, Dobbs LJ Jr. Primary meningeal rhabdomyosarcoma in a child with hypomelanosis of Ito. Arch Pathol Lab Med 2000;124(5):762–765

■ SECTION X ■

Pituitary Tumors

35

The Role of Surgery in Nonfunctioning Pituitary Macroadenomas

Kaisorn L. Chaichana, Brian Yu-Jin Hwang, Shaan M. Raza, and Alfredo Quiñones-Hinojosa

Pituitary adenomas are relatively common tumors that are found in 10 to 27% of the general population.[1,2] These benign tumors account for 8 to 10% of all intracranial tumors.[3,4] Pituitary adenomas arise from the epithelial pituitary cells of the adenohypophysis, which itself develops from the Rathke pouch.[5] Tumors exceeding 10 mm in diameter are defined as macroadenomas, and those smaller than 10 mm are termed microadenomas.

Clinical presentation of pituitary adenomas largely depends on the size, direction of growth, and functional status of the tumor. The tumor may grow within the sella and cause erosion and remodeling of the floor of the sella and posterior clinoid processes. It often extends superiorly into the suprasellar cistern and may compress the optic pathways, particularly the optic chiasm. This can lead to visual deficits, namely bitemporal hemianopsia. Further cephalad growth may cause compression of the hypothalamus or, if large enough, may obstruct the third ventricle, leading to hydrocephalus. Though uncommon, tumors can grow inferiorly into the sphenoid sinus, leading to cerebrospinal fluid (CSF) leakage and meningitis. Lateral extension out of the sella into the cavernous sinus can cause cranial neuropathies, and further lateral growth can lead to temporal lobe dysfunction. Endocrine abnormalities associated with pituitary adenomas are due to either hypopituitarism or excess secretion of a particular pituitary hormone.[6] A less common complication is pituitary apoplexy, which results from spontaneous hemorrhage or infarction of the tumor. Apoplexy can precipitate an acute endocrine crisis, which constitutes a medical emergency.[7]

Approximately 80% of macroadenomas are nonfunctioning tumors.[8,9] A majority of nonfunctioning pituitary adenomas (NFPAs) are of gonadotrophic cell origin but are rarely associated with signs and symptoms of gonadotropin excess.[10] Patients with NFPA may be asymptomatic ("incidentaloma") or may present with complaints due to mass effects (i.e., visual failure, hypothalamic syndrome, hypopituitarism, etc.) from compression of the surrounding structures. Visual impairment is the most common presenting symptom, with some degree of field defect seen in up to 60 to 80% of patients at initial diagnosis.[11–13] The incidence of pituitary apoplexy is relatively rare in NFPAs, where it is the presenting sign in 0.6 to 10.0% of patients with known pituitary tumors and is higher in patients with larger tumors.[14,15] Incidence in patients without known tumors is estimated to be less than 18 per 1 million people.[14,15] Treatment options for pituitary adenomas include medical therapy, surgery (transsphenoidal vs transcranial approaches), and radiotherapy.[16] Medical treatment is generally not effective in reducing the size of NFPAs. Therefore, microsurgical decompression by the transsphenoidal approach remains the treatment of choice. This chapter reviews the role of surgery and the currently available data in the surgical management of NFPAs.[10,14]

■ Surgery for Nonfunctioning Pituitary Adenomas

Surgery is the primary treatment modality for NFPAs that cause compression of adjacent neural structures, including the optic chiasm, other cranial nerves, hypothalamus, and third ventricle (**Fig. 35.1**).[10,14] For incidentally discovered macroadenomas, young age and large size as well as proximity to eloquent structures such as the optic chiasm also favor surgery over observation. The goals of surgery are typically to (1) achieve maximal degree of tumor resection, (2) relieve compression on adjacent structures, and (3) obtain a definitive tissue diagnosis. In transsphenoidal surgery (TSS), the pituitary fossa and tumor are accessed through the sphenoid sinus using an endonasal or a sublabial approach. Recently, the endonasal transsphenoidal approach has been preferred by most surgeons, primarily because of the ease of sphenoidal sinus access, lack of a sublabial incision, and improved wound healing.[17] Regardless of approach, TSS has been shown to be an effective and safe treatment option for local tumor control and symptom relief.[17,18] In this approach, tumors with suprasellar extension can often be coaxed into the pituitary fossa by removing the sellar component of the tumor or intraoperatively elevating the intracranial pressure. Most tumors (> 95%), even those with a significant suprasellar component, can be safely debulked or removed with this approach. However, in some circumstances, tumors that extend into the suprasellar space cannot be adequately removed using TSS. These rare tumors remain in the suprasellar space and do not descend into the sella. This is typically seen in fibrous tumors and tumors with significant

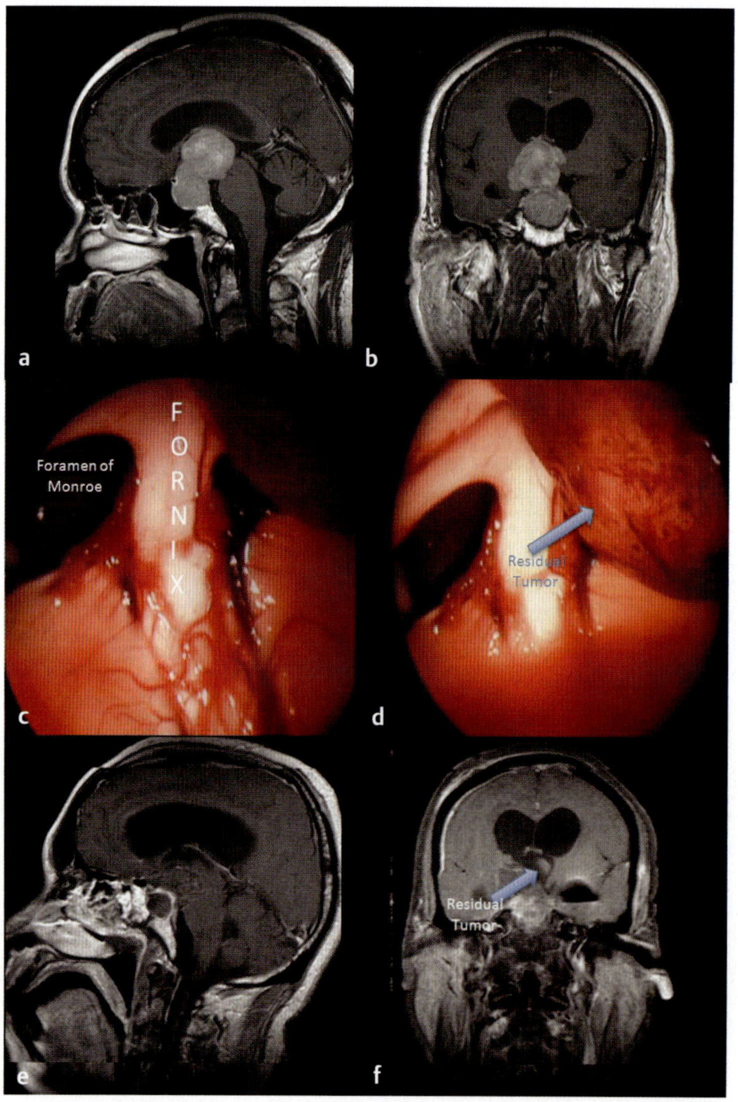

Fig. 35.1 A 65-year-old male with symptomatic pituitary macroadenoma with optic chiasm compression. **(a,b)** The lesion abuts the optic chiasm, hypothalamus, and fornix, with invasion into the bilateral cavernous sinus. Given the size and presence of compression, endoscopic endonasal surgery was pursued **(c,d)** and a small residual tumor was left behind because there was not a good plane of dissection with intracranial venous structures (*arrow* in **d** and **e**). **(e,f)** Good postoperative decompression of the intracranial structures with a small residual that was followed over time with no evidence of growth.

suprasellar extension to the subfrontal or petroclival regions. These tumors are typically approached first with TSS, and then followed with an intracranial approach for removal of residual tumor.[17–20]

Does TSS Lead to Improvement in Neurological Symptoms in Patients with NFPA? What Are the Most Common Postoperative Complications after TSS?

Level I and Level II Evidence

No Level I or Level II studies exist on this subject matter.

Level III and Level IV Evidence

TSS leads to improved visual function in a majority of patients. Over all, complete recovery of visual function is seen in 35 to 39%, and improvement in 50 to 60% of patients.[21–23] Visual recovery may be detected as early as a few days after surgery and can continue up to 3 to 5 years postoperatively in some patients.[21] Worsening of vision is reported in only 0.5 to 2.4% of patients.[23] Headache is another common symptom seen in 25 to 50% of patients, and surgery leads to its near complete resolution in a majority of patients.[11,24–27]

TSS is generally well tolerated and has an associated mortality of less than 1%.[2,23] The most common early complication after surgery is diabetes insipidus, which occurs in up to 15% of patients. However, only 0.9 to 2.0% of cases become permanent.[10,28] Other complications include transient isolated hyponatremia, cranial nerve palsy, sellar hematoma, subarachnoid hemorrhage, meningitis, and CSF leaks.[10] Parameters associated with unfavorable outcomes after surgery include cavernous sinus or temporal lobe involvement, large tumor size, requirement for transcranial approach, and presence of tumor apoplexy at the time of surgery.[23,29,30]

Is Surgery Indicated for Patients with Large Tumors without Neurological Findings?

Level I and Level II Evidence

No Level I or Level II studies exist on this subject matter.

Level III and Level IV Evidence

Previous studies on NFPAs without clinical symptoms are limited. The majority of patients that make up observational studies actually had clinical symptoms that ranged from visual dysfunction to pituitary dysfunction.[31,32] Therefore, all patients should undergo a complete history and physical examination, laboratory screening for hormone hypersecretion and for hypopituitarism, and visual field examination. Patients with symptoms associated with their pituitary adenoma should undergo surgery.

The role of surgical intervention for incidental NFPAs, however, is less well characterized. In long-term studies, microadenomas enlarge in 10.6% of patients.[31,32] These patients can generally be followed with repeat imaging every 1 to 2 years or longer to detect tumor enlargement.[31,32] Surgery is typically performed only with significant tumor enlargement.[31,32] However, the rate of growth of microadenomas is typically slow, so that the decision to pursue surgery depends on the rate and amount of growth as well as if there are clinical manifestations.[31,32]

Unlike microadenomas, macroadenomas will enlarge in 24.1% of patients.[31,32] Also, unlike microadenomas, the management of incidental macroadenomas is more controversial. Some advocate surgical intervention for patients with macroadenomas, even in the absence of symptoms, given that these tumors have already demonstrated growth.[31,33] Likewise, many surgeons advocate for surgery in tumors abutting the optic chiasm without symptoms.[31,33] However, if surgery is declined, patients with macroadenomas, especially those > 2.5 cm, should be followed closely, with repeated clinical examinations, including visual field testing, serial neuroimaging, and laboratory evaluation at more frequent intervals (i.e., 6 months).[31,33] Lesions that grow or cause clinical symptoms will require surgical intervention. The use of medical therapy with a dopamine agonist or octreotide is sometimes tried when surgery is deferred, but only 10 to 20% of patients will have a decrease in tumor size following medical therapy.[34]

Can TSS Improve Pituitary Dysfunction in Patients with NFPA?

Level I and Level II Evidence

No Level I and Level II studies exist on this subject matter.

Level III and Level IV Evidence

Results concerning pituitary function after surgery remain controversial (**Table 35.1**). Complete recovery of impaired pituitary function after surgery is less likely, with variable degrees of improvement seen in 15 to 50% of patients.[35] Several studies have demonstrated improvement in pituitary function after surgery, whereas others did not to show significant improvement or even reported a further decline in pituitary function.[11–14,24,25,29,30,36] This variability is likely due to the discrepancies in diagnostic criteria for hypopituitarism, patient characteristics, degree and duration of preoperative pituitary dysfunction, as well as surgical approach and techniques.[10] Nevertheless, a significant proportion of patients continue to have pituitary dysfunction after surgery (**Table 35.1**). For instance, Nomikos et al reported pituitary function remained unchanged in 48.9% and worsened in 1.9% of patients.[30] Dekkers et al showed that 83%, 60%, and 30% of patients continued to have growth hormone (GH) deficiency, gonadotropin deficiency, and adrenocorticotropic hormone (ACTH) deficiency after surgery, respectively.[14] Therefore, we recommend that the objective of surgery for NFPA should be improvement of compressive clinical symptoms (e.g., visual field defects) rather than recovery of pituitary function.

Which Surgical Approach Is Preferred for Patients with NFPAs?

Level I and Level II Evidence

No Level I or Level II studies exist on this subject matter.

Level III and Level IV Evidence

Surgical approaches to pituitary adenomas can be divided into extracranial and transcranial approaches. Regardless of approach, these tumors pose potential risks because of their invasiveness, size, and proximity to critical neurovascular structures, including the internal carotid arteries, optic nerve and chiasm, and cavernous sinus and associated cranial nerves, among others. The choice of approach should be tailored for the patient, characteristics of the tumor, goals of surgery, and surgeon's experience.[16–18] The extracranial approaches include the endonasal transsphenoidal and extended endonasal approaches (**Fig. 35.2**).[16–19,37] These approaches take advantage of the close proximity of the sella and pituitary tumor to the sphenoidal sinus. Transcranial approaches include the classic frontotemporal sphenoidal craniotomy for a lateral approach, and supraciliary or eyebrow as well as the transciliary or eyelid approach for a more midline, subfrontal approach.[17,18,38–40]

Both extracranial and transcranial approaches can reach the sella, but most surgeons prefer the extracranial approach because of the fewer side effects with this approach as compared with the transcranial approach.[27,41] The transsphenoidal approach offers a direct midline approach to the sella, usually with sufficient but limited tumor exposure.[17,18,42,43] This approach also allows for tumor exposure without necessitating brain retraction,

Table 35.1 Impact of transsphenoidal surgery on pituitary function for patients with nonfunctioning pituitary adenomas

Study	Level of evidence	No. patients	Follow-up (mo)	GH deficiency (%)		LH/FSH deficiency (%)		TSH deficiency (%)		ACTH deficiency (%)		Hypopituitarism (%)	
				Preop	Postop	Preop	Postop	Preop	Postop	Preop	Postop	Preop	Postop
Comtois et al 1991[11]	III/IV	126	–	–	–	75	70	18	31	36	29	–	–
Marazuela et al 1994[12]	III/IV	35	2 to 6	88	82	69	48	23	20	29	13	69	–
Arafah 1986[24]	III/IV	26	0.2	100	85	96	65	81	35	62	38	–	–
Greenman et al 2003[29]	III/IV	26	3 to 6	–	–	78	46	23	12	43	50	89	65
Nomikos et al 2004[30]	III/IV	660	12	–	–	77	65	19	16	35	18	85	72
Wichers-Rother et al 2004[13]	III/IV	109	1 to 6	85	78	61	50	31	34	32	25	–	–
Alameda et al 2005[8]	III/IV	51	–	80	88	62	57	21	27	19	19	85	89
Dekkers et al 2006[14]	III/IV	109	6	77	83	75	90	43	57	53	60	83	94

Abbreviations: ACTH, adrenocorticotropic hormone; GH, growth hormone; FSH, follicle-stimulating hormone; LH, luteinizing hormone; TSH, thyroid-stimulating hormone.

optic nerve manipulation, and vascular exposure.[1,44] This approach is therefore associated with relatively rapid recovery times and lower surgical morbidity and mortality rates.[1,44] The transsphenoidal approach is particularly well suited for intrasellar macroadenomas, extrasellar macroadenomas with slight suprasellar extension, and extrasellar macroadenomas with significant downward extension into the sphenoid sinus.[17,18,42,43] A modification of the endonasal transsphenoidal approach is sometimes referred to as the expanded endonasal approach.[20,37] This approach involves utilizing both nostrils to maximize exposure of the sella and potentially improved tumor resection, but it is associated with longer surgical times and postoperative sinusitis.[20,37] These extracranial approaches have become even safer with advances in intraoperative technology, including the binocular operating microscope, endoscopes, and navigation, among others.[17,18,42,43] Despite these advances, these tumors often cannot be completely resected because of their large size and parasellar extension, with recurrence rates up to 60% in some series.[11,14,25,29,45,46] Transcranial approaches are usually advocated for ir-

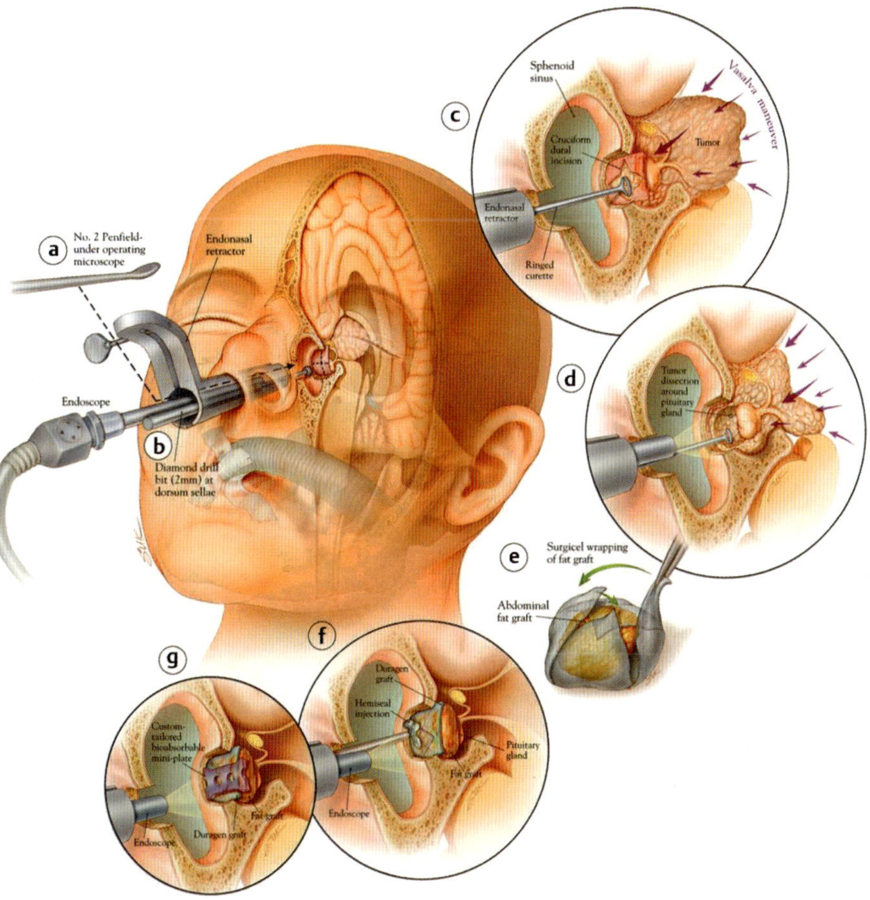

Fig. 35.2 Illustration of steps for the endonasal endoscopic approach to pituitary tumors. **(a)**The intranasal speculum is in place as a working corridor for the endoscope only if needed. **(b)** A 2-mm diamond burr in a minimal-angle drill handle is used to drill the anterior wall of the sella. **(c)** A cruciform dural incision is performed that is started at the center and guided by anatomical landmarks as well as surgical navigation if necessary, especially in redo cases where the anatomy can be distorted. **(d)** A ringed curette upgoing, downgoing, and with different angles and sizes is used for tumor removal after the dural incision with identification of the pituitary gland. Intraoperative maneuvers to push the tumor down from the suprasellar region include Valsalva maneuver. **(e)** The closure of the defect can be aided by the use of harvested fat, and for hemostasis the adipose tissue can be wrapped in Surgicel (Ethicon, Somerville, NJ). **(f)** Placement of the fat graft into the sella and sphenoid sinus followed by the placement of Duragen (Integra, Plainsboro, NJ) if there is a concern for a cerebrospinal fluid leak. **(g)** In this case, we illustrate the placement of the Synthes bioabsorbable miniplate (Synthes, East West Chester, PA, catalog #851.009.01S) with the subsequent use of fibrin glue (Tisseel, Baxter, Deerfield, IL) for reinforcement. (From Frazier JL, Chaichana K, Jallo GI, Quiñones-Hinojosa A. Combined endoscopic and microscopic management of pediatric pituitary region tumors through one nostril: technical note with case illustrations. Childs Nerv Syst 2008;24(12):1469–1478.)

regular multinodular tumors, with eccentric extensions into the frontal, temporal, or posterior fossa.[38,39,47,48] This approach is also used for macroadenomas with a hard or cartilaginous consistency, which is initially found during a transsphenoidal approach.[49] A transcranial approach is typically used here as a staged procedure, where it is the second stage.[49] The typical approach is the frontotemporal sphenoidal craniotomy, which provides a lateral approach to the sella.[17,18,38–40] A more direct path involves a subfrontal approach involving a supraciliary or transciliary approach.[17,18,38–40] The choice of transcranial approach depends on the surgeon's experience, location of the chiasm in relation to the infundibulum, and the size of the frontal sinus.[17,18,38–40]

Despite no randomized, controlled trials of extracranial versus transcranial approaches, the transsphenoidal approach is typically preferred because it requires no brain retraction and poses little risk to neurovascular structures.[17,42] However, it is difficult to achieve total tumor removal because of the limited surgical exposure.[17,42] The transcranial approach is used for extensive tumor removal but is associated with more surgical morbidity and mortality.[49] Therefore, the transsphenoidal approach is typically used in the first stage.[39,40,47–49] For significant residual tumor or progressive recurrence, the transcranial approach is sometimes used when a repeat transsphenoidal approach will have low yield.[39,40,47–49]

Is Total or Near-Total Resection Associated with Improved Recurrence-Free Survival as Compared with Partial Resection?

Level I and Level II Evidence

No Level I or Level II studies exist on this subject matter.

Level III and Level IV Evidence

Surgical techniques for the removal of NFPAs have become markedly refined over time. However, a significant proportion of NFPAs are large and invasive at diagnosis, rendering total resection difficult to achieve.[10] These lesions often extend into the suprasellar space near the third ventricle, as well as laterally into the cavernous sinus. These areas make it more difficult to achieve extensive resection. Radiographic cure is attained in ~ 30 to 40% of patients, although up to 70% has been reported by high-volume centers with highly experienced teams.[14,23,25,29,30,42,50,51]

Radiographic recurrence has become more common since the advent of magnetic resonance imaging (MRI), which is the imaging modality of choice for postoperative surveillance. Radiological recurrence of tumor is generally defined as either (1) appearance of pathological tissue not present on earlier postoperative MRI or (2) enlargement of known residual tumor remnant on postsurgical MRI. Overall reported recurrence rate of NFPAs after TSS alone generally ranges between 12 and 45%.[11,23,50,52] With residual NFPA, the risk of tumor regrowth is generally high, at 13 to 58% at long-term follow-up (**Table 35.2**).[11,14,25,29,45,46] Gross total resection, in comparison, has been associated with lower recurrence risk of 0 to 20% (**Table 35.2**). Total excision, however, may not independently predict the risk of recurrence because it is strongly influenced by the size and degree of invasiveness of the tumor.[53] Other risk factors for increased risk of recurrence include young age, large tumor size at diagnosis, invasion into the cavernous sinus, and suprasellar extension of the remnant tumor after surgery.[29,53] Nevertheless, recurrence rates reported in the literature continue to remain variable, and risk factors for recurrence remain unclear.[14] This is largely due to the discrepancies in follow-up duration, definitions of total resection and recurrence, and patient characteristics. Also, prospective data with predetermined surveillance interval are currently lacking.

Should Surgery Be Performed by an Experienced Surgeon and/or at a High-Volume Center?

Level I and Level II Evidence

No Level I or Level II studies exist on this subject matter.

Level III and Level IV Evidence

In recent years, there has been an emphasis on performing specific surgeries for relatively rare pathology at high-volume centers.[54] This includes pituitary surgery.[55–57] There have been multiple studies that have shown that experienced surgeons and surgery in high-volume centers are associated with lower morbidity and mortality for patients with pituitary adenomas.[55–57] Barker et al in 2003 performed a volume–outcome relationship analysis for transsphenoidal pituitary tumor surgery using the Nationwide Inpatient Sample from 1996 to 2000.[55] They found that both higher-volume surgeons and higher-volume centers were associated with lower mortality, shorter length of stay, and less complications as compared with both lower-volume surgeons and lower-volume centers.[55] Similar results have been documented for patients with acromegaly and Cushing disease.[56,57] Access to high-volume surgeons

Table 35.2 Recurrence rates of nonfunctioning pituitary adenoma after transsphenoidal surgery without radiation

Study	Level of evidence	No. patients	Mean follow-up (years)	Residual tumor		No residual tumor	
				Recurrence (%)	Mean time to detection (years)	Recurrence (%)	Mean time to detection (years)
Soto-Ares et al[83]	III/IV	51	5.6	13/34 (38)	2.2 ± 1.4	0/17 (0)	–
Greenman et al 2003[29]	III/IV	108	4.2	41/78(53)	2.2 ± 1.1	6/30 (20)	5 ± 2
Ferrante et al 2006[25]	III/IV	150	5.7	45/77 (58)	5.3 ± 4	14/73 (19)	7.5 ± 2.6
Dekkers et al 2006[14]	III/IV	97	6.0	9/70 (13)	6.3	0/27 (0)	–
Van den Bergh et al 2007[46]	III/IV	28	6.8	16/28 (57)	2.5	–	–
O'Sullivan et al 2009[45]	III/IV	126	5.7	53/100 (53)	–	0/26 (0)	–

Abbreviations: –, not mentioned.

and pituitary centers, however, is not uniform.[16] Mukherjee et al performed an analysis of the National Inpatient Sample between 1988 and 2005.[16] African Americans, Hispanics, and Asians had less access to high-volume centers (> 25 pituitary surgeries/year) as compared with whites.[16] Patients with less income also had less access to these high-volume centers.[16] As already stated, patients will generally have better outcomes with high-volume surgeons and high-volume centers; however, not all patients have access to these amenities.

Is There a Difference in Outcomes for Different Approaches to the Sella?

Level I and Level II Evidence

No Level I or Level II studies exist on this subject matter.

Level III and Level IV Evidence

There are several different approaches to the sella to remove NFPAs. These approaches can be divided into open craniotomy and transsphenoidal approaches. Open craniotomy involves removing the calvarium to access the sella from above, whereas transsphenoidal approaches involve accessing the sella inferiorly.[18] Transsphenoidal approaches include endonasal and sublabial approaches and can involve the use of endoscopy, microscopy, or both.[18] The theoretical advantage of the transsphenoidal approach is that it allows direct access to the sella. Open craniotomy approaches rely on a more circuitous approach to the sella in the midline by a lateral or subfrontal approach, which often requires brain manipulation.[18,58]

Komotar et al performed a review of the literature and found 11 studies on giant pituitary adenomas, which included a large proportion of secretory tumors.[58] In this study, 66, 304, and 106 patients underwent open craniotomy, sublabial transsphenoidal approach, and endonasal transsphenoidal approach, respectively.[58] Patients who underwent a transsphenoidal approach had higher incidences of gross total resection and lower recurrence rates as compared with patients who underwent open craniotomy.[58] The rate of CSF leakage was highest in the open cranial group, followed by the transsphenoidal sublabial group, and it was the least in the endonasal transsphenoidal group.[58] This same group used these same studies, as well as five more, to compare the endoscopic endonasal approach to microscopic transsphenoidal and open transcranial approaches.[19] They found that the endoscopic cohort had higher rates of gross total resection and improved visual outcome as compared with the open transcranial approach and microscopic transsphenoidal group.[19] Patients who underwent an endoscopic transsphenoidal approach had no CSF leaks and less surgical morbidity as compared with the open transcranial approach.[19] D'Haens et al performed an institutional study of 60 patients who underwent a complete endoscopically assisted resection and compared them with 60 patients who underwent microscopically assisted resection.[59] All of these patients had hormonally active tumors.[59] In the subset of patients with macroadenomas without cavernous sinus involvement, they found that remission rates were higher among patients who underwent endoscopically assisted as compared with microscopically assisted resection (78% vs 43%).[59] There were no differences seen in patients who had microadenomas.[59] CSF leaks, however, most commonly occurred in the endoscopically assisted cohort.[59] Kabil and colleagues reported similar findings.[37] Goudakos et al also performed a meta-analysis of 806 patients, of whom 369 had endoscopic surgery and 437 had microscopic surgery.[60] They found no difference in extent of resection, hormone remission rates, or CSF leaks among the groups.[60] Patients undergoing endoscopic resection, however, had shorter hospital stays, fewer intranasal and intracranial complications, and lower incidence of diabetes insipidus.[60] No studies have been restricted to patients with nonfunctioning pituitary adenomas.

Should Surgery Be Pursued for Recurrent or Residual Tumor?

Level I and Level II Evidence

No Level I or Level II studies exist on this subject matter.

Level III and Level IV Evidence

Gross total resection of NFPAs is achieved only in ~ 30 to 40% of patients, although rates up to 70% have been reported by high-volume centers with highly experienced teams.[14,23,25,29,30,42,50,51] The recurrence rate is 17% for patients with initial gross total resection of the tumor, and tumor enlargement is detected in 43% of patients who had residual mass after surgery.[61] Younger age, cavernous sinus invasion, extent of suprasellar extension of the residual tumor, and follow-up duration were all associated with increased recurrence and/or progression.[61] The optimal management of residual tumor as well as tumor recurrence is poorly understood because of a lack of prospective studies and randomized, controlled trials. It is generally accepted by most surgeons that, for NFPAs, residual tumor can be followed with serial physical examinations, including visual field testing and MRI.[33] For residual tumor with increased growth or tumor recurrence, the optimal management is less well defined. There has been increasing evidence that radiation may control recurrent disease, with 97 to 100% control rates in some series.[23,53,62,63] Radiation, however, is associated with significant side effects, including hypopituitarism, excess mortality, cerebrovascular disease, secondary tumors, optic nerve atrophy, and neurocognitive changes.[61] Therefore, many surgeons advocate for surgical intervention for younger patients with recurrence or progression.[64,65] Rudnik et al evaluated 20 cases of recurrent pituitary disease.[65] They found no increase in perioperative morbidity and mortality as compared with initial surgeries using the transsphenoidal approach.[65] McLaughlin et al evaluated the efficacy of resecting residual or recurrent sellar lesions using the supraorbital approach.[66] Only one patient in 11 developed complications.[66] Surgery should therefore be considered for younger patients with recurrence or progression to avoid radiation-associated side effects.

Does Postsurgical Adjuvant Radiotherapy Lead to Improved Recurrence-Free Survival?

Level I and Level II Evidence

No Level I or Level II studies exist on this subject matter.

Level III and Level IV Evidence

Postoperative radiotherapy can be administered as an adjuvant therapy, particularly after subtotal resection of NFPAs.[67,68] However, the effectiveness of radiotherapy for local tumor control currently remains controversial (**Table 35.3**).[14,23,25,29,46,50,53,62,69] Several studies have demonstrated a significant decrease in tumor regrowth rate in patients who underwent radiation after surgery as compared with those who were observed.[23,53] However, others have shown that long-term, tumor-free survival can be attained in a majority of patients with residual tumor without prophylactic radiotherapy (**Fig. 35.1**).[14] It is difficult to draw conclusions from the currently available data due to discrepancies among the studies in their indications for radiotherapy, treatment protocols, timing, and study designs, including follow-up duration. Furthermore, there has yet to be a prospective clinical trial or study that examines the impact of radiotherapy on the rate of tumor recurrence or regrowth. Of note, radiotherapy is not without side effects. Studies have reported radiation-associated pituitary dysfunction, optic nerve atrophy, worsening visual deficits, and increased cumulative risk of developing a second brain tumor within 20 years after treatment.[70–74] Given the risks, radiotherapy should be considered in selected patients with large residual tumor burden or panhypopituitarism. Many of the downsides of radiotherapy may be overcome with the use of stereotactic radiosurgery, which has the possible advantage of minimizing radiation exposure to the optic nerves and the pituitary gland while delivering maximal radiation to the tumor. Recent studies have reported good results with gamma knife radiosurgery for the treatment of residual NFPAs.[75,76] It appears likely that radiosurgery will play an important adjuvant role in the surgical management of NFPAs.[75,76]

Should Surgery Be Pursued for Elderly Patients?

Level I and Level II Evidence

No Level I or Level II studies exist on this subject matter.

Level III and Level IV Evidence

Populations in developed countries are progressively aging. Traditionally, 65 years of age has been used to designate elderly patients, but this cutoff has been increasing, especially with advances in medical and surgical therapies.[22] In the past, elderly patients were often denied aggressive surgeries because of their presumed high risk of surgery-related morbidity and mortality. The incidence of pituitary adenomas among elderly patients ranges from 11 to 14%.[77] Furthermore, elderly patients typically present with more advanced disease, with decreased visual acuity, more visual field loss, and larger tumors than found in younger patients.[78] Perioperative mortality for elderly patients has been as high as 11% in some series.[79] The factors associated with outcome in a study by Pietilä et al were the preoperative cerebrovascular condition and existence of multiple concomitant disease.[79] Moreover, Grossman et al performed a review of the National Inpatient Sample, where 8,400 patients were identified who underwent pituitary tumor surgery.[22] Inpatient mortality was 3.8%, and the factors independently associated with increased mortality were age > 80 and a Charlson comorbidity score.[22] Elderly patients who underwent craniotomy had significantly higher mortality than elderly patients who underwent TSS.[22]

There are a few studies on surgery for elderly patients with pituitary adenomas, and no randomized, controlled trials on surgery versus observation. Given the relatively low morbidity and mortality, most surgeons advocate operating on elderly patients with NFPA with tumors that have compressive pathology.[22,43,80,81] For incidentally discovered macroadenomas without compressive pathology, options include observation with serial neuroimaging or surgery depending on the patient's Charlson score, operative risk, and estimated survival.[22,43,80,81] Studies on the use of radiotherapy without surgery for elderly patients are limited.[82] Radiotherapy is usually not employed as a first-line treatment of pituitary adenomas because of the complications associated with radiation and a limited ability to shrink tumor.[82]

Table 35.3 Recurrence rates of nonfunctioning pituitary adenoma after transsphenoidal surgery with and without adjuvant radiation therapy

				Adjuvant radiation		No radiation	
Study	**Level of evidence**	**No. patients**	**Mean follow-up (years)**	**Recurrence (%)**	**5-year growth-free survival (%)**	**Recurrence (%)**	**5-year growth-free survival (%)**
Ebersold et al[43]	III/IV	100	6.1	18/58 (31)	–	12/42 (28)	–
Woollons et al 2000[50]	III/IV	72[a]	5.3	26/50 (52)	72	10/22 (46)	34
Greenman et al 2003[29]	III/IV	108	4.2	5/14 (35)	48[b]	47/108 (43)	48[b]
Ferrante et al 2006[25]	III/IV	150	5.7	14/76 (18)	–	59/150 (39)	–
Dekkers et al 2006[14]	III/IV	97	6.0	0/6 (0)	100	11/91 (11)	94
Losa et al 2008[23]	III/IV		4.4	1/81 (1)	–	216/355 (61)	–
Van den Bergh 2007[46]	III/IV	122	6.8	4/79 (5)	–	17/43 (40)	–
Park et al 2004[62]	III/IV	176	4.3	2/44 (5)	98	20/132 (15)	85
Brochier et al 2010[53]	III/IV	142	6.9	1/15 (6)	–	56/127 (44)	–

[a] Includes four patients operated by transcranial approach.
[b] No separated data.

Expert Recommendations

1. Patents who present with nonfunctioning pituitary adenomas should undergo a thorough history and physical examination, visual field examination, endocrine studies, and MRI (Grade 1C Recommendation, Level II/III Evidence).
2. Patients with nonfunctioning pituitary adenomas who present with clinical symptoms and/or who have compression of the optic nerve should be offered surgical resection. Other patients should be closely followed with serial MRI and visual examinations (Grade 1C Recommendation, Level II/III Evidence).
3. Transphenoidal surgery is typically the approach used for patients with nonfunctioning pituitary adenomas because it offers a midline approach to the tumor without needed brain manipulation (Grade 1C Recommendation, Level II/III Evidence).
4. Transphenoidal surgery leads to clinical improvements in the majority of patients, but rarely improves endocrine function (Grade 1C Recommendation, Level II/III Evidence).
5. High-volume centers with high-volume surgeons have improved outcomes as compared to low-volume centers and/or low-volume surgeons. (Grade 1C Recommendation, Level II/III Evidence).
6. Extent of surgical resection is associated with prolonged recurrence free time (Grade 1C Recommendation, Level II/III Evidence).
7. Recurrence or progression should be treated surgically for younger patients, while radiation should be offered to older patients or patients with more medical co-morbidities (Grade 1C Recommendation, Level II/III Evidence).
8. Elderly patients with low operative risk can benefit from surgical intervention similar to younger patients (Grade 1C Recommendation, Level II/III Evidence).

■ Summary and Conclusions

Nonfunctioning pituitary adenomas are a common type of pituitary tumor that frequently present with signs and symptoms secondary to compression on local neural structures. The mainstay treatment for these lesions is surgery, with the goal of complete resection when possible. The transsphenoidal surgical approach is the approach of choice for these lesions. Gross total resection can be achieved in 30 to 70% of cases depending on tumor characteristics and surgeon experience. Neurological symptoms from mass effect often improve after surgery, but recovery of impaired pituitary function is less likely and variable at best. Although controversial, postoperative radiotherapy can be considered in cases of residual tumors to decrease the risk of regrowth and progression. There has been an increasing trend toward employing multimodality management, with surgery, radiotherapy, and/or stereotactic radiosurgery for patients with these tumors, and this may contribute to improved outcome and quality of life. Nevertheless, large, prospective studies with long-term follow-up are needed to demonstrate the effectiveness of adjuvant therapies.

■ References

1. Black PM, Zervas NT, Candia G. Management of large pituitary adenomas by transsphenoidal surgery. Surg Neurol 1988; 29(6):443–447
2. Ciric I, Ragin A, Baumgartner C, Pierce D. Complications of transsphenoidal surgery: results of a national survey, review of the literature, and personal experience. Neurosurgery 1997; 40(2):225–236
3. Chanson P, Brochier S. Non-functioning pituitary adenomas. J Endocrinol Invest 2005;28(11, Suppl International):93–99
4. Ezzat S, Asa SL, Couldwell WT, et al. The prevalence of pituitary adenomas: a systematic review. Cancer 2004;101(3): 613–619
5. Asa SL. Practical pituitary pathology: what does the pathologist need to know? Arch Pathol Lab Med 2008;132(8): 1231–1240
6. Menucci M, Quiñones-Hinojosa A, Burger P, Salvatori R. Effect of dopaminergic drug treatment on surgical findings in prolactinomas. Pituitary 2011;14(1):68–74
7. Biousse V, Newman NJ, Oyesiku NM. Precipitating factors in pituitary apoplexy. J Neurol Neurosurg Psychiatry 2001; 71(4):542–545
8. Feldkamp J, Santen R, Harms E, Aulich A, Mödder U, Scherbaum WA. Incidentally discovered pituitary lesions: high frequency of macroadenomas and hormone-secreting adenomas—results of a prospective study. Clin Endocrinol (Oxf) 1999;51(1):109–113
9. McComb DJ, Ryan N, Horvath E, Kovacs K. Subclinical adenomas of the human pituitary: new light on old problems. Arch Pathol Lab Med 1983;107(9):488–491
10. Greenman Y, Stern N. How should a nonfunctioning pituitary macroadenoma be monitored after debulking surgery? Clin Endocrinol (Oxf) 2009;70(6):829–832
11. Comtois R, Beauregard H, Somma M, Serri O, Aris-Jilwan N, Hardy J. The clinical and endocrine outcome to trans-sphenoidal microsurgery of nonsecreting pituitary adenomas. Cancer 1991;68(4):860–866
12. Marazuela M, Astigarraga B, Vicente A, et al. Recovery of visual and endocrine function following transsphenoidal surgery of large nonfunctioning pituitary adenomas. J Endocrinol Invest 1994;17(9):703–707
13. Wichers-Rother M, Hoven S, Kristof RA, Bliesener N, Stoffel-Wagner B. Non-functioning pituitary adenomas: endocrinological and clinical outcome after transsphenoidal and transcranial surgery. Exp Clin Endocrinol Diabetes 2004; 112(6):323–327

14. Dekkers OM, Pereira AM, Roelfsema F, et al. Observation alone after transsphenoidal surgery for nonfunctioning pituitary macroadenoma. J Clin Endocrinol Metab 2006;91(5): 1796–1801
15. Nielsen EH, Lindholm J, Bjerre P, et al. Frequent occurrence of pituitary apoplexy in patients with non-functioning pituitary adenoma. Clin Endocrinol (Oxf) 2006;64(3):319–322
16. Mukherjee D, Zaidi HA, Kosztowski T, et al. Predictors of access to pituitary tumor resection in the United States, 1988-2005. Eur J Endocrinol 2009;161(2):259–265
17. Sanai N, Quiñones-Hinojosa A, Narvid J, Kunwar S. Safety and efficacy of the direct endonasal transsphenoidal approach for challenging sellar tumors. J Neurooncol 2008;87(3): 317–325
18. Frazier JL, Chaichana K, Jallo GI, Quiñones-Hinojosa A. Combined endoscopic and microscopic management of pediatric pituitary region tumors through one nostril: technical note with case illustrations. Childs Nerv Syst 2008;24(12): 1469–1478
19. Komotar RJ, Starke RM, Raper DM, Anand VK, Schwartz TH. Endoscopic endonasal compared with microscopic transsphenoidal and open transcranial resection of giant pituitary adenomas. Pituitary 2012;15(2):150–159
20. Xia X, Ramanathan M, Orr BA, et al. Expanded endonasal endoscopic approach for resection of a growth hormone-secreting pituitary macroadenoma coexistent with a cavernous carotid artery aneurysm. J Clin Neurosci 2012;19(10):1437–1441
21. Gnanalingham KK, Bhattacharjee S, Pennington R, Ng J, Mendoza N. The time course of visual field recovery following transphenoidal surgery for pituitary adenomas: predictive factors for a good outcome. J Neurol Neurosurg Psychiatry 2005;76(3):415–419
22. Grossman R, Mukherjee D, Chaichana KL, et al. Complications and death among elderly patients undergoing pituitary tumour surgery. Clin Endocrinol (Oxf) 2010;73(3): 361–368
23. Losa M, Mortini P, Barzaghi R, et al. Early results of surgery in patients with nonfunctioning pituitary adenoma and analysis of the risk of tumor recurrence. J Neurosurg 2008;108(3): 525–532
24. Arafah BM. Reversible hypopituitarism in patients with large nonfunctioning pituitary adenomas. J Clin Endocrinol Metab 1986;62(6):1173–1179
25. Ferrante E, Ferraroni M, Castrignanò T, et al. Non-functioning pituitary adenoma database: a useful resource to improve the clinical management of pituitary tumors. Eur J Endocrinol 2006;155(6):823–829
26. Mathioudakis N, Pendleton C, Quinones-Hinojosa A, Wand GS, Salvatori R. ACTH-secreting pituitary adenomas: size does not correlate with hormonal activity. Pituitary 2012;15(4): 526–532
27. Mortini P, Barzaghi R, Losa M, Boari N, Giovanelli M. Surgical treatment of giant pituitary adenomas: strategies and results in a series of 95 consecutive patients. Neurosurgery 2007;60(6):993–1002
28. Nemergut EC, Zuo Z, Jane JA Jr, Laws ER Jr. Predictors of diabetes insipidus after transsphenoidal surgery: a review of 881 patients. J Neurosurg 2005;103(3):448–454
29. Greenman Y, Ouaknine G, Veshchev I, Reider-Groswasser II, Segev Y, Stern N. Postoperative surveillance of clinically nonfunctioning pituitary macroadenomas: markers of tumour quiescence and regrowth. Clin Endocrinol (Oxf) 2003; 58(6):763–769
30. Nomikos P, Ladar C, Fahlbusch R, Buchfelder M. Impact of primary surgery on pituitary function in patients with nonfunctioning pituitary adenomas—a study on 721 patients. Acta Neurochir (Wien) 2004;146(1):27–35
31. Freda PU, Beckers AM, Katznelson L, et al; Endocrine Society. Pituitary incidentaloma: an Endocrine Society clinical practice guideline. J Clin Endocrinol Metab 2011;96(4):894–904
32. Sanno N, Oyama K, Tahara S, Teramoto A, Kato Y. A survey of pituitary incidentaloma in Japan. Eur J Endocrinol 2003;149(2):123–127
33. Molitch ME. Pituitary tumours: pituitary incidentalomas. Best Pract Res Clin Endocrinol Metab 2009;23(5):667–675
34. Dekkers OM, Pereira AM, Romijn JA. Treatment and follow-up of clinically nonfunctioning pituitary macroadenomas. J Clin Endocrinol Metab 2008;93(10):3717–3726
35. Molitch ME. Nonfunctioning pituitary tumors and pituitary incidentalomas. Endocrinol Metab Clin North Am 2008; 37(1):151–171, xi
36. Alameda C, Lucas T, Pineda E, et al. Experience in management of 51 non-functioning pituitary adenomas: indications for post-operative radiotherapy. J Endocrinol Invest 2005; 28(1):18–22
37. Kabil MS, Eby JB, Shahinian HK. Fully endoscopic endonasal vs. transseptal transsphenoidal pituitary surgery. Minim Invasive Neurosurg 2005;48(6):348–354
38. Raza SM, Boahene KD, Quinones-Hinojosa A. The transpalpebral incision: its use in keyhole approaches to cranial base brain tumors. Expert Rev Neurother 2010;10(11):1629–1632
39. Raza SM, Garzon-Muvdi T, Boaehene K, et al. The supraorbital craniotomy for access to the skull base and intraaxial lesions: a technique in evolution. Minim Invasive Neurosurg 2010;53(1):1–8
40. Raza SM, Quinones-Hinojosa A, Lim M, Boahene KD. The transconjunctival transorbital approach: a keyhole approach to the midline anterior skull base. World Neurosurg 2012
41. Mortini P, Losa M, Barzaghi R, Boari N, Giovanelli M. Results of transsphenoidal surgery in a large series of patients with pituitary adenoma. Neurosurgery 2005;56(6):1222–1233
42. Chang EF, Zada G, Kim S, et al. Long-term recurrence and mortality after surgery and adjuvant radiotherapy for nonfunctional pituitary adenomas. J Neurosurg 2008;108(4): 736–745
43. Ebersold MJ, Quast LM, Laws ER Jr, Scheithauer B, Randall RV. Long-term results in transsphenoidal removal of nonfunctioning pituitary adenomas. J Neurosurg 1986;64(5):713–719
44. Persky MS, Brunner E, Cooper PR, Cohen NL. Perioperative complications of transseptosphenoidal excision for pituitary adenomas. Skull Base Surg 1996;6(4):231–235
45. O'Sullivan EP, Woods C, Glynn N, et al. The natural history of surgically treated but radiotherapy-naïve nonfunctioning pituitary adenomas. Clin Endocrinol (Oxf) 2009;71(5): 709–714
46. van den Bergh AC, van den Berg G, Schoorl MA, et al. Immediate postoperative radiotherapy in residual nonfunctioning pituitary adenoma: beneficial effect on local control without additional negative impact on pituitary function and life expectancy. Int J Radiat Oncol Biol Phys 2007;67(3):863–869
47. Komotar RJ, Starke RM, Raper DM, Anand VK, Schwartz TH. Endoscopic endonasal compared with microscopic transsphenoidal and open transcranial resection of craniopharyngiomas. World Neurosurg 2012;77(2):329–341
48. Spallone A, Vidal RV, Gonzales JG. Transcranial approach to pituitary adenomas invading the cavernous sinus: a modification of the classical technique to be used in a low-technology environment. Surg Neurol Int 2010;1:25. doi: 10.4103/2152-7806.65054
49. King WA, Rodts GE, Becker DP, Mc Bride DQ. Microsurgical management of giant pituitary tumors. Skull Base Surg 1996;6(1):17–26

50. Woollons AC, Hunn MK, Rajapakse YR, et al. Non-functioning pituitary adenomas: indications for postoperative radiotherapy. Clin Endocrinol (Oxf) 2000;53(6):713–717
51. Zhang X, Fei Z, Zhang J, et al. Management of nonfunctioning pituitary adenomas with suprasellar extensions by transsphenoidal microsurgery. Surg Neurol 1999;52(4):380–385
52. Turner HE, Stratton IM, Byrne JV, Adams CB, Wass JA. Audit of selected patients with nonfunctioning pituitary adenomas treated without irradiation—a follow-up study. Clin Endocrinol (Oxf) 1999;51(3):281–284
53. Brochier S, Galland F, Kujas M, et al. Factors predicting relapse of nonfunctioning pituitary macroadenomas after neurosurgery: a study of 142 patients. Eur J Endocrinol 2010; 163(2):193–200
54. Birkmeyer JD, Stukel TA, Siewers AE, Goodney PP, Wennberg DE, Lucas FL. Surgeon volume and operative mortality in the United States. N Engl J Med 2003;349(22):2117–2127
55. Barker FG II, Klibanski A, Swearingen B. Transsphenoidal surgery for pituitary tumors in the United States, 1996-2000: mortality, morbidity, and the effects of hospital and surgeon volume. J Clin Endocrinol Metab 2003;88(10):4709–4719
56. Gittoes NJ, Sheppard MC, Johnson AP, Stewart PM. Outcome of surgery for acromegaly—the experience of a dedicated pituitary surgeon. QJM 1999;92(12):741–745
57. Rees DA, Hanna FW, Davies JS, Mills RG, Vafidis J, Scanlon MF. Long-term follow-up results of transsphenoidal surgery for Cushing's disease in a single centre using strict criteria for remission. Clin Endocrinol (Oxf) 2002;56(4):541–551
58. Komotar RJ, Starke RM, Raper DM, Anand VK, Schwartz TH. Endoscopic skull base surgery: a comprehensive comparison with open transcranial approaches. Br J Neurosurg 2012;26(5):637–648
59. D'Haens J, Van Rompaey K, Stadnik T, Haentjens P, Poppe K, Velkeniers B. Fully endoscopic transsphenoidal surgery for functioning pituitary adenomas: a retrospective comparison with traditional transsphenoidal microsurgery in the same institution. Surg Neurol 2009;72(4):336–340
60. Goudakos JK, Markou KD, Georgalas C. Endoscopic versus microscopic trans-sphenoidal pituitary surgery: a systematic review and meta-analysis. Clin Otolaryngol 2011;36(3): 212–220
61. Greenman Y, Stern N. Non-functioning pituitary adenomas. Best Pract Res Clin Endocrinol Metab 2009;23(5):625–638
62. Park P, Chandler WF, Barkan AL, et al. The role of radiation therapy after surgical resection of nonfunctional pituitary macroadenomas. Neurosurgery 2004;55(1):100–106
63. Sheehan JP, Kondziolka D, Flickinger J, Lunsford LD. Radiosurgery for residual or recurrent nonfunctioning pituitary adenoma. J Neurosurg 2002;97(5, Suppl):408–414
64. Alahmadi H, Dehdashti AR, Gentili F. Endoscopic endonasal surgery in recurrent and residual pituitary adenomas after microscopic resection. World Neurosurg 2012;77(3-4): 540–547
65. Rudnik A, Zawadzki T, Gałuszka-Ignasiak B, et al. Endoscopic transsphenoidal treatment in recurrent and residual pituitary adenomas—first experience. Minim Invasive Neurosurg 2006; 49(1):10–14
66. McLaughlin N, Ditzel Filho LF, Shahlaie K, Solari D, Kassam AB, Kelly DF. The supraorbital approach for recurrent or residual suprasellar tumors. Minim Invasive Neurosurg 2011; 54(4):155–161
67. Sun DQ, Cheng JJ, Frazier JL, et al. Treatment of pituitary adenomas using radiosurgery and radiotherapy: a single center experience and review of literature. Neurosurg Rev 2010; 34(2):181–189
68. Zeng J, See AP, Aziz K, et al. Nelfinavir induces radiation sensitization in pituitary adenoma cells. Cancer Biol Ther 2011; 12(7):657–663
69. Ebersold MJ, Quast LM, Laws ER Jr, Scheithauer B, Randall RV. Long-term results in transsphenoidal removal of nonfunctioning pituitary adenomas. J Neurosurg 1986;64(5):713–719
70. al-Mefty O, Kersh JE, Routh A, Smith RR. The long-term side effects of radiation therapy for benign brain tumors in adults. J Neurosurg 1990;73(4):502–512
71. Brada M, Rajan B, Traish D, et al. The long-term efficacy of conservative surgery and radiotherapy in the control of pituitary adenomas. Clin Endocrinol (Oxf) 1993;38(6):571–578
72. Littley MD, Shalet SM, Beardwell CG, Ahmed SR, Applegate G, Sutton ML. Hypopituitarism following external radiotherapy for pituitary tumours in adults. Q J Med 1989;70(262): 145–160
73. Minniti G, Traish D, Ashley S, Gonsalves A, Brada M. Risk of second brain tumor after conservative surgery and radiotherapy for pituitary adenoma: update after an additional 10 years. J Clin Endocrinol Metab 2005;90(2):800–804
74. Tsang RW, Brierley JD, Panzarella T, Gospodarowicz MK, Sutcliffe SB, Simpson WJ. Radiation therapy for pituitary adenoma: treatment outcome and prognostic factors. Int J Radiat Oncol Biol Phys 1994;30(3):557–565
75. Loeffler JS, Shih HA. Radiation therapy in the management of pituitary adenomas. J Clin Endocrinol Metab 2011; 96(7):1992–2003
76. Marek J, Jezková J, Hána V, et al. Is it possible to avoid hypopituitarism after irradiation of pituitary adenomas by the Leksell gamma knife? Eur J Endocrinol 2011;164(2):169–178
77. Kurosaki M, Saeger W, Lüdecke DK. Pituitary tumors in the elderly. Pathol Res Pract 2001;197(7):493–497
78. Cohen DL, Bevan JS, Adams CB. The presentation and management of pituitary tumours in the elderly. Age Ageing 1989;18(4):247–252
79. Pietilä TA, Stendel R, Hassler WE, Heimberger C, Ramsbacher J, Brock M. Brain tumor surgery in geriatric patients: a critical analysis in 44 patients over 80 years. Surg Neurol 1999;52(3):259–263
80. Ferrante L, Trillò G, Ramundo E, et al. Surgical treatment of pituitary tumors in the elderly: clinical outcome and long-term follow-up. J Neurooncol 2002;60(2):185–191
81. Sheehan JM, Douds GL, Hill K, Farace E. Transsphenoidal surgery for pituitary adenoma in elderly patients. Acta Neurochir (Wien) 2008;150(6):571–574
82. Petrovich Z, Yu C, Giannotta SL, Zee CS, Apuzzo ML. Gamma knife radiosurgery for pituitary adenoma: early results. Neurosurgery 2003;53(1):51–59
83. Soto-Ares G, Cortet-Rudelli C, Assaker R, et al. MRI protocol technique in the optimal therapeutic strategy of nonfunctioning pituitary adenomas. Eur J Endocrinol 2002;146(2): 176–186

36

The Role of Inferior Petrosal Sinus Sampling for Cushing Disease with Modern Dynamic Magnetic Resonance Imaging

Roukoz Chamoun and William T. Couldwell

Cushing syndrome refers to the constellation of signs and symptoms caused by chronic glucocorticoid excess. It can be spontaneous or induced iatrogenically, usually related to the treatment of inflammatory and autoimmune diseases with glucocorticoids. Spontaneous Cushing syndrome can be adrenocorticotropic hormone (ACTH)-dependent (typically caused by overproduction of ACTH by a pituitary tumor or by an ectopic source) or ACTH-independent (usually caused by adrenal tumors or hyperplasia) (**Table 36.1**). *Cushing disease* refers to the hypersecretion of ACTH by a pituitary tumor (usually an adenoma) and represents the most common cause of spontaneous Cushing syndrome (60 to 70%).[1]

Table 36.1 Causes of Cushing syndrome

Iatrogenic	Iatrogenic administration of glucocorticoids	
Spontaneous	ACTH-dependent	Pituitary tumor (Cushing disease)
		Ectopic secretion of ACTH
		Hypothalamic cause
	ACTH-independent	Adrenal tumor
		Adrenal hyperplasia
		Other adrenal diseases (e.g., dysplasia, primary pigmented nodular)

Abbreviation: ACTH, adrenocorticotropic hormone.

Although Harvey Cushing recognized a pituitary origin of Cushing disease almost a century ago,[2] the diagnosis and management of this disease still pose formidable challenges. Current diagnosis of Cushing disease relies on a combination of routine laboratory tests, suppression tests, brain imaging, and invasive measurements, such as bilateral inferior petrosal sinus sampling (BIPSS). To date, diagnostic and management strategies are far from ideal, and failure rates are still significant.[3] This chapter sheds light on some of the challenges associated with the diagnosis and treatment of Cushing disease and focuses on the role of BIPSS in modern medical practice, especially in view of the wide availability of high-quality dynamic magnetic resonance imaging (MRI).

■ Presentation

Glucocorticoid excess results in a myriad of clinical manifestations and is associated with a high rate of mortality and morbidity, underscoring the importance of an accurate diagnosis and efficacious treatment.[4] Classic manifestations include centripetal fat deposition with secondary weight gain, moon facies, and buffalo hump; hirsutism and skin thinning with secondary striae; and ecchymosis. Cushing disease also leads to osteoporosis that can predispose the patient to pathological fractures, a state of immunosuppression, hypertension, diabetes, cardiovascular diseases, infertility, and psychiatric disturbances.[5,6]

Cardiovascular complications, infections, and suicide due to depression or psychotic symptoms remain the leading life-threatening conditions associated with Cushing disease.[7]

■ Stepwise Diagnosis of Cushing Disease

The diagnosis of Cushing disease is done in a systematic stepwise fashion (**Table 36.2**). The first step in diagnosing the condition involves recognizing the characteristics of the disease in a comprehensive medical history and physical examination findings. The clinician should keep in mind that not all patients present with the complete classic picture of Cushing disease; some have atypical or incomplete clinical manifestation that can vary widely in severity.[8] The second step is to confirm a state of hypercortisolism and impaired physiological feedback of the hypothalamic–pituitary–adrenal axis, thus establishing the diagnosis of Cushing syndrome. This can usually be done through 24-hour urinary free cortisol levels, late-night salivary cortisol levels, and low-dose dexamethasone suppression tests. Step three involves investigation of the cause of Cushing syndrome, starting with differentiating whether the condition is ACTH-dependent or ACTH-independent. This can be done through measurements of ACTH plasma levels. Elevated ACTH levels typically indicate an ACTH-dependent cause, whereas suppressed levels point to an adrenal cause. In questionable cases, a corticotropin-releasing hormone (CRH) stimulation test can be performed: a brisk rise of ACTH indicates a pituitary origin, whereas a blunted response is expected in adrenal causes. The fourth step is to differentiate between pituitary (Cushing disease) and ectopic hypersecretion in ACTH-dependent cases. This is usually done through a high-dose dexamethasone suppression test. Cortisol levels are expected to be suppressed in patients with Cushing disease and refractory in ectopic cases. An MRI scan of the pituitary should also be performed to look for a pituitary tumor. The role and value of BIPSS in determining a pituitary origin of ACTH hypersecretion and in lateralizing the location of an adenoma within the pituitary gland are discussed in detail in a separate section of this chapter.

■ Surgical Outcome of Cushing Disease

Transsphenoidal surgery for resection of the ACTH-secreting tumor is currently the treatment of choice for Cushing disease. Immediate postoperative remission rates vary widely in the published literature, ranging from 42 to 98%,[9–11] mostly because of the heterogeneity of the disease, the variability in the diagnostic and therapeutic approaches, and the lack of a universally accepted definition for remission.[12,13] Ciric et al[10] recently reported a series of 136 patients with Cushing disease treated by transsphenoidal surgery. The overall immediate postoperative biochemical remission was 83.4% (89.8% for microadenomas and 30.7% in macroadenomas). After a mean follow-up of 68.4 months, the incidence of recurrence was 9.7%. In a large series of 426 patients reported by Hofmann et al,[14] the remission rate was 77.9% for microadenomas and 59% for macroadenomas. The recurrence rate was 15.2% for microadenomas and 13% for macroadenomas. In 57 patients, no adenoma was found; 29 of these patients had a hemihypophysectomy, leading to a remission rate of 38% in these cases.

Table 36.2 Stepwise diagnosis of Cushing disease

Step		Tests
Step 1	Clinical suspicion of Cushing	Careful history and physical examination
Step 2	Confirm a state of hypercortisolism (Cushing syndrome)	24-hour urinary free cortisol level Late night salivary cortisol level Low-dose dexamethasone suppression test
Step 3	Confirm ACTH-dependent status	ACTH plasma level CRH stimulation test
Step 4	Confirm a pituitary origin (Cushing disease)	High-dose dexamethasone suppression test Pituitary magnetic resonance imaging BIPSS

Abbreviations: ACTH, adrenocorticotropic hormone; BIPSS, bilateral inferior petrosal sinus sampling; CRH, corticotropin-releasing hormone.

Impact of Magnetic Resonance Imaging on Surgical Outcome

MRI is the gold-standard imaging modality for the pituitary gland. Because MRI offers superior resolution compared with other modalities, such as computed tomography, visualization of microadenomas is usually possible using MRI technology. The impact of using preoperative MRI on the surgical outcome is still disputed, however, with contradictory published reports in the medical literature. Although most series found a higher remission rate when the MRI is positive,[10,15,16] some found no such correlation.[14] Ciric et al[10] found that a positive MRI clearly portended a more favorable prognosis. When the MRI was positive, there was a higher likelihood of finding an adenoma during surgery (95% vs 52%) and a four times greater chance of achieving an immediate postoperative biochemical remission. In the series reported by Hofmann et al,[14] on the other hand, early remission was observed in 72.3% of patients with a positive MRI compared with 64.7% with a negative MRI; this difference was not statistically significant. This finding was attributed by the authors to the large experience of the primary surgeons in a meticulous and systematic exploration of the pituitary gland.

The real challenge with the interpretation of the MRI results in Cushing disease results from the high rate of false-positive and false-negative findings. A normal-looking MRI scan does not obviously exclude the presence of a pituitary tumor. ACTH-secreting tumors tend to be microadenomas, and some are so small that they can escape the resolution of the MRI. Jagannathan et al[17] found that, in 90% of patients (113 out of 125 patients) with negative MRI findings, a pituitary adenoma was removed during surgery and confirmed by histological evaluation. The overall remission rate in negative MRI cases in their series was 95%. On a few occasions, the lesion removed was not identified as an adenoma by histological examination; nevertheless, patients experienced an endocrinological remission. Interestingly, the authors found that the maximum tumor diameter of the adenoma found at surgery in the negative MRI cases was 5 mm; eight were consistent with macroadenomas involving the entire gland and not discernible as abnormal on the MRI scan because of their symmetric and homogeneous appearance. Similarly, the presence of a pituitary adenoma on the MRI scan does not prove that it is ACTH-secreting. In fact, pituitary incidentalomas are so prevalent that the coexistence of a small ACTH-secreting tumor and an incidental adenoma is plausible. It is estimated that the prevalence of pituitary incidentalomas is on the order of 15 to 20% according to postmortem and imaging studies.[18,19]

Dynamic Magnetic Resonance Imaging

The concept of dynamic MRI is based on the difference in enhancement patterns between the tumor and the normal pituitary gland. Both tumoral and normal pituitary tissues enhance after gadolinium injection; however, the former enhances more slowly than the latter, thus increasing the sensitivity of the MRI in the detection of microadenomas. Although a routine precontrast/postcontrast MRI scan may miss the abnormal focus, the dynamic MRI relies on serial acquisition within seconds after gadolinium injection to capture the timing of maximal contrast between the tumor and the gland.[20] In an interesting study, 26 patients with Cushing disease and 10 control normal subjects underwent conventional and dynamic MRIs.[21] The pre- and postcontrast images were initially reviewed, and then the dynamic sequences were interpreted by two radiologists who were blinded to the diagnosis. The results were then correlated against the surgical results and pathological reports. This study found that the sensitivity of dynamic MRI was greater than that of conventional MRI (0.67 vs 0.57). Unsurprisingly, it also found more false-positive findings with dynamic MRI because it can detect more incidental lesions, resulting in a decrease in specificity. Of note, a 1.0 tesla magnet was used in this study.[21] In a larger and more recent study of 87 patients, including a control group of 22 patients in whom the diagnosis was initially inferred clinically but then excluded after appropriate workup, the dynamic MRI (using a 1.5 tesla magnet) had a sensitivity of 0.96, a specificity of 0.84, a negative predictive value of 0.94, and a positive predictive value of 0.88.[22] **Table 36.3** summarizes the results of studies comparing dynamic and conventional MRI.

■ Role of Bilateral Inferior Petrosal Sinus Sampling in Cushing Disease

Despite the relatively high sensitivity and specificity of dynamic MRI, a negative finding does not exclude the diagnosis of Cushing disease, and a positive finding is certainly not sufficient to confirm it. This also applies to the panel of biochemical tests available.[22] As a result, the diagnosis typically relies on critical evaluation of all the tests available. This situation has created the need for an additional reliable test, especially for use in equivocal cases and when other diagnostic modalities lead to discordant results.

Table 36.3 Studies comparing dynamic and conventional magnetic resonance imaging

Study	No. patients	No. control participants	MRI sensitivity among patients	False-positive/incidentalomas among control participants	Magnet used
Kucharczyk et al 1994[28]	18	13	CMRI: 10 out of 18 DMRI: 23 out of 18	CMRI: 0 out of 13 DMRI: 4 out of 13	N/A
Bishop et al 1994[29]	10	0	CMRI: 8 out of 10 DMRI: 8 out of 10	N/A	N/A
Tabarin et al 1998[21]	26 (21 CD, 5 ectopic)	10	CMRI: 11 out of 21 DMRI: 14 out of 21	CMRI: 0 out of 10 DMRI: 3 out of 10	1.0 tesla

Abbreviations: CD, Cushing disease; CMRI, conventional MRI; DMRI, dynamic MRI.

Rationale for the Use of Bilateral Inferior Petrosal Sinus Sampling

To accurately diagnose Cushing disease, there is a need to establish a pituitary source of excessive ACTH secretion. It has been postulated that in this disease the ACTH concentration would be higher in the venous drainage of the pituitary gland than in the systemic circulation. The hypophyseal veins drain laterally into the cavernous sinuses, which drain posteriorly into the inferior petrosal sinus (IPS) that joins the internal jugular vein at the level of the jugular foramen. The idea is to measure simultaneously ACTH levels in the IPS bilaterally and in the peripheral blood (P). An IPS:P ratio of ACTH ≥ 2 would confirm the presence of Cushing disease. A side-to-side gradient (≥ 1.4) would also theoretically allow the lateralization of the adenoma because the drainage of the pituitary gland usually occurs predominantly via the ipsilateral IPS.[23,24] Corticotropin-releasing hormone (CRH) is most commonly used as a stimulating agent to increase the sensitivity of the test (after CRH injection, an IPS:P ratio ≥ 3 is used to indicate Cushing disease). Alternatively, desmopressin injections have been used for the same reason. On the other hand, additional measurements of prolactin have been used to normalize ACTH ratios.[23,24]

Anatomical Considerations

A thorough knowledge of the anatomy of the sellar and parasellar region is paramount for correct interpretation of the results and clear appreciation of the limitations of BIPSS. The cavernous sinuses are interconnected by four pathways: the anterior, posterior, and inferior intercavernous sinuses as well as the basilar sinus, which represents the largest communication in most cases.[23] These anatomical variations, with a high degree of communication between the cavernous sinuses, and the significant interpersonal differences in the venous drainage pose significant challenges to data interpretation and can result in false-negative and false-positive findings with respect to determination of laterality. In addition, there is significant interpersonal anatomical variability of the IPS outflow; four variants have been described[25]:

1. Type 1 (most common type, nearly 45% of the cases). IPS drains directly into the internal jugular bulb. No communication with the anterior condylar vein;
2. Type 2 (~ 24%). IPS anastomoses with the anterior condylar vein before draining into the internal jugular vein;
3. Type 3 (~ 24%). IPS drains into the internal jugular vein as a plexus of veins rather than as a single vein;
4. Type 4 (< 7%). IPS drains solely or predominantly into the vertebral venous plexus (and not the internal jugular vein) via the anterior condylar vein.

It is important to realize that a type 4 or even type 3 connection may render direct access to the IPS almost impossible. On the other hand, a prominent connection with the condylar vein may dilute the IPS sampling with systemic venous blood. In addition, symmetric IPS with ipsilateral drainage of the gland is found in < 60% of cases, further complicating the task of adenoma lateralization.[23]

Role of Bilateral Inferior Petrosal Sinus Sampling and Its Diagnostic Accuracy Evidence

In a landmark study published by Oldfield et al[26] in 1991, the authors prospectively studied 281 patients with Cushing syndrome to evaluate the value of BIPSS. The diagnostic criteria used were IPS:P ratio ≥ 2 before CRH and ≥ 3 after CRH administration.

The diagnosis of Cushing disease was considered established if there was histological confirmation of a surgical specimen or clinical remission after surgery (even in the absence of histopathological proof). The study found that the sensitivity of BIPSS was 95%, and its specificity was 100% before CRH. With CRH administration, they found a sensitivity and specificity of 100%. A difference of 1.4-fold or more between the two sinuses predicted the location of the adenoma in 65% and 67% of cases before and after CRH, respectively.[26] Since then, however, a large number of studies have sought to replicate these results in the diagnosis of Cushing disease. Using the same criteria, it has become increasingly apparent that the procedure can lead to false-negative and false-positive results. We conducted a PubMed search and reviewed the studies in the English literature that evaluated the role of BIPSS in Cushing disease. Papers where the primary goal was to determine the accuracy, sensitivity, and specificity of BIPSS were reviewed in detail. **Table 36.4** summarizes the findings of these studies.

Level I and Level II Evidence

None of the studies would qualify as Level I or II evidence.

Level III Evidence

All available studies evaluating the role of BIPSS have a very similar design. They consist of case series of patients suspected to have Cushing disease based on clinical presentation and biochemical evaluation. Pituitary MRI was part of the workup in all of these patients. In most of the studies, BIPSS was done in the case of negative or equivocal MRI findings, whereas in others it was performed for all patients. To determine the sensitivity and specificity, the results of BIPSS were compared with the surgical results. A diagnosis of Cushing disease was confirmed when there was postoperative clinical remission or histological proof. Except for the study by Oldfield et al,[26] all of the series have been retrospective studies. As shown in **Table 36.4**, after administration of CRH (and/or desmopressin), the sensitivity of the procedure varied between 90 and 100%, and the specificity between 60 and 100%. The accuracy of lateralization varied between 60 and 80% in the majority of the studies.

Published Guidelines

There are no clear guidelines or recommendations regarding the indications for the use of BIPSS or the

Table 36.4 Summary of studies evaluating the sensitivity and specificity of IPSS

Authors	No. patients	Before CRH/desmopressin		After CRH/desmopressin		Accuracy of lateralization (%)
		Sensitivity (%)	Specificity (%)	Sensitivity (%)	Specificity (%)	
Oldfield et al 1991[26]	281	95	100	100	100	67
López et al 1996[30]	32	90	N/A	95.8	N/A	66.7
Kaltsas et al 1999[31]	128	72.5	100	97	100	83
Bonelli et al 2000[32]	92	92.2	100	92.2	90	70
Colao et al 2001[33]	74	85	90	90	100	No correlation
Lefournier et al 2003[34]	86	N/A	N/A	N/A	N/A	57 (increased to 71 if venogram is symmetric)
Liu et al 2004[35]	95	93	100	95	100	67
Swearingen et al 2004[36]	179	85	67	90	67	N/A
Kaskarelis et al 2006[37]	78	N/A	N/A	94	62.5	N/A
Machado et al 2007[38]	56	N/A	N/A	92.1	100	78.7
Tsagarakis et al 2007[39]	54	61.7	100	97.9	100	N/A
Lin et al 2007[40]	18	89	N/A	94	N/A	59
Jehle et al 2008[41]	105	N/A	N/A	N/A	N/A	66
Andereggen et al 2012[42]	23	82.4	67	94	67	100

Abbreviations: CRH, corticotropin-releasing hormone; N/A, not available.

interpretation of the results. In practice, some centers reserve the use of BIPSS for cases with negative or equivocal MRI findings, whereas others recommend it in all patients with ACTH-dependent Cushing syndrome. After a workshop sponsored jointly by the Pituitary Society, the European Neuroendocrine Association, and the Italian Society of Endocrinology, a consensus statement was published in 2003.[27] It stated that BIPSS should be recommended in patients with ACTH-dependent Cushing syndrome whose clinical, biochemical, or radiological studies are discordant or equivocal. It also stated that the use of BIPSS for the localization of the microadenoma to the right or the left side of the gland is controversial and its accuracy is disputed.

Expert Recommendations

1. BIPSS is not a first-line diagnostic modality for Cushing disease (Grade 1C Recommendation, Level III Evidence).
2. Cushing syndrome is diagnosed in a systematic stepwise fashion, and BIPSS has an important role in evaluating ACTH-dependent Cushing syndrome to differentiate between a pituitary and an ectopic source (reported sensitivity > 90%; reported specificity varies between 60 and 100%) (Grade 1C Recommendation, Level III Evidence).
3. The role of BIPSS in lateralization of the adenoma to the right or the left of the gland is highly debatable because of anatomical variability. Reported accuracies often range between 60 and 80% (Grade 1C Recommendation, Level III Evidence).

■ Summary and Conclusions

Cushing syndrome is associated with a high mortality and morbidity. Cushing disease (the most common cause of ACTH-dependent Cushing syndrome) is potentially curable by surgery. To date, no single test is able to identify surgical candidates with certainty, and management decisions rely on a thorough understanding of the disease and critical interpretation of biochemical tests, brain imaging, and invasive testing. BIPSS has emerged as one of the most sensitive and specific diagnostic modalities available. Although many centers reserve its use for patients with negative and equivocal MRI findings, it has been our practice to use BIPSS in almost all cases because of the high incidence of incidentalomas on pituitary MRI and because of the high reported rates of treatment failures and recurrences. We believe that gathering data from all available tests up front maximizes the chances for optimal surgical indications and better surgical outcome.

■ References

1. Bertagna X, Guignat L, Groussin L, Bertherat J. Cushing's disease. Best Pract Res Clin Endocrinol Metab 2009;23(5):607–623
2. Cushing H. The basophil adenomas of the pituitary body and their clinical manifestations (pituitary basophilism). Bull Johns Hopkins Hosp 1932;50:137–195
3. Liu JK, Fleseriu M, Delashaw JB Jr, Ciric IS, Couldwell WT. Treatment options for Cushing disease after unsuccessful transsphenoidal surgery. Neurosurg Focus 2007;23(3):E8
4. Ross EJ, Linch DC. Cushing's syndrome—killing disease: discriminatory value of signs and symptoms aiding early diagnosis. Lancet 1982;2(8299):646–649
5. Nieman LK, Biller BM, Findling JW, et al. The diagnosis of Cushing's syndrome: an Endocrine Society Clinical Practice Guideline. J Clin Endocrinol Metab 2008;93(5):1526–1540
6. Findling JW, Raff H. Cushing's syndrome: important issues in diagnosis and management. J Clin Endocrinol Metab 2006;91(10):3746–3753
7. Etxabe J, Vazquez JA. Morbidity and mortality in Cushing's disease: an epidemiological approach. Clin Endocrinol (Oxf) 1994;40(4):479–484
8. Boscaro M, Barzon L, Sonino N. The diagnosis of Cushing's syndrome: atypical presentations and laboratory shortcomings. Arch Intern Med 2000;160(20):3045–3053
9. Trainer PJ, Lawrie HS, Verhelst J, et al. Transsphenoidal resection in Cushing's disease: undetectable serum cortisol as the definition of successful treatment. Clin Endocrinol (Oxf) 1993;38(1):73–78
10. Ciric I, Zhao JC, Du H, et al. Transsphenoidal surgery for Cushing disease: experience with 136 patients. Neurosurgery 2012;70(1):70–80
11. Weber A, Trainer PJ, Grossman AB, et al. Investigation, management and therapeutic outcome in 12 cases of childhood and adolescent Cushing's syndrome. Clin Endocrinol (Oxf) 1995;43(1):19–28
12. Arnott RD, Pestell RG, McKelvie PA, Henderson JK, McNeill PM, Alford FP. A critical evaluation of transsphenoidal pituitary surgery in the treatment of Cushing's disease: prediction of outcome. Acta Endocrinol (Copenh) 1990;123(4):423–430
13. Pieters GF, Hermus AR, Meijer E, Smals AG, Kloppenborg PW. Predictive factors for initial cure and relapse rate after pituitary surgery for Cushing's disease. J Clin Endocrinol Metab 1989;69(6):1122–1126
14. Hofmann BM, Hlavac M, Martinez R, Buchfelder M, Müller OA, Fahlbusch R. Long-term results after microsurgery for Cushing disease: experience with 426 primary operations over 35 years. J Neurosurg 2008;108(1):9–18
15. Bochicchio D, Losa M, Buchfelder M. Factors influencing the immediate and late outcome of Cushing's disease treated by transsphenoidal surgery: a retrospective study by the European Cushing's Disease Survey Group. J Clin Endocrinol Metab 1995;80(11):3114–3120
16. Rees DA, Hanna FW, Davies JS, Mills RG, Vafidis J, Scanlon MF. Long-term follow-up results of transsphenoidal surgery for Cushing's disease in a single centre using strict criteria for remission. Clin Endocrinol (Oxf) 2002;56(4):541–551
17. Jagannathan J, Smith R, DeVroom HL, et al. Outcome of using the histological pseudocapsule as a surgical capsule in Cushing disease. J Neurosurg 2009;111(3):531–539
18. Gross BA, Mindea SA, Pick AJ, Chandler JP, Batjer HH. Diagnostic approach to Cushing disease. Neurosurg Focus 2007;23(3):E1
19. Sivakumar W, Chamoun R, Nguyen V, Couldwell WT. Incidental pituitary adenomas. Neurosurg Focus 2011;31(6):E18
20. Sakamoto Y, Takahashi M, Korogi Y, Bussaka H, Ushio Y. Normal and abnormal pituitary glands: gadopentetate dimeglumine-enhanced MR imaging. Radiology 1991;178(2):441–445

21. Tabarin A, Laurent F, Catargi B, et al. Comparative evaluation of conventional and dynamic magnetic resonance imaging of the pituitary gland for the diagnosis of Cushing's disease. Clin Endocrinol (Oxf) 1998;49(3):293–300
22. Friedman TC, Zuckerbraun E, Lee ML, Kabil MS, Shahinian H. Dynamic pituitary MRI has high sensitivity and specificity for the diagnosis of mild Cushing's syndrome and should be part of the initial workup. Horm Metab Res 2007;39(6):451–456
23. Deipolyi A, Karaosmanoğlu A, Habito C, et al. The role of bilateral inferior petrosal sinus sampling in the diagnostic evaluation of Cushing syndrome. Diagn Interv Radiol 2012; 18(1):132–138
24. Lad SP, Patil CG, Laws ER Jr, Katznelson L. The role of inferior petrosal sinus sampling in the diagnostic localization of Cushing's disease. Neurosurg Focus 2007;23(3):E2
25. Shiu PC, Hanafee WN, Wilson GH, Rand RW. Cavernous sinus venography. Am J Roentgenol Radium Ther Nucl Med 1968;104(1):57–62
26. Oldfield EH, Doppman JL, Nieman LK, et al. Petrosal sinus sampling with and without corticotropin-releasing hormone for the differential diagnosis of Cushing's syndrome. N Engl J Med 1991;325(13):897–905
27. Arnaldi G, Angeli A, Atkinson AB, et al. Diagnosis and complications of Cushing's syndrome: a consensus statement. J Clin Endocrinol Metab 2003;88(12):5593–5602
28. Kucharczyk W, Bishop JE, Plewes DB, Keller MA, George S. Detection of pituitary microadenomas: comparison of dynamic keyhole fast spin-echo, unenhanced, and conventional contrast-enhanced MR imaging. AJR Am J Roentgenol 1994;163(3):671–679
29. Bishop J, Henkelman RM, Plewes DB. Dynamic spin-echo imaging: theoretical assessment and implementation. J Magn Reson Imaging 1994;4(6):843–852
30. López J, Barceló B, Lucas T, et al. Petrosal sinus sampling for diagnosis of Cushing's disease: evidence of false negative results. Clin Endocrinol (Oxf) 1996;45(2):147–156
31. Kaltsas GA, Giannulis MG, Newell-Price JD, et al. A critical analysis of the value of simultaneous inferior petrosal sinus sampling in Cushing's disease and the occult ectopic adrenocorticotropin syndrome. J Clin Endocrinol Metab 1999;84(2):487–492
32. Bonelli FS, Huston J III, Carpenter PC, Erickson D, Young WF Jr, Meyer FB. Adrenocorticotropic hormone-dependent Cushing's syndrome: sensitivity and specificity of inferior petrosal sinus sampling. AJNR Am J Neuroradiol 2000;21(4):690–696
33. Colao A, Faggiano A, Pivonello R, Pecori Giraldi F, Cavagnini F, Lombardi G; Study Group of the Italian Endocrinology Society on the Pathophysiology of the Hypothalamic-Pituitary-Adrenal Axis. Inferior petrosal sinus sampling in the differential diagnosis of Cushing's syndrome: results of an Italian multicenter study. Eur J Endocrinol 2001;144(5):499–507
34. Lefournier V, Martinie M, Vasdev A, et al. Accuracy of bilateral inferior petrosal or cavernous sinuses sampling in predicting the lateralization of Cushing's disease pituitary microadenoma: influence of catheter position and anatomy of venous drainage. J Clin Endocrinol Metab 2003;88(1):196–203
35. Liu C, Lo JC, Dowd CF, et al. Cavernous and inferior petrosal sinus sampling in the evaluation of ACTH-dependent Cushing's syndrome. Clin Endocrinol (Oxf) 2004;61(4):478–486
36. Swearingen B, Katznelson L, Miller K, et al. Diagnostic errors after inferior petrosal sinus sampling. J Clin Endocrinol Metab 2004;89(8):3752–3763
37. Kaskarelis IS, Tsatalou EG, Benakis SV, et al. Bilateral inferior petrosal sinuses sampling in the routine investigation of Cushing's syndrome: a comparison with MRI. AJR Am J Roentgenol 2006;187(2):562–570
38. Machado MC, de Sa SV, Domenice S, et al. The role of desmopressin in bilateral and simultaneous inferior petrosal sinus sampling for differential diagnosis of ACTH-dependent Cushing's syndrome. Clin Endocrinol (Oxf) 2007;66(1): 136–142
39. Tsagarakis S, Vassiliadi D, Kaskarelis IS, Komninos J, Souvatzoglou E, Thalassinos N. The application of the combined corticotropin-releasing hormone plus desmopressin stimulation during petrosal sinus sampling is both sensitive and specific in differentiating patients with Cushing's disease from patients with the occult ectopic adrenocorticotropin syndrome. J Clin Endocrinol Metab 2007;92(6):2080–2086
40. Lin LY, Teng MM, Huang CI, et al. Assessment of bilateral inferior petrosal sinus sampling (BIPSS) in the diagnosis of Cushing's disease. J Chin Med Assoc 2007;70(1):4–10
41. Jehle S, Walsh JE, Freda PU, Post KD. Selective use of bilateral inferior petrosal sinus sampling in patients with adrenocorticotropin-dependent Cushing's syndrome prior to transsphenoidal surgery. J Clin Endocrinol Metab 2008; 93(12):4624–4632
42. Andereggen L, Schroth G, Gralla J, et al. Selective inferior petrosal sinus sampling without venous outflow diversion in the detection of a pituitary adenoma in Cushing's syndrome. Neuroradiology 2012;54(5):495–503

37

The Role of Surgery for Recurrent Cushing's Disease

Garni Barkhoudarian and Edward R. Laws Jr.

Pituitary basophilism as an etiology of polyglandular disease was first characterized by Dr. Harvey Cushing in 1932.[1] He had first written about this disorder in 1912, but the pituitary gland was not thought to be the culprit.[2] Although he had not operated on a single patient with this disorder, through his efforts describing the clinical features and the pituitary histopathology of these patients, he significantly contributed to the understanding of the condition that bears his moniker, Cushing's disease.[3]

■ Cushing's Disease

Cushing's disease (CD) occurs in the setting of adrenocorticotropic hormone (ACTH) hypersecretion from a pituitary or hypothalamic source. The resultant hypercortisolemia causes most of the clinical manifestations of CD. This disorder falls under the more general condition, Cushing's syndrome—pertaining to any cause of symptomatic hypercortisolemia, most commonly exogenous corticosteroid administration. CD is a rare condition, affecting ~ 1 to 2 patients per million people. Peak incidence occurs between the third and fifth decades of life, with a strong predilection toward women.[4] Because of the many systems affected and the nonspecific nature of most symptoms, the diagnosis of this condition is often quite difficult and can take many years from onset of symptoms.

Clinically, patients with CD can present with weight gain, truncal obesity, moon facies, dorsocervical and supraclavicular fat-pad deposition, abdominal striae, hirsutism, hypertension, and insulin-resistant diabetes mellitus. The skin can become myxedematous and tough. Hair thinning or overt hair loss can occur. Hyperpigmentation can be present, particularly over the knuckles and other joint surfaces. Cognitive deficits, mood swings, and cerebral atrophy have also been reported.[5] If left untreated, CD can result in significant deleterious effects on overall health and survival.

In the setting of these clinical features, the diagnosis of CD is confirmed with laboratory confirmation of hypercortisolemia. Typically, serum cortisol is elevated, with an inappropriately normal or moderately elevated ACTH level. Midnight serum or salivary cortisol levels are more sensitive in confirming this, taking advantage of the diurnal cycle of serum cortisol levels. Elevated 24-hour urine free cortisol (UFC) is the gold standard for establishing the diagnosis of Cushing's syndrome.[6] The low-dose dexamethasone suppression test can help confirm hypercortisolemia. The high-dose dexamethasone suppression test is used to differentiate CD from nonpituitary sources of elevated circulating cortisol.[7]

With clinical and laboratory evidence of CD, dedicated neuroimaging is helpful to identify a pituitary lesion. Thin-cut coronal and sagittal sequences on magnetic resonance imaging (MRI) are necessary to identify microadenomas. Pre- and postcontrast SPGR

T1 sequences are particularly sensitive and are bolstered with dynamic postcontrast imaging. Neuroimaging can identify an adenoma in 60% of patients; of these, 10% are macroadenomas.[8]

In the setting of ambiguous imaging or laboratory findings, direct sampling of the cavernous sinus via inferior petrosal sinus sampling (IPSS) can confirm the source of ACTH secretion.[9] Some studies suggest that the laterality of stimulated ACTH sampling can help determine the location of the microadenoma.[10,11] The predictive value of this technique remains equivocal (57 to 71%) and does not preclude intraoperative thorough gland exploration.[12]

At present, the best initial therapy for CD is surgical resection of the pituitary adenoma. Postoperative remission rates have been reported as 70 to 93%. Remission rates are higher for microadenomas (82 to 93%) than for macroadenomas (40 to 86%).[13] Tumor recurrence after clinical remission has been detected in up to 26% of cases with long-term (20 years) follow-up.[14,15] Favorable factors predicting remission include the identification of a microadenoma on an MRI scan.[16,17] Negative ACTH immunocytochemical staining of resected tissue was still associated with a 66% remission rate.[18] Macroadenomas that are not pseudoencapsulated are more likely to invade the cavernous sinus and are more difficult to cure surgically.[19–21] Baseline preoperative serum cortisol and ACTH levels do not predict surgical outcomes.[22]

Radiotherapy and stereotactic radiosurgery are typically not utilized as primary therapy. They are useful adjuncts after noncurative surgical resection and should be reserved for persistent or recurrent disease.[18,23,24] Nevertheless, primary radiosurgery has been reported for CD, with clinical remission occurring in 49% of patients at an average of 7.5 months after onset of therapy.[24] The lengthy interval of active disease for this modality prolongs the patients' exposure to hypercortisolemia and its deleterious effects. Medications, such as ketoconazole, metyrapone, octreotide, and bromocriptine, can be used to suppress hypercortisolemia in CD but are not curative and are most efficacious after surgical resection.[25] Pasireotide and mifepristone have recently been approved for CD; however, long-term outcomes are still pending.[26,27]

The goal of surgery for CD is to achieve gross total resection of the pituitary adenoma when safely possible. Preservation and protection of normal structures, including the anterior and posterior lobes of the pituitary gland, the optic apparatus, and the cavernous sinus contents, are imperative to preventing significant morbidity. When possible, extracapsular dissection can be helpful to prevent future recurrence.[19,20,28] Routine examination of the entire gland and surrounding dura can detect satellite or multiple microadenomata, pituitary hyperplasia, or dural invasion. Careful postoperative monitoring and treatment of hypocortisolism, diabetes insipidus, hyperglycemia, and hypertension are critical to prevent postoperative complications.

Over all, this operation is relatively safe, with an operative mortality of 0.9%. Regardless, complication rates can be as high as 15%.[17] The increased rate of morbidity compared with other pituitary lesions is due to the increased medical comorbidities that occur in patients with CD. Obesity, diabetes, hypertension, and coronary artery disease contribute to these factors. Deep vein thrombosis (DVT) is disproportionately present postoperatively in these patients relative to other pituitary disorders.[29]

Close postoperative follow-up is necessary, regardless of clinical outcome. If in remission, patients are profoundly hypocortisolemic and require judicious exogenous corticosteroid supplementation.[30] Patients can typically be weaned off these steroids between 3 and 12 months following resection. Subsequently, routine cortisol assays, such as fasting morning cortisol, evening salivary cortisol, or 24-hour UFC, should be closely followed. A baseline MRI scan obtained at 3 months following surgery is helpful to compare future imaging in the setting of recurrence.[31] Earlier imaging can be distorted due to inflammation and scar formation.

Evidence-Based Management of Recurrent Cushing's Disease

CD can be difficult to cure, and remission does not guarantee recurrence-free survival. Postoperative data suggest disease recurrence in 5 to 27% of patients with long follow-up (33 to 59 months) who had achieved clinical remission following pituitary adenomectomy.[22,32–36] In a long-term study with a mean follow-up of 49 months, Patil et al report a recurrence rate of 17.4%.[37] The mean time to recurrence was 39 months.

When there is recurrence of CD, the most helpful information is the patient's symptoms and complaints. Patients typically can detect their own disease recurrence before overt manifestations of the disease occur. This can be confirmed with rising serum or salivary cortisol levels. Twenty-four-hour UFC levels are most specific for the diagnosis of recurrent disease. Once recurrence is suspected, dedicated pituitary MRI should be repeated and compared with the baseline postoperative images. Recurrent tumor can sometimes be difficult to differentiate from scar tissue, fat graft, or normal gland (**Figs. 37.1** and **37.2**). A thorough review of preoperative laboratory results, IPSS data, imaging, and histopathology can direct further studies or therapies. With equivocal laboratory or imaging findings, these studies should be repeated—particularly petrosal sinus sampling to detect the source of excess ACTH secretion.

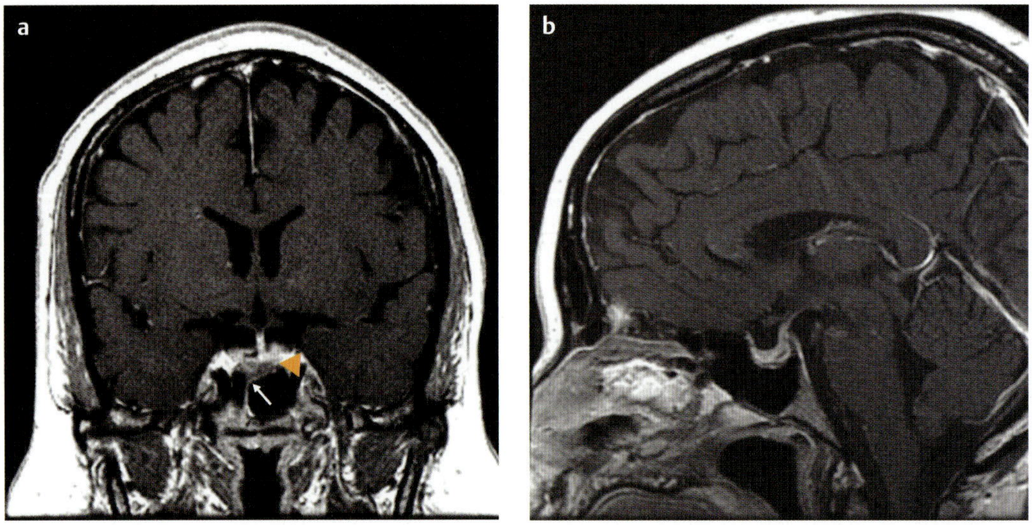

Fig. 37.1 **(a)** Coronal and **(b)** sagittal T1 postcontrast magnetic resonance imaging in a 32-year-old female with two previous microscopic transsphenoidal operations for microadenectomy. The interface between the normal gland and recurrent tumor can be seen (*arrowheads*). A large bony septation is present overlying the recurrent tumor (*arrow*). Postresection, the patient achieved early remission with a nadir cortisol of 2.8 mg/dL.

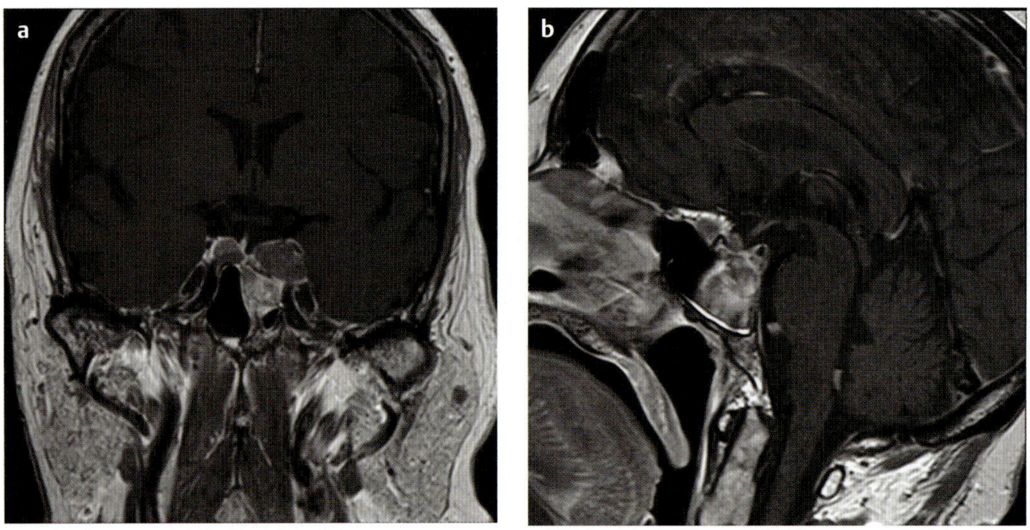

Fig. 37.2 **(a)** Coronal and **(b)** sagittal T1 postcontrast magnetic resonance imaging in a 64-year-old female who had a previous resection and postoperative radiation for her recurrent macroadenoma. Postresection, the patient achieved early remission with a nadir cortisol of 4.2 mg/dL.

Level I and II Evidence

There are no Level I or II evidence-based studies that compare management techniques for recurrent CD.

Level III and IV Evidence

Reoperative management of patients with recurrent CD from an identified ACTH-secreting adenoma, when possible, is ideal. Locatelli et al advocate immediate postoperative reexploration when the postoperative cortisol remains above 2 mg/dL. They reported a 67% remission rate in 12 patients, without additional therapy.[38] Others reported a 53 to 70% remission rate with this approach.[34,39] Hemihypophysectomy or total hypophysectomy may be indicated for refractory patients, although tumors demonstrating invasion on imaging or histopathology are not as likely to benefit from hypophysectomy.[40,41]

Repeat surgery should always be considered before proceeding to radiosurgery or other irreversible therapies. Generally, if a recurrent tumor can be identified, is not invasive, and can be safely resected, then reoperation should be recommended. Remission rates range from 31 to 73% (**Table 37.1**).[42–45] If previous operative pathology or IPSS is positive, remission can be achieved in ~ 55% of patients.[44] Certainly, the overall condition of the patient should be assessed because significant medical comorbidities can increase the risk of surgical mortality.

Medical therapy can help suppress circulating cortisol levels in these patients. It is important to remember that medical agents are not curative and can be associated with long-term toxicity. The cortisol synthesis inhibitors metyrapone and ketoconazole are frequently prescribed for refractory disease. Metyrapone works well to decrease cortisol levels but has significant androgenous side effects, including hirsutism and acne. Although efficacious in decreasing cortisol levels, ketoconazole is associated with a 5 to 10% risk of reversible hepatotoxicity, with occasional serious hepatic injury.[46] Pasireotide, a synthetic somatostatin analogue, has recently been approved for treatment of CD. It provides control in ~ 20% of patients but is associated with aggravation of diabetes mellitus.[27]

Stereotactic radiosurgery and fractionated stereotactic radiotherapy are frequently administered for refractory, surgically incurable CD. Given its delayed onset of action, concurrent medical therapy may be necessary for disease control. Sheehan et al report a 63% clinical remission at 12 months following gamma-knife radiosurgery (Gamma Knife, Electa, Atlanta, GA). In their series of 43 patients, they encountered new endocrine deficits in 16% of patients and one patient with new visual loss.[18]

The employment of progressively more radical surgical approaches (adenomectomy, hypophysectomy, and/or adrenalectomy) is tempered by the patient's severity of illness. Bilateral adrenalectomy is reserved for the most ill of patients who have failed surgical resection and radiosurgery. When this operation is done, circulating cortisol levels diminish consistently. Patients do report increased fatigue, and cortisol and mineralocorticoid replacement are necessary. Because this operation can now be performed laparoscopically, complication rates have diminished, with significant morbidity at 7.5 to 12%.[47,48] Preoperative pituitary radiosurgery is often advised to help prevent the development of Nelson's syndrome.[42]

In the setting of IPSS-confirmed recurrent disease and ambiguous or equivocal neuroimaging, the overall status of the patient should be considered. If the CD is causing uncontrollable medical conditions, particularly diabetes mellitus and hypertension, then hypophysectomy should be considered. The IPSS is unreliable in the postsurgical sella to lateralize ACTH secretion due to possible alterations in venous drainage of the pituitary gland. The decision for hemihypophysectomy or total hypophysectomy should be made based on imaging findings, intraoperative clues, and the patient's ability to undergo another operation for completion hypophysectomy.

Table 37.1 Remission rates for early and late surgery for recurrent Cushing's disease

Study	Title	No. patients	Length of follow-up (months)	Range of follow-up (months)	Remission rate (%)	Evidence level
Early reoperation						
Ram et al 1994[34]	Early Repeat Surgery for Persistent Cushing's Disease	29	34	4 to 84	71	IV
Locatelli et al 2005[38]	Clinical Review: The Strategy of Immediate Reoperation for Transsphenoidal Surgery for Cushing's Disease	12	27	4 to 76	67	IV
Reoperation for recurrent Cushing's disease						
Laws et al 1985[44]	Reoperation for Pituitary Adenomas	4	37	Not reported	25	IV
Friedman et al 1989[43]	Repeat Transsphenoidal Surgery for Cushing's Disease	33	11	0.5 to 39.0	73	IV
De Tommasi et al 2005[42]	Surgical Management of Adrenocorticotropic Hormone-Secreting Macroadenomas: Outcome and Challenges in Patients with Cushing's Disease or Nelson's Syndrome	26	Not reported	1.5 to 12.0	31	IV
Patil et al 2008[45]	Outcomes after Repeat Transsphenoidal Surgery for Recurrent Cushing's Disease	36	36	2 to 126	61	IV

Expert Recommendations

1. Reoperation for recurrent CD should be considered if a target can by identified by MRI or IPSS (Grade 1C Recommendation, Level IV Evidence).
2. Stereotactic radiosurgery or fractionated stereotactic radiotherapy should be utilized if there is no identifiable surgical target (Grade 1C Recommendation, Level IV Evidence).
3. Medication therapy is a useful adjunct to temporize the effects of hypercortisolemia as the patient undergoes further workup or as the delayed effects of radiotherapy take place (Grade 2C Recommendation, Level V Evidence).
4. Bilateral adrenalectomy should be reserved for significantly ill patients who have failed the foregoing strategies. Radiation to the sella should be applied to help prevent Nelson's syndrome (Grade 1C Recommendation, Level IV Evidence).

Therapeutic Nuances

Currently, our practice is to recommend repeat surgical excision whenever a safe target is found. If the tumor can only be debulked, this can still be helpful in decreasing the overall ACTH exposure and improving the efficacy of medical and radiosurgical therapies. Intraoperatively, we do not rely on frozen-section analysis of the resected tissue. Often, these are incongruous with the final immunohistopathological analysis, and some patients achieve cure with negative histopathological findings. Intraoperative ACTH analysis is also unreliable and does not reliably direct further surgical resection. Conversely, it is important to carefully document intraoperative findings because these can guide future radiosurgery targets that are not evident on imaging. If radiosurgery is initiated, patients should be treated with ketoconazole or other cortisol-suppressing agents until the radiosurgical effects take place.

■ Summary and Conclusions

Refractory CD remains one of the more difficult neuroendocrine entities to treat successfully. Surgery plays an important role in the management of this condition and is bolstered with medical and radiosurgical therapies. The general health implications require diligent and long-term management of these patients.

■ References

1. Cushing H. Further notes on pituitary basophilism. JAMA 1932;99:281–284
2. Cushing H. The Pituitary Body and Its Disorders: Clinical States Produced by Disorders of the Hypophysis Cerebri. New York, NY: Lippincott; 1912
3. Mehta GU, Lonser RR, Oldfield EH. The history of pituitary surgery for Cushing disease. J Neurosurg 2012;116(2): 261–268
4. Laws ER Jr, Jane JA Jr, Thapar K. Diagnostic considerations and surgical results for hyperfunctioning pituitary adenomas. In: Kaye AH, Laws ER, eds. Brain Tumors: An Encyclopedic Approach. 3rd ed. New York, NY: Elsevier; 2012:692–722
5. Patil CG, Lad SP, Katznelson L, Laws ER Jr. Brain atrophy and cognitive deficits in Cushing's disease. Neurosurg Focus 2007;23(3):E11
6. Nieman LK, Biller BM, Findling JW, et al. The diagnosis of Cushing's syndrome: an Endocrine Society Clinical Practice Guideline. J Clin Endocrinol Metab 2008;93(5):1526–1540
7. Findling JW, Raff H. Diagnosis and differential diagnosis of Cushing's syndrome. Endocrinol Metab Clin North Am 2001;30(3):729–747
8. Blevins LS Jr, Christy JH, Khajavi M, Tindall GT. Outcomes of therapy for Cushing's disease due to adrenocorticotropin-secreting pituitary macroadenomas. J Clin Endocrinol Metab 1998; 83(1):63–67
9. Kaskarelis IS, Tsatalou EG, Benakis SV, et al. Bilateral inferior petrosal sinuses sampling in the routine investigation of Cushing's syndrome: a comparison with MRI. AJR Am J Roentgenol 2006;187(2):562–570
10. Oldfield EH, Chrousos GP, Schulte HM, et al. Preoperative lateralization of ACTH-secreting pituitary microadenomas by bilateral and simultaneous inferior petrosal venous sinus sampling. N Engl J Med 1985;312(2):100–103
11. Oldfield EH, Doppman JL, Nieman LK, et al. Petrosal sinus sampling with and without corticotropin-releasing hormone for the differential diagnosis of Cushing's syndrome. N Engl J Med 1991;325(13):897–905
12. Lefournier V, Martinie M, Vasdev A, et al. Accuracy of bilateral inferior petrosal or cavernous sinuses sampling in predicting the lateralization of Cushing's disease pituitary microadenoma: influence of catheter position and anatomy of venous drainage. J Clin Endocrinol Metab 2003;88(1):196–203
13. Hassan-Smith ZK, Sherlock M, Reulen RC, et al. Outcome of Cushing's disease following transsphenoidal surgery in a single center over 20 years. J Clin Endocrinol Metab 2012; 97(4):1194–1201
14. Estrada J, Boronat M, Mielgo M, et al. The long-term outcome of pituitary irradiation after unsuccessful transsphenoidal surgery in Cushing's disease. N Engl J Med 1997;336(3):172–177
15. Leinung MC, Kane LA, Scheithauer BW, Carpenter PC, Laws ER Jr, Zimmerman D. Long term follow-up of transsphenoidal surgery for the treatment of Cushing's disease in childhood. J Clin Endocrinol Metab 1995;80(8):2475–2479
16. Prevedello DM, Pouratian N, Sherman J, et al. Management of Cushing's disease: outcome in patients with microadenoma detected on pituitary magnetic resonance imaging. J Neurosurg 2008;109(4):751–759
17. Semple PL, Laws ER Jr. Complications in a contemporary series of patients who underwent transsphenoidal surgery for Cushing's disease. J Neurosurg 1999;91(2):175–179
18. Sheehan JM, Vance ML, Sheehan JP, Ellegala DB, Laws ER Jr. Radiosurgery for Cushing's disease after failed transsphenoidal surgery. J Neurosurg 2000;93(5):738–742

19. Jagannathan J, Smith R, DeVroom HL, et al. Outcome of using the histological pseudocapsule as a surgical capsule in Cushing disease. J Neurosurg 2009;111(3):531–539
20. Monteith SJ, Starke RM, Jane JA Jr, Oldfield EH. Use of the histological pseudocapsule in surgery for Cushing disease: rapid postoperative cortisol decline predicting complete tumor resection. J Neurosurg 2012;116(4):721–727
21. Lonser RR, Ksendzovsky A, Wind JJ, Vortmeyer AO, Oldfield EH. Prospective evaluation of the characteristics and incidence of adenoma-associated dural invasion in Cushing disease. J Neurosurg 2012;116(2):272–279
22. Bochicchio D, Losa M, Buchfelder M. Factors influencing the immediate and late outcome of Cushing's disease treated by transsphenoidal surgery: a retrospective study by the European Cushing's Disease Survey Group. J Clin Endocrinol Metab 1995;80(11):3114–3120
23. Jagannathan J, Sheehan JP, Pouratian N, Laws ER, Steiner L, Vance ML. Gamma Knife surgery for Cushing's disease. J Neurosurg 2007;106(6):980–987
24. Devin JK, Allen GS, Cmelak AJ, Duggan DM, Blevins LS. The efficacy of linear accelerator radiosurgery in the management of patients with Cushing's disease. Stereotact Funct Neurosurg 2004;82(5-6):254–262
25. Morris D, Grossman A. The medical management of Cushing's syndrome. Ann N Y Acad Sci 2002;970(1):119–133
26. Sartor O, Cutler GB Jr. Mifepristone: treatment of Cushing's syndrome. Clin Obstet Gynecol 1996;39(2):506–510
27. Boscaro M, Ludlam WH, Atkinson B, et al. Treatment of pituitary-dependent Cushing's disease with the multireceptor ligand somatostatin analog pasireotide (SOM230): a multicenter, phase II trial. J Clin Endocrinol Metab 2009;94(1):115–122
28. Oldfield EH, Vortmeyer AO. Development of a histological pseudocapsule and its use as a surgical capsule in the excision of pituitary tumors. J Neurosurg 2006;104(1):7–19
29. Hofmann BM, Hlavac M, Martinez R, Buchfelder M, Müller OA, Fahlbusch R. Long-term results after microsurgery for Cushing disease: experience with 426 primary operations over 35 years. J Neurosurg 2008;108(1):9–18
30. Simmons NE, Alden TD, Thorner MO, Laws ER Jr. Serum cortisol response to transsphenoidal surgery for Cushing disease. J Neurosurg 2001;95(1):1–8
31. Atkinson AB, Kennedy A, Wiggam MI, McCance DR, Sheridan B. Long-term remission rates after pituitary surgery for Cushing's disease: the need for long-term surveillance. Clin Endocrinol (Oxf) 2005;63(5):549–559
32. Chen JC, Amar AP, Choi S, Singer P, Couldwell WT, Weiss MH. Transsphenoidal microsurgical treatment of Cushing disease: postoperative assessment of surgical efficacy by application of an overnight low-dose dexamethasone suppression test. J Neurosurg 2003;98(5):967–973
33. Hammer GD, Tyrrell JB, Lamborn KR, et al. Transsphenoidal microsurgery for Cushing's disease: initial outcome and long-term results. J Clin Endocrinol Metab 2004;89(12):6348–6357
34. Ram Z, Nieman LK, Cutler GB Jr, Chrousos GP, Doppman JL, Oldfield EH. Early repeat surgery for persistent Cushing's disease. J Neurosurg 1994;80(1):37–45
35. Rees DA, Hanna FW, Davies JS, Mills RG, Vafidis J, Scanlon MF. Long-term follow-up results of transsphenoidal surgery for Cushing's disease in a single centre using strict criteria for remission. Clin Endocrinol (Oxf) 2002;56(4):541–551
36. Utz AL, Swearingen B, Biller BM. Pituitary surgery and postoperative management in Cushing's disease. Endocrinol Metab Clin North Am 2005;34(2):459–478, xi
37. Patil CG, Prevedello DM, Lad SP, et al. Late recurrences of Cushing's disease after initial successful transsphenoidal surgery. J Clin Endocrinol Metab 2008;93(2):358–362
38. Locatelli M, Vance ML, Laws ER. Clinical review: the strategy of immediate reoperation for transsphenoidal surgery for Cushing's disease. J Clin Endocrinol Metab 2005;90(9):5478–5482
39. Trainer PJ, Lawrie HS, Verhelst J, et al. Transsphenoidal resection in Cushing's disease: undetectable serum cortisol as the definition of successful treatment. Clin Endocrinol (Oxf) 1993;38(1):73–78
40. Robert F, Hardy J. Cushing's disease: a correlation of radiological, surgical and pathological findings with therapeutic results. Pathol Res Pract 1991;187(5):617–621
41. Thomas JP, Richards SH. Long term results of radical hypophysectomy for Cushing's disease. Clin Endocrinol (Oxf) 1983;19(5):629–636
42. De Tommasi C, Vance ML, Okonkwo DO, Diallo A, Laws ER Jr. Surgical management of adrenocorticotropic hormone-secreting macroadenomas: outcome and challenges in patients with Cushing's disease or Nelson's syndrome. J Neurosurg 2005;103(5):825–830
43. Friedman RB, Oldfield EH, Nieman LK, et al. Repeat transsphenoidal surgery for Cushing's disease. J Neurosurg 1989;71(4):520–527
44. Laws ER Jr, Fode NC, Redmond MJ. Transsphenoidal surgery following unsuccessful prior therapy. An assessment of benefits and risks in 158 patients. J Neurosurg 1985;63(6):823–829
45. Patil CG, Veeravagu A, Prevedello DM, Katznelson L, Vance ML, Laws ER, Jr. Outcomes after repeat transsphenoidal surgery for recurrent Cushing's disease. Neurosurgery 2008;63(2):266–270
46. Lewis JH, Zimmerman HJ, Benson GD, Ishak KG. Hepatic injury associated with ketoconazole therapy: analysis of 33 cases. Gastroenterology 1984;86(3):503–513
47. Gagner M, Pomp A, Heniford BT, Pharand D, Lacroix A. Laparoscopic adrenalectomy: lessons learned from 100 consecutive procedures. Ann Surg 1997;226(3):238–246
48. Henry JF, Defechereux T, Raffaelli M, Lubrano D, Gramatica L. Complications of laparoscopic adrenalectomy: results of 169 consecutive procedures. World J Surg 2000;24(11):1342–1346

38

Management of Pituitary Apoplexy (Early versus Delayed Surgery)

Michael Schiraldi and Chirag G. Patil

Pituitary apoplexy is a clinical syndrome classically characterized by the sudden onset of severe headache, emesis, visual deficits, and in some cases cranial nerve palsy and decreased consciousness caused by hemorrhage and/or infarction of the pituitary gland (**Fig. 38.1**). Apoplexy manifests in up to 17% of patients with macroadenomas as the presenting condition.[1,2] Rarely, hemorrhage into normal pituitary is the culprit.[3] Compromise of pituitary function requires expeditious administration of corticosteroids and analysis of endocrine status, but the subsequent management of this entity remains debated. Many neurosurgeons agree that early operative decompression is optimal and yields the best visual outcomes.[4–8] On the other hand, several authors have advocated for delayed decompression (> 8 days postpresentation) reporting effective restoration of vision by such means.[6,9] Conservative management with steroids, bromocriptine, or radiosurgery has also been utilized, and still other patients achieve spontaneous symptomatic improvement without surgical or medical interventions.[10–13]

This chapter examines available reports related to the controversy surrounding optimal treatment of apoplectic patients with particular attention to timing of decompressive surgery and suggests evidenced-based recommendations for treatment.

■ Diagnosis and Evaluation

The sudden onset of headache, visual disturbance, and subsequent loss of consciousness is many times the manner in which apoplectic patients present. Visual symptoms are most common; ophthalmoplegia may be unilateral or bilateral and occurs more often than interruption of visual pathways. Of course, increases in intracranial pressure may lead to altered mental status ranging from lethargy to coma. Hypothalamic dysfunction also contributes to impaired mentation in some patients.

The tumor capsule may be compromised during episodes of apoplexy leading to subarachnoid hemorrhage with resultant meningismus, photophobia, nausea, and vomiting. Acute hydrocephalus may also occur secondary to suprasellar involvement. With hypothalamic involvement, patients are at risk of experiencing decreased blood pressure, abnormal thermoregulation, arrhythmias, aberrant respiratory patterns, and diabetes insipidus (DI).

Diagnosis is confirmed with neuroimaging including computed tomography (CT) or magnetic resonance imaging (MRI) (**Fig. 38.1**). Hemorrhage is best detected with MRI, which will also often reveal third ventricle distortion.[6] In some cases it will be difficult

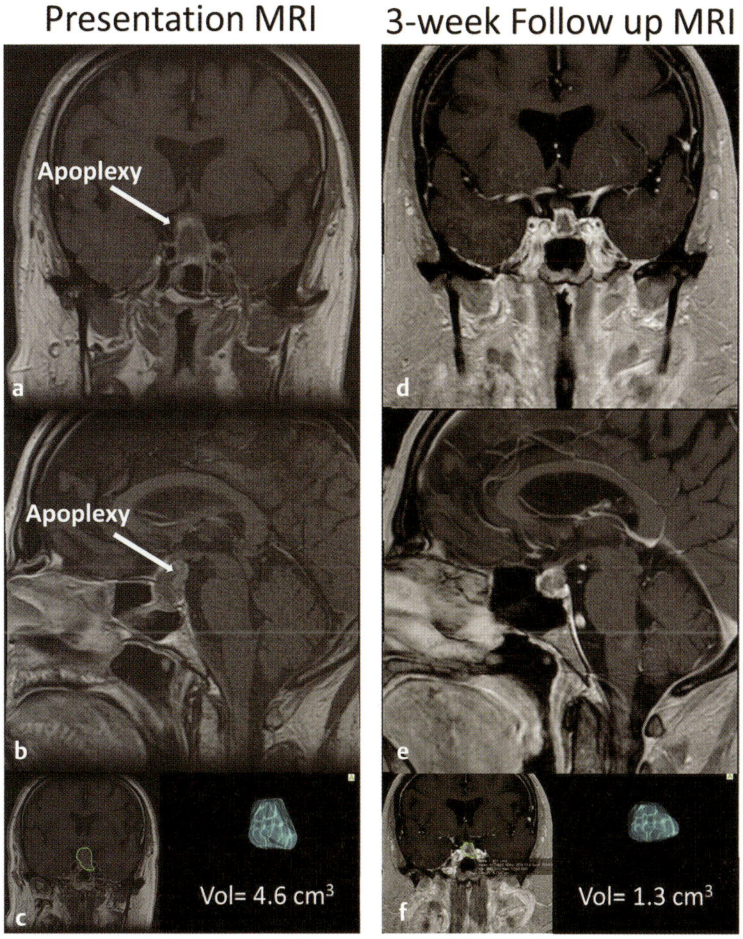

Fig. 38.1 A 73-year-old man within 48 hours of sudden onset of headache, vomiting, double vision, and sixth nerve palsy on the left eye but no decrement in visual acuity. The first magnetic resonance imaging (MRI) scan without contrast was obtained in **(a)** coronal and **(b)** sagittal views and demonstrated a sellar/suprasellar lesion with evidence of a T1 bright signal in the pituitary area and involvement of the left cavernous sinus consistent with pituitary apoplexy. The volumetric measurements **(c)** demonstrated that the lesion was ~ 4.6 cm^3. During the past 3 years the patient had a history of fatigue, difficulty focusing on his work, cold intolerance, and decrease in libido but no change in his weight and no galactorrhea. The endocrine workup revealed a nonfunctioning macroadenoma compressing the optic chiasm, with panhypopituitarism. The patient was managed medically with Synthroid (Abbott Laboratories, Abbott Park, IL), Testim (Auxilium Pharmaceuticals, Malvern, PA), and hydrocortisone and was asked to follow up with a neurosurgeon as an outpatient. By the time he presented to the office, his double vision and level of energy had markedly improved and a follow-up MRI with contrast ~ 3 weeks later demonstrated in **(d)** coronal and **(e)** sagittal views a much smaller lesion with decreased compression of the optic chiasm. The follow-up volumetric measurements **(f)** demonstrated that the lesion was ~ 1 cm^3. Neuro-ophthalmological exam demonstrated marked improvement of diplopia and sixth nerve palsy to almost normal. (Image courtesy of Drs. Quiñones-Hinojosa and Ignacio Jusué-Torres, Johns Hopkins University.)

to distinguish pituitary apoplexy from aneurysmal bleeding, and cerebral angiography will be necessary. Evaluation of endocrine function with emphasis on rapid correction of corticosteroid deficiency is also of paramount importance.

■ Treatment

The goals of treatment of any pituitary lesion include correction of hormonal imbalances secondary to pathological increases or decreases in gland secretion, as well as physical decompression of surrounding structures when necessary. In the case of pituitary apoplexy, immediate efforts are focused on stabilization of hemorrhage and expeditious correction of hormonal deficiency.

Surgical decompression is generally necessary for patients who experience sudden decreases in visual acuity, onset of field cuts, or neurological decline in the setting of hydrocephalus. Decompression of key structures, including the pituitary gland, optic pathways, cavernous sinus, and third ventricle, is the goal of operation, the optimal timing of which remains debated.

Conservative Management

Although surgery was at one time thought to provide the “only hope” for restoring vision in apoplectic patients,[14] conservative management has been utilized to greater degrees, especially in stable or improving patients.[10,12,15,16] In such cases, surgery is replaced by hormonal replacement and hemodynamic stabilization or no treatment at all. Several authors have demonstrated no untoward effects on vision or overall outcome when surgery was withheld, yet such an approach remains controversial.[17] Although the potential complications of surgery may be avoided by less aggressive management of patients experiencing apoplexy, operative decompression remains a mainstay of treatment for defensible reasons, including replicable demonstration of vision preservation.[6,9,18] Studies that advocate for conservative management of apoplexy have been summarized in **Table 38.1**.

Table 38.1 Studies advocating conservative management of apoplexy

Study	Level of evidence	N	Result
Maccagnan et al 1995[12]	II	5 surgically treated 7 conservative management	6 of 7 conservatively managed patients exhibited recovery of ophthalmoplegia
Ayuk et al 2004[10]	III	15 surgically treated 18 conservative management	No difference in tumor regrowth rates or need for hormone replacement between groups
Gruber et al 2006[27]	III	10 surgically treated 20 conservative management	No difference in visual or hormonal end points between groups
Leyer et al 2011[16]	III	19 surgically treated 24 conservative management	No difference in visual or hormonal end points between groups
Sibal et al 2004[8]	III	22 surgically treated 18 conservative management	No difference in visual or hormonal end points between groups
Lubina et al 2005[28]	IV	34 surgically treated 6 conservative management	4 of 6 conservatively managed patients experienced tumor shrinkage but only 2 had visual improvement
Santos et al 2011[15]	IV	2 conservatively managed	Resolution of hypopituitarism without surgery

Surgery

For cases requiring surgery, decompression is most often achieved by the transsphenoidal approach, although transcranial access is employed when appropriate. Studies advocating surgical treatment of apoplexy are summarized in **Table 38.2**. For decades, such means of treating apoplexy have been advocated repeatedly,[6,14,18,19] with much emphasis being placed on the rapid movement of patients to the operating room following presentation.[20–22] Early attention to physical decompression may not only preserve structures affected by mass effect but also protect patients from further deterioration secondary to expansion of hemorrhage.

The bulk of studies advocating surgery over conservative management do conclude that early decompression is best, but the definition of *early* differs among authors. Most often 7 or 8 days is the cutoff between early and late surgery as defined by published series,[2,4,7,9,23] but some studies argue in favor of decompression within 24 or 48 hours.[24–26] Favorable outcomes have also been reported when surgical evacuation was accomplished within 3.5 days of presentation.[5]

Table 38.2 Studies advocating early surgery for apoplexy

Study	Timing of surgery	Level of evidence	N	Result
Zhang et al 2007[25]	24 hours	III	65	Improved acuity in 88.4% of patients; improved visual fields in 92.7% of patients
Seuk et al 2011[24]	48 hours	III	21 treated within 48 hours 8 treated after 48 hours	Statistically significant improvements in visual fields and acuity when surgery was within 48 hours
Chuang et al 2006[5]	3.5 days	III	6 treated within 3.5 days 7 treated after 3.5 days (average 8 days)	Statistically significant advantage to early surgery in terms of visual fields and need for hormonal therapy
Bills et al 1993[4]	7 days	III	37	Delays beyond 1 week retard visual improvements
Randeva et al 1999[7]	8 days	III	35	100% of patients treated within 8 days had restoration of acuity versus 46% of patients treated after 8 days
Agrawal and Mahapatra 2005[23]	7 days	IV	23	Visual and hormonal improvements noted, but no comparison to delayed surgery
Muthukumar et al 2008[9]	7 days	IV	4	Visual and hormonal improvements noted, but no comparison to delayed surgery

Level I Evidence

There are no Level I evidence studies comparing treatment approaches to pituitary apoplexy.

Level II Evidence

The body of literature addressing treatment approaches to pituitary apoplexy contains one Level II evidence paper. Maccagnan et al advocate for conservative management of apoplectic patients in their 2005 prospective series. The authors analyzed 12 cases of patients presenting with sudden-onset headache, visual impairment, or ophthalmoplegia with CT scan confirmed diagnoses of pituitary apoplexy. Eleven of the patients in this series were initially treated with intravenous dexamethasone. Surgery was reserved for patients who failed to demonstrate visual or mental status improvement. Six of seven conservatively managed patients experienced complete recovery of ophthalmoplegia, whereas the seventh did recover partially. Recurrence occurred in one patient in each of the two treatment groups. Ultimately, the authors suggest that conservative management should be utilized when clinical and imaging findings are appropriate.[12]

Level III Evidence

The majority of literature addressing pituitary apoplexy argues for early surgical treatment.[20–22] Among Level III evidence studies, most define early surgery as that taking place within the first week following presentation,[2,4,7] but the cutoff ranges from 48 hours to 8 days, with one paper utilizing 3.5 days.[5,24]

Seuk et al compared outcomes between patients treated surgically within 48 hours and after this time point. Their retrospective analysis included 29 patients, 21 of whom were decompressed within 48 hours. There was a statistically significant advantage to early surgery as measured by both acuity and visual field outcomes.[24]

A retrospective study of 13 patients with pituitary apoplexy published in 2006 defined early surgery as that occurring within 3.5 days of presentation. In this series, statistically significant advantages were demonstrated when early operative management was chosen.[5]

In 1993, Bills et al published a retrospective series of 37 patients with pituitary apoplexy and conclude that surgery within 1 week of presentation is optimal. Significant improvements in visual function were observed when the 1-week benchmark was met, whereas delays beyond 1 week did have deleterious effects in some cases.[4] Randeva et al also reached the conclusion that surgery within 1 week is best, via their retrospective analysis of 35 cases occurring between 1985 and 1996. They too demonstrate statistically significant differences in acuity and visual field outcomes between patients treated before and after the 1-week time-point.[7] Most recently, Turgut and colleagues published an overview of 186 cases of apoplexy published in the last century. Their conclusion is that, although emergent surgery is not necessary to achieve the best outcomes, patients should be taken for operation within 1 week.[2]

Conservative management in the face of pituitary apoplexy is also gaining support.[8,10,16,27] In a retrospective analysis of 33 patients, Ayuk et al conclude that, when visual symptoms are stable or improving, surgery can be avoided. In such patients, there is no statistically significant difference in hormone replacement needs.[10]

Gruber and colleagues also conclude that surgery is not always necessary for apoplectic patients in their 2006 retrospective review of 30 patients. Ten patients were taken to surgery shortly after presentation, whereas the remaining 20 were treated conservatively. The authors conclude that there was no evidence of benefit when surgical management was employed, as measured by both visual and hormonal end points.[27] Similar results were observed by Sibal et al in 2004, in their report of 45 cases, 18 of which were treated conservatively. Still, conservative management was again reserved for the stable or improving patient.[8]

Most recently, a series of 45 patients hospitalized for pituitary apoplexy was published by Leyer et al and also advocates conservative management. Over half of their patients were not taken to the operating room and only six required high-dose steroids. At their mean follow-up point of 21 months, they showed no statistically significant advantage to surgical treatment.[16]

Level IV Evidence

In their retrospective analysis of 65 cases of apoplexy treated emergently by surgical means, Zhang et al[25] report positive results in the large majority of patients. The authors report on 49-month follow-up for 54 cases. Acuity improved in over 88% of cases and visual field cuts improved in over 92%. Choudhry et al also advocated for surgery within the first 24 hours of presentation in their 2011 retrospective chart review of four patients, but this paper did not compare early to late intervention.[26]

Both Muthukumar et al[9] and Agrawal and Mahapatra[23] have advocated for surgical intervention before the 1-week time point in case series of four and 23 patients, respectively. Both papers demonstrate visual and hormonal improvements in the majority of patients treated, but they lack significance because there is no comparison to alternative approaches.

There are also case series that support conservative management of pituitary apoplexy.[15,28] In a series of 40 patients reported by Lubina et al, six were treated conservatively. Whereas four of these patients experienced tumor shrinkage, only two had visual improvement.[28] Finally, a recent report of two cases of nonfunctioning macroadenomas and apoplexy treated conservatively also demonstrated favorable outcomes.[15]

Consensus Statement

The Society of Endocrinology formed the Pituitary Apoplexy Guidelines Development Group in 2009. This group has published a consensus statement regarding the approach to management of this controversial disease process in their "UK Guidelines." Though not intended to define the standard of care for apoplectic patients, this work aims to provide guidance to the multidisciplinary teams treating this disease both in the acute setting as well as after stabilization, when endocrine treatments become of increasing importance. Surgery is encouraged in patients with worsening neurological function, but the group's work is inconclusive with regard to conservative versus surgical management in stable patients. The authors of course argue for the further study of this disease process and trials to optimize treatment strategies.[29]

Expert Recommendations

1. In carefully selected, neurologically improving patients, conservative management with hormonal supplementation may be employed and surgery reserved for those who fail to show visual or mental status improvement (Grade 1B Recommendation, Level II Evidence).
2. When surgical treatment is employed for pituitary apoplexy, patients should be taken to the operating room early (within 48 hours to 1 week) to achieve the higher rates of visual and endocrinological improvement (Grade 1C Recommendation, Level III Evidence).

■ Summary and Conclusions

Pituitary apoplexy is a rare but potentially catastrophic complication of pituitary adenoma, most commonly seen in patients with nonfunctioning tumors. Visual impairment, manifest as ophthalmoplegia as well as decreased visual acuity, is often present, and the correction of such effects is an important goal of treatment. The rapid identification of endocrine abnormalities and equally expeditious correction of hormonal deficiencies is of urgent concern to the physician treating pituitary apoplexy.

Early surgery, though heterogeneously defined, is advocated by most reports comparing it to delayed operation. Surgery within 24 hours has been proposed as optimal by some authors, but a 1-week cutoff may actually suffice at providing favorable outcomes. Surgery probably should not be delayed beyond 1 week, but a definitive conclusion cannot be made at this time without better studies comparing surgical time points.

In certain cases it is reasonable to avoid surgery and manage patients medically or with observation. This approach should be reserved for stable or clinically improving patients but can indeed result in favorable outcomes at long-term follow-up. Although rare, the potentially devastating neurological impairments associated with pituitary apoplexy warrant its further study. Large, prospective, randomized trials should be undertaken to further optimize treatment guidelines.

Acknowledgments

We thank Dr. Quiñones-Hinojosa and Dr. Ignacio Jusué-Torres from Johns Hopkins University School of Medicine for their kind preparation of **Fig. 38.1** from their image bank and from the database from Dr. Quiñones-Hinojosa.

■ References

1. Wakai S, Fukushima T, Teramoto A, Sano K. Pituitary apoplexy: its incidence and clinical significance. J Neurosurg 1981;55(2):187–193
2. Turgut M, Ozsunar Y, Başak S, Güney E, Kir E, Meteoğlu I. Pituitary apoplexy: an overview of 186 cases published during the last century. Acta Neurochir (Wien) 2010;152(5):749–761
3. Laws ER. Pituitary tumor apoplexy: a review. J Intensive Care Med 2008;23(2):146–147
4. Bills DC, Meyer FB, Laws ER Jr, et al. A retrospective analysis of pituitary apoplexy. Neurosurgery 1993;33(4):602–608
5. Chuang CC, Chang CN, Wei KC, et al. Surgical treatment for severe visual compromised patients after pituitary apoplexy. J Neurooncol 2006;80(1):39–47
6. Onesti ST, Wisniewski T, Post KD. Clinical versus subclinical pituitary apoplexy: presentation, surgical management, and outcome in 21 patients. Neurosurgery 1990;26(6):980–986
7. Randeva HS, Schoebel J, Byrne J, Esiri M, Adams CB, Wass JA. Classical pituitary apoplexy: clinical features, management and outcome. Clin Endocrinol (Oxf) 1999;51(2):181–188
8. Sibal L, Ball SG, Connolly V, et al. Pituitary apoplexy: a review of clinical presentation, management and outcome in 45 cases. Pituitary 2004;7(3):157–163
9. Muthukumar N, Rossette D, Soundaram M, Senthilbabu S, Badrinarayanan T. Blindness following pituitary apoplexy: timing of surgery and neuro-ophthalmic outcome. J Clin Neurosci 2008;15(8):873–879

10. Ayuk J, McGregor EJ, Mitchell RD, Gittoes NJ. Acute management of pituitary apoplexy—surgery or conservative management? Clin Endocrinol (Oxf) 2004;61(6):747–752
11. Cardoso ER, Peterson EW. Pituitary apoplexy: a review. Neurosurgery 1984;14(3):363–373
12. Maccagnan P, Macedo CL, Kayath MJ, Nogueira RG, Abucham J. Conservative management of pituitary apoplexy: a prospective study. J Clin Endocrinol Metab 1995;80(7):2190–2197
13. McFadzean RM, Doyle D, Rampling R, Teasdale E, Teasdale G. Pituitary apoplexy and its effect on vision. Neurosurgery 1991;29(5):669–675
14. Epstein S, Pimstone BL, De Villiers JC, Jackson WP. Pituitary apoplexy in five patients with pituitary tumours. BMJ 1971;2(5756):267–270
15. Santos AB, França MM, Hirosawa RM, Marivo M, Zanini MA, Nunes VS. Conservative management of pituitary tumor apoplexy. Arq Bras Endocrinol Metabol 2011;55(5):345–348
16. Leyer C, Castinetti F, Morange I, et al. A conservative management is preferable in milder forms of pituitary tumor apoplexy. J Endocrinol Invest 2011;34(7):502–509
17. Semple PL, Webb MK, de Villiers JC, Laws ER Jr. Pituitary apoplexy. Neurosurgery 2005;56(1):65–72
18. da Motta LA, de Mello PA, de Lacerda CM, Neto AP, da Motta LD, Filho MF. Pituitary apoplexy: clinical course, endocrine evaluations and treatment analysis. J Neurosurg Sci 1999;43(1):25–36
19. Bonicki W, Kasperlik-Załuska A, Koszewski W, Zgliczyński W, Wisławski J. Pituitary apoplexy: endocrine, surgical and oncological emergency. Incidence, clinical course and treatment with reference to 799 cases of pituitary adenomas. Acta Neurochir (Wien) 1993;120(3-4):118–122
20. Woo HJ, Hwang JH, Hwang SK, Park YM. Clinical outcome of cranial neuropathy in patients with pituitary apoplexy. J Korean Neurosurg Soc 2010;48(3):213–218
21. Zhang F, Chen J, Lu Y, Ding X. Manifestation, management and outcome of subclinical pituitary adenoma apoplexy. J Clin Neurosci 2009;16(10):1273–1275
22. Deb S. Clinical significance of pituitary apoplexy. J Indian Med Assoc 1998;96(10):302–303, 307
23. Agrawal D, Mahapatra AK. Visual outcome of blind eyes in pituitary apoplexy after transsphenoidal surgery: a series of 14 eyes. Surg Neurol 2005;63(1):42–46
24. Seuk JW, Kim CH, Yang MS, Cheong JH, Kim JM. Visual outcome after transsphenoidal surgery in patients with pituitary apoplexy. J Korean Neurosurg Soc 2011;49(6):339–344
25. Zhang X, Fei Z, Zhang W, et al. Emergency transsphenoidal surgery for hemorrhagic pituitary adenomas. Surg Oncol 2007;16(2):115–120
26. Choudhry OJ, Choudhry AJ, Nunez EA, et al. Pituitary tumor apoplexy in patients with Cushing's disease: endocrinologic and visual outcomes after transsphenoidal surgery. Pituitary 2012;15(3):428–435
27. Gruber A, Clayton J, Kumar S, Robertson I, Howlett TA, Mansell P. Pituitary apoplexy: retrospective review of 30 patients—is surgical intervention always necessary? Br J Neurosurg 2006;20(6):379–385
28. Lubina A, Olchovsky D, Berezin M, Ram Z, Hadani M, Shimon I. Management of pituitary apoplexy: clinical experience with 40 patients. Acta Neurochir (Wien) 2005;147(2):151–157
29. Rajasekaran S, Vanderpump M, Baldeweg S, et al. UK guidelines for the management of pituitary apoplexy. Clin Endocrinol (Oxf) 2011;74(1):9–20

39

Stereotactic Radiosurgery for Functioning and Nonfunctioning Pituitary Adenomas

Jason Sheehan and Zhiyuan Xu

Pituitary adenomas are relatively common tumors, and they are found in 10 to 27% of the general population.[1,2] Pituitary adenomas represent one of the most challenging clinical entities. Other than for prolactinomas, where medical management is the first treatment, microsurgical resection, usually through a transsphenoidal approach, is the initial treatment for most patients. Nevertheless, pituitary adenomas remain difficult to cure with microsurgical techniques alone. Incomplete resection or tumor recurrence can be the case for many pituitary adenoma patients. Pituitary adenomas often require multimodality treatment, which includes stereotactic radiosurgery (SRS). Nearly a century ago, Harvey Cushing recognized the limitations of conventional surgical approaches for treating intracranial tumors like pituitary adenomas. Cushing and his colleagues used a radium bomb to deliver a single session of focused radiation to intracranial tumors.[3,4] Since then, neurosurgeons and radiation oncologists have utilized ionizing radiation to treat patients with recurrent or residual pituitary adenomas.

Great effort in the field of SRS has been placed on preservation of surrounding critical structures, including cranial nerves, normal pituitary gland, and intracranial vessels. In the past 2 decades, technical refinements for radiosurgical treatment of pituitary adenoma patients have been achieved secondary to advances in radiobiology, neuroimaging, medical physics, and engineering. This chapter reviews the role of, and evidence for, SRS in the treatment of pituitary adenoma patients.

■ Presentation

Microadenomas, which are defined as tumors < 1 cm in maximum dimension, are typically diagnosed incidentally during brain magnetic resonance imaging (MRI) or due to hormone hypersecretion. Macroadenomas, which are tumors ≥ 1 cm in dimension, are typically diagnosed as a result of mass effect leading to hypopituitarism, elevation in prolactin output (i.e., stalk effect), or a focal neurological deficit (e.g., cranial nerve dysfunction). The division between functioning and nonfunctioning adenomas is split evenly for microadenomas. For macroadenomas, nonfunctioning tumors represent the majority (~ 80%).[1] Common presenting symptoms of pituitary adenoma include headache (40 to 60%), visual disturbance, hypopituitarism, or rarely apoplexy.[1,2]

■ Pathology

Pituitary adenomas have different histopathological features that vary depending upon the subtype. A detailed description of the neuropathological features of pituitary adenomas goes beyond the scope of this chapter. However, a brief overview of the subject seems in order.

Growth hormone–producing adenomas are considered functioning somatotroph adenomas. Somatotroph cells are acidophilic and usually are arranged in sinusoidal, diffuse, or trabecular architecture. Prolactinomas are functioning lactrotroph adenomas. Lactotrophs are most commonly organized in trabeculae, papillae, or solid sheets; they may exhibit pseudorosettes around vascular spaces. Thyrotroph adenomas are made up of chromophobic cells. The cellular borders tend be less distinct, and cells may exhibit atypia as well as nuclear pleomorphism. Corticotroph adenomas frequently have three cellular variants that include Crooke cells, densely packed granulated corticotroph adenomas, and sparsely packed corticotroph adenomas.

Nonfunctioning pituitary adenomas may be composed of silent somatroph, lactotroph, corticotroph, and gonadotroph cells. Cells are commonly seen in nests or sheetlike arrangement and demonstrate copious granular eosinophilic cytoplasm.

■ Stereotactic Radiosurgery: The Fundamental Concept and Basic Techniques

Lars Leksell devised the concept of SRS in 1951. He described it as the "closed skull destruction of an intracranial target using ionizing radiation."[5] Seventeen years later, Leksell treated the first pituitary adenoma patient with the Gamma Knife (Elekta, Atlanta, GA). Over the ensuing years, SRS has been utilized to treat thousands of patients with pituitary adenomas.

SRS delivers a highly focused and large dose of radiation to the target while sparing surrounding structures from appreciable doses of radiation. SRS is characterized by a steep fall-off of the radiation dose to the surrounding critical structures. Radiosurgery is usually delivered in a single session but may be delivered in up to five sessions.[6] For cobalt-based SRS devices, which principally are the Gamma Knife (Elekta), the steepest fall-off is achieved at approximately a 50% isodose line, whereas for linear accelerator (LINAC)-based systems, it is usually achieved at an 80 to 90% isodose line. Thus the Gamma Knife (Elekta) will have more dose heterogeneity to the target volume than LINAC-based treatments. The advantages and disadvantages of "hot spots" (i.e., inhomogeneous doses within the target volume) continue to be the source of debate.

For radiosurgery, accurate mapping of the target and collateral structures is required. Each patient undergoes at least one type of stereotactic neuroimaging. For pituitary adenoma patients, this is most frequently stereotactic MRI or stereotactic computed tomography (CT), or both. During radiosurgical delivery, semirigid or rigid target immobilization is utilized. Patients are immobilized using rigid frames fixed to the skull or other immobilization devices (e.g., thermoplastic masks or bite blocks). Each immobilization device has its own stereotactic coordinate system. Radiosurgery is image guided and reliably achieves submillimeter accuracy in the intracranial space. Onboard imaging systems may be used to further track and adjust for sources of error (e.g., set-up error, patient movement, etc.).

There are several types of radiosurgical delivery devices, including the Gamma Knife (Elekta), modified LINACs, or proton beam units. Single-session radiosurgical doses to the tumor margin for nonfunctioning adenomas range from 12 to 18 Gy and 15 to 30 Gy for functioning adenomas. For multisession radiosurgery, these doses may be divided over two to five sessions or fractions.

Gamma knife radiosurgery utilizes multiple isocenters to achieve a dose plan that conforms to the target volume. The number and beam composition of the isocenters vary based upon the size, shape, and location of the pituitary adenoma. In the current version of the Gamma Knife known as the Perfexion (Elekta), each isocenter is composed of eight independent sectors of beams and each sector is composed of no more than 192 simultaneous beams. Beam sizes for the current Gamma Knife Perfexion (Elekta) unit vary from zero (i.e., blocked) to 16 mm. Other cobalt-based radiosurgical devices are also in use and include the Infini system (Masep Infini Medical Science Technology Development Co., City of Industry, CA) and the Rotating Gamma System (American Radiosurgery, San Diego, CA).

LINAC-based radiosurgery (e.g., Cyberknife, Accuray, Sunnyvale, CA; TrueBeam STX, Varian Medical Systems, Palo Alto, CA; Trilogy, Varian; Tomotherapy, Accuray; and Axesse, Elekta) uses multiple radiation arcs to crossfire photon beams at a target.[7] Most systems use nondynamic techniques in which the arc is moved around its radius to deliver radiation that enters from many different vantage points. Technical improvements with LINAC-based radiosurgery include beam shaping, intensity modulation, minileaf collimation, adaptive planning, and onboard CT or fluoroscopic imaging for targeting tracking.

Proton therapy has been utilized as a radiosurgical tool for intracranial pathology, including pituitary adenomas. Proton beam radiosurgery has an inherent superior dose distribution of protons compared with photons because of the Bragg-peak phenomenon.[8] Currently, there are just a few centers using proton beam technology to perform radiosurgery (one- to five-session treatment) or radiation therapy (> 5 fractions) in the United States and abroad. Some proton beam centers can modulate the beam, thereby providing intensity-modulated proton therapy. The number of proton beam centers is increasing as the technology becomes more cost-effective and the indications for protons expand beyond the intracranial space (e.g., prostate cancer, pediatric cancer, etc.).

Stereotactic Radiosurgery for Pituitary Adenomas

Level I and Level II Evidence

There are no Level I or Level II studies supporting the role of stereotactic radiosurgery for the treatment of pituitary adenomas.

Level III and Level IV Evidence

As with many areas of neurosurgery, the level of evidence to support the use of SRS is largely retrospective cohort studies and systematic reviews of the same. These studies constitute Level III evidence (**Tables 39.1, 392., 39.3**). Although ideally there would be more rigorous evidence to support its use, SRS for pituitary adenomas has become a mainstay of treatment throughout the world. The lack of clinical equipoise within the neurosurgery and radiation oncology communities will likely preclude a randomized, prospective trial of radiosurgery versus radiotherapy or repeat resection. Nevertheless, what follows constitutes 1C+ recommendations derived from overwhelming evidence from observational studies extending over a nearly 40-year radiosurgical experience.

Table 39.1 Summary of the literature review for the radiosurgical management of nonfunctioning pituitary adenomas

Study	Patients (N)	Mean/median follow-up (months)	Mean/median margin dose (Gy)	Radiological control of tumor (%)	Neurological deficit (%)	Delayed hypopituitarism (%)
Feigl et al 2002[10]	61	55.2	15	94	NR	40
Sheehan et al 2002[11]	42	31.2	16	97.6	4.8	0
Wowra and Stummer 2002[12]	30	57.7	16	93.3	0	10
Petrovich et al 2003[13]	52	34	15	100	3	NR
Losa et al 2004[14]	54	41.1	16.6	96.3	0	9.3
Muacevic et al 2004[15]	51	21.7	16.5	95	0	3.9
Kajiwara et al 2005[16]	14	32.1	12.6	92.9	7.1	7.1
Picozzi et al 2005[17]	51	40.6	16.5	96.1	NR	NR
Iwai et al 2005[18]	28	36.4	12.3	93	0	7
Mingione et al 2006[19]	100	46.4	18.5	92.2	0	25
Voges et al 2006[20]	37	56.6	13.4	100	4.2	12.3
Liscák et al 2007[21]	140	60	20	100	0	1.4
Pollock et al 2008[22]	62	64	16	96.8	1.6	27
Höybye and Rähn 2009[9]	23	78	20	100	4.3	0
Kobayashi 2009[23]	71	50.2	NR	96.7	2.8	8.2
Castro et al 2010[24]	14	42	12.5	100	0	0
Hayashi et al 2010[25]	43	36	18.2	100	0	0
Gopalan et al 2011[26]	48	95	18.4	83	6.3	39
Iwata et al 2011[27]	100	33	21 Gy/3 Fr 25 Gy/5 Fr	98	1	2
Park et al 2011[28]	125	62	13	90	2.4	24
Total/average	1146	48.66	15.9	95.7	2.1	12.0

Abbreviations: NR, not reported; Fr, fraction.

Table 39.2 Summary of the literature review for the radiosurgical management of Cushing syndrome

Study	Patients (N)	Mean/median margin dose (Gy)	Mean/median follow-up (months)	Biochemical remission (%)	Neurological deficit (%)	Hypopituitarism (%)
Izawa et al 2000[30]	12	23.8	26.4	16.7	0	0
Sheehan et al 2000[31]	43	20	39.1	63	2.3	16
Shin et al 2000[32]	7	32.3	88.2	50	6.3	16.7
Höybye et al 2001[33]	18	NR	16.8	44	0	68.8
Feigl et al 2002[10]	4	15	55.2	60	NR	40
Kobayashi et al 2002[34]	20	28.7	64	23.3	NR	NR
Laws et al 2002[35]	40	20	NR	74	2.5	24
Pollock et al 2002[36]	9	20	42.4	78	22.2	16
Choi et al 2003[37]	7	28.5	42.5	55.6	0	0
Petrovich et al 2003[13]	3	15	34	NR	3	NR
Wong et al 2003[38]	5	NR	38	100	0	20
Witt 2003[39]	8	24	24	0	0	NR
Devin et al 2004[40]	35	14.7	42	49	0	40
Kajiwara et al 2005[16]	2	26	38.5	50	0	50
Voges et al 2006[20]	17	16.4	58.7	52.9	4.2	12.3
Castinetti et al 2007[41]	40	29.5	54.7	42.5	5	15
Jagannathan et al 2007[42]	90	23	45	54	5	22
Petit et al 2007[43]	33	20	62	52	0	52
Pollock et al 2008[44]	8	20	73	87	0	36
Tinnel et al 2008[45]	12	25	37	50	0	50
Castinetti et al 2009[46]	18	28	94	50	5.3	21
Wan et al 2009[47]	68	23	67.3	27.9	2.9	1.7
Kobayashi 2009[23]	30	28.7	64.1	35	NR	NR
Hayashi et al 2010[25]	13	25.2	36	38	15.4	0
Sheehan et al 2011[31]	82	24	31	54	NR	22
Total/average	624	23	48.9	49.9	3.4	23.6

Abbreviations: NR, Not reported; Fr, fraction.

Stereotactic Radiosurgery and Nonfunctioning Pituitary Adenomas

After a resection, long-term control of a pituitary tumor will be achieved in 50 to 80% of macroadenomas.[9] For those with pituitary adenoma recurrence, SRS serves as an excellent treatment approach. It can also be utilized in patients with evidence of residual tumor and for whom tumor progression is likely (e.g., patients with silent adrenocorticotropic hormone [ACTH] or TSH adenomas). Based upon the literature, radiosurgery affords long-term tumor control (i.e., tumor stabilization or regression) in the vast majority of patients with nonfunctioning adenomas and does so with a low rate of complications.[9]

Table 39.3 Summary of the literature review for the radiosurgical management of acromegaly

Study	Patients (N)	Mean/median follow-up (months)	Mean/median margin dose (Gy)	Biochemical remission (%)	Neurological deficit (%)	Hypopituitarism (%)
Izawa et al 2000[30]	29	26.4	23.8	41.4	0	0
Shin et al 2000[32]	6	42.7	34.4	66.7	6.3	0
Zhang et al 2000[50]	68	34	31.3	36.8	2.9	0
Fukuoka et al 2001[51]	9	42	20	50	0	0
Ikeda et al 2001[52]	17	55.8	25	82	0	0
Feigl et al 2002[10]	9	55.2	15	60	NR	40
Pollock et al 2002[36]	26	42.4	20	42	0	16
Attanasio et al 2003[53]	30	46	20	23	0	6.6
Choi et al 2003[37]	9	42.5	28.5	50	0	0
Muramatsu et al 2003[54]	4	30	27.5	50	0	0
Petrovich et al 2003[13]	5	34	15	NR	3	NR
Witt 2003[39]	4	24	24	25	0	NR
Castinetti et al 2005[55]	82	49.5	25	17	0	17.1
Gutt et al 2005[56]	44	22.8	18	47.7	0	NR
Kajiwara et al 2005[16]	2	53.5	13.5	0	0	0
Kobayashi et al 2005[57]	67	63.3	18.9	4.8	11.1	14.6
Jezková et al 2006[58]	96	53.7	35	50	0	26
Voges et al 2006[20]	64	54.3	16.5	37.5	4.2	12.3
Pollock et al 2007[59]	46	63	20	50	2.2	33
Roberts et al 2007[60]	9	25.4	21	44.4	0	33.3
Vik-Mo et al 2007[61]	61	66	26.5	17	3.3	13.1
Jagannathan et al 2008[62]	95	57	22	53	4.2	34
Losa et al 2008[63]	83	69	21.5	60.2	0	8.5
Pollock et al 2008	27	46.9	20	67	0	36
Tinnel et al 2008[45]	9	35	25	44.4	11	22
Castinetti et al 2009[46]	43	102	24	42	5.3	21
Wan et al[a] 2009[47]	103	67.3	21.4	36.9	1	1.7
Ronchi et al 2009[64]	35	120	20	46.0	0	40
Iwai et al 2010[65]	26	84	20	38.0	0	8
Hayashi et al 2010[25]	25	36	25.2	40.0	0	0
Poon et al 2010[66]	40	73.8	20–35	75	0	11.4[b]; 27.3[c]
Sheehan et al 2011[31]	130	31	24	53	NR	34
Total/average	1,303	51.5	22.6	43.6	1.8	14.9

Abbreviations: NR, Not reported.

[a] MASEP gamma knife surgery.

[b] Initial gamma knife surgery.

[c] Repeat gamma knife surgery.

Some of the major radiosurgical series since 2002 that describe outcomes for nonfunctioning adenoma patients are listed in **Table 39.1**.[9–28] Single session radiosurgery margin doses of 12 to 18 Gy are frequently used for patients with nonfunctioning adenomas. Tumor control rates range from 83 to 100% (average, 95.7%) (**Table 39.1**). Neurological deficits are rare (average, 2.1%, range 0 to 7.1%). The most frequent side effect from radiosurgery in pituitary adenoma patients is delayed hypopituitarism (average, 12%; range, 0 to 39%). However, hormonal deficits can be replaced with hormonal supplementation, thereby allowing a patient to have normal neuroendocrine function.

At our institution, in an early report, we demonstrated a 90% rate of local tumor control in a series of 100 patients with nonfunctioning pituitary adenomas with a mean follow-up of 44.9 months.[19] Tumor control was statistically lower when the margin dose to the adenoma was reduced below 12 Gy.[19] In a more recent publication from our group, we examined the outcomes of a smaller group of patients with a minimum follow-up of 4 years after radiosurgery. The overall progression-free survival was 83%; the vast majority of patients (75%) demonstrated a marked decrease in the volume of their adenoma after SRS.[26] This same study demonstrated that long-term tumor control was related to adenoma volume. Those patients with an adenoma volume of < 5 mL were far more likely to have tumor control after radiosurgery. This study finding emphasizes the importance of a maximal, safe tumor resection prior to radiosurgery.

Stereotactic Radiosurgery and Cushing Disease

In the vast majority (i.e., 80% or more) of cases, endogenous Cushing syndrome results from excessive production of ACTH, with the majority of these being related to a pituitary adenoma.[29] Although resection remains the primary treatment for Cushing disease, many adenomas demonstrate invasion of the dura or cavernous sinus or are difficult to delineate on MRI scans, thereby making a cure after resection less likely. Radiosurgery is an invaluable treatment approach for patients with persistent Cushing disease after a resection.

Table 39.2 details the major radiosurgical series for patients with Cushing disease since 2000.[10,13,16,20,23,25,30–48] Most authors utilized a 24-hour urine free cortisol or serum cortisol to denote an endocrine remission. In addition, the radiosurgical margin doses ranged from 18 Gy to as high as 30 Gy to the adenomas of patients with persistent Cushing disease.

Most series demonstrated achievement of remission in the majority of patients (i.e., > 50%). Remission rates after radiosurgery ranged from 16.7 to 87% (**Table 39.2**). Regrettably, the endocrine remission rates after radiosurgery do not equal the high rates of tumor control seen in purely nonfunctioning adenomas. At our institution, endocrine remission of Cushing disease was achieved at a mean time of 12 months after SRS.[42] In most series, the rates of newly developed or worsened cranial neuropathies after radiosurgery, including visual deterioration, are fairly low (average, 3.4%; **Table 39.2**). Hypopituitarism after radiosurgery for Cushing disease appears slightly higher (average, 24.9%; **Table 39.2**) as compared with nonfunctioning adenoma series. This increased rate of hypopituitarism in patients with Cushing disease as compared with those with nonfunctioning adenomas may be a result of higher margin doses delivered to a functioning adenoma and consequently the resulting higher dose to collateral structures, such as the normal pituitary gland and stalk. Late recurrences of Cushing disease after a period of radiosurgically induced endocrine remission were also demonstrated in several Cushing disease series.[42,45] This finding underscores the need for long-term follow-up in radiosurgical patients.

Stereotactic Radiosurgery and Acromegaly

Acromegaly is the second most common type of functioning adenoma, and it occurs with a prevalence of ~ 60 per million.[49] Uncontrolled acromegaly causes significant morbidity (e.g., hypertension, diabetes, cardiomyopathy, and sleep apnea) and a shortened life expectancy for afflicted patients.[49] Resection, if successful, offers an immediate endocrine remission for patients and as such is the preferred first-line treatment for patients with acromegaly. However, similar to those with Cushing disease, those with acromegaly may have a tumor that invades the cavernous sinus or dura and is difficult to cure with a resection. In addition, many patients with acromegaly have macroadenomas, and complete resection of these large adenomas is not always feasible.

Table 39.3 details recent radiosurgical series for patients with acromegaly.[10,13,16,20,25,30,32,36,37,39,44–48,50–66] Margin doses of 18 to 30 Gy are routinely delivered to the adenoma during radiosurgery. After radiosurgery, endocrine remission is achieved in an average of 43.6% of patients with acromegaly (range, 0 to 82%; **Table 39.3**; **Fig. 39.1**). Neurological deficits and hypopituitarism occur in an average 1.8% (range, 0 to 11%) and 15.3% (range, 0 to 40%), respectively (**Table 39.3**). The temporary cessation of antisecretory medications around the time of radiosurgery yielded a

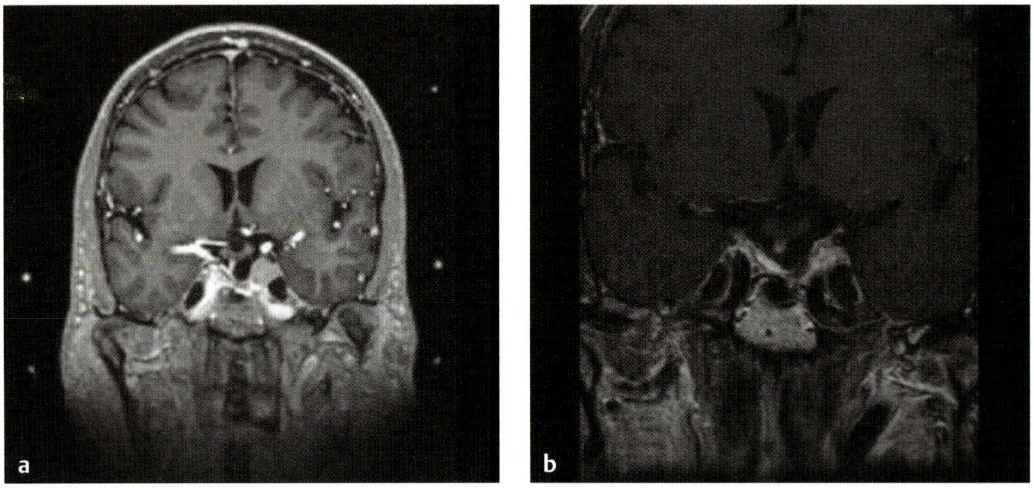

Fig. 39.1 Postcontrast, coronal magnetic resonance imaging: **(a)** A 42-year-old male presenting with persistent acromegaly after prior resection. **(b)** The patient underwent stereotactic radiosurgery (SRS) in which 25 Gy was delivered to the adenoma margin. Six months later, he achieved an endocrine remission. At 5 years after SRS, the pituitary adenoma remains shrunken, and the patient remains in remission.

higher chance of remission in patients with acromegaly treated at our center and others.[48] Also, those patients with an adenoma < 3 mL were more likely to achieve endocrine remission after radiosurgery.[48] Again, even if there is clear cavernous sinus invasion by the adenoma, a safe cytoreductive surgery seems prudent for patients with acromegaly; such a resection seems to increase the chance of endocrine remission after radiosurgery.

At our center, the mean time to endocrine remission after radiosurgery for patients with acromegaly was 24 months. This is twice as long as that for patients with Cushing. This and similar findings suggest a differential response of secretory pituitary adenomas to radiosurgery. We believe that the differential sensitivity of functioning adenoma subtypes to radiosurgery warrants further investigation. The underlying radiobiological difference and ways to enhance the effects of radiosurgery in specific types of functioning pituitary adenomas could be exploited for therapeutic gains.[44]

Stereotactic Radiosurgery–Induced Biochemical Remission and Late Recurrence

SRS results in endocrine remission within a period of time that is substantially longer than that achieved after resection.[67] It is generally advisable to bridge patients with suppressive medications after radiosurgery. After radiosurgery, patients can be taken off of the antisecretory medication periodically and endocrine testing performed to detect if a remission has been achieved. Antisecretory medications can be halted when a postradiosurgery endocrine remission has been achieved. The time interval in which remission after radiosurgery occurs ranges from 3 months to 8 years.[31,32,59] Most series demonstrate endocrine remission in patients with Cushing disease and acromegaly within 1 to 3 years after radiosurgery.

Certain factors have been shown to influence the likelihood of achieving remission. Pollock et al[59] evaluated 46 patients with growth hormone (GH)-secreting adenomas and identified two significant associations. A preradiosurgical immunoglobulin F-1 (IGF-1) level greater than 2.25 times the upper limit of normal range was significantly associated with a lower rate of endocrine remission (hazard ratio [HR], 2.9; 95% confidence interval [CI], 1.2 to 6.9). Another report by Castinetti and colleagues[55] showed similarly significant associations between preoperative GH and IGF-1 levels and the eventual achievement of post-SRS remission.

The use of tumor suppressive medications around the time of radiosurgery has been shown to influence remission.[59] In patients with IGF-1 levels < 2.25 times the upper limit of normal and those who were off somatostatin agonists at the time of radiosurgery, the rate of biochemical remission after radiosurgery exceeded 80%. A similar observation was reported by Landolt et al,[68] who showed that the post-SRS remission rates decreased from 60 to 11% when patients were given octreotide during the periradiosurgical period. Antisecretory medications may decrease radiosensitivity of adenoma cells by causing decreased cell cycling through the G1/M phase. Additionally, octreotide can serve as a free radical scavenger and reduce the DNA damage following ionizing radiation.

The lowering of endocrine remission rates in patients on antisecretory medications is not limited to those with acromegaly. Landolt and Lomax[69] found worse outcomes in patients treated with radiosurgery for prolactinomas while on dopamine agonists. Pouratian et al,[70] in their analysis of 23 patients with aggressive prolactinomas, demonstrated a significant increase in the rate of remission in those patients off dopamine agonists at the time of radiosurgery. We noted a similar improvement in endocrine remission in patients with acromegaly who were systematically taken off suppressive medications at the time of gamma knife radiosurgery.[62]

The actual effect of pituitary suppressive medications on endocrine outcomes after radiosurgery remains controversial. Reports in the literature have not been entirely consistent regarding the importance of a temporary cessation of suppressive medications at the time of radiosurgery.[36,53,55,59,68,69] Two different groups analyzed remission rates after radiosurgery in the setting of somatostatin agonists, and they failed to identify an effect on endocrine remission outcomes.[53,55] Although it is true that the literature is inconsistent and that positive findings are derived exclusively from Level III evidence, it is the practice at many centers to discontinue the administration of suppressive medications for 6 to 8 weeks around the period of radiosurgery. The precise duration of cessation from suppressive medication should be based upon the specific pharmacokinetics of the substance utilized. Most patients can easily tolerate a brief period off suppressive medications during their radiosurgery. Any step that does not harm the patient and may increase the chance of endocrine remission would seem worthwhile.

The overall extent and time period to achieve endocrine remission vary widely across series. As previously noted, there does appear to be a differential radiosensitivity between the various types of secretory pituitary adenomas.[20,23,44] In general, Cushing disease demonstrates the highest rates of biochemical remission, followed by acromegaly, prolactinomas, and Nelson syndrome. Pollock et al[44] reviewed a retrospective series of 46 patients who were similar in terms of their preradiosurgical attributes. The study demonstrated wide variations in endocrine remission after SRS for the various types of secretory adenomas. Although this study and others suggest a differential radiosensitivity for secretory adenomas, the underlying causes for this disparity remain unclear.

A few cases of recurrence following radiosurgically induced remission have been reported.[36,42] These reports serve to emphasize the importance of long-term radiographic and endocrine follow-up after SRS.

Complications after Stereotactic Radiosurgery

Complications following radiosurgery for a pituitary adenoma are uncommon. Hypopituitarism is the most frequently occurring unintended side effect of radiosurgery for a pituitary adenoma. Approximately 30% of pituitary adenoma patients will eventually develop some form of anterior pituitary deficiency after radiosurgery. New onset or worsening of existing hypopituitarism has been correlated to the treatment volume, with those patients having a tumor volume ≤ 4.0 mL exhibiting an 18% 5-year risk of hypopituitarism as compared with 58% for those with larger adenoma volumes.[22] Hypopituitarism after radiosurgery is also likely to be related to the preradiosurgical status of the normal pituitary gland, type and timing of prior treatments, patient age, dose per volume delivered to the normal gland, dose delivered to the pituitary stalk, and rigorousness and length of the endocrine follow-up. An absolutely safe radiosurgical dose to use that will avoid hypopituitarism probably does not exist. Some have advocated placement of a spacer between the residual adenoma and pituitary gland if radiosurgery is being considered after a resection.[71] However, one should not compromise delivery of an optimal dose to the target volume because of a desire to avoid hypopituitarism. Adenoma progression or persistence of a hormonal overproduction by a functioning adenoma is a substantially greater threat to a patient's life expectancy and quality of life than delayed hypopituitarism. With the help of an astute neuroendocrinologist, hypopituitarism can be fully managed with hormonal supplementation.

The next most common side effect of radiosurgery is a cranial neuropathy. Cranial nerves are located in either the adjacent parasellar (III, IV, V, and VI) or suprasellar (II) space and, therefore, are at potential risk of injury from radiosurgery. Cranial neuropathies after radiosurgery occur in 2% or fewer of all patients (**Tables 39.1, 39.2, 39.3**). Improved targeting, greater conformality, steeper dose gradients, and enhanced shielding strategies help minimize this risk.[72] There are reports of improvements in cranial nerve function in patients with pituitary adenoma after radiosurgically induced shrinkage of an adenoma, particularly one that extends into the parasellar or suprasellar space.

Other fairly rare complications include radiation necrosis of the adjacent parenchyma (e.g., temporal lobe or hypothalamus),[20,36,44,47] stenosis of the cavernous segment of the carotid artery,[36,73] and secondary tumor formation.[74] Regarding radiosurgery-induced tumor formation after treatment of a pituitary tumor, no such cases have been reported to date after

SRS. In short, the risk of serious and irreversible complications after radiosurgery for a pituitary adenoma appears to be exceedingly low.

Other Areas of Controversy

Radiotherapy versus Radiosurgery

In the modern era, most patients with pituitary adenoma in the United States are treated with SRS. For those with a larger-volume tumor, a more diffusely infiltrative one, or one with suprasellar or brainstem extension, fractionated external beam radiotherapy (EBRT) can be considered so as to minimize the risk of complications.[75] The local tumor control rate after conventional fractionated EBRT for nonfunctioning pituitary adenomas is > 90% in most series. The rate of endocrine remission of functioning tumors after EBRT is longer and the overall extent of remission seems less than that achieved with SRS.[76] Hypopituitarism after EBRT ranges from 50 to 100% depending upon the length and rigorousness of endocrine follow-up.[77,78] EBRT carries a 1 to 3% risk of optic neuropathy.[77,78] Other serious complications include a 2.7% risk of radiotherapy-induced tumor formation at 10 years after EBRT and a 4% risk at 5 years of stroke after EBRT; such complications seem to exceed comparable risks from SRS.[79] As such, contemporary management for pituitary adenomas favors an approach of resection followed by radiosurgery.

Up-Front Treatment with Radiosurgery

SRS is performed as an up-front treatment for some patients with pituitary adenomas. Radiosurgery is rarely used as the initial treatment for patients with pituitary adenomas. In general, resection offers the following benefits: (1) histological confirmation of tumor type; (2) rapid remission for those with functioning adenomas; and (3) reduction in target volume and clearance from critical structures if radiosurgery is contemplated afterward. Although some patients may have comorbidities that may preclude a craniotomy, few patients with adenomas cannot undergo a safe and beneficial transsphenoidal resection as an up-front treatment.

In rare instances where a nearly definitive diagnosis can be made on the basis of endocrine and radiological studies and the patient is unfit for an initial resection, radiosurgery can be used as an up-front treatment for pituitary adenoma. Results for up-front treatment with radiosurgery for patients with nonfunctioning adenoma who were radiologically diagnosed appear comparable to those who underwent radiosurgery after a previous resection.[19] Based upon the available literature, radiosurgery as an up-front treatment for pituitary adenomas should be used sparingly. Up-front treatment with radiosurgery merits further investigation.

Expert Recommendations

1. Stereotactic radiosurgery (SRS) should be used as an adjunct following incomplete or failed resection of functioning and nonfunctioning pituitary adenomas. Adenoma volume is directly linked to complications and inversely related to success (Grade 1C Recommendation, Level III–V Evidence).
2. Higher radiosurgical doses should be utilized for functioning adenomas than for nonfunctioning ones (Grade 1C Recommendation, Level III–V Evidence).
3. Doses to critical or at risk structures including the optic pathways should be carefully limited to avoid radiosurgically induced complications (Grade 1C Recommendation, Level III–V Evidence).
4. Endocrine testing should be performed in the years following SRS so as to detect delayed hypopituitarism and permit replacement of deficient hormones (Grade 1C Recommendation, Level III–V Evidence).
5. Pituitary suppressive medications appear to alter the radiosensitivity of a functioning adenoma and should be temporarily discontinued when possible during the periradiosurgery period (Grade 1C Recommendation, Level III–V Evidence).

■ Summary and Conclusions

SRS plays an important role in the management of patients with pituitary adenomas. SRS is typically recommended in patients with substantial residual tumor or tumor recurrence after resection. Radiosurgery is also recommended for those with functioning adenomas that fail to achieve endocrine remission after resection. Neurological function after SRS is typically preserved or even improved. Delayed hypopituitarism is the most common complication but is manageable with hormone replacement under the guidance of a neuroendocrinologist. Other serious complications appear exceedingly rare. Pituitary adenoma patients undergoing radiosurgery should have long-term follow-up.

■ References

1. Dekkers OM, Pereira AM, Romijn JA. Treatment and follow-up of clinically nonfunctioning pituitary macroadenomas. J Clin Endocrinol Metab 2008;93(10):3717–3726
2. Vance ML. Treatment of patients with a pituitary adenoma: one clinician's experience. Neurosurg Focus 2004;16(4):E1
3. Seymour ZA, Cohen-Gadol AA. Cushing's lost cases of "radium bomb" brachytherapy for gliomas. J Neurosurg 2010; 113(1):141–148
4. Schulder M, Loeffler JS, Howes AE, Alexander E III, Black PM. Historical vignette: The radium bomb: Harvey Cushing and the interstitial irradiation of gliomas. J Neurosurg 1996; 84(3):530–532
5. Leksell L. The stereotaxic method and radiosurgery of the brain. Acta Chir Scand 1951;102(4):316–319
6. Barnett GH, Linskey ME, Adler JR, et al; American Association of Neurological Surgeons; Congress of Neurological Surgeons Washington Committee Stereotactic Radiosurgery Task Force. Stereotactic radiosurgery—an organized neurosurgery-sanctioned definition. J Neurosurg 2007;106(1):1–5
7. Friedman WA, Foote KD. Linear accelerator radiosurgery in the management of brain tumours. Ann Med 2000;32(1): 64–80
8. Chen CC, Chapman P, Petit J, Loeffler J. Proton radiosurgery in neurosurgery. Neurosurg Focus 2007;23(6):E5
9. Höybye C, Rähn T. Adjuvant gamma knife radiosurgery in non-functioning pituitary adenomas; low risk of long-term complications in selected patients. Pituitary 2009;12(3): 211–216
10. Feigl GC, Bonelli CM, Berghold A, Mokry M. Effects of gamma knife radiosurgery of pituitary adenomas on pituitary function. J Neurosurg 2002;97(5, Suppl):415–421
11. Sheehan JP, Kondziolka D, Flickinger J, Lunsford LD. Radiosurgery for residual or recurrent nonfunctioning pituitary adenoma. J Neurosurg 2002;97(5, Suppl):408–414
12. Wowra B, Stummer W. Efficacy of gamma knife radiosurgery for nonfunctioning pituitary adenomas: a quantitative follow up with magnetic resonance imaging-based volumetric analysis. J Neurosurg 2002;97(5, Suppl):429–432
13. Petrovich Z, Jozsef G, Yu C, Apuzzo ML. Radiotherapy and stereotactic radiosurgery for pituitary tumors. Neurosurg Clin N Am 2003;14(1):147–166
14. Losa M, Valle M, Mortini P, et al. Gamma knife surgery for treatment of residual nonfunctioning pituitary adenomas after surgical debulking. J Neurosurg 2004;100(3):438–444
15. Muacevic A, Uhl E, Wowra B. Gamma knife radiosurgery for nonfunctioning pituitary adenomas. Acta Neurochir Suppl (Wien) 2004;91:51–54
16. Kajiwara K, Saito K, Yoshikawa K, et al. Image-guided stereotactic radiosurgery with the CyberKnife for pituitary adenomas. Minim Invasive Neurosurg 2005;48(2):91–96
17. Picozzi P, Losa M, Mortini P, et al. Radiosurgery and the prevention of regrowth of incompletely removed nonfunctioning pituitary adenomas. J Neurosurg 2005;102(Suppl):71–74
18. Iwai Y, Yamanaka K, Yoshioka K, et al. The usefulness of adjuvant therapy using gamma knife radiosurgery for the recurrent or residual nonfunctioning pituitary adenomas. No Shinkei Geka 2005;33(8):777–783
19. Mingione V, Yen CP, Vance ML, et al. Gamma surgery in the treatment of nonsecretory pituitary macroadenoma. J Neurosurg 2006;104(6):876–883
20. Voges J, Kocher M, Runge M, et al. Linear accelerator radiosurgery for pituitary macroadenomas: a 7-year follow-up study. Cancer 2006;107(6):1355–1364
21. Liscák R, Vladyka V, Marek J, Simonová G, Vymazal J. Gamma knife radiosurgery for endocrine-inactive pituitary adenomas. Acta Neurochir (Wien) 2007;149(10):999–1006
22. Pollock BE, Cochran J, Natt N, et al. Gamma knife radiosurgery for patients with nonfunctioning pituitary adenomas: results from a 15-year experience. Int J Radiat Oncol Biol Phys 2008;70(5):1325–1329
23. Kobayashi T. Long-term results of stereotactic gamma knife radiosurgery for pituitary adenomas. Specific strategies for different types of adenoma. Prog Neurol Surg 2009;22:77–95
24. Castro DG, Cecílio SA, Canteras MM. Radiosurgery for pituitary adenomas: evaluation of its efficacy and safety. Radiat Oncol 2010;5:109
25. Hayashi M, Chernov M, Tamura N, et al. Gamma knife robotic microradiosurgery of pituitary adenomas invading the cavernous sinus: treatment concept and results in 89 cases. J Neurooncol 2010;98(2):185–194
26. Gopalan R, Schlesinger D, Vance ML, Laws E, Sheehan J. Long-term outcomes after gamma knife radiosurgery for patients with a nonfunctioning pituitary adenoma. Neurosurgery 2011;69(2):284–293
27. Iwata H, Sato K, Tatewaki K, et al. Hypofractionated stereotactic radiotherapy with CyberKnife for nonfunctioning pituitary adenoma: high local control with low toxicity. Neuro-oncol 2011;13(8):916–922
28. Park KJ, Kano H, Parry PV, et al. Long-term outcomes after gamma knife stereotactic radiosurgery for nonfunctional pituitary adenomas. Neurosurgery 2011;69(6):1188–1199
29. Biller BMK, Grossman AB, Stewart PM, et al. Treatment of adrenocorticotropin-dependent Cushing's syndrome: a consensus statement. J Clin Endocrinol Metab 2008;93(7): 2454–2462
30. Izawa M, Hayashi M, Nakaya K, et al. Gamma knife radiosurgery for pituitary adenomas. J Neurosurg 2000;93(Suppl 3): 19–22
31. Sheehan JM, Vance ML, Sheehan JP, Ellegala DB, Laws ER Jr. Radiosurgery for Cushing's disease after failed transsphenoidal surgery. J Neurosurg 2000;93(5):738–742
32. Shin M, Kurita H, Sasaki T, et al. Stereotactic radiosurgery for pituitary adenoma invading the cavernous sinus. J Neurosurg 2000;93(Suppl 3):2–5
33. Höybye C, Grenbäck E, Rähn T, Degerblad M, Thorén M, Hulting AL. Adrenocorticotropic hormone-producing pituitary tumors: 12- to 22-year follow-up after treatment with stereotactic radiosurgery. Neurosurgery 2001;49(2):284–291
34. Kobayashi T, Kida Y, Mori Y. Gamma knife radiosurgery in the treatment of Cushing disease: long-term results. J Neurosurg 2002;97(5, Suppl):422–428
35. Laws ER, Reitmeyer M, Thapar K, Vance ML. Cushing's disease resulting from pituitary corticotrophic microadenoma. Treatment results from transsphenoidal microsurgery and gamma knife radiosurgery. Neurochirurgie 2002;48(2-3 Pt 2):294–299
36. Pollock BE, Nippoldt TB, Stafford SL, Foote RL, Abboud CF. Results of stereotactic radiosurgery in patients with hormone-producing pituitary adenomas: factors associated with endocrine normalization. J Neurosurg 2002;97(3):525–530
37. Choi JY, Chang JH, Chang JW, Ha Y, Park YG, Chung SS. Radiological and hormonal responses of functioning pituitary adenomas after gamma knife radiosurgery. Yonsei Med J 2003;44(4):602–607
38. Wong GK, Leung CH, Chiu KW, et al. LINAC radiosurgery in recurrent Cushing's disease after transsphenoidal surgery: a series of 5 cases. Minim Invasive Neurosurg 2003;46(6): 327–330
39. Witt TC. Stereotactic radiosurgery for pituitary tumors. Neurosurg Focus 2003;14(5):e10
40. Devin JK, Allen GS, Cmelak AJ, Duggan DM, Blevins LS. The efficacy of linear accelerator radiosurgery in the management of patients with Cushing's disease. Stereotact Funct Neurosurg 2004;82(5-6):254–262
41. Castinetti F, Nagai M, Dufour H, et al. Gamma knife radiosurgery is a successful adjunctive treatment in Cushing's disease. Eur J Endocrinol 2007;156(1):91–98

42. Jagannathan J, Sheehan JP, Pouratian N, Laws ER, Steiner L, Vance ML. Gamma knife surgery for Cushing's disease. J Neurosurg 2007;106(6):980–987
43. Petit JH, Biller BMK, Coen JJ, et al. Proton stereotactic radiosurgery in management of persistent acromegaly. Endocr Pract 2007;13(7):726–734
44. Pollock BE, Brown PD, Nippoldt TB, Young WF Jr. Pituitary tumor type affects the chance of biochemical remission after radiosurgery of hormone-secreting pituitary adenomas. Neurosurgery 2008;62(6):1271–1276
45. Tinnel BA, Henderson MA, Witt TC, et al. Endocrine response after gamma knife-based stereotactic radiosurgery for secretory pituitary adenoma. Stereotact Funct Neurosurg 2008;86(5):292–296
46. Castinetti F, Morange I, Dufour H, Regis J, Brue T. Radiotherapy and radiosurgery in acromegaly. Pituitary 2009;12(1):3–10
47. Wan H, Chihiro O, Yuan S. MASEP gamma knife radiosurgery for secretory pituitary adenomas: experience in 347 consecutive cases. J Exp Clin Cancer Res 2009;28:36
48. Sheehan JP, Pouratian N, Steiner L, Laws ER, Vance ML. Gamma knife surgery for pituitary adenomas: factors related to radiological and endocrine outcomes. J Neurosurg 2011;114(2):303–309
49. Melmed S. Medical progress: Acromegaly. N Engl J Med 2006;355(24):2558–2573
50. Zhang N, Pan L, Wang EM, Dai JZ, Wang BJ, Cai PW. Radiosurgery for growth hormone-producing pituitary adenomas. J Neurosurg 2000;93(Suppl 3):6–9
51. Fukuoka S, Ito T, Takanashi M, Hojo A, Nakamura H. Gamma knife radiosurgery for growth hormone-secreting pituitary adenomas invading the cavernous sinus. Stereotact Funct Neurosurg 2001;76(3-4):213–217
52. Ikeda H, Jokura H, Yoshimoto T. Transsphenoidal surgery and adjuvant gamma knife treatment for growth hormone-secreting pituitary adenoma. J Neurosurg 2001;95(2):285–291
53. Attanasio R, Epaminonda P, Motti E, et al. Gamma-knife radiosurgery in acromegaly: a 4-year follow-up study. J Clin Endocrinol Metab 2003;88(7):3105–3112
54. Muramatsu J, Yoshida M, Shioura H, et al. Clinical results of LINAC-based stereotactic radiosurgery for pituitary adenoma. Nippon Igaku Hoshasen Gakkai Zasshi 2003;63(5):225–230
55. Castinetti F, Taieb D, Kuhn J-M, et al. Outcome of gamma knife radiosurgery in 82 patients with acromegaly: correlation with initial hypersecretion. J Clin Endocrinol Metab 2005;90(8):4483–4488
56. Gutt B, Wowra B, Alexandrov R, et al. Gamma-knife surgery is effective in normalising plasma insulin-like growth factor I in patients with acromegaly. Exp Clin Endocrinol Diabetes 2005;113(4):219–224
57. Kobayashi T, Mori Y, Uchiyama Y, Kida Y, Fujitani S. Long-term results of gamma knife surgery for growth hormone-producing pituitary adenoma: is the disease difficult to cure? J Neurosurg 2005;102(Suppl):119–123
58. Jezková J, Marek J, Hána V, et al. Gamma knife radiosurgery for acromegaly—long-term experience. Clin Endocrinol (Oxf) 2006;64(5):588–595
59. Pollock BE, Jacob JT, Brown PD, Nippoldt TB. Radiosurgery of growth hormone-producing pituitary adenomas: factors associated with biochemical remission. J Neurosurg 2007;106(5):833–838
60. Roberts BK, Ouyang DL, Lad SP, et al. Efficacy and safety of CyberKnife radiosurgery for acromegaly. Pituitary 2007;10(1):19–25
61. Vik-Mo EO, Oksnes M, Pedersen P-H, et al. Gamma knife stereotactic radiosurgery for acromegaly. Eur J Endocrinol 2007;157(3):255–263
62. Jagannathan J, Sheehan JP, Pouratian N, Laws ER Jr, Steiner L, Vance ML. Gamma knife radiosurgery for acromegaly: outcomes after failed transsphenoidal surgery. Neurosurgery 2008;62(6):1262–1269
63. Losa M, Gioia L, Picozzi P, et al. The role of stereotactic radiotherapy in patients with growth hormone-secreting pituitary adenoma. J Clin Endocrinol Metab 2008;93(7):2546–2552
64. Ronchi CL, Attanasio R, Verrua E, et al. Efficacy and tolerability of gamma knife radiosurgery in acromegaly: a 10-year follow-up study. Clin Endocrinol (Oxf) 2009;71(6):846–852
65. Iwai Y, Yamanaka K, Yoshimura M, Kawasaki I, Yamagami K, Yoshioka K. Gamma knife radiosurgery for growth hormone-producing adenomas. J Clin Neurosci 2010;17(3):299–304
66. Poon TL, Leung SC, Poon CY, Yu CP. Predictors of outcome following gamma knife surgery for acromegaly. J Neurosurg 2010;113(Suppl):149–152
67. Jagannathan J, Smith R, DeVroom HL, et al. Outcome of using the histological pseudocapsule as a surgical capsule in Cushing disease. J Neurosurg 2009;111(3):531–539
68. Landolt AM, Haller D, Lomax N, et al. Octreotide may act as a radioprotective agent in acromegaly. J Clin Endocrinol Metab 2000;85(3):1287–1289
69. Landolt AM, Lomax N. Gamma knife radiosurgery for prolactinomas. J Neurosurg 2000;93(Suppl 3):14–18
70. Pouratian N, Sheehan J, Jagannathan J, Laws ER Jr, Steiner L, Vance ML. Gamma knife radiosurgery for medically and surgically refractory prolactinomas. Neurosurgery 2006;59(2):255–266
71. Taussky P, Kalra R, Coppens J, Mohebali J, Jensen R, Couldwell WT. Endocrinological outcome after pituitary transposition (hypophysopexy) and adjuvant radiotherapy for tumors involving the cavernous sinus. J Neurosurg 2011;115(1):55–62
72. Jagannathan J, Yen CP, Pouratian N, Laws ER, Sheehan JP. Stereotactic radiosurgery for pituitary adenomas: a comprehensive review of indications, techniques and long-term results using the gamma knife. J Neurooncol 2009;92(3):345–356
73. Lim YJ, Leem W, Park JT, Kim TS, Rhee BA, Kim GK. Cerebral infarction with ICA occlusion after gamma knife radiosurgery for pituitary adenoma: a case report. Stereotact Funct Neurosurg 1999;72(Suppl 1):132–139
74. Loeffler JS, Niemierko A, Chapman PH. Second tumors after radiosurgery: tip of the iceberg or a bump in the road? Neurosurgery 2003;52(6):1436–1440
75. Mitsumori M, Shrieve DC, Alexander E III, et al. Initial clinical results of LINAC-based stereotactic radiosurgery and stereotactic radiotherapy for pituitary adenomas. Int J Radiat Oncol Biol Phys 1998;42(3):573–580
76. Landolt AM, Haller D, Lomax N, et al. Stereotactic radiosurgery for recurrent surgically treated acromegaly: comparison with fractionated radiotherapy. J Neurosurg 1998;88(6):1002–1008
77. Zierhut D, Flentje M, Adolph J, Erdmann J, Raue F, Wannenmacher M. External radiotherapy of pituitary adenomas. Int J Radiat Oncol Biol Phys 1995;33(2):307–314
78. Becker G, Kocher M, Kortmann RD, et al. Radiation therapy in the multimodal treatment approach of pituitary adenoma. Strahlenther Onkol 2002;178(4):173–186
79. Brada M, Burchell L, Ashley S, Traish D. The incidence of cerebrovascular accidents in patients with pituitary adenoma. Int J Radiat Oncol Biol Phys 1999;45(3):693–698

■ SECTION XI ■

Craniopharyngiomas

40

Controversies in the Surgical Treatment of Craniopharyngiomas

Tong Yang and Theodore H. Schwartz

Craniopharyngioma, a term first used by Cushing in 1932, denotes a relatively rare form of extra-axial, pathologically benign central nervous system neoplasm of epithelial origin. Craniopharyngiomas are typically located in the sellar and parasellar region, resulting commonly in adherence to the pituitary stalk, optic chiasm and apparatus, vessels of the circle of Willis, and hypothalamus and floor of the third ventricle. Because of their unique anatomical location, craniopharyngiomas and their treatment can produce severe, devastating symptoms in patients, in spite of the benign pathology. Treatment, in the form of surgery and radiation either alone or in combination, is routinely necessary to alleviate symptoms and prevent the disease process from causing further deterioration in the patient's condition.[1]

This chapter focuses on both the decision to proceed with, and the optimal approach for, surgical treatment. As such, the first controversy centers on the relative merits of surgery compared with radiotherapy, and the second controversy is the choice of surgical approach, namely transsphenoidal versus transcranial. Whether the transsphenoidal approach is performed using an endonasal endoscopic or a microscopic sublabial approach is not important because the principle behind both surgical techniques is similar, albeit the endonasal endoscopic approach may utilize more extended transplanum openings and increase the applicability of the transsphenoidal approach. The best available evidence is presented in the hope of providing some guidance to daily clinical practice.

■ Epidemiology and Pathology

Craniopharyngiomas represent 2 to 5% of all intracranial neoplasms and 5.6 to 15.0% of pediatric neoplasms. The reported incidence is 0.13 cases per 100,000 person-years with no sex predilection. There is a bimodal age distribution of occurrences, with peak age ranges between 5 and 14 and 50 and 74 years.[1]

Histologically, there are two major subtypes of craniopharyngiomas: the adamantinomatous type is more prevalent in children, and it is theorized to arise from neoplastic transformation of epithelial rest cells within the remnant craniopharyngeal duct; the papillary type is almost exclusively found in adults and is hypothesized to derive from metaplastic changes of epithelial cells within the pituitary stalk or adenohypophysis.[2] Craniopharyngioma is classified as a World Health Organization (WHO) grade I neoplasm, with rare malignant transformations reported.[1] Mutations in the Wnt signaling pathway protein β-catenin have been found only in the adamantinomatous subtype of tumors, suggesting a distinction between the two subtypes at the molecular level.[3]

■ Clinical Presentations and Imaging Characteristics

Considering the underlying pathogenic processes already mentioned, it is not surprising that most craniopharyngiomas are located in the sellar and parasellar region. As many as 94 to 95% of craniopharyngiomas have a suprasellar component. Of these, 20 to 41% occur in a purely suprasellar location, whereas 53 to 75% have both intra- and suprasellar components. Occasionally the tumor can extend into neighboring cranial fossa locations or even be found in ectopic locations.[4] Common presenting symptoms are related to increased intracranial pressure from ventricular obstruction and hydrocephalus (such as headaches, nausea/vomiting, papilledema), visual dysfunction from compression of the optic chiasm and nerve or tract (such as visual field defects or decreased visual acuity), hormonal disequilibrium from pituitary stalk infiltration (all hypophyseal hormones can be affected, including both anterior and posterior lobes), and behavioral/developmental abnormalities from hypothalamic injury in children (such as excessive food-seeking behaviors, or precocious puberty).[4]

The majority (58 to 76%) of reported cases have a tumor size that ranges between 2 and 4 cm. Craniopharyngiomas often have irregular borders with a cystic component (46 to 64% are mainly cystic, 18 to 39% are mainly solid, and 8 to 36% are mixed). The cystic component tends to be hyperintense on T2-weighted magnetic resonance imaging (MRI). On postcontrast MRI scans, the cystic component often enhances along the cyst wall. The solid lesions tend to have a heterogeneous enhancement pattern. The adamantinomatous type usually shows calcifications on plain head computed tomography (CT) and also frequently contains cystic components. MRI can provide invaluable information on the relationships between the lesion and the chiasm, adjacent blood vessels, pituitary stalk, and floor of the third ventricle, which is critical for surgical planning as well as radiation dosing[4] (**Fig. 40.1**).

■ Literature Review

Surgery versus Radiation

Although craniopharyngiomas are benign neoplasms, most patients present with debilitating symptoms at the time of their discovery. It is generally accepted that some form of intervention is needed once the tumor is found. However, the type of intervention to use has been a topic of ongoing debate. A large body of literature exists to support either of two main treatment strategies. The first is aggressive surgical resection with the goal of gross total resection (GTR). Surgery was first attempted by pioneering neurosurgeons when craniopharyngiomas became a recognized clinical entity. With the advent of modern microsurgical techniques, imaging modalities, and perioperative steroid and vasopressin use, GTR became possible with reasonably low mortalities and morbidities, and it has been advocated as a curative measure. Reports have shown that GTR (radiographically confirmed) is associated with a 10-year recurrence rate of 0 to 62% versus 25 to 100% with subtotal resection (STR).[4] Repeat surgery for recurrence is generally considered more difficult due to interruption of the arachnoid plane as well as scarring between the tumor and the adjacent critical

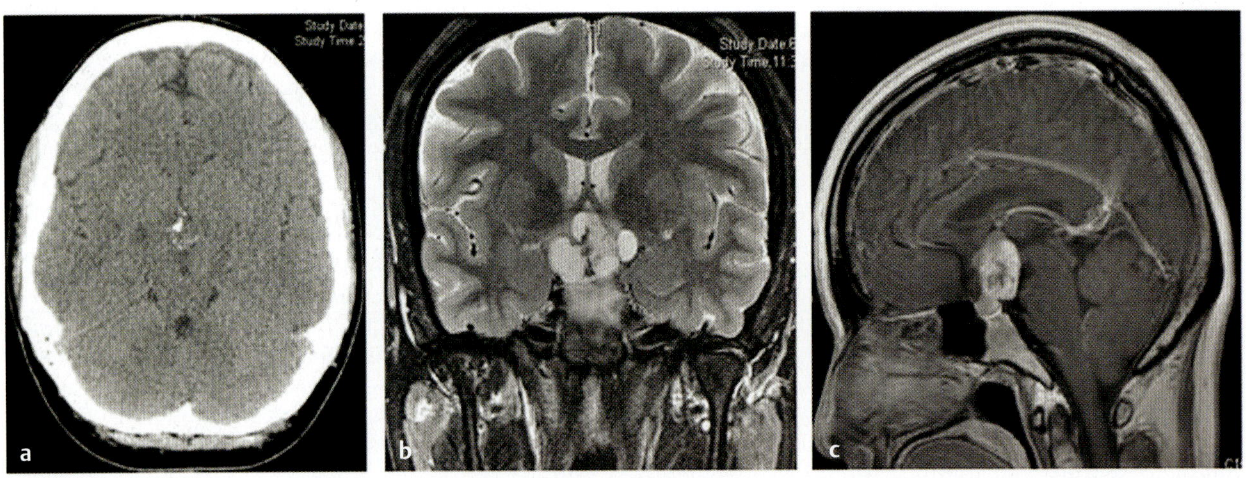

Fig. 40.1 Classic radiographic characteristics of craniopharyngiomas. **(a)** Plain computed tomographic scan showing calcification of a suprasellar lesion. **(b)** Coronal T2 magnetic resonance imaging (MRI) sequence showing a suprasellar lesion with multiple cystic components. **(c)** Sagittal T1 postcontrast MRI sequence showing a suprasellar enhancing lesion with upward displacement of the optic chiasm and extension to the floor of the third ventricle.

structures. These factors render surgical treatment of recurrent disease less successful and more morbid. In Yaşargil's hands, surgical mortality in children was 11.8% with 72.5% good outcome for primary surgery versus 42.1% with 31.6% good outcome for secondary surgery. In adults, mortality was 8.2% with 80.3% good outcome in primary surgery versus 38.5% with 38.5% good result in secondary surgery.[5]

The second option is limited surgical resection/decompression with adjuvant radiation treatment. Radiotherapy was added to the treatment regime for craniopharyngiomas more recently than surgery. The rationale for using this approach is to avoid potential surgery-related complications that may significantly affect quality of life (QOL), especially in children.[6,7] Considering most of the patients will survive long after the initial diagnosis in the modern era (10-year survival rate 83 to 92.7%),[4] the issue of QOL is pertinent to the patient's well-being. However, there was initial doubt about the effectiveness of radiation on a histologically benign (fewer cell divisions and DNA replications) process. In addition, there has always been concern over the long-term side effects of radiation, especially in children. A summary of the literature on treatment modalities for craniopharyngiomas is listed in **Table 40.1**.

Level I and Level II Evidence

There is no study available in the literature that qualifies as either Level I or Level II evidence to evaluate the role of surgery alone compared with surgery with radiotherapy for craniopharyngiomas.

Level III Evidence

Because of the unique characteristics of craniopharyngioma with respect to anatomical location, patients' symptoms, and technical demands, most of the available data in the literature are case series from large centers accumulated over a long period of time, many of which predate the era when modern imaging modalities were commonly used. Hence, the extent of resection was often based on the surgeon's estimate, which is known to be inaccurate. In addition, both radiation delivery as well as microsurgical technique have improved over the past 50 years; thus the available reports are markedly heterogeneous, usually without control groups, or with historical controls or comparisons with other published series. Few reports include patients with radiation as the primary mode of treatment. Typically radiotherapy was used as an adjuvant therapy after patients had undergone surgery. Although tumor size, location, and patients' presenting symptoms play important roles in shaping the choice of treatment modality, many reports have not included explicit descriptions of these characteristics, making direct comparisons difficult. Due to concerns for the side effects of radiation in children, age of the patient can also bias the strategy for treatment selection.

Discussion of the relative merits of the various radiation modalities is presented elsewhere and is beyond the scope of this chapter. **Table 40.1**[8–13] includes an overview of the Level III evidence comparing surgery and radiation in disease control in specific clinical situations.

Level IV Evidence

There are a large number of case series in the literature reporting an institutional or individual surgeon's experience with craniopharyngiomas. Too numerous to all be listed, we tabulated some notable and frequently cited large surgical series are shown in **Table 40.1**. Yaşargil et al[5] reported 144 (70 children) patients treated with microsurgery (CT scans available since 1976) between 1967 and 1989. GTR was achieved in 90% of cases. The recurrence rate was 7%. "Good" results were achieved in 67.4% of patients. In a pediatric series of 50 patients treated from 1975 to 1989,[14] a 90% (45/50) rate of GTR (surgeon's estimate) was achieved with a 34% recurrence rate. A French group[15] reported on 122 patients (29 children) treated between 1975 and 2000 with GTR in 59% (surgeon's estimate). Mortality was 2.5% with 85% achieving excellent functional result. Recurrence rate was 23.8% (29/122). Another series[16] of 121 (32 children) patients treated from 1974 to 1991 showed a GTR rate of 57% (69/121, based on imaging). "Good outcome" was found in 60.3%, with a 24% (29/121) recurrence rate. Another pediatric series[17] of 66 patients treated from 1984 to 2001 showed a 50% GTR rate. Recurrence was 53% (35/66), with 76% displaying normal development out of 45 patients available for interview. Another 22 children were followed prospectively from 2002 to 2004 and preoperative evaluation of hypothalamic injury was used to decide the goals of surgery.[17] GTR was achieved in only 23%, but no QOL-related deteriorations were evident postoperatively. Fahlbusch's group[18] reported 168 (148 for primary surgery, 30 children) patients treated between 1983 and 1997. For primary surgery, 49.3% had a GTR. Mortality was 1.1% for primary transcranial cases and 10.5% for recurrent cases. Overall survival was 92.7% 10 years after primary surgery. The majority of the patients (79%) were independent without impairment. The same group[19] recently published 73 patients treated between 1997 and 2005. Using stringent patient selection criteria, they achieved GTR in 83.1% without any mortality.

Conclusion

The various surgical series, predominantly those already listed, have shown that, with modern surgical techniques coupled with careful patient selection

Table 40.1 Evidence for treatment strategies for craniopharyngiomas

Level of evidence	Studies	Description
Level I or II	No studies	
Level III	Rajan et al 1993[8]	173 patients (45% children) treated at Royal Marsden Hospital with external beam XRT alone or after surgery from 1950 to 1986. Extent of surgery does not affect survival or PFS. Age and XRT technique are significant prognostic factors for survival. No radiation optic neuropathy noted.
	Fischer et al1985[9]	37 children treated at Boston Children's Hospital from 1972 to 1981, either with surgery or with radiation (some had BX, cyst aspiration, or shunt placement). Extent of third ventricle deformity and tumor size are compared. Radiation is at least similar to surgery at tumor control. Long-term QOL effect is also studied.
	Fischer et al 1990[10]	61 children treated at Boston Children's Hospital from 1970 to 1990.10-year PFS is 100% for XRT-alone group, 86% for surgery+XRT group, and 31% for surgery-alone group. More patients presented with visual deficits in the surgery-alone group preoperatively.
	Scott et al 1994[11]	121 patients (35% children) treated at Churchill Hospital from 1964 to 2003. 10-year PFS is 100% for patients with GTR or GTR+XRT, 77% for PR+XRT, 38% for PR only.
	Karavitaki et al 2005[12]	Systematic review of the literature, 274 studies, comparing patients with GTR, STR, or STR+XRT. No significant difference found between GTR and STR+XRT group in PFS or OS.
	Yang et al 2010[13]	35 (from 95 treated from 1959 to 1982) patients treated at Boston Children's Hospital were given psychophysiological tests. Surgical group showed more frontal lobe and visual perceptual dysfunction. Both groups have different extent of short-term memory and manual dexterity deficits. IQ was not affected significantly in either group.
	Cavazzuti et al 1983[6] Merchant et al 2006[7]	28 patients enrolled in phase 2 CRT study at St. Jude's Hospital were divided into "minimally invasive," "moderately invasive," and "extensive" groups based on the extent of surgical interventions received prior to CRT. An almost 10 point drop in IQ between patients with minimal surgical intervention versus those with extensive surgeries (worse) was found.
Level IV	Yaşargil et al 1990[5]	144 (70 < 16 yo) patients from 1967 to 1989 treated with microsurgery (CT scans available since 1976). GTR using various surgical approaches. Recurrence rate is 7%. 67.4% had "good" results.
	Hoffman et al 1992[14]	50 children treated at Sick Children's Hospital in Toronto from 1/1975 to 12/1989. All had surgery, with 90% (45/50) GTR (surgeon's estimate), 34% recurrence.
	Van Effenterre and Boch 2002[15]	122 (29 <16 yo) patients treated from 1975 to 2000 in Paris. GTR 59% (surgeon's estimate). GTR was 84% based on postoperative CT (higher than surgeon's estimate), likely because of residual observed microscopic disease below the resolution of the CT scan. Mortality 2.5%. 85% excellent functional result. 23.8% (29/122) recurrence.
	Duff et al 2000[16]	121 (32 ≤ 16 yo) patients treated at Mayo Clinic from 1974 to 1991. GTR 57% (69/121, based on imaging). 60.3% "good outcome." 24% (29/121) recurrence.
	Puget et al 2007[17]	66 children treated at Necker-Enfants from 1984 to 2001. 50% GTR. 53% recurrence (35/66). 76% with normal development out of 45 patients available for interview. 22 children collected prospectively from 2002 to 2004. Preop evaluation of hypothalamic injury to decide extent of surgery. 23% GTR. No QOL-related deterioration in the prospective group.
	Fahlbusch et al 1999[18]	168 (148 for initial surgery, 30 children) patients treated in Germany from 1983 to 1997. 49.3% GTR for primary surgery. Mortality 1.1% for primary transcranial cases and 10.5% for recurrent cases. OS 92.7% after 10 years for primary surgery. 79% are independent without impairment.
	Hofmann et al 2012[19]	73 patients treated in the same institution as above from 5/1997 to 1/2005. Patients with preoperative hypothalamic damage or HCP were excluded from open surgery unless conditions were resolved. GTR 83.1%. No mortality.

Abbreviations: BX, biopsy; CRT, conformal radiation therapy; GTR, gross total resection; HCP, hydrocephalus; IQ, intelligence quotient; PFS, progression-free survival; OS, overall survival; PR, partial resection; QOL, quality of life; STR, subtotal resection; XRT, radiotherapy; yo, years old.

based on preoperative symptoms and tumor anatomy, GTR can be achieved with excellent outcome in the majority of adult patients, especially in experienced hands. Tumor recurrence is significantly higher following subtotal resection without adjuvant radiotherapy. A recent prospective pediatric trial has shown an 80% risk reduction for recurrence with complete resection versus incomplete resection.[20] However, radiotherapy is also an effective strategy for treating craniopharyngiomas. Radiation-related side effects are rare with modern technology. Although there is still no unequivocal evidence available to support a single treatment strategy for craniopharyngiomas, the general consensus[21,22] is that surgical excision should be pursued to the minimum extent to alleviate any mass effect–related symptoms and to the maximum extent that will not cause irreversible harm to the patient. Given the ease with which hormones can be replaced with medical therapy, an endocrinological deficit may be acceptable to achieve GTR and possible cure. However, STR followed by adjuvant radiotherapy may be an equally successful strategy, particularly in the pediatric population, where hypothalamic injury is not well tolerated. Whether to administer radiation immediately after STR or at the time of recurrence is also a matter of debate and is not discussed in this chapter.

Regardless of the treatment strategy, hypopituitarism is common among craniopharyngioma patients. There is no Level I evidence favoring any treatment modality, except that symptomatic diabetes insipidus (DI) may be more common in surgically treated patients.[4] Preoperative hormonal deficits seldom recover after treatment. Although visual improvement is commonly reported postsurgery, treatment-related visual deterioration is not negligible. Hypothalamic injury can be a devastating complication (particularly in children), an important factor that has led the medical community toward a more conservative surgical approach to spare children from unacceptable neuropsychological morbidity.

For recurrent craniopharyngioma, the choice of treatment modality is also a matter of debate. The same principle of minimal surgery to alleviate mass effect holds true, and perhaps a lower threshold to administer radiotherapy instead of attempting a GTR may apply, given the higher surgery-related morbidity in these cases.

Other treatment modalities, including intracystic implantation of radioactive or chemotherapeutic agents,[4] are discussed in Chapters 41 and 42.

Surgical treatment is necessary to relieve preoperative symptoms for most craniopharyngioma patients. The extent of surgery should be gauged by avoidance of significant postoperative deficits (although pituitary dysfunction may be acceptable), especially hypothalamic injuries. Radiotherapy is an effective strategy to treat the tumor, although for patients at a very young age, this approach may not be optimal. One should consider both surgery and radiation as useful tools to be used judiciously, instead of as competing modalities, in the armamentarium against craniopharyngiomas.

Transsphenoidal versus Transcranial Approaches

Craniopharyngiomas are typically located in the sellar and parasellar area. To reach this area surgically, two main strategies can be considered: transcranial or transsphenoidal. Yaşargil et al[5] listed six common configurations of craniopharyngiomas and used different surgical approaches or combinations of them for tumor resections. Several subsequent publications have also classified craniopharyngiomas, mostly based on their relationships to the sella, the chiasm, and the floor of the third ventricle, to guide surgical approach selection. One group[17] has devised a grading system of hypothalamic involvement based on preoperative MRI and used the grade to determine the aggressiveness of the planned surgery. Multiple standard open craniotomy approaches (such as subfrontal with or without translaminal, frontotemporal (pterional) with or without orbitozygomatic osteotomy, transcallosal or transcortical-transventricular) have been used alone or in combination and each has its pros and cons[23,24] (**Fig. 40.2**). The transsphenoidal approach was traditionally used only for small intrasellar and infradiaphragmatic tumors.[5] However, with the advent of extended transsphenoidal approaches using standard microscope and microsurgical techniques, as well as the more recent use of the endoscope with its ability to increase the intrasphenoidal field of view, the variety of craniopharyngiomas in different locations and sizes that can be removed with a transsphenoidal approach have expanded significantly.[25–28] Lack of pneumatization of the sphenoid sinus in children as well as concerns for cerebrospinal fluid (CSF) leak have been addressed with satisfaction with continued improvement of transsphenoidal endoscopic techniques.[29,30] (**Figs. 40.3** and **40.4**)

Although there is a large body of literature reporting surgical results on craniopharyngiomas, all the reports are case series (some are large from high-volume centers) without control or controls that are not comparable. This reflects the relatively rare nature of the disease as well as the surgical challenge the tumor presents to preclude a unified approach to the lesion. The selection of a particular surgical approach is typically based on the preference of the surgeon, the size and the anatomy of the tumor, and the presumed limitations of a particular surgical approach in relation to the characteristics of the tumor. Studies with some internal control (open microsurgery vs microscopic transsphenoidal approach), although not completely comparable, as well as two systematic re-

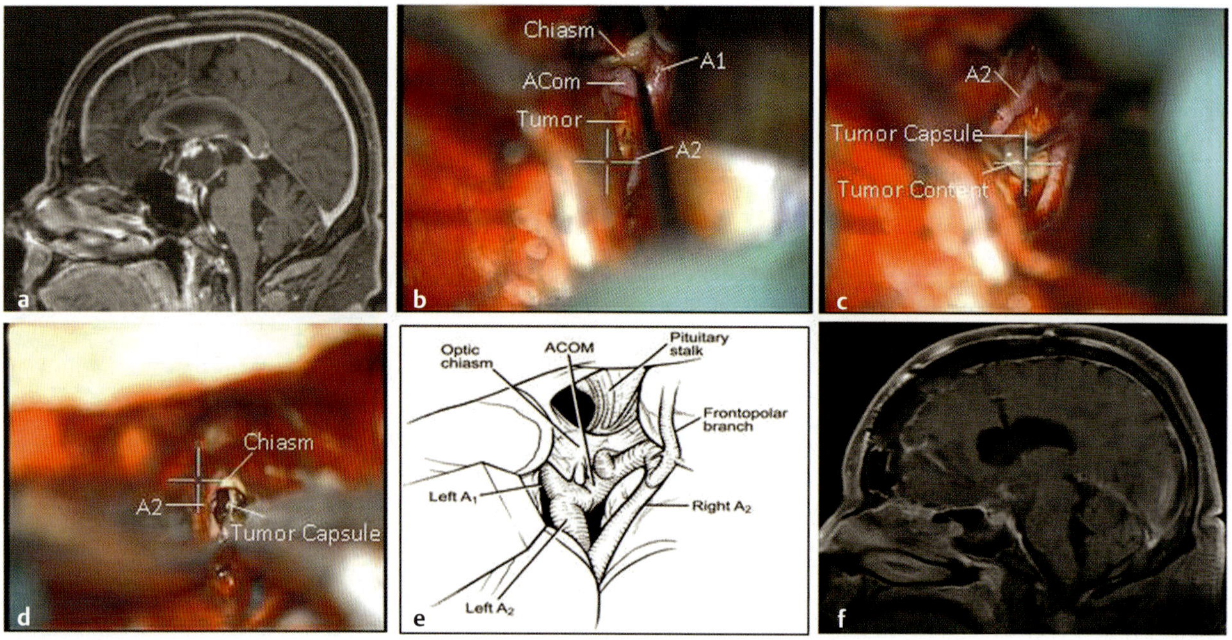

Fig. 40.2 An example of open craniotomy (frontal craniotomy with interhemispheric and translaminal approach) using a microscope. **(a)** Preoperative sagittal T1 postcontrast magnetic resonance imaging (MRI) sequence showing a heterogeneously enhancing suprasellar lesion with invasion into the third ventricle. **(b)** Intraoperative view showing the tumor and its relationship to the surrounding neurovascular structures (optic chiasm and anterior cerebral artery branches). **(c)** Intraoperative view showing tumor content after the tumor capsule was opened. **(d)** Intraoperative view showing removal of the tumor capsule from the lamina terminalis area. **(e)** Diagram showing surgical anatomy from the interhemispheric approach. **(f)** Postoperative sagittal T1 postcontrast MRI sequence showing near total resection of the suprasellar lesion. (Used with permission from Dr. Laligam N. Sekhar (LNS), University of Washington, Department of Neurosurgery, Seattle, Washington. LNS has the copyright to the diagram in **(e)**.)

views,[31,32] are listed in **Table 40.2**. All the other major series are included in the references of the two review articles. There is no reported series that compares the microscopic versus the endoscopic transsphenoidal approach directly. The endoscopically assisted microscopic transsphenoidal approach is considered a microscopic transsphenoidal approach.

Level I–Level III Evidence

There is no publication available to qualify as Level I, II, or III evidence to compare transcranial versus microscopic or endoscopic transsphenoidal approaches.

Level IV Evidence

There are two systematic reviews comparing open craniotomy versus a transsphenoidal approach.[31,32] Elliot et al[31] have performed a meta-analysis of series (1990 to 2010) with significant numbers of children treated with either a transcranial (TC) or a transsphenoidal (TS) approach. They have identified 48 studies with 2,955 patients for a TC approach and 13 studies with 373 patients for a TS approach (microscopic or endoscopic). The TC group has had "less visual loss, more frequent hydrocephalus and increased intracranial pressure, larger tumors, and more suprasellar disease" preoperatively. Postoperatively, they tend to have "lower rates of GTR, more frequent recurrence after GTR, higher neurological morbidity, more frequent diabetes insipidus, less improvement, and greater deterioration in vision." No difference was found in "operative mortality, obesity/hyperphagia, or overall survival percentages." The authors felt that it was not valid to compare the two approaches directly; rather, each has its own use depending on the clinical characteristics of the tumor.

Another systematic review[28] looked at the outcome of open transcranial (OT) versus transsphenoidal microscopic (TM) versus endoscopic endonasal (EE) transsphenoidal approach. This study included 88 papers with 3,470 patients from 1995 to 2010 (55 OT, 14 TM, and 19 EE). The average size of the tumor was 3.9 cm for OT and 2.5 and 2.9 for TM and EE, respectively, although this difference was not statistically significant. Range of follow-up was 13 to 133 months, 7 to 122 months, and 4 to 48 months for OT, TM, and EE, respectively. No difference in outcomes between the TM or EE approach was found. However, GTR rates for the transsphenoidal approach groups (EE: 66.9%; TM: 69.1%) were significantly higher than for the OT group (48.3%). The EE group also had a significantly

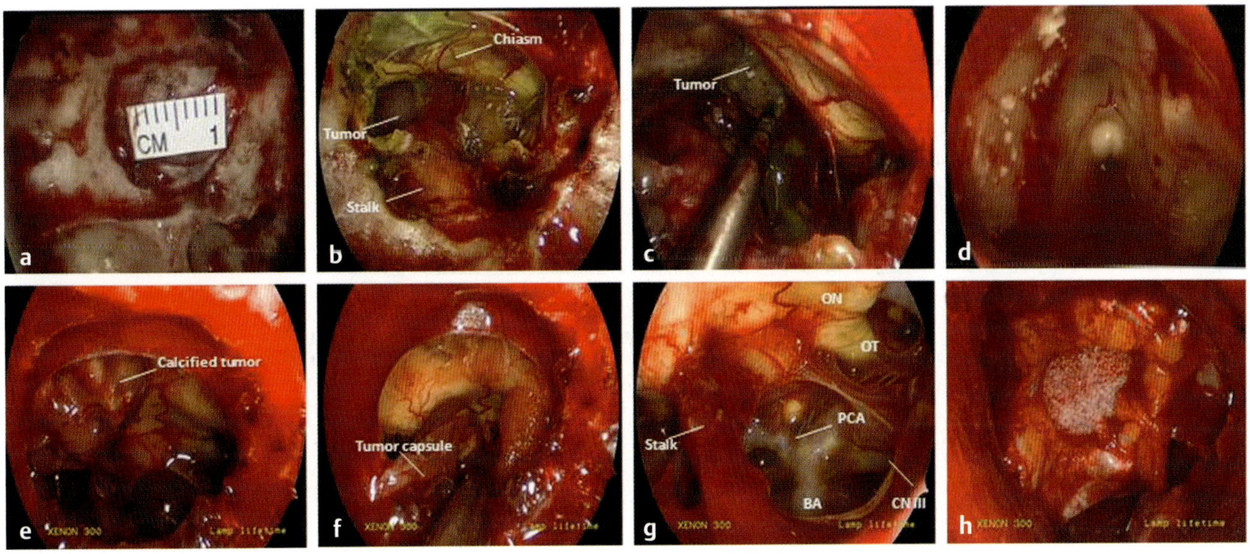

Fig. 40.3 Illustrative cases of craniopharyngiomas resected using an endoscopic transnasal approach, intraoperative views. Case 1: **(a)** Intraoperative view of the bony opening including the top of the sella, tuberculum sellae, and planum sphenoidale bone removal. **(b)** Intraoperative view after dural opening and dissection of arachnoid membranes from the tumor. The optic chiasm, infiltrated pituitary stalk, and portions of the calcified tumor are shown. **(c)** Use of the NICO Myriad device (NICO, Indianapolis, IN) for tumor removal. **(d)** View of the resection cavity including the floor of the third ventricle at the end of complete tumor resection. Note that there are small remnants of calcification adherent to the walls of the third ventricle/ hypothalamus, which are left in place to avoid hypothalamic injury. Case 2: **(e)** Intraoperative view showing the chiasm and a portion of the calcified tumor abutting the chiasm. **(f)** View of the tumor capsule being removed from the chiasm after removal of the majority of the tumor. **(g)** After removal of the tumor, a view of the resection cavity showing the preserved pituitary stalk, optic nerve and tract (ON and OT), basilar artery (BA), posterior cerebral artery (PCA), and cranial nerve III (CNIII). **(h)** "Gasket-seal" closure of the skull base defect after tumor removal using Medpor (Porex Corp., Newnan, GA) over the fascia lata, prior to overlay of a nasoseptal graft.

Table 40.2 Evidence for surgical approaches for craniopharyngiomas

Level of evidence	Studies	Description
Level I, II, or III	No studies	
Level IV	Elliott et al 2011[31]	Meta-analysis of series of pediatric patients treated with either transcranial or transsphenoidal approach for craniopharyngioma. Tumor anatomy and patients' symptoms differ between the two populations preoperatively. Concluded that it's not valid to compare the two approaches directly.
	Komotar et al 2012[32]	Systematic review of the literature on transcranial versus microscopic transnasal versus endoscopic transnasal approach for craniopharyngiomas. Although not statistically significant, transcranial series tend to have larger tumors. No difference in outcomes between microscopic or endoscopic transnasal approach. Endoscopic series have shorter follow-up time. Transnasal approach group has higher rate of GTR and higher rate of CSF leak compared with open group.
	Maira et al 1995[33]	Report on 57 patients: 61% transsphenoidal (microscopic) and 39% pterional. If a tumor is entirely or partially intrasellar, then transnasal, if completely suprasellar, then pterional. 66% GTR in TS group with 100% good outcome, 94% GTR in pterional group with 91% good outcome.
	Fahlbusch et al 1999[18]	148 patients: 23.6% had transsphenoidal (microscopic). 60% of TS cases are < 2 cm in size versus 22.3% in the open group. 85.7% GTR for TS and 45.7% for open after primary surgery.
	Hofmann et al 2012[19]	73 patients (same group as above, later series), 26 (35.6%) had TS. TS is used if tumor is subdiaphragmatic. Major suprasellar calcification is contraindication for TS. GTR 88.5% in TS group and 79.5% in open.
	Karavitaki et al[12]	121 patients, TS (microscopic) used in 26 cases. 31% GTR versus 15% in open. TS only used on intrasellar lesions.
	Chakrabarti et al 2005[34]	86 patients treated from 1984 to 1994 at USC. 18 treated with open craniotomy for purely suprasellar tumors. Extended TS approach (microscopic) is used if tumor is purely intrasellar, intrasellar with suprasellar extension and predominantly cystic, or purely suprasellar and cystic. Good outcome was obtained with extended TS approach on selected patients.

Abbreviations: CSF, cerebral spinal fluid; GTR, gross-total resection; TS, transsphenoidal; USC, University of Southern California.

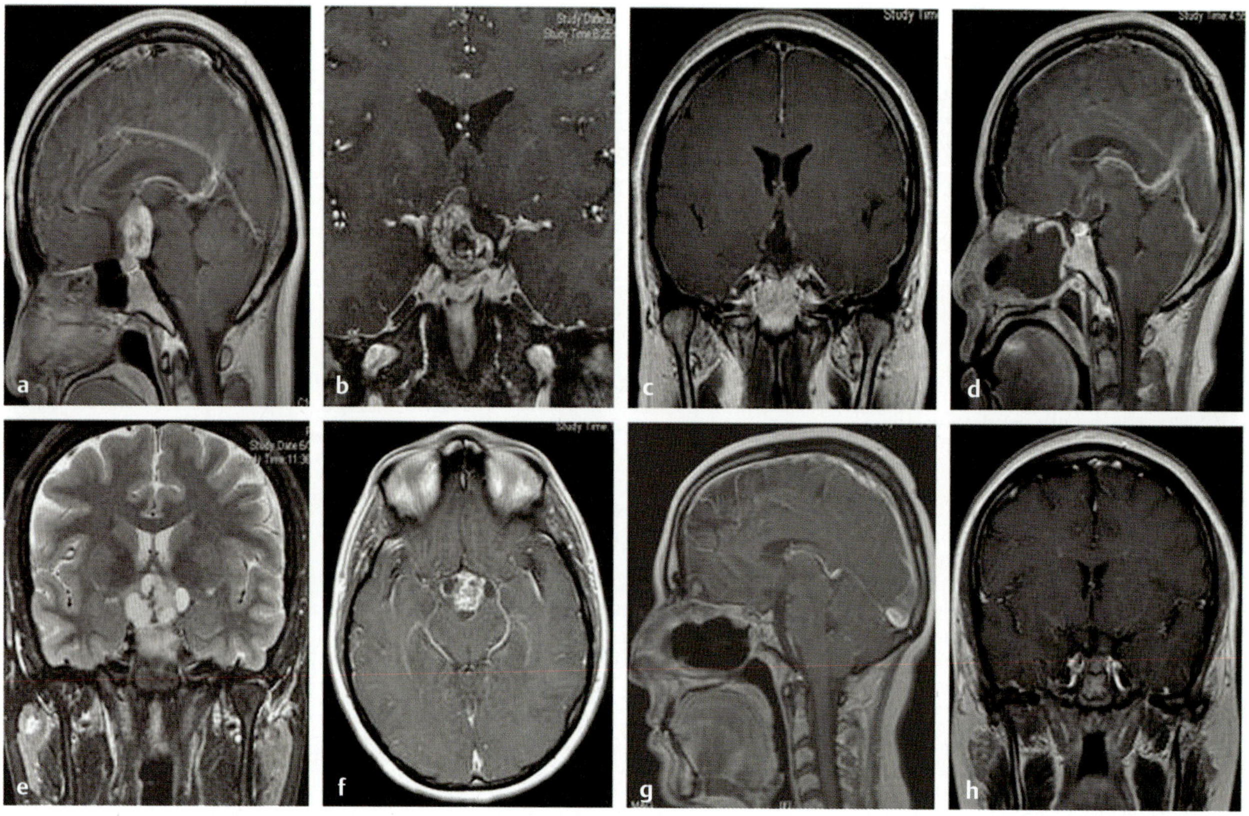

Fig. 40.4 Illustrative cases of craniopharyngiomas resected using an endoscopic transnasal approach, radiographic images. Case 1: **(a)** Preoperative magnetic resonance imaging (MRI) T1 postcontrast sagittal view of the tumor, showing suprasellar extension into the third ventricle with chiasmal compression/displacement. **(b)** Preoperative MRI T1 postcontrast coronal view of the tumor. **(c)** Postoperative MRI T1 postcontrast coronal view showing complete resection of the tumor and relief of the chiasmal compression. **(d)** Postoperative MRI T1 postcontrast sagittal view again showing complete resection, with the nasoseptal flap overlying the skull base defect. Case 2: **(e)** Preoperative MRI T2 coronal view showing a multicystic lesion in the suprasellar region. **(f)** Preoperative MRI T1 postcontrast axial view showing an enhancing suprasellar lesion. **(g)** Postoperative MRI T1 postcontrast sagittal view showing complete resection of the tumor. **(h)** Postoperative MRI T1 postcontrast coronal view again showing complete resection of the tumor and decompression of the chiasm.

higher rate of visual improvement (56.2%) versus the OT group (33.1%). Although there was a lower seizure rate in the transsphenoidal groups, the rate of CSF leaks (EE: 18.4%; TM: 9.0%) was significantly higher in the transsphenoidal groups compared with the open group (2.6%). However, more recent EE reports have shown much lower rates (3.8%) of postoperative CSF leaks.[30] These authors, in contrast to the first review, concluded that expanded endonasal endoscopic surgeries may offer certain benefits over craniotomy in the resection of craniopharyngiomas, particularly by reducing the rate of brain retraction, contusion, and the risk of seizures; increasing visual improvement with less optic nerve manipulation; and increasing rates of GTR in well-selected cases through increased visualization of the walls of the third ventricle.

Few reports are available in which the same series contain significant numbers of both OT and TM cases. Endoscopic series tend to have exclusively EE cases. A report[33] on 57 patients (61% TM and 39% pterional) in which TM was used if the tumor was entirely or partially intrasellar and pterional was used if the tumor was completely suprasellar, showed GTR in 66% of the TM group with 100% good outcome, and GTR in 94% of the pterional group with 91% good outcome. Another series[18] with 148 patients (23.6% with TM) reported 60% of the TM cases with tumor size < 2 cm versus 22.3% in the OT cases (i.e., smaller tumors in the TM group). GTR was 85.7% for TM and 45.7% for OT cases after primary surgery. The same group has published a more recent series of 73 patients[19] in which 26 (35.6%) were treated with TM. TM was used if the tumor was subdiaphragmatic. Significant suprasellar calcification was considered a contraindication for TM. GTR was 88.5% in the TM group and 79.5% in the OT group. Another large series of 121

Table 40.3 Factors influencing choice of surgical approach

	Location			Consistency			Ca^{2+}		Medical comorbidity	
Approach	**I**	**I+S**	**S**	**Cystic**	**Mixed**	**Solid**	**Sig**	**No**	**Sig**	**No**
TC	X	Y	P	Z	Z	Z	P	Z	D	Z
TS	P	P	Y	F	F	F	Y	Z	Y	Z
IV	X	X	P	P	D	X	X	Z	P	Z

Abbreviations: Ca^{2+}, calcifications; D, makes approach more difficult; F, can be a factor if location is not favorable; I, intrasellar; I+S, intrasellar with suprasellar extension; IV, intraventricular fenestration; P, preferred approach; S, purely suprasellar; Sig, significant; TC, transcranial; TS, transsphenoidal; X, approach should be avoided ; Y, depends on experience of the surgeon; Z, not an influence on approach.

patients[12] in which TM was used in 26 cases reported GTR in 31% for TM versus 15% in OT cases. TM was used, however, only on intrasellar lesions. Chakrabarti et al[34] reported 86 patients treated from 1984 to 1994. Eighteen were treated with an OT approach for purely suprasellar tumors. Extended TM was used if the tumor was "purely intrasellar, intrasellar with suprasellar extension and predominantly cystic, or purely suprasellar and cystic." Good outcome was obtained with an extended TM approach on selected patients even with suprasellar extension.

Expert Recommendations

Surgery versus Radiation

1. Surgical treatment is necessary to relieve preoperative symptoms for most patients (Grade 1C Recommendation, Level III/IV Evidence).
2. The extent of surgery should be gauged by avoidance of significant postoperative deficits (although pituitary dysfunction may be acceptable), especially hypothalamic injuries (Grade 1C Recommendation, Level III/IV Evidence).
3. Radiotherapy is an effective strategy to treat the tumor, although for patients at a very young age, this approach may not be optimal (Grade 1C Recommendation, Level III/IV Evidence).
4. Both surgery and radiation are useful tools to be used judiciously to treat craniopharyngiomas (Grade 1C Recommendation, Level III/IV Evidence).

Transsphenoidal versus Transcranial

1. Transsphenoidal and open transcranial approaches (microscopic or endoscopic) are both useful for craniopharyngioma treatment. There are no unequivocal data to favor either approach (Grade 2C Recommendation, Level IV Evidence).
2. Both are effective and should be complementary to each other depending on the anatomical characteristics of the tumor and the experience and comfort level of the surgeon (Grade 2C Recommendation, Level IV Evidence).

Summary and Conclusions

Transsphenoidal and open transcranial approaches (microscopic or endoscopic) are both useful for craniopharyngioma treatment. With the advancement of closure techniques for expanded endonasal endoscopic approaches, the CSF leak rate is now less than 5% for experienced teams,[30] making the EE approach an attractive option for suitable craniopharyngiomas, and the size and location of tumors suitable for this approach are expanding. The main limitation for the endoscopic transsphenoidal approach is significant tumor lateral to the carotid arteries. There are, however, no unequivocal data to favor either approach; rather, both are effective and should be complementary to each other depending on the anatomical characteristics of the tumor and the experience and comfort level of the surgeon. Because of the relatively recent development of the expanded EE techniques, the follow-up for this group is shorter compared with the OT group. Hence, conclusions about long-term tumor control cannot be made. Although the average time to recurrence is 1.0 to 4.3 years, delayed recurrences beyond 20 to 30 years have been reported.[4] It is foreseeable that, with longer follow-up, we may see more recurrence with the EE group. Likewise, many of the OT series were collected over a long period of time, and many contain cases predating the time when modern imaging was routinely obtained. The extent of resection in these series was frequently based on surgeon's estimate, which may have erroneously overestimated the number of GTR cases and subsequently also overestimated the rate of recurrence after presumed GTR.

For craniopharyngiomas in a predominantly ventral midline location without significant lateral extension beyond the carotid arteries, the transsphenoidal expanded endoscopic endonasal approach offers certain advantages in experienced hands, such as the lack of brain and optic nerve retraction/manipulation and a wide panoramic view of the undersurface of the chiasm and floor/walls of the third ventricle. Likewise, patients with medical comorbidities, who may not tolerate a craniotomy but need tumor debulking, may benefit from an endonasal approach. Tumors with significant lateral extent, vascular encasement, or multicompartmental location may preferentially benefit from a transcranial approach. Likewise, tumors with largely solid or calcified components may be more difficult to remove endonasally depending on the experience of the surgeon and the degree of exposure achieved with the approach. Alternative surgical strategies, such as endoscopic intraventricular cyst fenestration to relieve pressure followed by radiotherapy, may also be considered for largely cystic tumors that present to the ventricular surfaces. Some of the clinical factors guiding our choice of surgical approach are listed in **Table 40.3**.

References

1. Karavitaki N, Wass JAH. Craniopharyngiomas. Endocrinol Metab Clin North Am 2008;37(1):173–193, ix–x
2. Prabhu VC, Brown HG. The pathogenesis of craniopharyngiomas. Childs Nerv Syst 2005;21(8-9):622–627
3. Sekine S, Shibata T, Kokubu A, et al. Craniopharyngiomas of adamantinomatous type harbor β-catenin gene mutations. Am J Pathol 2002;161(6):1997–2001
4. Karavitaki N, Cudlip S, Adams CBT, Wass JAH. Craniopharyngiomas. Endocr Rev 2006;27(4):371–397
5. Yaşargil MG, Curcic M, Kis M, Siegenthaler G, Teddy PJ, Roth P. Total removal of craniopharyngiomas. Approaches and long-term results in 144 patients. J Neurosurg 1990;73(1):3–11
6. Cavazzuti V, Fischer EG, Welch K, Belli JA, Winston KR. Neurological and psychophysiological sequelae following different treatments of craniopharyngioma in children. J Neurosurg 1983;59(3):409–417
7. Merchant TE, Kiehna EN, Kun LE, et al. Phase II trial of conformal radiation therapy for pediatric patients with craniopharyngioma and correlation of surgical factors and radiation dosimetry with change in cognitive function. J Neurosurg 2006;104(2, Suppl):94–102
8. Rajan B, Ashley S, Gorman C, et al. Craniopharyngioma—long-term results following limited surgery and radiotherapy. Radiother Oncol 1993;26(1):1–10
9. Fischer EG, Welch K, Belli JA, et al. Treatment of craniopharyngiomas in children: 1972-1981. J Neurosurg 1985;62(4):496–501
10. Fischer EG, Welch K, Shillito J Jr, Winston KR, Tarbell NJ. Craniopharyngiomas in children: long-term effects of conservative surgical procedures combined with radiation therapy. J Neurosurg 1990;73(4):534–540
11. Scott RM, Hetelekidis S, Barnes PD, Goumnerova L, Tarbell NJ. Surgery, radiation, and combination therapy in the treatment of childhood craniopharyngioma—a 20-year experience. Pediatr Neurosurg 1994;21(Suppl 1):75–81
12. Karavitaki N, Brufani C, Warner JT, et al. Craniopharyngiomas in children and adults: systematic analysis of 121 cases with long-term follow-up. Clin Endocrinol (Oxf) 2005;62(4):397–409
13. Yang I, Sughrue ME, Rutkowski MJ, et al. Craniopharyngioma: a comparison of tumor control with various treatment strategies. Neurosurg Focus 2010;28(4):E5
14. Hoffman HJ, De Silva M, Humphreys RP, Drake JM, Smith ML, Blaser SI. Aggressive surgical management of craniopharyngiomas in children. J Neurosurg 1992;76(1):47–52
15. Van Effenterre R, Boch A-L. Craniopharyngioma in adults and children: a study of 122 surgical cases. J Neurosurg 2002;97(1):3–11
16. Duff JM, Meyer FB, Ilstrup DM, Laws ER Jr, Schleck CD, Scheithauer BW. Long-term outcomes for surgically resected craniopharyngiomas. Neurosurgery 2000;46(2):291–302
17. Puget S, Garnett M, Wray A, et al. Pediatric craniopharyngiomas: classification and treatment according to the degree of hypothalamic involvement. J Neurosurg 2007;106(1, Suppl):3–12
18. Fahlbusch R, Honegger J, Paulus W, Huk W, Buchfelder M. Surgical treatment of craniopharyngiomas: experience with 168 patients. J Neurosurg 1999;90(2):237–250
19. Hofmann BM, Höllig A, Strauss C, Buslei R, Buchfelder M, Fahlbusch R. Results after treatment of craniopharyngiomas: further experiences with 73 patients since 1997. J Neurosurg 2012;116(2):373–384
20. Müller HL, Gebhardt U, Schröder S, et al; Study Committee of KRANIOPHARYNGEOM 2000/2007. Analyses of treatment variables for patients with childhood craniopharyngioma—results of the multicenter prospective trial KRANIOPHARYNGEOM 2000 after three years of follow-up. Horm Res Paediatr 2010;73(3):175–180
21. Rutka JT. Craniopharyngioma. J Neurosurg 2002;97(1):1–2
22. Boop FA. Craniopharyngioma. J Neurosurg 2007;106(1 Suppl):1–2
23. Komotar RJ, Roguski M, Bruce JN. Surgical management of craniopharyngiomas. J Neurooncol 2009;92(3):283–296
24. Liu JK, Cole CD, Kestle JRW, Brockmeyer DL, Walker ML. Cranial base strategies for resection of craniopharyngioma in children. Neurosurg Focus 2005;18(6A):E9
25. Schwartz TH, Fraser JF, Brown S, Tabaee A, Kacker A, Anand VK. Endoscopic cranial base surgery: classification of operative approaches. Neurosurgery 2008;62(5):991–1002
26. Cappabianca P, Cavallo LM, Colao A, et al. Endoscopic endonasal transsphenoidal approach: outcome analysis of 100 consecutive procedures. Minim Invasive Neurosurg 2002;45(4):193–200
27. Jane JA Jr, Kiehna E, Payne SC, Early SV, Laws ER Jr. Early outcomes of endoscopic transsphenoidal surgery for adult craniopharyngiomas. Neurosurg Focus 2010;28(4):E9
28. Frank G, Pasquini E, Doglietto F, et al. The endoscopic extended transsphenoidal approach for extrasellar craniopharyngiomas. Neurosurgery 2006;59(Suppl 1):75–83
29. Gardner PA, Prevedello DM, Kassam AB, Snyderman CH, Carrau RL, Mintz AH. The evolution of the endonasal approach for craniopharyngiomas. J Neurosurg 2008;108(5):1043–1047
30. Leng LZ, Greenfield JP, Souweidane MM, Anand VK, Schwartz TH. Endosocpic, endonasal resection of craniopharyngiomas: analysis of outcome including extent of resection, cerebrospinal fluid leak, return to preoperative productivity, and body mass index. Neurosurgery 2011;70:110–124
31. Elliott RE, Jane JA Jr, Wisoff JH. Surgical management of craniopharyngiomas in children: meta-analysis and comparison of transcranial and transsphenoidal approaches. Neurosurgery 2011;69(3):630–643
32. Komotar RJ, Starke RM, Raper DM, Anand VK, Schwartz TH. Endoscopic endonasal compared with microscopic transsphenoidal and open transcranial resection of craniopharyngiomas. World Neurosurg 2012;77(2):329–341
33. Maira G, Anile C, Rossi GF, Colosimo C. Surgical treatment of craniopharyngiomas: an evaluation of the transsphenoidal and pterional approaches. Neurosurgery 1995;36(4):715–724
34. Chakrabarti I, Amar AP, Couldwell W, Weiss MH. Long-term neurological, visual, and endocrine outcomes following transnasal resection of craniopharyngioma. J Neurosurg 2005;102(4):650–657

41

Use of Radiotherapy in Optimizing Management of Craniopharyngioma

Lawrence Kleinberg

Craniopharyngioma[1,2] is an uncommon benign tumor occurring in an estimated 350 patients each year in the United States. Nevertheless, it is a subject of interest because it occurs frequently in children, it has a high rate of long-term survival, and both the tumor and treatment may cause significant long-term morbidity and disability. Craniopharyngioma is thought to develop from embryological remnants of the Rathke pouch, a precursor of the pituitary gland. Even though the disease is generally benign and indolent, therapy is challenging because the tumor is located in the parasellar region, resulting in risk to the optic nerves, tract, and chiasm, and the hypothalamus, circle of Willis, and nearby brain tissue. In recent years there has been increasing recognition that radiation, especially with current precision techniques, has an important role to play not only in controlling residual or recurrent tumor but also in minimizing the need for the most aggressive resection when consequent morbidity is likely.

The rarity of the tumor has thus far limited the opportunity for prospective study powered to provide key information needed to optimize patient care. Most of the evidence that guides management is therefore Level IV (observational and may have been accumulated over a substantial time period) with some Level III prospectively collected data. Recently there have been attempts at more rigorous prospective uncontrolled phase 2 studies that might provide more robust information, but evidence is still subject to much interpretation and ambiguity given the lack of good historical comparative data and the small cohort sizes. Although the available data do suffer from these weaknesses, the information can be utilized to develop sound strategies to manage patients today even while efforts are underway to learn more, including a recently initiated randomized trial described below.

Controversies related to the use of radiotherapy for this illness, the subject of this chapter, include the following: (1) Is the long-term control with subtotal resection and radiation high enough to justify abandoning the goal of gross total resection when the risk of injury is significant? (2) After a subtotal resection, is immediate radiation optimal or is it appropriate to delay radiation until tumor growth is confirmed? (3) When radiotherapy is indicated, what is the optimal technique for radiation to maintain control and minimize the risks of later toxicity? Selected important data bearing on these controversies are reviewed below and provide guidance on how to optimally utilize radiotherapy in achieving high rates of tumor control while best maintaining quality of life for the long term.

■ Is Subtotal Resection Followed by Radiation an Appropriate Alternative to Gross Total Resection?

Maintaining Quality of Life: Using Radiotherapy to Allow Less Extensive Resections

Level I and Level II Evidence

There are no Level I or Level II evidence studies comparing gross total resection to subtotal resection with or without radiation.

Level III and Level IV Evidence

Historically, the optimal therapy has been considered to be a gross total resection, which leads to a high rate of long-term control and survival. It was observed that when patients do undergo a more limited subtotal resection, the control rates with the addition of subsequent radiotherapy appear to be similar to those achieved with a more complete removal. Given the potential morbidity of gross total resection when tumor infiltrates the hypothalamus or optic pathways, there is an increasing expert sentiment that maximal "safe" resection with a plan for radiation to control residual disease may be a desirable therapy. The available data, reviewed in this chapter, do suggest that control rates are favorable with this approach. Morbidity, at least in the early years after treatment, also appears to be reduced, despite the addition of radiotherapy to the management. Therefore, this conservative approach, while exposing patients to both surgery and radiation, may be optimal when the goal of gross total resection carries high risk. However, the available follow-up may not, in most studies, be long enough to include the effects of the very-long-term risks of radiation or the long-term morbidity and mortality that may result from morbid obesity occurring after hypothalamic injury that can occur during attempted gross total resection[3]

A recent meta-analysis[4] examined the issue of outcome after subtotal resection in a dataset derived from the published literature of 8,058 patients described in 274 papers. The study set was confined to 442 patients operated after 1990, including patients for whom specific information about control and morbidity was provided rather than aggregate data only, which may create a bias. Results of this crude analysis are summarized in **Table 41.1** and do demonstrate similar progression-free survival with gross total resection and subtotal resection plus radiotherapy.

Table 41.1 Progression-free survival (PFS) and overall survival (OS) outcomes of therapy from published literature with gross total resection (GTR), subtotal resection (STR), and STR with radiotherapy (RT)

	2-year PFS	5-year PFS	5-year OS	10-year OS
GTR (256)	88	67	98	98
STR (101)	67	34	96	93
	$p < 0.001$	$p < 0.0001$	p = not significant	$p = 0.054$
STR/RT (85)	91%	69%	99%	95%

Source: Yang I, Sughrue ME, Rutkowski MJ, et al. Craniopharyngioma: a comparison of tumor control with various treatment strategies. Neurosurg Focus 2010;28(4):E5.

The various groups described, with a mean follow-up of 54 months, were assessed not only for outcome but also for morbidity[5] in a related publication. New neurological deficits reportedly occurred in 5% undergoing any surgery and 2% of those getting limited resection and radiotherapy. The relative risk for any endocrinopathy for patients undergoing a gross total resection was 52% versus 19% and 20% for subtotal resection with or without radiotherapy, respectively. For a group treated with stereotactic radiosurgery, the rate was similar, at 18%. The most common deficit after gross total resection was pituitary dysfunction. Vascular injury was an uncommon result of resection (< 1%) and was not observed after radiation, although this would be expected to be a very long-term complication that is known to occur after cranial irradiation, especially in childhood. Visual deterioration, permanent decline in acuity or a field cut, was 3.5% after gross total resection, 2.1% after subtotal resection, and 6.4% after subtotal resection plus radiotherapy 6.4 (p = ns). Although these data suggest good control rates and perhaps improved quality of life outcome with subtotal resection compared with more aggressive gross total resection, the data are subject to many biases and the limitations of retrospective review.

The results of some larger single-institution reports are concordant with the results of the rough meta-analysis just presented. For example, Schoenfield et al,[6] from the University of California–San Francisco, described 113 patients in a series with median follow-up of 56 months (19 to 144) treated between 1980 and 2009. The results are summarized in **Table 41.2**. Gross total resection was associated with significantly greater risk of developing diabe-

Table 41.2 Progression-free survival (PFS) and overall survival (OS) outcomes of therapy at the University of California–San Francisco with gross total resection (GTR), subtotal resection (STR), and STR with radiotherapy (RT)

	2-year PFS	10-year OS
GTR (30)	75%	96
STR (37)	36% ($p > 0.001$)	80 ($p = 0.066$)
STR/RT (46)	73% ($p < 0.001$)	96 ($p = 0.05$ vs STR) ($p = 0.066$ vs GTR)

Source: Schoenfeld A, Pekmezci M, Barnes MJ, et al. The superiority of conservative resection and adjuvant radiation for craniopharyngiomas. J Neurooncol 2012;108(1):133–139.

tes insipidus (56.3 vs 13.3% with subtotal resection and radiotherapy, $p < 0.001$) and panhypopituitarism (54.8 vs 26.7% with subtotal resection plus radiotherapy, $p = 0.014$). After radiation, there were three later strokes and one later malignancy, all potentially treatment related.

Similar results were observed in a series of 121 adult and childhood[7] patients treated at Oxford University from 1964 to 2003 who were reported with a mean follow-up of 103 months (0.3 to 468). Local control at 20 years of follow-up was 100% in those with a gross total resection (19 patients, including three who were later irradiated) at up to 20-year follow-up, but control was only 38% and 32% at 10 and 20 years, respectively, after partial resection alone. The control results for subtotal resection when radiation was added were 77% at 10 and 20 years. This outcome, at least through the first decade of follow-up, was similar to that for those operated before and after 1980 and 1990, addressing the concern that reported results frequently span several eras of radiation and surgical technique. The 10-year disease-related survival was 90% at 10 and 20 years and 84% at 30 years. The deaths considered tumor related included perioperative, tumor effects on brainstem, and fatal seizures. Death potentially related to late effects of the tumor and treatments, such as obesity-related illness, were not described. There were no meaningful or statistically significant differences in control or survival for adult onset or childhood onset with respect to tumor-related survival.

Puget et al[8] proposed a preoperative grading system to determine surgical morbidity risk and have begun a prospective study to validate whether use of this system to guide extent of surgical resection would improve quality of life outcome. Their study was motivated by the recognition that there are quality of life problems resulting from surgery for craniopharyngioma that may not be fully captured in the usual end points of mortality, vision status, and endocrine function. These include the effects of hypothalamic injury, such as hyperphagia with obesity, and neuropsychological disorders causing social difficulties, including food-seeking rage, injuries thought to be more common and significant in the pediatric population.

The retrospective component of Puget et al's analysis included patients treated from 1984 to 2001. Tumors were classified according to radiological findings: grade 0: no hypothalamic involvement; grade 1, negligible hypothalamic damage or residual tumor displacement and hypothalamus; and grade 2, significant hypothalamic damage (floor of the third ventricle not identifiable). With a median follow-up of 7 years, body mass index (BMI) was related to magnetic resonance imaging (MRI) grade and surgeon experience, whereas health-related quality of life related to MRI grade and hydrocephalus.

Based on this, the following strategy was proposed: grade 0, complete excision and repeat excision if not complete; grade 1, attempt excision and if incomplete assess for repeat excision or not; grade 2, planned subtotal removal with hypothalamic preservation. After incomplete resection, radiotherapy is recommended for patients older than 5 years. The cohort prospectively treated according to this algorithm had 22 patients with a mean follow-up 14 months. The mean BMI was +1.3 standard deviation (SD) compared with +2.5 SD in the retrospective group. However, 27% still weighed above the 98th percentile. Overall health quality of life remained similar to results from preoperative testing in the prospective group. Although 18% of patients in the retrospective group developed uncontrollable hyperphagia/food rages, treatment guided by the prospective policy resulted in no such situations, with only manageable hyperphagia and no morbid obesity or substantial behavioral dysfunction. In addition, whereas 20% of patients in the unguided retrospective group had visual deterioration after surgery, this did not occur in the prospective group. This study appears to validate the concept that criteria can be developed to guide the surgical approach and optimize quality of life outcome, using radiotherapy when total resection is not achieved. A cross-sectional follow-up study involving 183 patients in Germany has, however, provided intriguing evidence that morbid obesity may substantially decrease long-term survival (20 years, $p = 0.034$), suggesting the possibility that using radiotherapy and limited surgery may even have the potential to improve very long-term all-cause survival.[3]

Another prospective study[9] that utilized the Children's Cancer Leukemia Group Guidelines to determine surgical approach also demonstrated favorable morbidity outcome when aggressive resection is deliberately replaced by subtotal removal and radiation under certain circumstances. Surgical risk was assessed, after any needed endoscopic cyst drainage, based on tumors > 4 cm, hydrocephalus, hypothalamic syndrome at diagnosis (and breach of floor of third ventricle). If all four factors were present, subtotal resection only was intended, with residual as needed to be left in and around the floor of the third ventricle and hypothalamus. In the risk group with two to three of these factors, a near total resection or subtotal resection was considered according to intraoperative findings. For medium- and low-risk patients (0 to 1 risk factors) with no hypothalamic involvement, the goal was complete resection. For the initial 20 patients enrolled, complete surgical excision occurred in 30%, near total in 25%, and subtotal in 45%. Except for one patient with a new visual field deficit, there were no new postoperative neurological deficits and no mortality. Hypothalamic function was stable in regard to weight, BMI, and thirst. There was frequently subsequent endocrine dysfunction, as expected. Of the nine patients with a subtotal resection, six received radiotherapy as per the guideline and two of three observed patients actually required radiotherapy for growth within 1 year of surgery without a need for further resection. With a short median follow-up of 3 years, survival is 100%.

A cautionary point about the retrospectively assessed favorable outcomes with all approaches is raised by reported results of the Kraniopharyngeom 2000 multinational, multi-institutional prospective observational trial, which has demonstrated lower control rates than many of the retrospective studies even after gross total resection.[3] This study accrued 57 patients in the interval between 2001 and 2004. Comparable with other reports, the 3-year overall survival of patients prospectively recruited for Kraniopharyngeom 2000 was excellent (0.97), but high rates of early events (recurrence or progression) were observed after incomplete resection (EFS 0.31) and after complete resection (event-free survival [EFS] 0.64) during the first 3 years of follow-up. The hazard rate was similar with incomplete resection followed by radiotherapy to that for complete resection. Hypothalamic injury, especially of the posterior hypothalamus, was associated with later morbid obesity, resulting in a recommendation against radical resection that may result in such an injury.[10] The authors speculate that the recurrence rates may appear higher than expected from the historical literature because this is a multi-institutional study, and rigorous follow-up with modern imaging is obtained as scheduled and reliably reported. Additional patients were enrolled and follow-up continues.

■ After Subtotal Resection, Should Radiotherapy Be Delayed until Recurrence?

Balancing Reduction in Recurrence Rate versus Treatment Burden and Toxicity

Level I and Level II Evidence

There is no Level I or Level II evidence comparing immediate radiotherapy after subtotal resection with radiation given only at the time of recurrence. A Level II randomized trial is ongoing.

Level III and Level IV Evidence

With many indolent "benign" intracranial tumors, a policy of immediate postoperative radiation after subtotal resections seemed desirable before the routine availability of modern imaging, as recurrence might only be detected after significant growth causing potentially permanent symptoms. Even though radiation is beneficial in preventing or delaying recurrence, it is not clear that there is a benefit to treating at diagnosis rather than waiting for early imaging signs of growth, this approach may delay any additional treatment-related morbidity. This is in contrast to malignant cancers, where residual untreated disease creates a constant risk of distant metastasis rather than just a risk of modest increase in local disease bulk.

Some retrospective studies have caused concern about delaying radiation by demonstrating decreased survival with this approach, although these studies were subject to the inherent bias of retrospective studies that may have spanned several decades. For example, Regine and colleagues[11,12] reported a 78% survival rate at 20 years in children who received immediate radiotherapy but 25% for those who received treatment at the time of recurrence. The experience from Oxford University[7] raised the question of reduced survival rates after treatment given at recurrence, with a 10-year survival of 70% for those with recurrence versus 99% for those without. This report involved a small number of patients with many potential important confounding factors. The data yet to be described here suggest that, in an era when patients can be routinely followed not only with neuro-ophthalmological exam but also with routine MRI, it may be feasible to delay until progression without much risk of injury or uncontrollable aggressive growth.

A relatively large series from the University of Heidelberg,[13] described in more detail in the next section about radiation technologies, included 40 patients. Twenty-eight patients were treated at the time of recurrence with fractionated stereotactic radiotherapy and 12 were treated after the initial surgery. Progression-free survival was 100% at 10 years after radiotherapy, demonstrating long-term efficacy even in the setting of recurrence when newer precision radiotherapy technologies are utilized.

An ongoing multi-institutional prospective randomized trial is now rigorously assessing the role of immediate versus delayed radiotherapy after subtotal resection of craniopharyngioma. In this trial, Kraniopharyngeom 2007,[14] patients are prospectively followed without adjuvant radiotherapy if they have had a complete resection or if they are < 5 years old with incomplete cognitive toxicity may be high in young children. Children 5 and older are randomized to observation or radiation if only a subtotal resection was performed. The primary objective is to assess quality of life outcome using a variety of measures, including extensive neurocognitive testing, evaluation of function, measures of hypothalamic function, vision testing, and endocrinologic status. Radiation is to be fractionated external beam treatment to a dose of 54 Gy at 1.8 Gy per day, with the at-risk area, clinical target volume (CTV), containing the gross tumor with a margin of 5 mm. An additional margin of 3 to 5 mm is to be added to create the planning target volume (PTV). In this study, the role of stereotactic radiosurgery and intracystic radiotherapy is considered too uncertain and it is recommended that these techniques be utilized only as appropriate for recurrence. This trial, if successfully completed, will provide important information about control rates, survival, and quality of life end points, and 111 of 150 patients had been accrued through early 2013.

■ Optimal Radiation Technique

Targeting of Disease While Limiting Dose to Uninvolved Tissues

Level I and Level II Evidence

There are no Level I or Level II evidence studies comparing outcome with different techniques for delivering radiotherapy, in terms of quality of life outcome, tumor control, or survival.

Level III and Level IV Evidence

The relative benefits of radiotherapy may have been improved by new highly conformal and/or image-guided techniques developed over the past 2 decades that ensure adequate delivery of radiation to the tumor, allow more limited exposure of normal tissues vulnerable to injury, and assess changes in cyst volume. Although definitive conclusions can't be reached from available data and follow-up, preliminary data and strong rationale indicate that craniopharyngioma is optimally treated with this approach. This tumor is generally not widely infiltrative and recurs at its primary location, so that conformal radiation technologies, such as three-dimensional planning, intensity-modulated radiotherapy, or even fractionated or single-dose stereotactic treatment, may result in improved therapeutic ratio by targeting more precisely defined volumes with assurance of dose delivery.

Single-fraction stereotactic radiosurgery was driven by the early precision technologies that required invasive immobilization unsuited to repetitive daily treatments and by the hypothesis that benign tumors might be most sensitive to a large fraction of radiation, similar to normal tissues. More recently, noninvasive radiation systems have allowed treatments to be administered with noninvasive repeated daily immobilization and with precision approaching that achieved with invasive systems. Fractionation may be optimal in this situation because the nearby optic pathways are easily injured by large single doses of radiation and therefore create a limit to the dose that can be administered to nearby tumor. However, the optic pathways are relatively less sensitive to fractionated radiation over 25 to 30 visits and are less of a barrier to full-dose treatment with that approach. Routine imaging during treatment may be an essential component when conformal fractionated plans are used because changes in cyst size over time can result in missing of tumor or altered doses to normal structures, which can be dealt with by cyst drainage or replanning of the radiotherapy. Proton therapy, which has physical properties allowing sharper dose reduction away from the target, is also being evaluated as an approach to administer fractionated treatment with further reduction in long-term risks. Finally, injection of radiosotope into a cyst can be a highly localized means of delivering treatment but is not effective for thicker adjacent solid components.

With the available data, the use of highly conformal fractionated radiotherapy technologies can be recommended. An example is illustrated in **Fig. 41.1**, which demonstrates a radiation plan that targets a cystic craniopharyngioma, subtotally resected, with

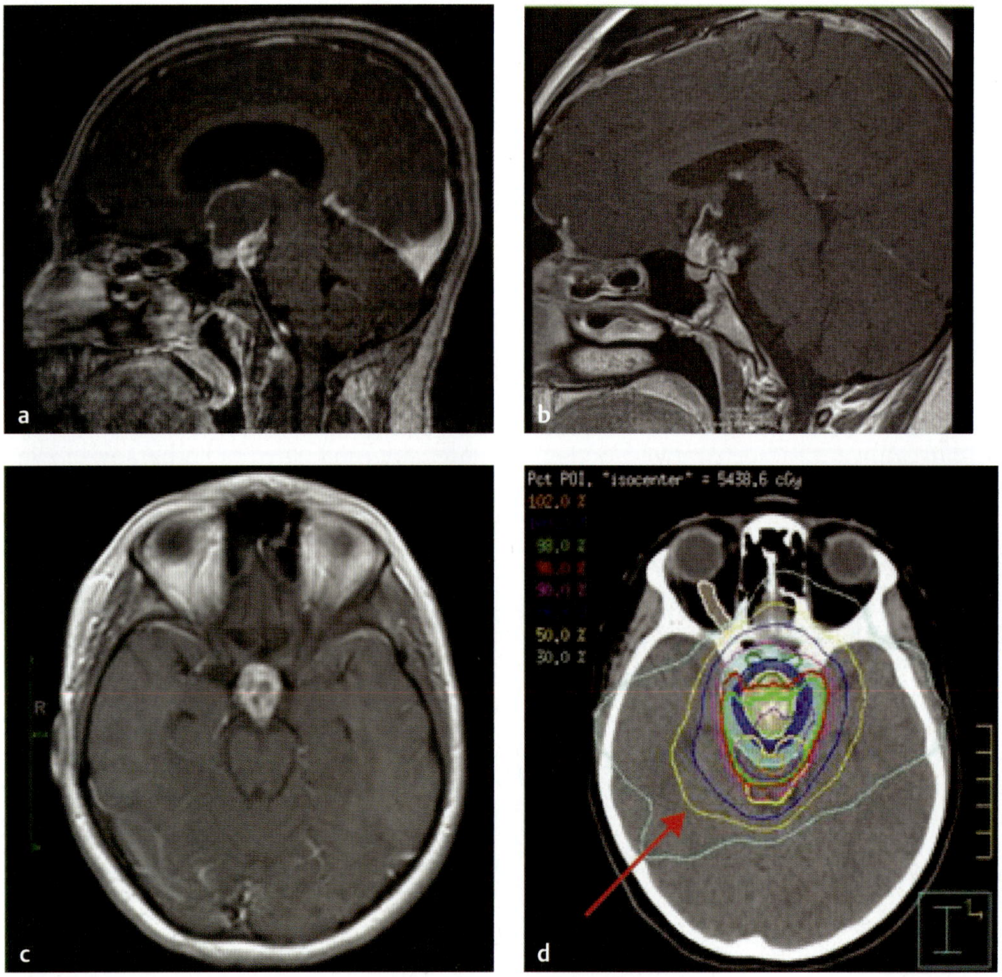

Fig. 41.1 Highly conformal radiation plan for a 14-year-old female treated after subtotal resection of a cystic craniopharyngioma. **(a)** Preoperative magnetic resonance imaging (MRI), **(b,c)** Postoperative MRI scans. **(d)** Radiation plan. The normal brain outside the line identified by the arrow receives 50% or less than the planned dose of 54 Gy.

a conformal dose distribution delivering a high dose to the target with a modest margin and delivering limited radiation to the remainder of the brain, including the bulk of the nearby temporal lobes. This approach has been adopted by the international Kraniopharyngeom 2007[14] randomized trial examining the role of radiation. The radiotherapy guidelines for this study were discussed previously. Although not addressed in those protocol guidelines, it is desirable to use imaging during treatment to monitor for cyst enlargement that can result in radiation underdosage to a portion of the disease. The key data supporting this approach are described later.

Highly Conformal Fractionated Radiation

Results from the University of Heidelberg[13] provide evidence about the potential for advanced radiation technology to improve outcome. Fractionated stereotactic radiotherapy was utilized to provide high precision, minimizing the margin needed for positioning and target definition uncertainties, and thereby potentially reducing the risk of meaningful toxicities and ensuring accurate aim to hit the target fully each day. A margin for positioning uncertainty of 2 mm was used beyond the imaging-identified tumor. The dose used was 50.4 to 55.6 Gy at 1.8 Gy to 2.0 Gy per day.

Forty patients were treated, with progression-free survival of 100% at 10 years after treatment, whether treatment was given at diagnosis or for a recurrence. With a median follow-up time of 98 months (2 to 326 months), 5- and 10-year survival was 97% and 89%, respectively, without suggestion of a difference for those treated initially or at recurrence. Hormone deficiencies prior to treatment were common, but only one patient developed a new hormone deficiency and another progressed from partial deficit to panhypopituitarism. Formal neuropsychological assessment was not performed on a regular basis in this series, but 38 patients did not demonstrate any decline in neuropsychological status during follow-up, whereas two patients developed major cognitive dysfunction.

Minniti et al[15] reported similar results in 39 patients (25 immediate, 14 at recurrence) treated with fractionated stereotactic conformal radiotherapy (50 Gy with conventional fractionation, 5 to 8 mm margin), with a local progression-free survival rate of 92% and an overall survival rate of 100% at 5 years. The issue of cyst control was directly addressed. Thirty percent had symptomatic cyst enlargement up to 8 months after treatment (seven during treatment, three after) treated by aspiration through existing or newly inserted Ommaya reservoirs, without reports of later occurrences, suggesting that this approach is indeed successful for cyst as well as solid tumor control.

Investigators at St. Jude Children's Research Hospital[16] rigorously assessed this approach in a prospective phase 2 trial of conformal radiation therapy (CRT) for craniopharyngioma to determine whether the irradiated volume could be safely reduced while maintaining control rates and decreasing effects on cognitive function. Twenty-eight pediatric patients (median age, 7.3 years) received radiotherapy, 54 to 55.8 Gy, to the gross tumor volume (GTV), including solid and cystic components surrounded by a 1-cm CTV margin to allow for unappreciated extension, plus an additional 5 mm PTV to allow for treatment inaccuracy related to positioning and imaging. It may have been important that repeat imaging was performed to have a stable med with MRI during weeks 3 and 5 of treatment to verify continued appropriate targeting of the tumor and cyst, which resulted in 13 patients undergoing a cyst aspiration during treatment and three requiring a revised plan to appropriately treat the enlarged altered volume.

Patients were evaluated serially with neuropsychometric testing to determine the effect of clinical factors and radiation dosimetry on intelligence quotient (IQ). After a median follow-up of 36.6 months (24.4 to 80.0 months), the 3-year progression-free survival rate was 90.3%. Cognitive outcome for patients was adversely affected by the following factors: age, more extensive surgery ($p = 0.014$), multiple surgical procedures, diabetes insipidus, hydrocephalus at diagnosis, cerebrospinal fluid shunt ($p = 0.005$), need for shunt revisions, Ommaya reservoir, and cyst aspirations. The percentage of total brain, supratentorial brain, or left temporal lobe volumes receiving a dose in excess of 45 Gy had a significant impact on IQ over time. Patients over 7.4 years old tended to have a stable IQ after treatment, but younger patients had a steady and substantial decline during the available follow-up of up to 4 years. These data provide prospective evidence that the use of a target of observed tumor with a 1-cm margin results in tumor control similar to that achieved using conventional radiotherapy, and they provide support for delaying radiation when possible in children < 5 to 7 years old.

Based on these good results, and an increasing capacity for adaptive radiation planning that allows dose delivery to be altered midtreatment in response to target changes, the St. Jude group has implemented a smaller CTV margin of 5 mm with a PTV margin of 3 mm and weekly MRI to assess for changes in cyst size and anatomy.[17] Planning was to be reperformed if the MRI showed that the GTV, as it changed during treatment, abutted or exceeded the PTV used for the original radiation planning. Using these criteria, replanning was found necessary in nine of 14 patients, and therefore repeat imaging during highly conformal treatment is warranted and has potential to further improve outcome for patients.

Proton radiotherapy may have the potential to further improve the therapeutic ratios compared with standard photon or X-ray treatment.[18] This technology allows the dose to be deposited with even greater precision because the beams have relatively sharp and predictable limits to the depth of penetration. A study compared plans using standard photon radiation with those using protons.[18] The plans demonstrated similarly excellent coverage of the target volume in comparison with the conformal conventional photon radiotherapy plans. There was a reduction in body dose and as well as in entire brain dose, which also may be of importance in the younger pediatric population but is likely of less meaningful benefit in adults. Meaningful clinical data are not yet available to assess the value of this promising approach.

Stereotactic Radiosurgery (Single Fraction)

Single-fraction stereotactic radiosurgery (SRS) is another high-precision radiation approach that has also been utilized. The advantages of SRS are not only completion of treatment in one session but also precision of the technology, which allows a lower dose to be delivered to normal tissues as well as a possible tumor control benefit in benign histologies with large, single radiation doses. The data using this approach in initial management do not provide convincing evidence that it is a superior approach. This may relate to the radiosensitivity of the nearby structures, including the optic nerves/chiasm, pituitary gland, and hypothalamus. These structures, especially the optic pathways, are at particular risk of injury from single-fraction treatment; therefore, their protection frequently requires constraining the dose delivered to nearby portions of the tumor. To maintain safety, the solid component without cyst wall has been utilized as the target volume, but equivalent long-term control has not been validated. In addition, a driving force for the utilization of single-dose SRS was the requirement for invasive immobilization, but the development of technologies that allow repeated noninvasive fractionated radiation with nearly the same precision allows protection of nearby normal tissues with a combination of precise targeting and division of treatment into multiple fractions.

Ulfarsson et al[19] reported results with a median follow-up period 16.8 years (6 to 34 years) for 21 patients who underwent gamma knife radiosurgery, including children and adults. There was a wide dose range, 3 to 25 Gy, reflecting uncertainty as to the optimal dose in the initial use of this technology for craniopharyngioma. Treatment failure occurred in 85% of patients (11/13) treated with < 6 Gy, a dose not generally now considered efficacious for any solid tumor. Failure was 33% (3/9) for patients treated with a higher dose. Deterioration of visual function was reported in eight patients (38%), and in seven it was thought attributable to tumor growth. More recent results have been reported from the University of Pittsburgh.[20] Forty-six patients were treated, 43 at recurrence, with gamma knife radiosurgery with a median marginal dose of 13 Gy but as low as 10 Gy when needed to protect the optic apparatus. The median volume was only 1 mL. In this population the 5-year survival was 97%, with 67% remaining recurrence free. The 5-year overall local control rate for solid tumors (n = 22), cystic tumors (n = 5), mixed solid and cystic tumors treated with complete radiosurgical coverage (n = 14), and mixed solid and cystic tumors treated only for the solid component (n = 10) was 77.5%, 100%, 64.3%, and 51.9%, respectively When the entire cyst was treated, the 5-year progression-free survival was 75%, versus 52% (p = 0.020) if only solid tumor was treated. This emphasizes the potential efficacy of radiation in controlling the cystic component and raises questions about the concept of treating the solid component only (especially given that salvage radiation in this critical region is risky under many circumstances). SRS may be useful for small solid residual craniopharyngiomas located ~ 5 mm or more away from the optic pathway because the pathway can be adequately shielded while still treating the entirety of the tumor.

Intracystic Radioisotopes (Brachytherapy)

Radioisotope instillation to treat the cyst component of a craniopharyngioma can be successful, but appropriateness in initial management may be limited to select cases given the advances in external beam radiation that may allow safe treatment of the entire volume at risk for progression. Significant radiation dose is primarily confined to the cyst wall itself, and therefore adequate control of the solid portion of the tumor is not frequently achieved. Radiosotopes may reduce cyst fluid production through effects on secretory cells and also through fibrosis/sclerosis of the cyst wall.[21] Phosphorus-32 (P32), yttrium-90, gold-198, and rhenium-186 have been used for this purpose because they create weakly penetrating beta irradiation.

Barriger et al[22] has reported a group of 22 patients treated after 1997 using P32 with 1-, 3-, and 5-year progression-free survival of 68%, 49%, and 31%, respectively. Julow et al[23] reported on 60 patients treated with yttrium for recurrent cyst after surgery (no prior radiation). Over 70% had an 80% reduction in cyst volume, but there were no 3-year survivors, and 10 patients reportedly died of progressive solid tumor. This therapy, it should be noted, would be appropriate only for carefully selected patients because it does not effectively deliver radiation to solid components and may potentially enhance the risk of later external beam radiotherapy if the optic pathways receive a significant dose. Other nonradioactive agents have demonstrated effectiveness for cyst therapy, including bleomycin and interferon. The appropriate role of, and optimal approach to, intracystic therapy remains controversial and is discussed elsewhere in this text.

■ Summary and Conclusions

Radiotherapy has an important role in optimizing therapy for craniopharyngioma. Although gross total resection leads to a high rate of 5- to 10-year control, invasion of nearby critical structures frequently causes gross total resection to be impossible or likely to cause unacceptable morbidity, including hypothalamic dysfunction, vision deficits, and endocrinopathy. Gross total resection may lead to a higher risk of hyperphagia and morbid obesity, especially in the pediatric population, sequelae that also pose substantial risk not only to quality of life but also to length of life. Subtotal resection or biopsy with the addition of radiation also leads to apparently similar control rates and may allow use of more limited surgery in situations where there is a high risk of injury to optic tracts or the hypothalamus. However, radiation is also associated with meaningful risk, especially in the pediatric population. These risks relate to long-term endocrinopathy, neurocognitive deficits, damage to visual pathways, and late stroke and malignancy. With imaging follow-up it may be possible to delay radiotherapy, with limited risk of substantial growth that would adversely affect outcome. The question of the relative quality of life and survival outcome with delayed versus early preventive irradiation is the subject of an ongoing international randomized trial, but there is a strong rationale for delaying radiation in children < 5 to 7 years old, where the risks of radiation-induced neurocognitive deficits might be quite high. There may be not only a quality of life but also a long-term survival impact from morbid obesity and other problems that result from gross total resection having an impact on the hypothalamus.

Questions relate not only to the optimal use of radiotherapy as part of an alternative to gross total resection but also to the optimal radiation technique, which can include conventionally fractionated radiation or SRS. Available data support limiting the extent of surgery to avoid morbidity, with favorable long-term results either with immediate radiation or with radiation when growth is identified. Because the tumor is generally well demarcated, highly conformal radiotherapy may be utilized, which may be especially important in reducing toxicities in children. Cyst monitoring to assess stability of targeted anatomy is desirable during radiation. Single-dose SRS may be useful for small solid lesions at a safe distance from the optic apparatus, and intracystic radiotherapy is appropriate for well-selected primarily cystic cases. These latter techniques are less well validated, and there is considerable controversy because they appropriately treat the entire extent of disease in only highly selected cases.

Expert Recommendations

1. Craniopharyngioma is uncommon and occurs in both children and adults. Numerous uncontrolled historical studies demonstrate a high chance of long-term survival through several decades of follow-up.
2. The typical location of craniopharyngioma, abutting the hypothalamus, the optic nerves and chiasm, the third ventricle, and the brain, results in a substantial chance of reduced quality of life that may result from either the tumor itself or therapy. The impacts of tumor- and treatment-related hypothalamic injury and the toxicities of radiation are more significant in pediatric than in adult patients.
3. Gross total resection results in a high rate of long-term control and survival. This is the primary objective when it is judged to be safe (Grade 1C Recommendation, Level III/IV Evidence).
4. When there is a significant risk of injury from gross total resection that may have a long-term impact on the quality of life, subtotal resection should be considered. Surgical risks appear high when there is invasion of the hypothalamus. Presence of hydrocephalus, breach of the floor of the fourth ventricle, and large tumor size may also be important (Grade 2C Recommendation, Level III/IV Evidence).
5. With availability of modern routine imaging, radiation may not only be administered after subtotal resection as part of an immediate initial therapeutic plan or at the time of tumor growth (Grade 1C Recommendation, Level IV Evidence).
   a. Children 5 to 7 years old are at high risk of significant neurocognitive toxicities resulting from radiation, and deferring radiation until tumor growth or until the child is older should be strongly considered.
   b. In the absence of robust data comparing survival and quality of life outcome with immediate and delayed radiation, either approach is reasonable to consider. A randomized trial is ongoing.
6. Conformal radiation techniques using conventional or stereotactic technologies lead to high control rates and may reduce the risks of toxicities compared with treatment of larger areas (Grade 1C Recommendation, Level III/IV Evidence).
   a. Margins of 2 to 5 mm appear acceptable using precision image-guided techniques with doses of 5,000 to 5,400 cGy at 180 to 200 cGy per day. Larger margins may be needed depending upon techniques utilized.
   b. Imaging during therapy is appropriate because changes in cyst size may alter the amount of radiation delivered to the tumor, especially when highly conformal radiation plans are used.
   c. Radiotherapy appears to result in good long-term control of craniopharyngioma cysts, but in the short term, attention to potential cyst growth is important.
   d. The role of stereotactic radiosurgery (single dose) is uncertain but can be appropriate under select limited clinical circumstances. Radiosurgery may be most useful for small craniopharyngiomas that can be completely encompassed within the treatment field, including cystic components, without risky dosing of optic nerves.
   e. The role of SRS (single dose) is uncertain but it can be appropriate under select limited clinical circumstances for cyst control. Rates of long-term control and vision outcome remain of concern depending upon individual circumstances.

■ References

1. Müller HL. Childhood craniopharyngioma. Pituitary 2013; 16(1):56–67
2. Müller HL. Diagnostics, treatment, and follow-up in craniopharyngioma. Front Endocrinol (Lausanne) 2011;2:70
3. Müller HL, Gebhardt U, Etavard-Gorris N, et al. Prognosis and sequela in patients with childhood craniopharyngioma – results of HIT-ENDO and update on KRANIOPHARYNGEOM 2000. Klin Padiatr 2004;216(6):343–348
4. Yang I, Sughrue ME, Rutkowski MJ, et al. Craniopharyngioma: a comparison of tumor control with various treatment strategies. Neurosurg Focus 2010;28(4):E5
5. Sughrue ME, Yang I, Kane AJ, et al. Endocrinologic, neurologic, and visual morbidity after treatment for craniopharyngioma. J Neurooncol 2011;101(3):463–476
6. Schoenfeld A, Pekmezci M, Barnes MJ, et al. The superiority of conservative resection and adjuvant radiation for craniopharyngiomas. J Neurooncol 2012;108(1):133–139
7. Karavitaki N, Brufani C, Warner JT, et al. Craniopharyngiomas in children and adults: systematic analysis of 121 cases with long-term follow-up. Clin Endocrinol (Oxf) 2005;62(4): 397–409
8. Puget S, Garnett M, Wray A, et al. Pediatric craniopharyngiomas: classification and treatment according to the degree of hypothalamic involvement. J Neurosurg 2007;106(1, Suppl): 3–12
9. Mallucci C, Pizer B, Blair J, et al. Management of craniopharyngioma: the Liverpool experience following the introduction of the CCLG guidelines. Introducing a new risk assessment grading system. Childs Nerv Syst 2012;28(8):1181–1192
10. Müller HL, Gebhardt U, Teske C, et al; Study Committee of KRANIOPHARYNGEOM 2000. Post-operative hypothalamic lesions and obesity in childhood craniopharyngioma: results of the multinational prospective trial KRANIOPHARYNGEOM 2000 after 3-year follow-up. Eur J Endocrinol 2011;165(1):17–24
11. Regine WF, Kramer S. Pediatric craniopharyngiomas: long term results of combined treatment with surgery and radiation. Int J Radiat Oncol Biol Phys 1992;24(4):611–617
12. Regine WF, Mohiuddin M, Kramer S. Long-term results of pediatric and adult craniopharyngiomas treated with combined surgery and radiation. Radiother Oncol 1993;27(1):13–21
13. Combs SE, Thilmann C, Huber PE, Hoess A, Debus J, Schulz-Ertner D. Achievement of long-term local control in patients with craniopharyngiomas using high precision stereotactic radiotherapy. Cancer 2007;109(11):2308–2314
14. German Society of Pediatric Oncology and Hematology. Kraniopharyngeom 2007 study protocol. 2007; this is an ongoing study available at kraniopharyngeom.net
15. Minniti G, Saran F, Traish D, et al. Fractionated stereotactic conformal radiotherapy following conservative surgery in the control of craniopharyngiomas. Radiother Oncol 2007; 82(1):90–95
16. Merchant TE, Kiehna EN, Kun LE, et al. Phase II trial of conformal radiation therapy for pediatric patients with craniopharyngioma and correlation of surgical factors and radiation dosimetry with change in cognitive function. J Neurosurg 2006;104(2, Suppl):94–102
17. Beltran C, Naik M, Merchant TE. Dosimetric effect of target expansion and setup uncertainty during radiation therapy in pediatric craniopharyngioma. Radiother Oncol 2010; 97(3):399–403
18. Beltran C, Roca M, Merchant TE. On the benefits and risks of proton therapy in pediatric craniopharyngioma. Int J Radiat Oncol Biol Phys 2012;82(2):e281–e287
19. Ulfarsson E, Lindquist C, Roberts M, et al. Gamma knife radiosurgery for craniopharyngiomas: long-term results in the first Swedish patients. J Neurosurg 2002;97(5, Suppl):613–622
20. Niranjan A, Kano H, Mathieu D, Kondziolka D, Flickinger JC, Lunsford LD. Radiosurgery for craniopharyngioma. Int J Radiat Oncol Biol Phys 2010;78(1):64–71
21. Szeifert GT, Bálint K, Sipos L, Sarker MH, Czirják S, Julow J. Pathological findings in cystic craniopharyngiomas after stereotactic intracavitary irradiation with yttrium-90 isotope. Prog Neurol Surg 2007;20:297–302
22. Barriger RB, Chang A, Lo SS, et al. Phosphorus-32 therapy for cystic craniopharyngiomas. Radiother Oncol 2011;98(2): 207–212
23. Julow J, Backlund EO, Lányi F, et al. Long-term results and late complications after intracavitary yttrium-90 colloid irradiation of recurrent cystic craniopharyngiomas. Neurosurgery 2007;61(2):288–295

42

Intra-Cyst Therapies for Craniopharyngiomas

Graeme F. Woodworth and Jon D. Weingart

Craniopharyngiomas (CPs) are slow-growing, histologically benign tumors arising from embryonic tissue in the region of the pituitary infundibulum. These tumors are most commonly found in children but can also present in adults later in life.[1] The complex epithelial, neuroectoderm-derived cells that constitute CPs lead to cystic, soft tissue, and calcified components. Approximately 90% of CPs have a significant cystic component, usually filled with a dark viscous fluid composed of cholesterol crystals, hemoglobin by-products, and epithelial cells.[2,3] This more cystic, often calcified, variant is labeled the adamantinomatous type, whereas the papillary form often has more soft tissue architecture and carries a lower risk of morbidity and recurrence.[4]

Another critical feature of CPs are the dense adhesions to nearby intracranial structures. As opposed to discrete extra-axial tumors separated by arachnoid planes, the CP capsule is often firmly attached to nearby sensitive neural and vascular structures, including the pituitary gland/stalk, hypothalamus, optic apparatus, and carotid arteries and branches. Therefore, although these tumors are generally histologically benign, they often behave in a more malignant fashion, leading to a high risk of neurological deficits and tumor recurrence.

Given the age distribution at presentation, tenuous attachments, and location of CPs, careful consideration of the treatment options for each patient is paramount. The primary goals of treatment are preservation of neurological function, the hypothalmic-pituitary axes, and gross total resection (GTR)/cure. At highest risk are hypothalamic function often leading to morbid obesity and personality changes (particularly in younger patients), vision loss, and pituitary dysfunction. Surgery, when possible, represents the first line of therapy and the best chance of complete tumor removal. However, GTR is often not possible due to the risk of neurological injury from attempts to dissect the capsule from crucial neurovascular structures. In numerous recent case series, GTR was achieved in only 50 to 80% of attempted complete resections.[5–7] Importantly, even in the setting of apparent GTR, recurrence has been observed in 10 to 30%.[6,8]

Fortunately, good options for adjuvant therapy exist to treat the residual tumor, including radiation (fractionated or intensity-modulated radiotherapy, stereotactic radiosurgery, proton beam therapy, et al) and intratumoral instillations for cystic lesions. This chapter focuses on the evidence for the use of intracystic therapies, including β-emitting radionuclides, bleomycin, and interferon-α, the main goals of this form of therapy being reduction of cyst volume and mass effect, and overall tumor-growth control.

■ Literature Review

Intracystic Beta-Emitting Radiation Sources

Level I Evidence

No prospective, randomized trials exist for the use of β-emitting radionuclides in CP.

Level II and Level IV Evidence

Beta-emission, like other forms of radiation, eventually leads to DNA damage causing cell death via apoptosis. Instillation of β-emitting substances directly into the tumor cyst offers the opportunity for direct local radiation treatment to the tumor. Numerous case-control and cohort studies exist that have explored the use of intracavitary radiation sources for the treatment of CP. Early studies with this approach began in the 1950s[9,10] and evolved into comparisons between various β-emitting radiation sources, including phosphorus-32, yttrium-90, rhenium-186, and aurum-198.[11,12] Histopathological changes following these treatments include fibrosis in the cyst wall, destruction of neoplastic epithelium, and local vasculopathy, confirming the powerful effects of β-emitting radiation.[13–15]

The results of these comparison studies show that, regardless of the radiation source used, intracavitary radiotherapy reduces the size of the cyst in 50 to 100% of cases (**Table 42.1**).[11,12,16,17,40] Patient survival at 10 years after this treatment type ranges from 45 to 80%; however, in one of the series with longer follow-up, Julow et al reported declining survival rates after 20 years.[17] Local radiation toxicity on surrounding structures following intra-cystic radiotherapy is a concern based on literature reports. Although new endocrinopathy is seen infrequently (< 1%), visual loss and hypothalamic damage have been reported in ~ 5% of patients. Regional vascular changes resulting in a moyamoya type vasculopathy, and even subarachnoid hemorrhage, have been reported.[17] Additional downsides of intracavitary radiotherapy are the logistical hurdles of obtaining, handling, and dosing the radioisotopes. Many centers find this additional complexity not worth the costs when suitable alternatives exist.

In 2005, the Children's Cancer and Leukaemia Group (CCLG) formulated guidelines for the management of pediatric CP.[18] The guidelines included limited surgery followed by up-front radiotherapy for large tumors with hypothalamic involvement, and a radical resection only for smaller tumors without hypothalamic involvement. To date, it is unclear if this management strategy leads to improved outcomes for children with CP.

Intracystic Bleomycin

Level I Evidence

No prospective, randomized trials exist for the use of bleomycin in CP.

Table 42.1 Comparison studies of intracavitary radiotherapy

Study	Radiation source	Dose	No. patients	Follow-up (months)	Cyst growth control	Mean survival (years)	Complications
Voges et al 1997[11]	Y-90 P-32 Re-186	NA	62	144	Y-90, P-32, 80% Re-186 0%	9 ± 0.9	VL 4/62 CN III 1/62 PI 3/62
Hasegawa et al 2004[40]	P-32	200 Gy	49	48	70%		VL 9/49 CN III 0/49 PI 5/17
Julow et al 2007[17]	Y-90	300 Gy	60	NA	100%	9.4	VL 3/60 CN III 6/60 PI 0/42
Derrey et al 2008[16]	Re-186	381 mBq	42	43	87%	NA	VL 2/42 CN III 0/42 PI 0/42

Abbreviations: CN, cranial nerve; mBq, megabecquerel; NA, not available; P, phosphorous; PI, pituitary insufficiency; Re, rhenium; VL, vision loss; Y, yttrium.

Level II to Level IV Evidence

Bleomycin has chemotherapeutic properties that serve to inhibit cell cycle growth arrest, cell death, and decreased fluid secretion in CP.[19] Bleomycin is used to treat numerous cancers and conditions, including squamous cell carcinoma, lymphoma, malignant pleural effusion, and others. In 1985, Takahashi et al reported the first use of intracystic bleomycin in CP and found good cyst control in four of seven children with cystic tumors receiving minimal initial excision.[20] Since then, numerous case-control and cohort studies have been performed evaluating local bleomycin treatment as initial therapy and in the setting of tumor recurrence.[21–23]

In 1996, Broggi and Franzini reported 100% cyst control rates in 14 patients receiving intracystic bleomycin after an average follow-up of 4 years.[24] These early studies led clinicians to believe that durable tumor control could be achieved with this therapy. Further studies by Mottolese et al, Hukin et al, and Park et al confirmed excellent earlier tumor control, but longer follow-up showed recurrence in 40 to 50% of patients at a median of 1 to 2 years following bleomycin treatment.[22,25,26]

Complications from intracystic bleomycin therapy have been a controversial topic. Linnert and Gehl reviewed the literature and found that most frequent adverse effects from local intracranial bleomycin instillation were transient fever, headaches, nausea and vomiting, lethargy, and peritumoral edema. Five out of 189 patients (3%) treated from 1973 to 2007 had severe, and six patients (3%) had moderate adverse effects. One death was directly related to this treatment, where the investigators reported use of a very high dose. Two patients (2%) developed loss of vision and two patients (2%) had hearing loss because of the treatment.[27] One key to minimizing complications is making sure all of the holes in the catheter tip are inside the tumor cyst and the catheter has a tight seal with the cyst capsule, to avoid drug leakage into the surrounding space and tissues. Although numerous dosing schemes have been suggested, the appropriate dose and frequency of intracystic bleomycin have not been defined scientifically. The usual dose per instillation has been reported between 2 and 5 mg, or 0.09 mg/mL/dose (range, 0.01 to 2.0 mg/mL/dose) administered multiple times per week. Lactate dehydrogenase levels in the cyst fluid gradually decrease with treatment and have been used by some investigators to determine when to stop bleomycin therapy.[26,28]

Given the relatively high incidence of unwanted side effects and late progression following treatment, intracystic bleomycin currently has a limited role in the management of cystic CPs. Many view this treatment as a stalling mechanism to control the cystic components for a variable period of time to allow delay of radiotherapy or further resection, which may be beneficial, particularly in young children. In other cases of large, challenging cystic tumors, reduction of the cyst volume and expansiveness may change the resectability of the tumor and enable more complete removal.

Recently, Fang et al reviewed this topic for the Cochrane Database series to establish guidelines for the use of intracystic bleomycin in CP. The summary statement reported no appropriate clinical trials from which to draw any definitive conclusions regarding the effects of intracystic bleomycin in these patients. Hence, based on the currently available evidence, no definitive recommendations for the use of intracystic bleomycin in the treatment of cystic CPs can be made at this time.[21]

Intracystic Interferon-α

Level I and Level II Evidence

No prospective, randomized trials exist for the use of intracystic interferon-α (IFN-α) in CP.

Level III and Level IV Evidence

IFN-α is an endogenous cytokine known to have antitumor properties related to its role in inflammation and immunomodulation.[29] Although the exact mechanism of action of IFN-α in CP control is not known, preliminary studies suggest that it may work by activating Fas-mediated apoptosis.[30] IFN-α has been shown to successfully treat squamous cell carcinoma, which originates from a similar cell type to CP.[31] Therefore, it was hypothesized that this therapy would have efficacy against CP as well. Prior to its investigation in treating CP, intracranial delivery of IFN-α had been studied for the treatment of glioma[32,33] and viral encephalitis,[34–36] where it was shown to have little benefit but a reasonable safety profile. In 2005, Cavalheiro et al first reported on the successful use of intracystic IFN-α in nine children with cystic craniopharyngiomas[37] and expanded this to a multicenter series with 60 patients.[38] Clinical and radiological improvement was achieved in 76% of the cases, whereas 30% had mild side effects, including headache and eyelid edema. New endocrinological deficits were observed in 13% of the cases.

More recently, Dastoli and colleagues reported their series of 19 patients with cystic CP receiving intratumoral IFN-α. These results corroborated the previous findings, showing a cyst volume reduction of at least 60% in all patients, and minimal treatment-related side effects.[39] Although it is still early in the evaluation of this treatment, intracystic IFN-α, like intracystic bleomycin, appears to provide short-term control of cystic CP and delay the timing of more definitive treatment aimed at longer-term control. In comparing these two temporizing treatment modalities, IFN-α appears to have similar advantages to intracystic bleomycin in terms of cyst control but does not appear to have the toxicity issues commonly seen with bleomycin, particularly if the latter spills into the subarachnoid space. However, longer follow-up is needed for patients receiving intracystic IFN-α to determine if this is a viable treatment option.

Currently, no published guidelines or consensus statements exist regarding the use of intracystic IFN-α.

General Considerations and Pearls

1. The Ommaya reservoir is useful for repeat treatments, as well as access to the cyst fluid for decompression if needed.
2. To confirm catheter seal and hole locations, radio-opaque dye can be instilled into the Ommaya reservoir and a computed tomographic scan performed
3. Multiple catheter placements/instillations may be necessary for multicystic tumors or loculated cysts.
4. Real-time ultrasonography, stereotaxis, and endoscopy are helpful in directing the catheter into the cyst, especially when the cyst wall is firm.

Expert Recommendations

1. Given the high morbidity of radical resection, adjuvant therapies, such as intra-cyst therapies, play a major role in management.
2. While shown to be effective in reducing cyst size, intra-cystic beta-emitting radiation sources are plagued by concerns of local radiation toxicity to surrounding neurovascular structures (Grade 1C Recommendation, Level II–IV Evidence).
3. A chemotherapeutic agent, intra-cyst bleomycin has been shown only to control cyst size and is currently viewed as a means to halt disease progression. Additionally, its use is associated with several undesirable side effects that are independent of dosing. Hence, this modality currently has a limited role in the multi-modality management of craniopharyngiomas (Grade 1C+ Recommendation, Level II–IV Evidence).
4. Interferon-α has been shown in Level III/IV studies to result in clinical and radiographic improvement with fewer and more tolerable side effects. However, similar to bleomycin, its use is currently limited to short-term control. Due to its more favorable side effect profile, interferon-α appears to be the preferred intra-cyst therapy. However, control studies directly comparing these agents have not yet been published (Grade 1C Recommendation, Level III–IV Evidence).

Summary and Conclusions

CP is a benign tumor histopathologically and in theory should be curable by complete resection. In reality, given the high morbidity of radical resection in many cases, adjuvant therapies for CP have emerged to play a major role in the clinical management. In complex cases where complete resection is not feasible, a multimodal therapeutic approach may provide the optimal outcome, balancing disease (tumor) control and maintenance of neurological function. As part of the multimodality armamentarium, intracystic therapies with bleomycin and more recently IFN-α have a role in conjunction with external radiotherapy, particularly in the predominantly cystic craniopharyngiomas. Currently, considering these intracystic modalities, IFN-α appears to have fewer side effects with similar tumor control rates compared to bleomycin and internal radiation, but more experience and longer follow-up are needed.

References

1. Mortini P, Losa M, Pozzobon G, et al. Neurosurgical treatment of craniopharyngioma in adults and children: early and long-term results in a large case series. J Neurosurg 2011;114(5):1350–1359
2. Alén JF, Boto GR, Lagares A, de la Lama A, Gómez PA, Lobato RD. Intratumoural bleomycin as a treatment for recurrent cystic craniopharyngioma. Case report and review of the literature. Neurocirugia (Astur) 2002;13(6):479–485
3. Szeifert GT, Julow J, Szabolcs M, Slowik F, Bálint K, Pásztor E. Secretory component of cystic craniopharyngiomas: a mucino-histochemical and electron-microscopic study. Surg Neurol 1991;36(4):286–293
4. Pekmezci M, Louie J, Gupta N, Bloomer MM, Tihan T. Clinicopathological characteristics of adamantinomatous and papillary craniopharyngiomas: University of California, San Francisco experience 1985-2005. Neurosurgery 2010; 67(5):1341–1349
5. Caldarelli M, Massimi L, Tamburrini G, Cappa M, Di Rocco C. Long-term results of the surgical treatment of craniopharyngioma: the experience at the Policlinico Gemelli, Catholic University, Rome. Childs Nerv Syst 2005;21(8-9):747–757
6. Fahlbusch R, Honegger J, Paulus W, Huk W, Buchfelder M. Surgical treatment of craniopharyngiomas: experience with 168 patients. J Neurosurg 1999;90(2):237–250
7. Zuccaro G. Radical resection of craniopharyngioma. Childs Nerv Syst 2005;21(8-9):679–690
8. Villani RM, Tomei G, Bello L, et al. Long-term results of treatment for craniopharyngioma in children. Childs Nerv Syst 1997;13(7):397–405
9. Wycis HT, Robbins R, Spiegeladolf M, Meszaros J, Spiegel EA. Studies in stereoencephalotomy III; treatment of a cystic craniopharyngioma by injection of radioactive P32. Confin Neurol 1954;14(4):193–202
10. Leksell L. The stereotaxic method and radiosurgery of the brain. Acta Chir Scand 1951;102(4):316–319
11. Voges J, Sturm V, Lehrke R, Treuer H, Gauss C, Berthold F. Cystic craniopharyngioma: long-term results after intracavitary irradiation with stereotactically applied colloidal

beta-emitting radioactive sources. Neurosurgery 1997;40(2): 263–269
12. Munari C, Landre E, Musolino A, Turak B, Habert MO, Chodkiewicz JP. Long term results of stereotactic endocavitary beta irradiation of craniopharyngioma cysts. J Neurosurg Sci 1989;33(1):99–105
13. Szeifert GT, Bálint K, Sipos L, Sarker MH, Czirják S, Julow J. Pathological findings in cystic craniopharyngiomas after stereotactic intracavitary irradiation with yttrium-90 isotope. Prog Neurol Surg 2007;20:297–302
14. Szeifert GT, Julow J, Slowik F, Bálint K, Lányi F, Pásztor E. Pathological changes in cystic craniopharyngiomas following intracavital 90yttrium treatment. Acta Neurochir (Wien) 1990;102(1-2):14–18
15. Szeifert GT, Sipos L, Horváth M, et al. Pathological characteristics of surgically removed craniopharyngiomas: analysis of 131 cases. Acta Neurochir (Wien) 1993;124(2-4):139–143
16. Derrey S, Blond S, Reyns N, et al. Management of cystic craniopharyngiomas with stereotactic endocavitary irradiation using colloidal ^{186}Re: a retrospective study of 48 consecutive patients. Neurosurgery 2008;63(6):1045–1052
17. Julow J, Backlund EO, Lányi F, et al. Long-term results and late complications after intracavitary yttrium-90 colloid irradiation of recurrent cystic craniopharyngiomas. Neurosurgery 2007;61(2):288–295
18. Mallucci C et al., Childs Nerv Syst 2012;28(8):1181–1192
19. Broggi G, Franzini A, Cajola L, Pluchino F. Cell kinetic investigations in craniopharyngioma: preliminary results and considerations. Pediatr Neurosurg 1994;21(Suppl 1):21–23
20. Takahashi H, Nakazawa S, Shimura T. Evaluation of postoperative intratumoral injection of bleomycin for craniopharyngioma in children. J Neurosurg 1985;62(1):120–127
21. Fang Y, Cai BW, Zhang H, et al. Intracystic bleomycin for cystic craniopharyngiomas in children. Cochrane Database Syst Rev 2012;4:CD008890
22. Mottolese C, Stan H, Hermier M, et al. Intracystic chemotherapy with bleomycin in the treatment of craniopharyngiomas. Childs Nerv Syst 2001;17(12):724–730
23. Takahashi H, Yamaguchi F, Teramoto A. Long-term outcome and reconsideration of intracystic chemotherapy with bleomycin for craniopharyngioma in children. Childs Nerv Syst 2005;21(8-9):701–704
24. Broggi G, Franzini A. Bleomycin for cystic craniopharyngioma. J Neurosurg 1996;84(6):1080–1081
25. Hukin J, Steinbok P, Lafay-Cousin L, et al. Intracystic bleomycin therapy for craniopharyngioma in children: the Canadian experience. Cancer 2007;109(10):2124–2131
26. Park DH, Park JY, Kim JH, et al. Outcome of postoperative intratumoral bleomycin injection for cystic craniopharyngioma. J Korean Med Sci 2002;17(2):254–259
27. Linnert M, Gehl J. Bleomycin treatment of brain tumors: an evaluation. Anticancer Drugs 2009;20(3):157–164
28. Buckell M, Crompton MR, Robertson MC, Barnes GK. Lactate dehydrogenase in cerebral cyst fluids; total activity and isoenzyme distributions as an index of malignancy. J Neurosurg 1970;32(5):545–552
29. Muro M, Naomoto Y, Orita K. Mechanism of the combined antitumor effect of natural human tumor necrosis factor-alpha and natural human interferon-alpha on cell cycle progression. Jpn J Cancer Res 1991;82(1):118–126
30. Ierardi DF, Fernandes MJ, Silva IR, et al. Apoptosis in alpha interferon (IFN-alpha) intratumoral chemotherapy for cystic craniopharyngiomas. Childs Nerv Syst 2007;23(9): 1041–1046
31. Jakacki RI, Cohen BH, Jamison C, et al. Phase II evaluation of interferon-alpha-2a for progressive or recurrent craniopharyngiomas. J Neurosurg 2000;92(2):255–260
32. Vaquero J, Martínez R. Intratumoral immunotherapy with interferon-alpha and interleukin-2 in glioblastoma. Neuroreport 1992;3(11):981–983
33. Martínez R, Vaquero J, Ramiro J, García Salazar F, De Oya S. Intratumoural and intraventricular human lymphoblastoid alpha interferon (HLBI) for treatment of glioblastoma multiforme. Acta Neurochir (Wien) 1989;100(1-2):46–49
34. O'Brien L, Perkins S, Williams A, et al. Alpha interferon as an adenovirus-vectored vaccine adjuvant and antiviral in Venezuelan equine encephalitis virus infection. J Gen Virol 2009;90(Pt 4):874–882
35. Lukaszewski RA, Brooks TJ. Pegylated alpha interferon is an effective treatment for virulent Venezuelan equine encephalitis virus and has profound effects on the host immune response to infection. J Virol 2000;74(11):5006–5015
36. Mayer V, Zachar V, Schmidtmayerová H, et al. Early intrathecal production of specific IgM and IgG antibodies and alpha-interferon in herpes simplex virus encephalitis. Acta Virol 1986;30(2):149–157
37. Cavalheiro S, Dastoli PA, Silva NS, Toledo S, Lederman H, da Silva MC. Use of interferon alpha in intratumoral chemotherapy for cystic craniopharyngioma. Childs Nerv Syst 2005;21(8-9):719–724
38. Cavalheiro S, Di Rocco C, Valenzuela S, et al. Craniopharyngiomas: intratumoral chemotherapy with interferon-alpha: a multicenter preliminary study with 60 cases. Neurosurg Focus 2010;28(4):E12
39. Dastoli PA, Nicácio JM, Silva NS, et al. Cystic craniopharyngioma: intratumoral chemotherapy with alpha interferon. Arq Neuropsiquiatr 2011;69(1):50–55
40. Hasegawa T, Kondziolka D, Hadjipanayis CG, Lunsford LD. Management of cystic craniopharyngiomas with phosphorus-32 intracavitary irradiation. Neurosurgery 2004;54(4): 813–820,

▪ SECTION XII ▪

Cranial Base Malignancies

43

Open versus Endoscopic Resection of Midline Anterior Cranial Base Malignancy

D. David Beahm, Tyler J. Kenning, Christopher J. Farrell, Marc R. Rosen, and James J. Evans

Anterior cranial base (ACB) malignancies typically arise from or are associated with the nasal cavity and paranasal sinuses. Sinonasal malignancies have historically presented unique challenges for treatment due to concerns with surgical access, proximity to vital neurological structures, reconstruction, rehabilitation, and cosmetic issues. Since the introduction of open craniofacial resection techniques by Ketcham et al, the "gold standard" for resection of sinonasal malignancies has been via the lateral rhinotomy, Weber-Ferguson incision, midface degloving, eyebrow and eyelid incisions, bicoronal incision, or a combination thereof. These surgical approaches have provided access to the nasal vault, paranasal sinuses, anterior cranial base, and craniocervical junction.[1] With the advent of endoscopic sinus surgery and the expansion of endoscopic techniques for resection of sinonasal pathology, debate has grown regarding the suitability of endoscopic approaches for managing sinonasal cancers. As the indications for endoscopic resection of tumors and expanded endonasal approaches (EEAs) to the cranial base have grown, the contraindications to these approaches have diminished. As with any emerging surgical technique or technology, many questions still surround EEA. Despite a growing repository of literature in support of it, the question of whether EEA is equivalent, or even superior, to open techniques remains unanswered. This chapter explores these questions and provides levels of evidence based on the current literature.

■ Epidemiology and Etiology

Sinonasal malignancies (SNMs) are relatively rare, representing less than 1% of cancers over all and ~ 3% of all malignancy arising within the upper respiratory tract. The annual incidence in the United States is estimated to be ~ 1 in 100,000 persons per year, whereas in Asia they are significantly more prevalent, second only to nasopharyngeal carcinoma as the most common head and neck malignancy in this region. Of the subsites of the nasal cavity and paranasal sinuses, tumors arise most commonly (60%) from the maxillary sinus. Twenty to thirty percent of SNMs originate from the nasal cavity, 10 to 15% from the ethmoid sinuses, and the remaining minority of tumors arise from the frontal or sphenoid sinuses. However, the epicenter of the tumor is often difficult to ascertain because multiple sites are usually involved in advanced-stage tumors. Males are slightly more affected, at a M:F ratio of 1.5. Adults are more commonly affected; 80% of SNMs occur in persons age 45 to 85 years, with the majority of these presenting in the fifth and sixth decades of life.[2,3]

SNMs present with various symptoms, including nasal obstruction, rhinorrhea, postnasal drip, and epistaxis. Advanced-stage neoplasms may present with symptoms indicative of invasion into adjacent structures, including diplopia, vision loss, facial numbness, trismus, or skin changes. Detecting SNMs can be particularly challenging to the clinician in the early stages because patients may remain relatively asymptomatic until the neoplasm becomes more advanced, or the symptoms may be mistaken for, and treated as, benign inflammatory disease, such as rhinosinusitis or nasal allergies.

Risk factors for SNM vary according to the specific pathology encountered. Chronic exposure to various environmental contaminants, such as wood dust, chemical irritants, chromium and nickel particles, isopropyl oil, dichlorodiethyl sulfide, mustard gas, and other fine particles, increases the risk of developing SNM. For example, wood dust exposure increases the risk of squamous cell carcinoma by over 20 times and increases the risk of adenocarcinoma by over 800 times. Certain industrial fields are known to have higher exposure rates to these carcinogens; thus, workers in the fields of furniture making, woodworking, and leather and textile manufacturing should be treated with a higher index of suspicion if presenting with sinonasal complaints.

■ Workup and Staging

All patients presenting with sinonasal complaints should undergo a careful and thorough history and complete head and neck examination, including thorough rhinoscopic endonasal evaluation. Imaging is often helpful for evaluation of the sinonasal anatomy, especially in those patients who have not previously had sinus surgery, because the paranasal sinuses are not readily evaluated with rhinoscopy. Computed tomography (CT) is superior in evaluating the bony sinonasal anatomy, whereas magnetic resonance imaging (MR) is superior in delineating soft tissue and neurovascular structures and brain. Positron-emission tomography (PET) may be beneficial in evaluating for regional and distant disease, including metastasis. Biopsy is often indicated prior to definitive treatment. However, it is often preferable to obtain imaging prior to biopsy of sinonasal masses to delineate the neurovascular relationships of the mass prior to biopsy.

Staging of SNM is based on the American Joint Committee on Cancer (AJCC) *Cancer Staging Manual*, currently in its seventh edition.[4] Additionally, staging for olfactory neuroblastoma and sinonasal undifferentiated carcinoma (SNUC) follows the modified Kadish or University of California–Los Angeles staging systems.[5–7]

■ Pathology

To evaluate open versus endoscopic resection of ACB malignancies it is important to recognize the diverse tumor pathologies that present in this location and how the individual tumor biology affects overall treatment. SNMs are a heterogeneous mix of epithelial, nonepithelial, and lymphoid malignancies, as delineated in **Table 43.1**.

Squamous Cell Carcinoma

Squamous cell carcinoma (SCCA) is the most common of all SNMs, constituting up to 80% of SNMs. An estimated 70% of all SCCA arise from the maxillary sinus, 12% from the nasal cavity, and the remainder from the nasal vestibule and the frontal, ethmoid, and sphenoid sinuses. Although many subtypes of SCCA occur within the sinonasal tract, they share a similar aggressive and infiltrative quality. Most SCCAs arising in the sinonasal tract are of the keratinizing type, a feature that adds to the relative ease of identification with hematoxylin and eosin staining.

Due to its aggressive nature, SCCA tends to display a moderately rapid growth pattern and invades adjacent structures. Unlike its counterparts in other subsites of the head and neck, sinonasal SCCA has a low incidence of lymph node involvement upon presentation (< 10%), and thus prophylactic lymphadenectomy is not typically necessary. Likewise, distant metastasis on initial presentation is rare. Although SCCA is an aggressive malignancy, prognosis is improved with detection of disease at an early stage, with disease arising from the ethmoid sinuses, and with tumors that are treated with multimodality therapy. Treatment of SCCA is generally multimodality, with surgical resection offered to those who are appropriate candidates followed by postoperative radiotherapy. Chemotherapy may be considered in advanced disease or other select cases.

Adenocarcinoma

Adenocarcinomas of the sinonasal tract are more prevalent in Europe and Asia, where they are the most common SNM. As a group, adenocarcinomas are the most common malignancies arising from the ethmoid sinuses and olfactory cleft, accounting for 40 to 60% of all tumors in this location, and thus they may frequently involve the anterior cranial base. Adenocarcinomas are most highly associated with environmental exposure to wood dust, varnishes, and various other organic compounds. Although not a primary risk factor for these tumors, smoking may have a synergistic effect in the pathogenesis of sinonasal adenocarcinomas. Adenocarcinomas are typically divided into intestinal and nonintestinal subtypes, with the latter being further divided into low or high grade. The histological subtype relates to overall prognosis and tumor aggressiveness. Regardless of histological type, treatment of sinonasal adenocarcinomas is

Table 43.1 Pathologies encountered in anterior cranial base malignancy

Neoplasm	Most common sinonasal location	Percentage of overall sinonasal malignancy
Epithelial		> 98%
– Squamous cell carcinoma	Maxillary sinus	80%
– Adenocarcinoma	Ethmoid sinus/olfactory cleft	10 to 20%
– Adenoid cystic carcinoma	Maxillary sinus	5%
– Melanoma	Nasal cavity	< 5%
– Esthesioneuroblastoma	Olfactory cleft	3 to 5%
– Undifferentiated carcinoma (SNUC)	Nasal cavity	< 1%
– Neuroendocrine carcinoma	Nasal cavity	< 1%
Nonepithelial	Mixed	< 1%
– Rhabdomyosarcoma		Rare[a]
– Leiomyosarcoma		Rare
– Fibrosarcoma		Rare
– Liposarcoma		Rare
– Angiosarcoma		Rare
– Myxosarcoma		Rare
– Hemangiopericytoma		Rare
– Chondrosarcoma		Rare
– Osteosarcoma		Rare
Lymphoreticular	Mixed/nasal cavity	< 1%
– Lymphoma		Rare[b]
– Plasmacytoma		Rare
– Giant cell tumor		Rare

[a] Rhabdomyosarcoma more prevalent in children/adolescents
[b] Sinonasal lymphoma, especially NK/T cell lymphoma, has higher prevalence in Asia and Latin American countries
Note: Included are the most common presenting locations and percentage of overall sinonasal malignancies when available.

surgical resection when possible, with postoperative radiotherapy. In select cases, systemic chemotherapy may be offered. Additionally, the application of topical 5-fluorouracil (5-FU) immediately following tumor resection has shown promise of possible improved tumor control and overall survival and thus may have a role in treatment of both primary and recurrent adenocarcinomas.[8]

Adenoid Cystic Carcinoma

Although many salivary gland malignancies may arise from the minor salivary glands within the nasal cavity or involve the sinonasal tract via direct superior extension from the hard and soft palates, adenoid cystic carcinoma is by far the most common salivary gland tumor found within the nasal cavity and paranasal sinuses. In fact, the sinonasal tract represents 11 to 29% of all primary locations of adenoid cystic carcinoma neoplasms. This tumor is typified by its neurotropic nature and propensity for delayed distant metastasis to bone, lung, or brain. Distant metastases often present 10 to 20 years following definitive treatment of the primary tumor. Adenoid cystic carcinomas typically display the characteristic histological appearance of small blue cells with the classic "Swiss cheese" cribriform appearance, with spaces filled with either eosinophilic hyaline or basophilic mucinous material. These neoplasms are categorized by subtype based on the pattern of growth: cribriform, tubular, or solid. It is speculated that the size of the primary lesion is a more important indicator of the overall prognosis than the histological grade. Treatment of choice for these tumors is surgical excision followed by postoperative radiotherapy. A high recurrence rate is noted due to difficulty in obtaining negative margins and the high rate of perineural invasion.[9]

Olfactory Neuroblastoma

Olfactory neuroblastoma (ONB) is a rare malignant neoplasm of neuroectodermal origin. Historically, this malignancy has been given many labels: esthesioneuroblastoma, esthesioneurocytoma, and esthesioneuroepithelioma. These tumors arise from the reserve cell that produces neuronal and sustentacular cells. Histological examination reveals a vascularized stroma infiltrated by nests and lobular growths of cells. A background of glandular structure representing pseudorosettes is often seen.[9]

Olfactory neuroblastomas have a slight female preponderance and a bimodal occurrence between 15 and 50 years of age.[9] Treatment relies upon aggressive surgical resection followed by radiotherapy. Unfortunately, ONB is an unpredictable disease, and, although early disease is associated with a higher 5-year survival, late recurrences and metastases may occur up to 20 years following treatment of the primary tumor.[9]

Melanoma

Mucosal melanomas are rare neoplasms, accounting for around 1% of all melanomas; ~ 50% of all mucosal melanomas occur within the sinonasal tract. Compared with cutaneous melanoma, mucosal melanomas have a much worse prognosis, with a recurrence rate between 60 and 80% and a 5-year survival of 10%. The fact that between one third to one half of sinonasal melanoma tumors lack pigment presents difficulty in diagnosis and surgical resection. Accordingly, immunohistochemical stains are often helpful in establishing the diagnosis. The treatment of choice is complete surgical resection whenever possible. Again, postoperative adjuvant radiotherapy is typically offered.[9]

Sinonasal Undifferentiated Carcinoma

SNUC is a rare and highly aggressive malignancy of the nasal cavity that is characterized by locally aggressive disease that rapidly progresses over weeks to months. SNUC has a predilection for rapid mucosal spread and invasion into lymphovascular spaces. Histologically, these small blue cell tumors are characterized by their hyperchromatic nuclei, ill-defined cell membranes, prominent nucleoli, and high nuclear to cytoplasmic ratios. Immunohistochemical stains are not typically helpful in establishing the diagnosis of SNUC, with the exception of helping to rule out other tumors.[10]

Treatment of SNUC is aimed at aggressive tumor resection followed by radiotherapy in patients deemed surgically resectable. Because SNUC has a propensity for lymphatic involvement, patients with presenting clinical lymphadenopathy should undergo neck dissection and patients without lymphadenopathy should receive prophylactic radiotherapy. Chemotherapy is typically offered for improved tumor control. In patients with unresectable disease, curative intent chemoirradiation may be offered; however, tumor control in these patients is much less likely. Despite aggressive treatment, the 2- and 5-year survival rates are low, with patients who present with lower clinical stage and aggressive multimodality treatment having better survival rates.[11]

■ Oncological Principles and Considerations

The oncological principles guiding the surgical treatment of midline anterior cranial base malignancies can be divided into those applying to cancer therapy in general and those that are disease specific. These surgical techniques include biopsy to obtain a proper histological diagnosis followed by cytoreduction of the tumor mass to the maximum possible extent with the ultimate goal being a total resection with negative margins. Surgery is performed while keeping in mind the need to preserve optimal function and the possible need for adjuvant therapies tailored to the specific clinical situation. The important functional considerations for these patients include preservation of neurological and sinonasal function, vision, swallowing, voice, and a normal physical appearance.

The optimum surgical procedure allows complete resection with microscopically negative margins. This requires meticulous documentation of biopsy points and intraoperative frozen pathology to achieve sound surgical margins. The use of a three-dimensional tumor map is helpful to record these areas as the tumor is removed. To achieve total tumor extirpation, knowledge of the growth patterns of individual pathologies of this region is essential. For example, it must be recognized that intranasal malignancies usually grow into the paranasal sinuses and cranial base by eroding these structures, rather than by direct invasion. Even when these tumors grow to an impressive size, there is often a small area of attachment/invasion that can be identified and resected, allowing for complete removal of the lesion.[12]

Using frozen sections as a guide, tumor resection should be performed to obtain negative surgical margins. With functional consideration an important, but secondary, concern, a stepwise surgical technique should be executed. This may require resection of intranasal and paranasal contents, including sphenoethmoidectomy, maxillary antrostomy, septectomy, frontal sinusotomy, and unilateral/bilateral orbital decompression. Direct extension into the orbit with invasion of the orbital soft tissue contents may necessitate orbital exenteration. Finally, when involved, the cranial base needs to be addressed. The need to resect the cribriform plate or ethmoid roof is generally decided intraoperatively based on tumor involvement or invasion. When the anterior cranial base is resected, the dura should also be sampled for frozen section and removed when tumor is detected. There should be no hesitancy in removing macroscopically involved tissue, including dura, periorbita, and other important structures. It has been shown repeatedly, however, that tumor invasion into the brain portends a poor prognosis, with limited survival regardless of histology.

Over all, it must be remembered that the treatment of cranial base tumors often requires an aggressive multimodal approach to achieve disease control while avoiding excessive morbidity and negatively affecting a patient's quality of life. For most pathologies, surgery remains the initial treatment of choice, and a complete extirpation and surgical cure should be attempted whenever feasible, accounting for histology, extent of disease, and the patient's preoperative clinical condition. The use of appropriate adjuvant therapy, however, is frequently required to achieve good oncological outcomes. Postoperative radiation therapy with or without chemotherapy is often required in patients with high-grade tumors, significant extent of disease, bone invasion, perineural spread, intracranial extension, dural or brain involvement, or positive margins.[13]

The choice of operative procedure depends on the location, size, gross characteristics, histological characteristics, and radiosensitivity of the tumor, as well as the preoperative neurological and medical condition of the patient. Both endoscopic and open approaches should be carefully considered for these lesions. Surgeons should be knowledgeable about, and competent in, both approaches. This allows the surgeon to devise the best strategy to achieve the desired surgical objective. Traditional open approaches and newer endoscopic techniques can be utilized in isolation or as a combination for a specific procedure. In general, the specific surgical approach utilized should be dictated by the pathology and its staging and ideally should not be dictated by any limitation of available surgical expertise and equipment.

■ Surgical Approaches

Traditional Open Approaches

Modern cranial base surgery has evolved over the past 30 years though the cooperation of multidisciplinary teams, including specialists in neurosurgery, otolaryngology, ophthalmology, oral maxillofacial surgery, and plastic surgery. Surgeons may approach the same anterior cranial base tumor very differently depending on their specialty, experience, familiarity with a given procedure, and available resources. Furthermore, some extensive tumors may require multiple approaches for resection. The philosophy of single-stage versus staged surgery plays an important role in these cases.

The literature is rich with many named approaches to anterior cranial base tumors. Each patient requires a very individually designed surgical approach depending on the tumor biology and location. There are many considerations in planning an anterior cranial base surgical approach, including preservation of the structure and function of uninvolved anatomy, utilization of the most direct route to the pathology while taking advantage of avenues provided by the pathway of tumor growth, using natural corridors to the tumor, minimizing brain and orbital retraction; preservation of tissue and pedicles for reconstruction flaps and the need to plan for repair while designing the approach, and taking advantage of early disruption of blood supply to the tumor to facilitate resection.

Traditional "open" approaches to midline anterior cranial base malignancies involve a transcranial route, a transfacial route, or both combined (**Figs. 43.1** and **43.2**). The general premise of the "open" approaches is to achieve maximal access to the tumor, allowing for an en bloc resection of the tumor contained within a margin of surrounding normal tissue. Proponents of the en bloc resection believe that these surgical approaches achieve complete removal and allow the greatest chance of cure.

The transfrontal route most often involves a coronal incision from zygoma to zygoma, and a bifrontal craniotomy above the frontal sinus or with cranialization of the frontal sinus. Dissection is maintained extradural unless the tumor involves the dura or brain. An orbitofrontal osteotomy may be added to minimize brain retraction for extensive tumors. Advantages of this approach are the wide exposure and the ability to combine with transfacial approaches. Also, there is access to ample amounts of pericranium for repair of the anterior cranial base defect. Drawbacks include the need to traverse normal, often uninvolved anatomy of the frontal bone/sinus and orbits, possible cosmetic deformity, and often anosmia. Less invasive techniques, such as a limited, unilateral fronto-orbital craniotomy via an eyelid or eyebrow incision, have also been reported alone or in combination with transfacial approaches.

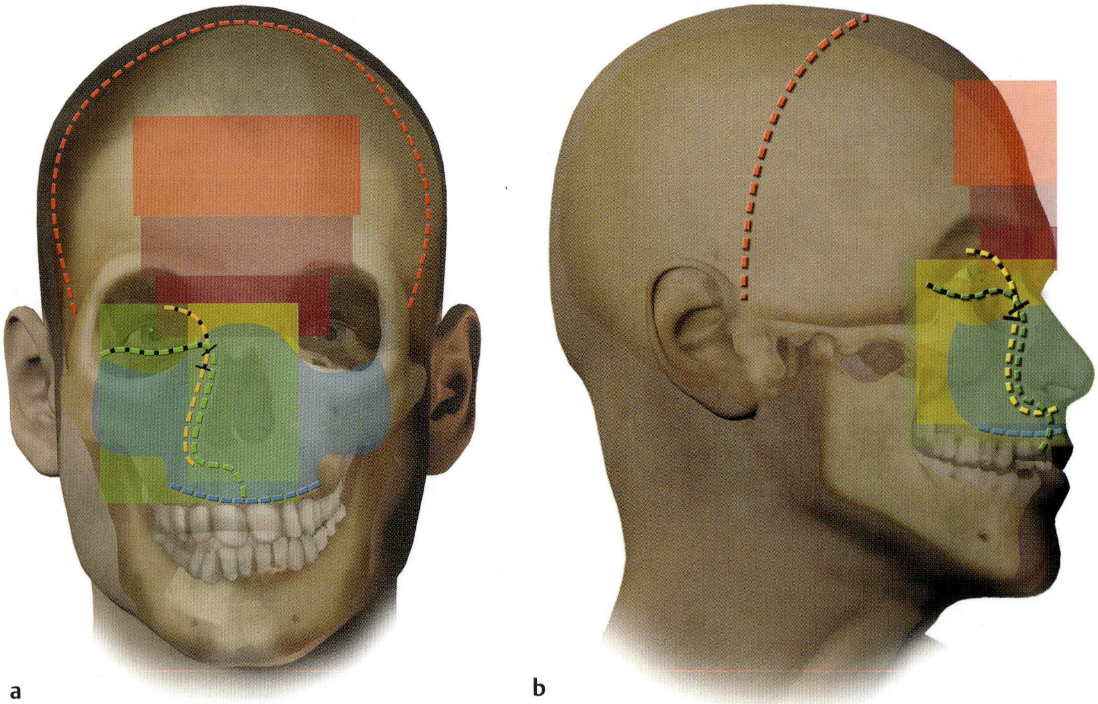

Fig. 43.1 Common open approaches to the anterior cranial base. **(a)** Coronal and **(b)** sagittal views of common incisions (*dashed lines*) with corresponding area of access provided to the nasal cavity, paranasal sinuses, and anterior cranial base (*shaded boxes*).

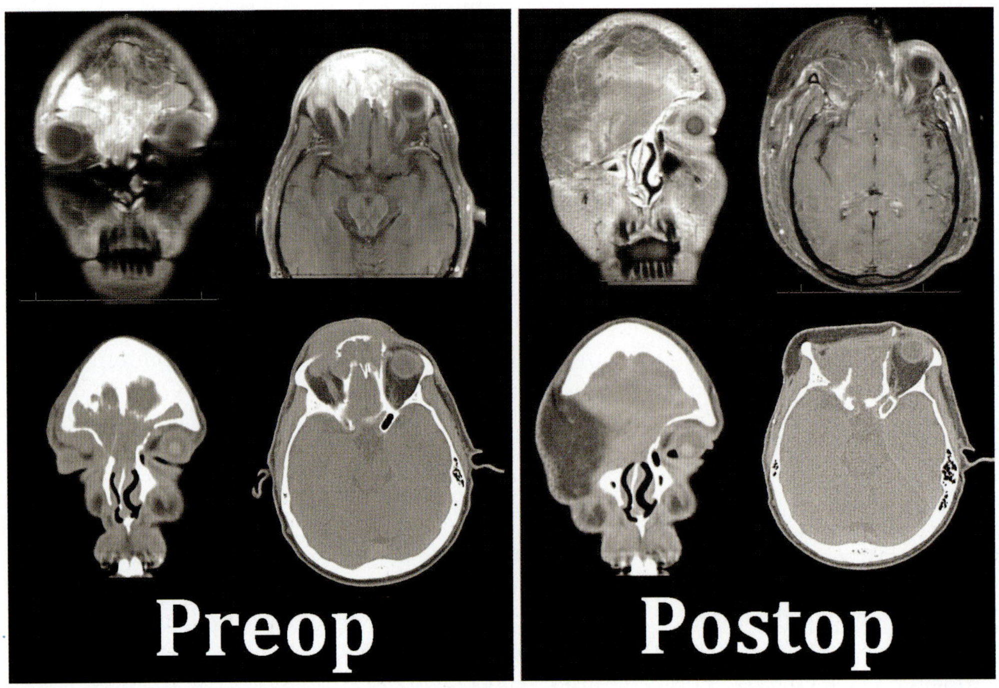

Fig. 43.2 Preoperative and postoperative computed tomographic and magnetic resonance images of a patient with adenocarcinoma of the anterior cranial base invading the orbit, anterior and posterior tables of the frontal sinus, cranial base, and dura treated with an open approach to craniofacial resection with microvascular free flap reconstruction and postoperative radiation and chemotherapy.

The transfacial procedures involve some form of nasofacial incision and an approach through the nasal cavity, paranasal sinuses, or orbit. The frontoethmoidectomy, initially described by Lynch in 1921, is essentially an approach through the lamina papyracea of the medial orbital wall to the ethmoid region. A curved vertical incision is made approximately 1 cm medial to the medial canthus, extending from the medial aspect of the eyebrow to the nasomaxillary groove. The anterior ethmoidal artery is divided, and the medial wall of the orbit is removed from that level down to the lacrimal duct. This approach provides unilateral access to the ethmoid and sphenoid sinuses, medial orbit, and unilateral anterior cranial base, and it can be extended superiorly to the ipsilateral frontal sinus. Risks include facial cosmetic deformity as well as damage to the medial canthal ligament or lacrimal duct.

For tumors with more extensive unilateral involvement of the nasal cavity, the lateral rhinotomy approach is used. The incision extends along the nasomaxillary groove inferior around the ala to the columella. Osteotomies are made between the infraorbital foramen, medial orbit, and nasion, preserving the lacrimal duct. This allows direct access to the ipsilateral nasal cavity and ethmoid region. If there is maxillary sinus involvement, the incision is carried vertically through the upper lip. Orbital involvement requires a Weber-Ferguson extension of the incision across the lower eyelid.

For midline cranial base malignancies extending inferiorly to involve the maxilla bilaterally, the midface degloving procedure and its many renditions have been developed. This involves a circumferential mucosal incision in the nares bilaterally followed by a complete transfixion incision. After intercartilaginous dissection of the upper and lower lateral nasal cartilage, a sublabial incision is made 5 mm above the labiogingival sulcus. Skin and soft tissue of the face are dissected in a subperiosteal fashion up to the inferior orbital rims, preserving the infraorbital nerves. A nasomaxillary osteotomy is made with a horizontal cut through the nasion and bilateral vertical cuts medial to the infraorbital foraminae. Next, a Le Fort I osteotomy is performed and the maxilla downfractured for full exposure of the bilateral nasal cavity, maxillary sinuses, ethmoid regions, and anterior cranial base.

Expanded Endoscopic Approaches

The endoscopic endonasal resection of sinonasal malignancies must adhere to the same oncological principles as open procedures; although the technical aspects of the resection are vastly different, the oncological principles of adequate resection with negative margins need to be followed at all times. Whereas the wide exposure afforded by open approaches allows for en bloc resection, the constraint of using the natural orifices of the nose often prevents complete visualization of all but the smallest tumors. Thus, tumor debulking is often employed to reduce the size of the tumor so that adequate visualization of the tumor margins is achieved. The surgeon must pay close attention to identify the tumor origin and any areas of invasion. The use of frozen sections is essential to obtain negative margins around the involved tissue, thus achieving an adequate oncological resection. If complete resection of the tumor with negative margins cannot be achieved during the endoscopic procedure, the surgeon must have the ability and proper informed consent to convert to an open procedure.

The unique biology of each tumor subtype and variability of sinonasal anatomy make complete standardization of endonasal resection somewhat difficult. Unlike traditional open approaches, where normal structures are typically systematically disrupted to reach the pathology as part of a defined approach, in endoscopic endonasal resections the location of the tumor dictates the appropriate approach and which structures are resected to obtain negative margins (**Figs. 43.3** and **43.4**). Because the tumor is encountered immediately in the approach, endoscopic endonasal resections rarely disrupt normal uninvolved structures as part of the approach. The major categories of endoscopic resections are based on the origin of the tumor. Thus, tumors that are primarily intranasal and are laterally based involving the maxillary sinus are treated by an endoscopic medial maxillectomy, whereas tumors that are primarily on the septum and adjacent nasal cavity can be resected with negative margins on the septum, without the need to disrupt normal adjacent facial structures. Neoplasms arising from the tissues along the anterior cranial base can be resected with either unilateral or bilateral endoscopic anterior craniofacial resection. Endoscopic resection of the anterior cranial base can be employed to resect the cribriform plate, crista galli, olfactory bulb, and dura of the anterior cranial base if necessary without the need to remove uninvolved frontal bone or sinus. However, with modifications made based on the tumor location, it is rare that one needs to perform a wide full resection of the anterior cranial base in each case, as may be done with open approaches. For neoplasms that extensively involve multiple structures or locations within the nasal cavity and paranasal sinuses, a combination of the foregoing approaches may be utilized. Although the technical aspects of these approaches are outside the scope of this chapter, they have been adequately described in recent literature.[14]

Although many neoplasms are amenable to endoscopic resection, several tumor locations are contraindications for purely endoscopic approach due to anatomical restrictions. These include neoplasms that involve the anterior wall of the frontal sinus, extend into the facial soft tissue, involve the anterior wall of the maxilla, involve the hard palate, and involve the orbital tissues with the need for orbital exenteration.

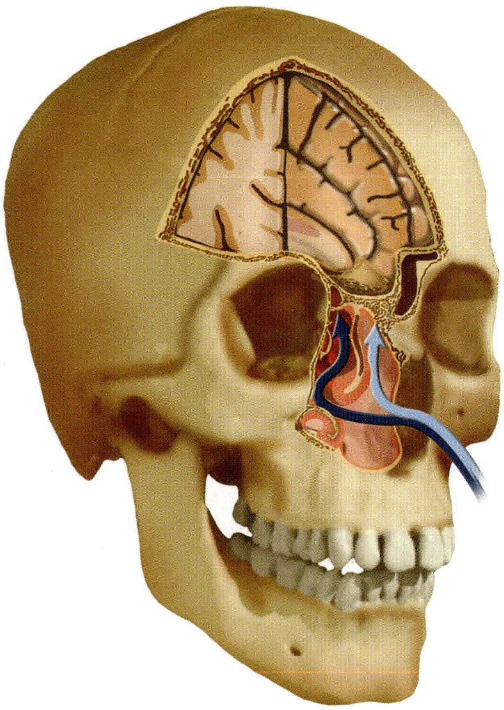

Fig. 43.3 Artist's depiction of endoscopic endonasal approaches to the nasal cavity, paranasal sinuses, and anterior cranial base. The lighter blue arrow illustrates an approach to the nasal corridor and cribriform, whereas the darker blue arrow illustrates an approach through the transethmoid corridor and fovea ethmoidalis.

An open approach or combined open-endoscopic technique is often required if any of these structures are found to be involved.[14]

■ Open versus Endoscopic Cranial Base Surgery

To critically evaluate open versus endoscopic cranial base techniques and approaches, several key factors are reviewed: ability for oncological resection of malignancy (en bloc versus piecemeal resection), surgical margins, morbidity and complications, and functional outcomes and quality of life.

En Bloc Oncological Resection

In the late 1800s, Halsted and others realized that tumor recurrence rates and thus survival dramatically improved when tumors were removed in an en bloc fashion without violating the tumor and while taking a generous cuff of normal tissue as a margin as well as any lymphatics in the general region. Over time, this technique was extrapolated to all oncological surgeries to become a basic tenet of sound oncological surgical resection. Traditional open cranial base technique is no exception, because many advocate complete en bloc resection as the standard for these approaches.[15] Recently, however, the concept of en bloc resection has been challenged in certain select instances, such as Mohs surgery for select cutaneous malignancies[16] and endoscopic conservation laryngeal surgery. Both are examples of accepted oncological surgical practices in which the neoplasm is not removed en bloc, and there does not seem to be any adverse oncological outcome.[12]

Level I and Level II Evidence

There is currently no Level I or II evidence that en bloc resection is superior to controlled tumor debulking followed by complete surgical extirpation.

Level III and Level IV Evidence

There is currently no Level III or IV evidence that en bloc resection is superior to controlled tumor debulking followed by complete surgical extirpation.

In the endoscopic technique, tumor debulking is often necessary to gain access to the nasal cavity and paranasal sinuses and to allow adequate visualization of the tumor origin for surgical resection. Although the nasal cavity and paranasal sinuses may be filled with a large exophytic neoplasm, it is often the case that the area of actual mucosal involvement is much less. Thus, tumor debulking is a common technique employed during endoscopic resections to isolate and visualize the involved structures or site of tumor origin. Once debulking is performed, it is often the case that the epicenter and involved surrounding structures may be resected similarly to an en bloc fashion. Although some argue that this may lead to a higher incidence of positive margins, systematic surgical resection and frozen section control can assist in complete tumor eradication with the ability to achieve negative margins.[12] Critics still doubt the soundness of the tumor debulking principle[15]; however, there currently is no evidence in the literature that tumor debulking prior to complete resection leads to unfavorable oncological outcomes.[12]

Finally, although en bloc tumor resection is certainly a goal of open techniques, it is not always possible. Due to lack of visualization and proximity to vital neurovascular structures, some degree of piecemeal resection is often necessary in open approaches.[17,18] In fact, in a recent review of open craniofacial resections involving transdural spread of tumor, close to one half (11/23) of patients could not have the tumor resected in the en bloc fashion due to risk to neurovascular structures. Analysis showed

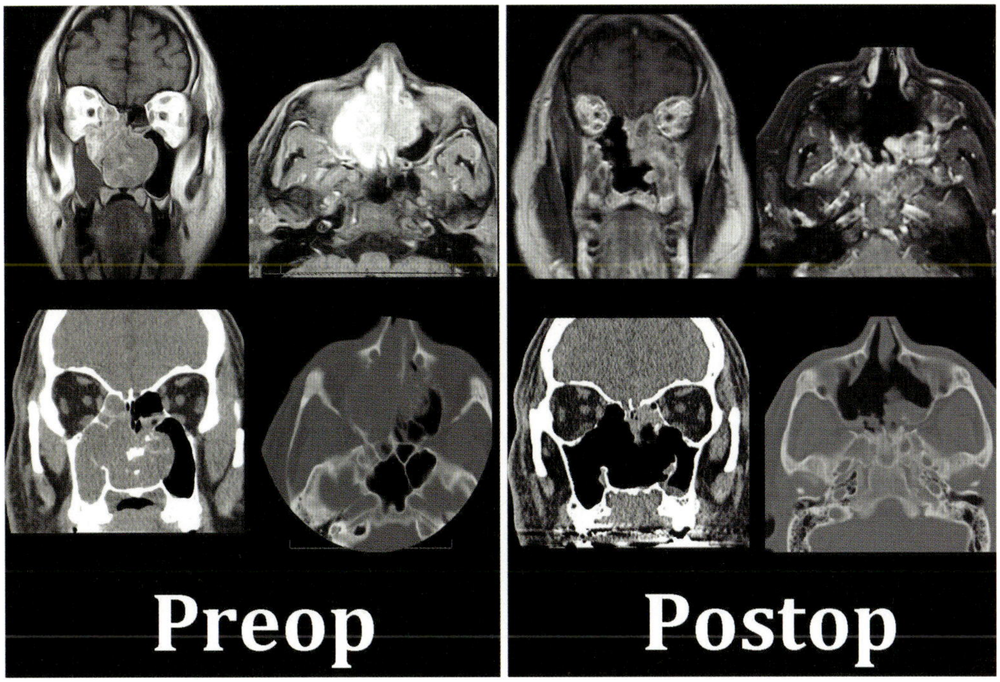

Fig. 43.4 Preoperative and postoperative computed tomographic and magnetic resonance images of a patient with squamous cell carcinoma of the ethmoid sinus extending to but not invading the orbit, with involvement of the anterior cranial base, treated with an endoscopic endonasal approach to tumor resection and postoperative radiation therapy. Note that the postoperative images demonstrate crusting, postoperative changes, and scar in the left ethmoid area that was closely monitored and not found to be tumor recurrence.

there was no statistical difference in overall survival or progression-free survival in patients who had en bloc resection versus patients who had piecemeal resections. No large study has addressed this question directly, but it is again suggested that en bloc resection may not be required and thus the "non–en bloc" techniques employed during endoscopic resection may be oncologically sound.[19]

Recommendation for Management of En Bloc Surgical Resection

En bloc resection may not be required for management of cranial base tumors as long as meticulous attention is given to ensure complete surgical extirpation (Grade 2C Recommendation, Level III/IV Evidence).

Margins

At the time of publication, no studies comparing the ability to obtain negative margins in open versus endoscopic resections could be identified in print. Thus the authors conclude that there is no Level I, II, III, or IV evidence to suggest that one is superior to the other.

Level I and Level II Evidence

Due to limitation in the ability to study margins in anterior cranial base malignancy resections, there is no Level I or II evidence to determine if margin status (positive or negative) influences survival outcomes.

Level III and Level IV Evidence

As indicated in the previous sections, resection with negative margins is a paramount goal in cranial base procedures, regardless of the approach utilized. In fact, multiple studies have shown a significant correlation between the involvement of the surgical margins and decreased survival for multiple pathologies, even if postoperative adjuvant therapy was given.

Feiz-Efran et al evaluated 28 patients who underwent cranial base resection for dural involvement from a variety of pathologies and reported that overall survival and progression-free survival were similar in patients with dural invasion to those in patients without dural invasion. Factors found to significantly influence OS and PFS included microscopically negative margins and brain invasion. Patients who did not have a gross total resection had a significantly lower overall survival. In subgroup analysis, those patients who were able to have gross total resection with negative margins had higher overall survival rates than those with microscopically positive margins.[19] Similarly, a recent review of both open and combined anterior cranial base resections in 282 patients at two institutions spanning over 35 years of treatment found that those patients with microscopically negative margins after resection had a significantly higher 5-year overall survival and disease-specific survival at 68% vs 49% ($p = 0.04$) and 73% vs 50% ($p = 0.004$), respectively.[20]

Recommendations for Management of Surgical Margins

1. There is no evidence to suggest that one approach is superior to the other in terms of ability to obtain negative margins with open versus endoscopic approaches.
2. Gross tumor resection with negative margins is superior to resections with microscopically positive margins as evidenced by higher overall survival and progression-free survival rates (Grade 1C Recommendation, Level III/IV Evidence).

Morbidity and Complications

The surgical treatment of midline ACB malignancies carries significant potential for morbidity. Complications can occur in many forms, involving the central nervous system, the orbit, and the nose and paranasal sinuses. In addition, both infectious and systemic difficulties can result. The reported complication rate is extremely variable and was as high as 33% in some series.

Level I and Level II Evidence

There is currently no Level I or II evidence directly comparing open versus endoscopic resection techniques with respect to morbidity and complications.

Level III and Level IV Evidence

There is currently no Level III or IV evidence directly comparing open versus endoscopic resection techniques with respect to morbidity and complications.

The comparison of complication rates between traditional open craniofacial approaches and endoscopic approaches for the resection of midline ACB malignancies is limited by significant variation in the literature. The use of open approaches has a much longer history; thus reviews of open techniques often span a longer follow-up period of time and include a greater number of patients. The largest series combine the results of multiple institutions and report an overall complication rate in roughly one third of those. Endoscopic approaches have become more frequently used only in the last 10 to 15 years, and an adequate analysis of their associated morbidity suffers from limited numbers. We have attempted to review the published complication rates associated with both open and endoscopic approaches in **Table 43.2**.[12,13,15,17,21–28]

Table 43.2 Morbidity of open versus endoscopic anterior cranial base resection

	Endoscopic endonasal					
	Hanna 2009[13]	Batra 2010[21]	Dave 2007[22]	Snyderman 2008[12]	Chen 2006[23]	Castelnuovo 2007[24]
Primary pathology	Esthesio (17%)	SCC (19%)	Esthesio (53%)	Esthesio (100%)	Adeno (57%)	Esthesio (100%)
N	93	31	19	23	7	10
Overall morbidity	NR	6 (19%)	12 (63%)	NR	0 (0%)	NR
Mortality	0 (0%)	0 (0%)	0 (0%)	0 (0%)	0 (0%)	0 (0%)
CNS complications	3 (3%)	2 (10%)	1 (5%)	4 (17%)	0 (0%)	0 (0%)
CSF leaks	3 (3%)	2 (10%)	1 (5%)	4 (17%)	0 (0%)	0 (0%)
Orbital complications	2 (2%)	NR	1 (5%)	NR	NR	NR
Systemic complications	NR	2 (10%)	NR	NR	NR	NR
Infectious complications	1 (1%)	1 (5%)	1 (5%)	NR	NR	NR
ENT complications	1 (1%)	1 (5%)	4 (21%)	11 (48%)	NR	10 (100%)

Abbreviations: AdenoCA, adenocarcinoma; NR, not reported; CNS, central nervous system complications, pneumocephalus, intracranial hypertension, stroke, seizures, confusion, pituitary deficiency, cerebral contusion; Orbital complications, epiphora, diplopia, visual loss, hematoma; Systemic complications, electrolyte abnormalities, cardiopulmonary failure, thromboembolic events, air embolus, pneumonia; Infectious complications, meningitis, infected bone flap, intracranial abscess/encephalitis, cellulitis/wound infection; ENT, ear, nose, and throat complications, sinusitis/mucocele, serous otitis media, hemorrhage, dacryocystitis, epistaxis, nasal crusting; SCC, squamous cell carcinoma.

It seems somewhat intuitive that endoscopic approaches are less invasive and would therefore impose less morbidity. With endoscopy, the concerns created by the approach portion of open craniofacial resections may be avoided, namely the cosmetic concerns raised by facial incisions or craniotomies, the potential neurological sequelae of brain retraction, and the resultant negative impact on functional outcome and quality of life. Unfortunately, reviews of either open or endoscopic resections of midline ACB malignancies have rarely addressed these issues, although their importance is being recognized more recently. These outcome measures are now being included in current reviews.

One complication that may be more often avoided with endoscopic approaches is that of infection, including meningitis, infected bone flap, intracranial abscess and/or encephalitis, cellulitis, and wound infection. A definitive conclusion may be not be possible due to the limited numbers, but endoscopic approaches report infectious complications in 0 to 5% of patients, whereas they occur in 6 to 26% of open approaches. Limiting the possibility of infection is essential in patients with malignancies because a delay in wound healing will likely delay the utilization of adjuvant therapy, including radiotherapy. Postoperative sinusitis and nasal crusting are included separately in this analysis because they rarely cause a delay in adjuvant therapy (see **Table 43.2**).

Critics of endoscopic resection of ACB malignancies, however, have questioned the ability to adequately manage significant intraoperative bleeding or repair cerebrospinal fluid leaks. In the limited data available, the complication rates associated with hemorrhage or spinal fluid leaks do not appear to be any higher with endoscopic approaches than with open techniques (see **Table 43.2**).

Although the large series reviewing the open craniofacial approaches reveal fairly high morbidity rates, many of the complications occurred early in these series. The reasons cited for this include increased experience with these techniques, better understanding of the pathology, and the availability of effective adjuvant therapy, namely radiotherapy. This has also coincided with the advent of endoscopic resection of ACB malignancies, resulting in more favorable complication rates in these more recent studies. Finally, a direct comparison of complications between open and endoscopic approaches may not be feasible because the latter are more often reserved for less extensive disease at many centers.

Recommendations for Management of Morbidity and Complications

1. There are no studies directly comparing open versus endoscopic resection of cranial base tumors in reference to morbidity and complications.
2. Endoscopic approaches may be less invasive and thus may cause less overall morbidity (Grade 2C Recommendation, Level V Evidence).

Open craniofacial					
Levine 1999[25]	Howard 2006[26]	Ganly 2005[27]	Kraus 1994[28]	McCaffrey 1994[17]	Patel 2003[15]
Esthesio (100%)	AdenoCA (62%)	AdenoCA (32%)	SCC (21%)	Esthesio (44%)	SCC (29%)
35	308	334	85	54	1,317
NR	99 (32%)	110 (33%)	33 (39%)	14 (26%)	433 (33%)
0 (0%)	5 (1.6%)	15 (4.5%)	2 (2%)	0 (0%)	56 (4%)
9 (25.7%)	29 (9.4%)	41 (12%)	9 (11%)	5 (9%)	193 (15%)
5 (14%)	8 (2.6%)	NR	2 (2%)	2 (3.7%)	NR
8 (22.9%)	21 (7%)	7 (2%)	1 (1%)	NR	20 (2%)
7 (20%)	4 (1%)	16 (5%)	5 (6%)	NR	57 (4%)
3 (8.6%)	19 (6.2%)	46 (14%)	22 (26%)	8 (15%)	237 (18%)
NR	21 (7%)	NR	2 (2%)	NR	NR

Functional Outcomes and Quality of Life

Functional outcomes and quality of life after anterior cranial base surgery are difficult to evaluate due to the inherent complexities of the various tumor pathologies and variations of surgical treatments employed for resection. Additionally, there is currently no single widely accepted and well validated disease-specific tool to administer to patients requiring cranial base surgeries.[29] However, there has been a recent interest in developing such a validated tool[30] as well as in the development of a widely accessible database system for the recording and study of such information.[31]

Level I and Level II Evidence

There is currently no Level I or II evidence directly comparing open versus endoscopic resection techniques and their impact on patient quality of life postmalignancy treatment.

Level III and Level IV Evidence

Few studies report on quality of life outcomes after resection of ACB malignancies. Fukuda et al reported on such a population with 13 patients undergoing open resection techniques for anterior cranial base malignancy. They report that 89% of the patients had complaints that included unsightly appearance and 69% of patients were dissatisfied with life postresection.[32] Similarly, Woertgen et al found low quality of life scores for survivors of ASM postsurgery, with only half of patients reporting normal quality of life scores. They found the lowest scores in the areas of job, health, and leisure.[33] Gil et al reported much better quality of life scores for patients with ACB pathology, with most patients (75%) reporting improvement or no change in quality of life postsurgery. To be noted, however, is the fact that the population studied included mostly patients with benign conditions. When analyzed for type of pathology, there were lower quality of life scores in patients with malignancy. Additionally, the authors found perioperative radiotherapy correlated with lower scores as well.[34] In a follow-up study, Gil et al found that clinician perceptions of quality of life post–open cranial base resection were grossly inaccurate when compared with patient and caregiver perceptions. This suggests that clinicians may underestimate the impact that treatment of cranial base lesions has on postresection quality of life.[35]

Endoscopic treatment of anterior cranial base malignancy often leads to nasal morbidity, including crusting, nasal discharge, change in sense of smell, and nasal obstruction. These morbidities are often proportional to the degree of surgical resection and need for perioperative radiotherapy. Almeida et al found that the most common morbidity is nasal crusting, which tends to decrease over time. Interestingly, they found that the degree of nasal crusting was related to the degree of the endonasal resection and significantly related to the method of reconstruction or use of pedicled nasoseptal flap or fat graft.[36] In a similar study, Pant et al reported an increase in sinonasal morbidity following endoscopic resection of ACB tumors. However, they also noted that morbidity decreased over time and thus resulted in very favorable quality of life scores 4 to 6 months postoperatively. Unfortunately, they did not define all pathologies treated and did not stratify results based on benign versus malignant disease.[37]

In a direct comparison of quality of life scores of patients who had open versus endoscopic resection of anterior cranial base tumors, Abergel et al reported higher scores in all areas studied in the endoscopic cohort. The advantage of endoscopic resection for quality of life was particularly noted in the impact on physical function and emotional state domains.[38]

Expert Recommendations

1. Quality of life is difficult to study in patients undergoing treatment for skull base tumors and may be grossly underestimated by treating clinicians.
2. Endoscopic approaches may be superior to open resection in terms of quality of life outcomes, particularly in physical function and emotional state domains (Grade 2C Recommendation, Level III/IV Evidence).

■ Summary and Conclusions

Despite a growing literature repository of articles in support of EEA, the question of whether EEA is equivalent, or even superior to, traditional open cranial base techniques remains unanswered. Due to the complexities and inherent difficulties in studying and comparing these surgical techniques, there is no Level I or II evidence from which to draw conclusions. Given the individual properties of various tumor pathologies, it may not be possible to conclude that either open or endoscopic cranial base approaches to tumor resection are superior. Rather, the modern cranial base surgical team should have the skill and resources to utilize both open and endoscopic techniques. Having reviewed the current available literature addressing open and endoscopic surgical approaches to ACB malignancies considering the ability for oncological resection, surgical margins, morbidity and complications, and functional outcomes with quality of life measures, we conclude that there is evidence in the current literature to support a class 2C recommendation that endoscopic approaches have distinct advantages in select clinical situations.

References

1. Van Buren JM, Ommaya AK, Ketcham AS. Ten years' experience with radical combined craniofacial resection of malignant tumors of the paranasal sinuses. J Neurosurg 1968;28(4):341–350
2. Cummings CW. Cummings Otolaryngology Head and Neck Surgery. 4th ed. Philadelphia, PA: Elsevier Mosby; 2005
3. Wenig BM. Atlas of Head and Neck Pathology. Philadelphia, PA: Saunders; 1993
4. Edge SB; American Joint Committee on Cancer. AJCC Cancer Staging Manual. 7th ed. New York, NY: Springer; 2010
5. Kadish S, Goodman M, Wang CC. Olfactory neuroblastoma: a clinical analysis of 17 cases. Cancer 1976;37(3):1571–1576
6 Morita A, Ebersold MJ, Olsen KD, Foote RL, Lewis JE, Quast LM. Esthesioneuroblastoma: prognosis and management. Neurosurgery 1993;32(5):706–714; discussion 714–715
7. Dulguerov P, Calcaterra T. Esthesioneuroblastoma: the UCLA experience 1970-1990. Laryngoscope 1992;102(8):843–849
8. Jardeleza C, Seiberling K, Floreani S, Wormald PJ. Surgical outcomes of endoscopic management of adenocarcinoma of the sinonasal cavity. Rhinology 2009;47(4):354–361
9. Richardson MS. Pathology of skull base tumors. Otolaryngol Clin North Am 2001;34(6):1025–1042, vii
10. Bridge JA, Bowen JM, Smith RB. The small round blue cell tumors of the sinonasal area. Head Neck Pathol 2010;4(1):84–93
11. Mendenhall WM, Mendenhall CM, Riggs CE Jr, Villaret DB, Mendenhall NP. Sinonasal undifferentiated carcinoma. Am J Clin Oncol 2006;29(1):27–31
12. Snyderman CH, Carrau RL, Kassam AB, et al. Endoscopic skull base surgery: principles of endonasal oncological surgery. J Surg Oncol 2008;97(8):658–664
13. Hanna E, DeMonte F, Ibrahim S, Roberts D, Levine N, Kupferman M. Endoscopic resection of sinonasal cancers with and without craniotomy: oncologic results. Arch Otolaryngol Head Neck Surg 2009;135(12):1219–1224
14. Rosen M, Schaberg M, Lynn M, Evans J. The endoscopic approach to sinonasal malignancy. Oper Tech Otolaryngol Head Neck Surg 2011;22(4):291–296
15. Patel SG, Singh B, Polluri A, et al. Craniofacial surgery for malignant skull base tumors: report of an international collaborative study. Cancer 2003;98(6):1179–1187
16. Nouri K, ed. Mohs Micrographic Surgery. New York, NY: Springer; 2012
17. McCaffrey TV, Olsen KD, Yohanan JM, Lewis JE, Ebersold MJ, Piepgras DG. Factors affecting survival of patients with tumors of the anterior skull base. Laryngoscope 1994;104(8 Pt 1):940–945
18. Batra PS, Citardi MJ. Endoscopic management of sinonasal malignancy. Otolaryngol Clin North Am 2006;39(3):619–637, x–xi
19. Feiz-Erfan I, Suki D, Hanna E, DeMonte F. Prognostic significance of transdural invasion of cranial base malignancies in patients undergoing craniofacial resection. Neurosurgery 2007;61(6):1178–1185
20. Gil Z, Fliss DM, Cavel O, Shah JP, Kraus DH. Improvement in survival during the past 4 decades among patients with anterior skull base cancer. Head Neck 2012;34(9):1212–1217
21. Batra PS, Luong A, Kanowitz SJ, et al. Outcomes of minimally invasive endoscopic resection of anterior skull base neoplasms. Laryngoscope 2010;120(1):9–16
22. Dave SP, Bared A, Casiano RR. Surgical outcomes and safety of transnasal endoscopic resection for anterior skull tumors. Otolaryngol Head Neck Surg 2007;136(6):920–927
23. Chen MK. Minimally invasive endoscopic resection of sinonasal malignancies and skull base surgery. Acta Otolaryngol 2006;126(9):981–986
24. Castelnuovo P, Bignami M, Delù G, Battaglia P, Bignardi M, Dallan I. Endonasal endoscopic resection and radiotherapy in olfactory neuroblastoma: our experience. Head Neck 2007;29(9):845–850
25. Levine PA, Gallagher R, Cantrell RW. Esthesioneuroblastoma: reflections of a 21-year experience. Laryngoscope 1999;109(10):1539–1543
26. Howard DJ, Lund VJ, Wei WI. Craniofacial resection for tumors of the nasal cavity and paranasal sinuses: a 25-year experience. Head Neck 2006;28(10):867–873
27. Ganly I, Patel SG, Singh B, et al. Craniofacial resection for malignant paranasal sinus tumors: Report of an international collaborative study. Head Neck 2005;27(7):575–584
28. Kraus DH, Shah JP, Arbit E, Galicich JH, Strong EW. Complications of craniofacial resection for tumors involving the anterior skull base. Head Neck 1994;16(4):307–312
29. Shah JP. Quality of life after skull base surgery: the patient's predicament. Skull Base 2010;20(1):3–4
30. Gil Z, Abergel A, Spektor S, Shabtai E, Khafif A, Fliss DM. Development of a cancer-specific anterior skull base quality-of-life questionnaire. J Neurosurg 2004;100(5):813–819
31. Patel SG. internet-based multi-institutional clinical research: a new method to conduct and manage quality of life studies. Skull Base 2010;20(1):23–26
32. Fukuda K, Saeki N, Mine S, et al. Evaluation of outcome and QOL in patients with craniofacial resection for malignant tumors involving the anterior skull base. Neurol Res 2000;22(6):545–550
33. Woertgen C, Rothoerl RD, Hosemann W, Strutz J. Quality of life following surgery for malignancies of the anterior skull base. Skull Base 2007;17(2):119–123
34. Gil Z, Abergel A, Spektor S, et al. Quality of life following surgery for anterior skull base tumors. Arch Otolaryngol Head Neck Surg 2003;129(12):1303–1309
35. Gil Z, Abergel A, Spektor S, Khafif A, Fliss DM. Patient, caregiver, and surgeon perceptions of quality of life following anterior skull base surgery. Arch Otolaryngol Head Neck Surg 2004;130(11):1276–1281
36. de Almeida JR, Snyderman CH, Gardner PA, Carrau RL, Vescan AD. Nasal morbidity following endoscopic skull base surgery: a prospective cohort study. Head Neck 2011;33(4):547–551
37. Pant H, Bhatki AM, Snyderman CH, et al. Quality of life following endonasal skull base surgery. Skull Base 2010;20(1):35–40
38. Abergel A, Cavel O, Margalit N, Fliss DM, Gil Z. Comparison of quality of life after transnasal endoscopic vs open skull base tumor resection. Arch Otolaryngol Head Neck Surg 2012;138(2):142–147

44

The Role of Craniofacial Resection in Anterior Skull Base Malignancies

Shaan M. Raza and Franco DeMonte

Malignant tumors of the anterior skull base represent a pathologically diverse group of neoplasms that pose a formidable management challenge to surgical and nonsurgical practitioners in many subspecialties. These tumors can arise from the bony skull base itself or secondarily involve the skull base, either by arising in the intracranial space or, as they more frequently do, from the subcranial soft tissue and aerodigestive tract. Specifically, the resection of malignancies arising from the paranasal sinuses has long challenged surgeons because of the multiple anatomical compartments involved, the critical neurovascular structures placed at risk by the tumor and the surgical resection and the obstacles of reconstruction, all in the context of maintaining an acceptable quality of life for the patient. Combined craniofacial resection was first described by Ketcham et al in the 1950s.[1] Since then, tremendous advancements in surgical access, anatomical understanding, and microvascular reconstruction have occurred in parallel with the development of radiotherapeutic and chemotherapeutic approaches. Consequently, the role of surgery has been extended and redefined in the context of multimodality treatment paradigms. This chapter briefly reviews surgical considerations while discussing relevant controversies that define the role of surgery in the management of malignancies invading the skull base.

Background and Principles of Management

Most malignancies of the nasal cavity and paranasal sinuses originate in the respiratory mucosa. Rare tumors of olfactory epithelial or soft tissue origins also occur and give rise to the myriad of neoplasms that are encountered in this region[2]; **Table 44.1** lists the most common malignancies encountered. Each histology has its own natural history and manage-

Table 44.1 Examples of commonly encountered skull base malignancies

Commonly Encountered Skull Base Malignances
Squamous cell carcinoma
Olfactory neuroblastoma (esthesioneuroblastoma)
Adenocarcinoma
Adenoid cystic carcinoma
Sinonasal undifferentiated carcinoma
Sarcoma
Basal cell carcinoma
Chordoma

ment paradigm, as is discussed later in this chapter; however, due to the rarity of these tumors, surgical studies predominantly lump these neoplasms into a single entity when assessing outcomes. Discussion of each histological entity is beyond the scope of this chapter but is available in the literature.

Early identification of the tumor pathology is imperative in ensuring patients are treated with the appropriate management paradigm. A representative biopsy of the neoplasm is typically obtained endonasally and evaluated by experts in head and neck pathology. Once the correct histological diagnosis is assigned, patients are further staged according to the tumor, node, metastasis (TNM) system, as shown in **Table 44.2**.[3] Tumor histology, stage, presence of nodal disease and/or metastases, applicability and potential success of adjuvant therapy, along with surgical resectability and cosmetic reconstruction, are considered by a multidisciplinary team (**Table 44.3**) to construct the optimal treatment paradigm.

A spectrum of management paradigms, consisting of combinations of surgical resection, chemotherapy, and radiotherapy, are employed depending on the histological diagnosis (**Table 44.4**). In general, surgery and some form of radiotherapy are combined, whereas other adjuvant therapies, such as radiosurgical boost and chemotherapy, may be added (**Fig. 44.1**). The most common paradigm is that of surgical resection followed by intensity-modulated radiotherapy.

Table 44.2 American Joint Committee on Cancer staging of carcinoma of the ethmoid sinus and nasal cavity

T-stage	Description
TX	Primary tumor cannot be assessed
T0	No evidence of primary tumor
Tis	Cancer cells are only in the innermost layer of mucosal epithelium; also known as carcinoma in situ
T1	Tumor is only in the nasal cavity or one of the ethmoid sinuses, although it may have grown into the bones of the sinus
T2	Tumor has grown into other nasal or paranasal cavities
T3	Tumor has grown into bone of orbit, hard palate, cribriform plate
T4a	Tumor has grown into other structures such as the eye, skin of the nose, skin of the cheek, sphenoid sinus, frontal sinus, or facial skeleton. (T4a cancers are considered resectable)
T4b	Tumor is growing into orbital apex, brain, dura, some parts of the cranial base (i.e., clivus, middle cranial fossa), cranial nerves, or nasopharynx

Table 44.3 Disciplines necessary for comprehensive care of patients with skull base tumors

Neurosurgery
Otolaryngology–head and neck surgery
Plastic surgery
Ophthalmology
Dental oncology
Diagnostic imaging
Pathology
Medical oncology
Radiation oncology

Table 44.4 Examples of different management paradigms

Surgical resection
Basal cell carcinoma
Low-grade chondrosarcoma
Desmoid fibromatosis
Particular low-grade sarcomas and low-grade adenocarcinomas
Surgical resection followed by postoperative radiation therapy
Olfactory neuroblastoma
Adenocarcinoma
Adenoid cystic carcinoma
Squamous cell carcinoma
Particular low-grade sarcomas
Pre- and postoperative chemotherapy, surgical resection and postoperative radiation therapy
Squamous cell carcinoma
High-grade sarcomas
Sinonasal undifferentiated carcinoma
Melanoma
Chemotherapy, radiation therapy, surgical resection, and stereotactic radiosurgery
Squamous cell carcinoma (particularly with perineural extension)
Adenoid cystic carcinoma (particularly with perineural extension)
Some high-grade sarcomas and sinonasal undifferentiated carcinoma

Source: Modified from DeMonte F. Evolving role of skullbase surgery for patients with low and high grade malignancies. J Neurooncol 2004;69(1-3):191–198.

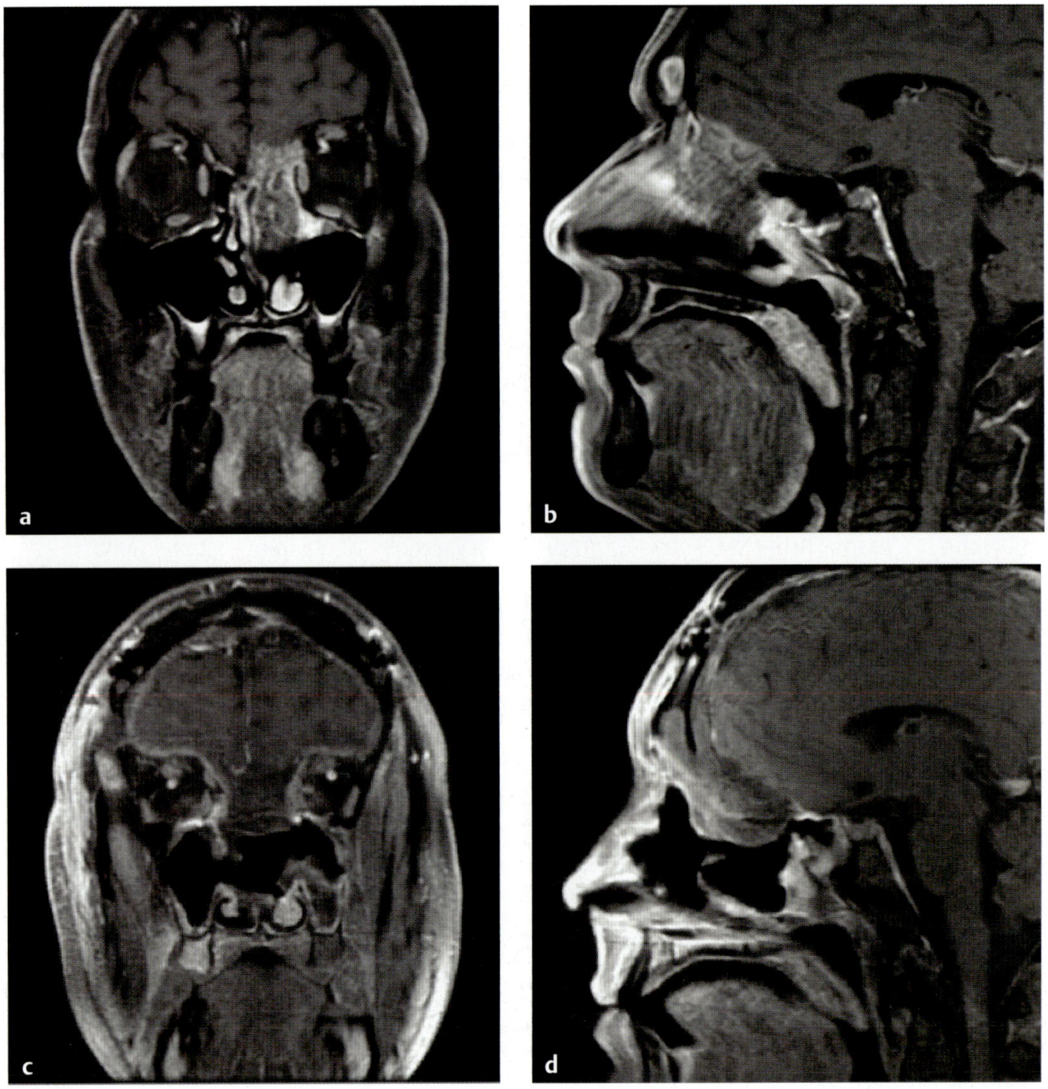

Fig. 44.1 49-year-old male with moderately differentiated SCC. Preoperative images **(a,b)** reveal intracerebral and left orbital invasion. Patient was treated with three courses of cisplatinum, taxotere, and 5-FU with stable appearing disease on postinduction MRI. A cranio-endoscopic approach was used to resect the tumor in its entirety including its intracerebral and intraorbital components **(c,d)**. Final pathology revealed extensive tumor necrosis with few remaining viable cells. Postoperative irradiation was given to 60Gy.

This is primarily recommended for olfactory neuroblastoma, adenocarcinoma, and adenoid cystic carcinoma, among many others.[4] Induction chemotherapy may be employed for histologies like squamous cell carcinoma, sinonasal undifferentiated carcinoma (SNUC), and some high-grade sarcomas.[5,6] Although surgery plays a role in the management of the majority of patients, an important subset of patients are best managed with nonsurgical therapies. Examples are patients with lymphoma, neuroendocrine carcinoma, Ewing sarcoma, and some patients with SNUC. Ultimately, as **Table 44.4** demonstrates, several treatment protocols are employed where surgical resection plays a significant role in oncological control; as such, it is imperative to understand not only the evidence behind surgery but also what the goals of any surgical intervention are based on in the published literature.

■ Surgical Considerations and Evolution in Techniques

It wasn't until the introduction of craniofacial resection that a significant improvement in long-term disease control was appreciated. Several studies have demonstrated a dismal natural history for malignancies of the paranasal sinuses affecting the skull base, with mean overall 5-year survival rates of ~ 30% without surgical intervention.[7] Since its introduction more than 50 years ago, craniofacial resection has remained the gold standard for anterior skull base malignancy resection. Combined craniofacial approaches for these tumors have evolved tremendously since their original description by Ketcham.[1] Initial reports of a single-stage craniofacial resection demonstrated that, although tumor access and resection could be achieved, relatively high rates of neurological and nonneurological morbidity and mortality were encountered. These major postoperative complications could be grouped into five classes: neurological/intracranial (contusion, tension pneumocephalus, etc.), wound/cosmetic (infection, flap necrosis, cerebrospinal fluid leaks, etc.), ocular (blindness, diplopia, hematoma), and systemic.[8]

Since these original reports, several key techniques and concepts have evolved over time to improve oncological and surgical outcomes. Improved understanding of complex cranial base anatomy has resulted in modifications to traditional surgical approaches. Examples of such modifications include the transbasal and subcranial approaches, extended bifrontal craniotomy with orbital osteotomies, and orbitozygomatic approaches.[9,10] When supplemented by an open transfacial or endoscopic approach, the surgical approach can now be tailored to the pathology to provide optimal access while minimizing unnecessary soft tissue morbidity.

In recent years, there has been a growing interest in endonasal approaches to the midline and paramedian skull base.[11] By working through natural corridors, endoscopic techniques can provide a direct surgical trajectory aimed at the epicenter of selected pathology. Primarily, this technique has been sought out as a replacement for transfacial approaches for either benign (i.e., pituitary adenomas) and/or extradural pathology (clival chordomas) where the overlying facial skeleton and soft tissue structures are not involved. More recently, an increasing number of reports describe outcomes subsequent to the use of pure endoscopic resection of cranial base malignancies. Although these reports demonstrate seemingly promising results, they are complicated by comparisons of endoscopic resection of low- and intermediate-stage pathology (T1 and T2) with craniofacial resection for more extensive disease (T3 and T4). In general, endoscopic approaches have proven efficacious with regard to oncological and surgical outcomes for malignancies primarily within the nasal cavity and paranasal sinuses with limited secondary skull base involvement (i.e., cribriform plate invasion but no significant dural involvement or intradural extension).[12] Purely endoscopic approaches are also thought to be limited with regard to disease extending lateral to the cribriform plate/optic nerves, significant neurovascular involvement, and involvement of the overlying facial soft tissue, and where there is a need for significant dural reconstruction. Ultimately, endoscopic approaches have provided an alternative to traditional craniofacial approaches for certain types of lesions. As more data are generated, it will be important to ensure these new techniques are assessed and compared with open approaches using the correct outcome measures (i.e., negative margins, complication rates, quality of life measures) and with correct control cohorts (i.e., controlling for histology, stage of disease, anatomical considerations, etc.).

Another advancement that has occurred to combat complications traditionally seen in skull base resection (either via open or endoscopic approaches) is the increasing focus on skull base reconstruction and separation of the intracranial contents from the nasal cavity and paranasal sinuses. Vascularized pedicled flaps, such as pericranial grafts, provide the necessary watertight closure to separate the different compartments while also reducing the risk of infection/meningitis.[13] Additionally, improvements in microvascular reconstruction provide for robust reconstruction in salvage situations or when local tissue is infiltrated with disease.[14,15] These flaps provide not only the bulk to fill dead space but also the vascularity needed for any soft tissue reconstruction to withstand adjuvant radiation and chemotherapy. Similar reconstructive advancements have been made with the use of endoscopic techniques. Although the nasoseptal flap is the most fundamental means of dural coverage, the development of multilayered grafts and fascial grafts (i.e., pericranial, temporal-parietal fascia) that can be endoscopically harvested have also provided alternate methods of dural coverage.[16]

Concurrent with the surgical advancements seen over the last several years, changes in treatment paradigms for sinonasal malignancies have evolved as we have gained more experience and additional understanding of these disease processes. As already discussed, induction chemotherapy can be used for pathologies like high-grade squamous cell carcinoma (SCC) and sarcomas and sinonasal undifferentiated carcinoma to help transform them from surgically and oncologically challenging lesions to more manageable entities. As these therapies evolve, it is imperative for skull base surgeons to understand their role and the context for surgery in these management paradigms.

■ Limitations in Interpreting the Literature

In interpreting the literature on this surgical area, several crucial points must be kept in mind prior to drawing any conclusions. Although there are several published studies on this subject matter, there is unfortunately a great deal of inconsistency with regard

Table 44.5 Studies representative of the literature focusing on sinonasal malignancies invading the skull base

Study	Level of evidence	No. patients	Most common histological types	Rates of negative margins (%)	Study conclusions
Patel et al 2003[8]	III	1,307	Squamous cell carcinoma (29%) Adenocarcinoma (16%)	54.3	Surgical margins shown to be an independent predictor of 5-year recurrence-free survival (64.1% vs 29.6%, $p < 0.0001$)
Cantu et al 2012[17]	III	366	Adenocarcinoma (48%) Squamous cell carcinoma (12%)	74	Positive surgical margins shown to be independent predictor of poorer 5-year recurrence (HR 2.34, $p < 0.001$) and overall survival rates (HR 2.65, $p < 0.001$)
Bentz et al 2003[18]	III	166	Squamous cell carcinoma (24%) Sarcoma (19%)	60	Surgical margins independently associated with 5-year recurrence-free survival (RR 1.43, 95% CI 1.15 to 1.79, $p = 0.001$) and overall survival
Feiz-Erfan et al 2007[19]	III	28	Olfactory neuroblastoma High-grade adenocarcinoma	79	Gross total resection—negative margins found to be significant predictor of overall survival in multivariate analysis (RR 5.7, 95% CI 1.2 to 26.7 $p = 0.03$)
Clayman et al 1995[15]	III	39	Squamous cell carcinomas (51%) Basal cell carcinomas (21%)	47	Negative margins associated with improved 5-year disease-specific survival (63% vs 0%)

not only to the primary outcomes employed but also to how they are assessed. Additionally, there is a major discrepancy among studies in terms of how tumors are classified (i.e., size vs T stage and histology), goals of surgery (i.e., gross total resection vs microscopic negative margins), and adjuvant therapy.

The primary outcomes/end points must first be defined according to the disease process and should be clinically relevant. In general, oncological outcomes such as overall survival, 5-year progression-free survival, and recurrence rates assess the impact of any intervention (surgery or adjuvant therapy or both). Furthermore, other outcomes that must also be assessed include neurological function and disease-specific quality of life measurements.

■ Controversies in the Surgical Management of Skull Base Malignancies

Does Surgery Make an Impact and What Are the Goals of Surgery?

The goal of surgical resection is negative margins.

Level I and Level II Evidence

No Level I or II studies exist evaluating the role of surgery.

Level III Evidence

There are numerous studies demonstrating the need for negative margins in the management of head and neck malignancies. Similarly, several studies in the literature address the goals of surgical management in patients with head and neck malignancies secondarily invading the skull base. It should be noted that some studies have found no association between margin status and survival. These studies, however, include small patient numbers and tend to be underpowered. **Table 44.5** highlights several selected studies that are representative of the literature. The importance of *histologically* negative margins during surgical resection cannot be overemphasized based on the published data.

In the largest series published to date on this disease entity, the International Collaborative Study reported outcomes from a large retrospective cohort study.[8] In a multi-institutional study involving over 17 centers, the safety and efficacy of craniofacial resection was assessed in over 1,300 patients with skull base malignancies operated on between October 1956 and January 2000. A variety of histological tumor types were included in the analysis (where the most common variants were squamous cell carcinoma and adenocarcinoma), and the majority (46.7%) were TNM stage IV cancers. With a median follow-up of 25 months, the 5-year overall survival was 53.6%, and recurrence-free survival was 41.7%. Intraoperatively verified histologically tumor-free margins were found to be statistically significant as a predictor of 5-year recurrence-free survival (64.1% vs 29.6%, $p < 0.0001$, RR 2.3, 95% CI 1.8 to 2.9). Representative of the overall literature, this is one of the largest studies to be published demonstrating that the goal of surgery is to obtain histologically negative margins.

The second-largest study published to date in this area, by Cantu et al,[17] retrospectively analyzed their monoinstitutional experience with malignant paranasal sinus tumors requiring craniofacial resection. Their cohort of 366 patients treated between 1987 and 2007 consisted of patients with intraorbital spread (29%), cribriform plate erosion (29%), intracranial–extradural extension (14%), and intradural extension (10.7%). As with many other series, the most common histologies treated were adenocarcinoma (48.6%), squamous cell carcinoma (12.0%), and sinonasal undifferentiated carcinoma (10.7%). All patients underwent a combined transcranial and transfacial approach consisting of a bifrontal craniotomy with a facial approach tailored to the tumor. With regard to surgical outcomes, negative margins (based on intraoperative frozen section) were obtained in 74.0%. Within the series, ~ 56% of patients underwent postoperative radiotherapy; the remainder had either received preoperative radiation or had died or refused further treatment. The 5-year recurrence rate was 38.4% and 5-year overall survival was 46.3%. A multivariate Cox analysis for both recurrence rates and overall survival indicated positive surgical margins to be statistically predictive of poorer outcomes (recurrence rates: HR 2.34, $p < 0.001$, overall survival: HR 2.65, $p < 0.001$).

Another study in this area by Bentz et al retrospectively assessed outcomes from anterior skull base resection performed at their institution over a 27-year period[18]; a majority of the 166 patients studied carried the diagnosis of squamous cell carcinoma (24%), followed by sarcoma (19%) and esthesioneuroblastoma (12%). The most commonly found epicenter for the tumors resected was the nasal cavity (38%), followed by the ethmoid sinus (26%). A majority of patients underwent a standard craniofacial resection (bifrontal craniotomy plus a transfacial approach), where the goal of intervention was gross total resection. Employing 5-year disease-specific and relapse-free survival for each histology, multivariate Cox proportional hazard analysis found that surgical margins had a significant impact.

In another single-institution study done by Feiz-Erfan et al, a retrospective analysis was performed of their experience with craniofacial malignancies with transdural spread (subdural tumor or brain invasion) with 28 patients.[19] Although the study was primarily designed to assess the prognostic significance of transdural tumor spread, a multivariate analysis further demonstrated gross total resection—negative margins as compared with other resection outcomes as a significant predictor of overall survival (RR 5.7; 95% CI 1.2 to 26.7, $p = 0.03$; adjusted for other variables RR 5.0; 95% CI 0.8 to 29.9; $p = 0.08$). Negative surgical margins were also identified as an independent predictor of improved progression-free survival (RR 5.4; 95% CI 1.1 to 28.5; $p = 0.05$). This analysis not only demonstrated the importance of surgically obtained negative margins but also demonstrated survival benefit with maximal safe resection even in the setting of an aggressive cancer invading the dura and brain.

Assessing their outcomes with extensive malignant tumors involving the skull base, upper head and neck, dura and intracranial space necessitating free tissue transfer for repair, Clayman et al demonstrated a similar role for surgery with regard to oncological outcomes.[15] In a cohort of 31 patients, resections were performed in the anterior (49%), middle (26%), and posterior fossa (8%). A third of the patients underwent radical orbitectomy as part of the surgical resection. As a result of the extensive defects created in the tumor resection, all patients in this study needed a microvascular free tissue transfer (97% success rate). Tumor-free margins were obtained in 47% of anterior cranial fossa resections, and in 30% of middle fossa resections. The overall 5-year disease-specific survival was 55% and was found to be positively correlated with tumor-free margins (63% vs 0%). Ultimately, this study not only highlighted the improved technique of soft tissue reconstruction but also demonstrated a role for aggressive surgical resection with the goal of negative margins, even with large, invasive skull base tumors requiring extensive reconstructions.

What Other Surgical Factors Affect Survival?

Factors such as dural/brain invasion, vascular involvement, and orbital involvement have been shown to affect resectability and oncological outcomes; en bloc surgical resection has not been shown to affect outcomes.

Level I and Level II Evidence

No Level I or II studies have been performed evaluating surgical variables affecting resection and oncological outcomes.

Level III Evidence

Although craniofacial resection has been demonstrated to have a positive impact on several outcomes in patients with paranasal sinus malignancies, several other surgical variables may not only independently affect surgical resection but also impact oncological outcomes. Variables like neoplastic invasion of brain and dura and orbital involvement have been shown to decrease survival in these patients.[20] However, it is not evident that these factors independently influence patient outcomes; there is currently a paucity of studies that address these issues in a multivariate analysis.

The depth of tumor invasion (i.e., dural vs subdural vs brain and/or perineural involvement) has been shown to be independently associated with overall and progression-free survival. Although the fraction of patients undergoing craniofacial resection for lesions with brain invasion is small (reported rates of 6.4% to 21.6% in larger series), the degree of invasion has traditionally been thought to be an obstacle to obtaining maximal resection while being associated with higher complication rates (i.e., neurovascular injury, CSF leak rates). Additionally, these lesions can invade the intracranial contents by infiltrating along cranial nerves—representing an additional obstacle to surgical resection and a source of postoperative morbidity. Furthermore, a high degree of invasion could be reflective of a biologically more aggressive tumor. Feiz-Erfan et al addressed this issue in their retrospective assessment of 28 patients from a prospectively collected database with evidence of transdural disease extension (subdural or brain invasion).[19] Based on operative records and pathology reports, they identified subdural extension only in 16 patients and brain invasion in 12 patients within the cohort. Accounting for factors known to affect survival (i.e., extent of resection), the authors found brain invasion to be a negative predictor for progression-free survival. Within this analysis, as discussed earlier, the authors still found a role for safe, aggressive surgical resection with the goal of gross total resection—negative histological margins.

The issue of vascular invasion (i.e., internal carotid artery involvement) is another controversy of growing importance because there has been a shift toward a more aggressive approach to cranial base malignancies. Factors limiting resection of such lesions have traditionally included either internal carotid artery or cavernous sinus invasion. In the context of the need for negative margins, some authors have advocated the use of carotid resection along with a high-flow vascular bypass to obtain a maximal resection.[21] On the other hand, reflecting on the thromboembolic and ischemic complications associated with vascular bypass grafts in general, others believe that maximal resection should be the goal as long as neurological and nonneurological morbidity is minimized.[22] In their retrospective analysis of their experience with anterolateral skull base malignancies, Hentschel et al demonstrated in a univariate analysis that internal carotid artery resection was associated with worsened overall median survival (5.3 vs 2.5 years).[23] Internal carotid artery resection was performed only in those patients with circumferential arterial involvement passing balloon test occlusion preoperatively. Although associated with noticeably lower rates of recurrence, patients undergoing internal carotid artery (ICA) resection ultimately succumbed to regional and distant tumor burden. Similar findings have been confirmed by other studies.[22] Hence we feel that tumor resection with vascular preservation carries the best chance of an optimal neurological outcome while obtaining acceptable oncological outcomes.

The last surgical issue is that of en bloc resection. The fundamental premise is that the primary goal of oncological surgery is complete excision of the neoplasm. With the concerns for tumor spread via a piecemeal resection, traditionally a monobloc resection has been the primary surgical goal to minimize the risk of local disease recurrence and improve overall survival. This was the primary impetus for larger open approaches even for focal (T1/T2) disease at the skull base. However, with the growing popularity of endoscopic approaches, the need for en bloc resection is now under systematic review, because endoscopic approaches rely on internal debulking during resection for larger tumors. Several studies specifically addressing head and neck malignancies with skull base involvement have assessed the impact of monobloc resection on overall survival and progression-free survival.[8,18,19,24] No study to date has found en bloc resection to be correlated with oncological outcomes (i.e., overall survival or progression-free survival). These data also have implications for pure endoscopic resections of sinonasal malignancies. In light of the current data, for larger lesions, our technique consists of debulking the tumor to identify critical neurovascular structures safely, followed by monobloc resection of the remaining tumor.

Expert Recommendations

1. Surgery has a demonstrated role in improving survival in craniofacial malignancies without distant metastases (Grade 1B Recommendation, Level II Evidence).
2. The goal of surgery is microscopically negative margins, which have been shown to be independently associated with improved overall survival and progression-free survival (Grade 1C+ Recommendation, Level II/III Evidence).
3. The depth of tumor invasion (i.e., subdural extension) has been shown to affect oncological outcomes and affects surgical resection; there is still a role for surgery with the goal of negative margins in these patients (Grade 1C Recommendation, Level II/III Evidence).
4. With carotid artery involvement, although a role for surgery exists, the goal should be maximal resection with preservation of the parent vessel (Grade 1C Recommendation, Level III–V Evidence).
5. The goal of surgical resection should be en bloc resection of the area of skull base involvement as long as surgical morbidity is minimized (Grade 1C Recommendation, Level III–V Evidence).
6. There is a need for prospective studies to evaluate this area with standardized and appropriate outcome measures that incorporate not only surgical and oncological outcomes but also quality of life and neurological outcomes.

Summary and Conclusions

Since the original introduction of craniofacial resection, the field of skull base surgery has evolved tremendously along with our understanding and nonsurgical management of sinonasal malignancies. Surgical concepts, such as modern skull base techniques with osteotomies to minimize neurological morbidity, endoscopic approaches to minimize soft tissue disruption, broad-spectrum antibiotics, and soft tissue and bony reconstructive techniques, have advanced. This has occurred in the context of adjuvant therapies that can be offered either pre- or postoperatively depending on tumor histology and increasing recognition of performance status, neurological function, and patient selection. Therefore, there is a need to continually reevaluate the role of surgery and factors that affect surgical outcomes and complications. Because this cohort of patients is difficult to study in large numbers or in a prospective, controlled fashion, a majority of studies in the area provide Level III evidence. As the literature is reviewed and evaluated, it is important to remember that the existing studies are limited; hence, for factors that are not statistically associated with improved outcomes (i.e., en bloc resection), good surgical sense and not just a statistical analysis should guide surgical decision making.

References

1. Ketcham AS, Wilkins RH, Vanburen JM, Smith RR. A combined intracranial facial approach to the paranasal sinuses. Am J Surg 1963;106:698–703
2. DeMonte F. Evolving role of skullbase surgery for patients with low and high grade malignancies. J Neurooncol 2004;69(1-3): 191–198
3. American Joint Committee on Cancer (AJCC). AJCC Staging Manual. Philadelphia, PA: Lippincott-Raven; 1997
4. Lund VJ, Chisholm EJ, Takes RP, et al. Evidence for treatment strategies in sinonasal adenocarcinoma. Head Neck 2012; 34(8):1168–1178
5. Choi KN, Rotman M, Aziz H, et al. Concomitant infusion cisplatin and hyperfractionated radiotherapy for locally advanced nasopharyngeal and paranasal sinus tumors. Int J Radiat Oncol Biol Phys 1997;39(4):823–829
6. Lee MM, Vokes EE, Rosen A, Witt ME, Weichselbaum RR, Haraf DJ. Multimodality therapy in advanced paranasal sinus carcinoma: superior long-term results. Cancer J Sci Am 1999; 5(4):219–223
7. Sisson GA Sr, Toriumi DM, Atiyah RA. Paranasal sinus malignancy: a comprehensive update. Laryngoscope 1989; 99(2):143–150
8. Patel SG, Singh B, Polluri A, et al. Craniofacial surgery for malignant skull base tumors: report of an international collaborative study. Cancer 2003;98(6):1179–1187
9. Conway JE, Raza SM, Li K, McDermott MW, Quiñones-Hinojosa A. A surgical modification for performing orbitozygomatic osteotomies: technical note. Neurosurg Rev 2010;33(4): 491–500
10. Feiz-Erfan I, Spetzler RF, Horn EM, et al. Proposed classification for the transbasal approach and its modifications. Skull Base 2008;18(1):29–47
11. Snyderman CH, Carrau RL, Kassam AB, et al. Endoscopic skull base surgery: principles of endonasal oncological surgery. J Surg Oncol 2008;97(8):658–664
12. Hanna E, DeMonte F, Ibrahim S, Roberts D, Levine N, Kupferman M. Endoscopic resection of sinonasal cancers with and without craniotomy: oncologic results. Arch Otolaryngol Head Neck Surg 2009;135(12):1219–1224
13. Rodrigues M, O'Malley BW Jr, Staecker H, Tamargo R. Extended pericranial flap and bone graft reconstruction in anterior skull base surgery. Otolaryngol Head Neck Surg 2004; 131(1):69–76
14. Hanasono MM, Silva A, Skoracki RJ, et al. Skull base reconstruction: an updated approach. Plast Reconstr Surg 2011; 128(3):675–686
15. Clayman GL, DeMonte F, Jaffe DM, et al. Outcome and complications of extended cranial-base resection requiring microvascular free-tissue transfer. Arch Otolaryngol Head Neck Surg 1995;121(11):1253–1257

16. Zanation AM, Carrau RL, Snyderman CH, et al. Nasoseptal flap reconstruction of high flow intraoperative cerebral spinal fluid leaks during endoscopic skull base surgery. Am J Rhinol Allergy 2009;23(5):518–521
17. Cantu G, Solero CL, Miceli R, et al. Anterior craniofacial resection for malignant paranasal tumors: a monoinstitutional experience of 366 cases. Head Neck 2012;34(1):78–87
18. Bentz BG, Bilsky MH, Shah JP, Kraus D. Anterior skull base surgery for malignant tumors: a multivariate analysis of 27 years of experience. Head Neck 2003;25(7):515–520
19. Feiz-Erfan I, Suki D, Hanna E, DeMonte F. Prognostic significance of transdural invasion of cranial base malignancies in patients undergoing craniofacial resection. Neurosurgery 2007;61(6):1178–1185
20. Howard DJ, Lund VJ, Wei WI. Craniofacial resection for tumors of the nasal cavity and paranasal sinuses: a 25-year experience. Head Neck 2006;28(10):867–873
21. Couldwell WT, Taussky P, Sivakumar W. Submandibular high-flow bypass in the treatment of skull base lesions: an analysis of long-term outcome. Neurosurgery 2012;71(3):645–650
22. Brisman MH, Sen C, Catalano P. Results of surgery for head and neck tumors that involve the carotid artery at the skull base. J Neurosurg 1997;86(5):787–792
23. Hentschel SJ, Vora Y, Suki D, Hanna EY, DeMonte F. Malignant tumors of the anterolateral skull base. Neurosurgery 2010;66(1):102–112
24. McCutcheon IE, Blacklock JB, Weber RS, et al. Anterior transcranial (craniofacial) resection of tumors of the paranasal sinuses: surgical technique and results. Neurosurgery 1996;38(3):471–479

▪ SECTION XIII ▪

Chordomas

45

The Role of Surgery in the Management of Skull Base Chordomas

Jacob Ruzevick, Shaan M. Raza, and Alfredo Quiñones-Hinojosa

Chordomas are rare, slow-growing tumors that originate from remnants of the notochord and can arise from the skull base, sacrococcygeal region, spheno-occipital region, and vertebrae.[1] Skull base chordomas in particular are rare, with an estimated incidence of 1 case per 2,000,000 individuals per year[2] and account for 0.1 to 0.2% of all intracranial neoplasms.[3] Although generally considered low-grade malignancies, most skull base chordomas eventually relapse because of the difficulty in achieving gross total resection, the high recurrence rate, and occasional metastases. Skull base chordomas arise from notochordal elements within bone, including the clivus, petrous apex, and craniocervical junction, but can involve multiple tissue types within the skull base, including brainstem, cranial nerves, and neurovascular structures, thus making complete surgical resection a formidable challenge, especially in the setting of recurrent disease.

Currently, there is no standard of care for chordoma, but the general rationale is maximal surgical resection followed by adjuvant radiation. As a result, adjuvant radiation is prescribed to aid in tumor control after resection, though radiation doses of 55 to 80 Gy are required to improve outcomes.[4] This radiation is typically applied in the form of charged-particle therapy (i.e., proton beam therapy) because its Bragg peak allows application of high doses of radiation relatively short distances away from critical neural structures, such as the brainstem.

In light of the high risk of surgery in this area, the anatomical complexity of chordomas, and the relative paucity of prospective data on these lesions, there is debate over the role of surgery in their management. Questions like, What is the goal of surgery? What is the role of open versus endoscopic surgery? and Is there a survival difference between different histological subtypes? as well as other questions remain unanswered because no prospective clinical study has been done with this disease entity. This chapter reviews and classifies the published literature to date in an effort to provide an evidence-based rationale for surgical decision making.

▪ Histology and Radiology

Believed to arise from notochordal remnants, chordomas are histologically notable for their physaliferous appearances and positive immunoreactivity for several markers: S-100, cytokeratin, and epithelial markers (i.e., epithelial membrane antigen—MUC1). Due to their similar appearance, certain subtypes of chordomas can be confused for chondrosarcoma—a critical mistake given that the management paradigms for the two are very different. As with other tumors, chordomas display varying degrees of histopathological features and are classified into one of three subtypes: classical (conventional), chondroid, or dedifferentiated. The classical variant microscopically appears as groups of cells separated by fibrous septa, where the cells have round nuclei, and abundant vacuolated cytoplasm that gives these tumors their physiliferous appearance. On the other hand, chondroid chordomas show histological features similar to both chordomas and chondrosarcomas, the malignant cartilage-forming skull base tumor. In light of the histological variety, there is a great deal of controversy regarding the impact of histologic subtype on survival and treatment paradigms.

Radiographically, chordomas are characterized by bony destruction on computed tomographic (CT) imaging of the skull base. Although they typically arise from the midline, their invasive nature facilitates their invasion into different contiguous compartments of the skull base. On magnetic resonance imaging (MRI), they are typically isointense on T1-weighted imaging and hyperintense on T2-weighted imaging, with minimal enhancement after gadolinium administration. With regard to surgical planning, there are several aspects of preoperative radiography that must be assessed. On CT imaging, the extent of skull base involvement should be assessed (i.e., involvement of the petrous bone beyond the clivus) to help determine if a midline versus lateral versus staged approach will be necessary for resection. Additionally, for lesions located in the lower clivus/craniocervical junction, the occipital condyles should be reviewed for secondary tumor erosion; with condylar involvement, the condyles are typically drilled to obtain maximal tumor resection and eradicate a potential epicenter of the tumor. These patients are also at risk for postoperative occipital-cervical instability. On MRI scans, the tumor should be examined for potential intradural extension, which would affect intraoperative skull base reconstruction. Additionally, because these tumors can be quite infiltrative, they can encase the vasculature. With vascular encasement, a conventional angiogram should be considered for balloon test occlusion to plan for a potential intraoperative catastrophe. Embolization is not the primary goal of angiography because these tumors do not have significant vascular pedicles.

■ Surgical Treatment of Chordomas

Skull base chordomas typically arise from the clivus but infiltrate other osseous compartments of the skull base (i.e., petrous bone) and envelop nearby cranial nerves, vascular structures, and brainstem.[5] Chordomas can extend outside the clivus in both the sagittal and coronal planes. Extension in the ventral direction, toward the anterior cranial fossa, and the caudal direction, toward the cervical spine, is common. Furthermore, lateral extension into the petrosphenoclival junction, petrous apex, occipital condyle, and jugular foramen requires the surgical team to be judicious in the surgical approach taken. Consequently, the surgical management of these lesions can often require a combination of surgical approaches in a single stage or over the course of multiple surgeries.

Prior to treatment, CT and MRI are required for localization of skull base chordomas because of both bony and potential soft tissue involvement. Typically, there is extensive lytic bone destruction with intratumoral calcifications. Chordomas are usually extradural tumors, though they can invade into or through the dura, causing direct brainstem compression. The extent of dural invasion can typically be seen with MRI, and when dural invasion is not present, various authors suggest using extradural approaches to decrease the risk of seeding a recurrent tumor into the intradural space.

The surgical treatment of clival chordomas has evolved over the years in parallel with the field of skull base surgery as new open and endoscopic approaches have been developed. With improvements in our anatomical understanding, numerous safe open approaches to all three cranial fossa have evolved. In the early management of these lesions, transfacial approaches were en vogue for lesions primarily located in the midline skull base. Such approaches permitted access to tumors through a natural corridor between the cranial nerves and internal carotid arteries. In fact, several early surgical series exclusively employed midfacial degloving/transfacial approaches for the management of clival chordomas. Although these techniques were successful for purely midline lesions, they were limited for lesions extending laterally beyond the neurovascular structures. Since these initial series, there has been growth in our anatomical knowledge, skull base approaches, and technology that has expanded the surgical management of these lesions.

The myriad of open skull base approaches includes midline ventral approaches (i.e., extended bifrontal, high transcervical), anterolateral approaches (i.e., orbitozygomatic, preauricular infratemporal fossa), and lateral approaches (i.e., posterior petrosal, far lateral transcondylar). With the introduction of endoscopy, transfacial approaches have been replaced by endoscopic approaches either through the nasal corridors (endonasal), maxillary sinuses (Caldwell-Luc), oropharynx (transoral), or cervical spine (transcervical).[2,5–18] As a result, in comparison to the traditional transfacial approaches, endoscopic approaches can provide similar, if not improved, access to the ventral midline skull base (from the anterior skull base inferiorly to the craniocervical junction) and parts of the facial skeleton. In addition, endoscopy improves illumination and visualization through a narrow corridor, facilitating surgical dissection.

In light of the numerous surgical options, selection of the correct surgical approach is an important factor in achieving the goals of surgery, which are discussed later. There are several other considerations that go into this decision-making process. Because chordomas are primarily extradural tumors, the dura can serve as an important barrier; hence an extradural route should be the primary approach to minimize the risk of postoperative cerebrospinal fluid (CSF) fistula or CSF seeding with the tumor. On occasion, these tumors transgress the dura, requiring an intradural approach as a second stage. The other anatomical factors to consider are the compartments of the skull base involved by the target lesion. These tumors are invasive and can involve multiple compartments of the skull base, intracranial space, and head/neck region. Al-Mefty and Borba[6] classify tumors based on patterns of extension to aid in surgical planning. Type I tumors are restricted to a single solitary anatomical area of the skull base. Type II are tumors that extend to two or more contiguous areas of the skull base where radical resection can be obtained via a single skull base approach. Type III lesions involve several contiguous anatomical compartments and will require two or more approaches/stages to achieve radical resection. As such, many patients may require a combination of approaches or surgical stages to achieve an acceptable tumor resection with minimal morbidity. For example, for clival lesions with significant lateral extension beyond the neurovasculature, one may use an initial ventral endoscopic approach followed by a lateral approach (transpetrosal, far lateral transcondylar) for judicious and efficient tumor resection (**Fig. 45.1**). The last major factor to consider is the reconstruction. Because these tumors can transgress the dura, the

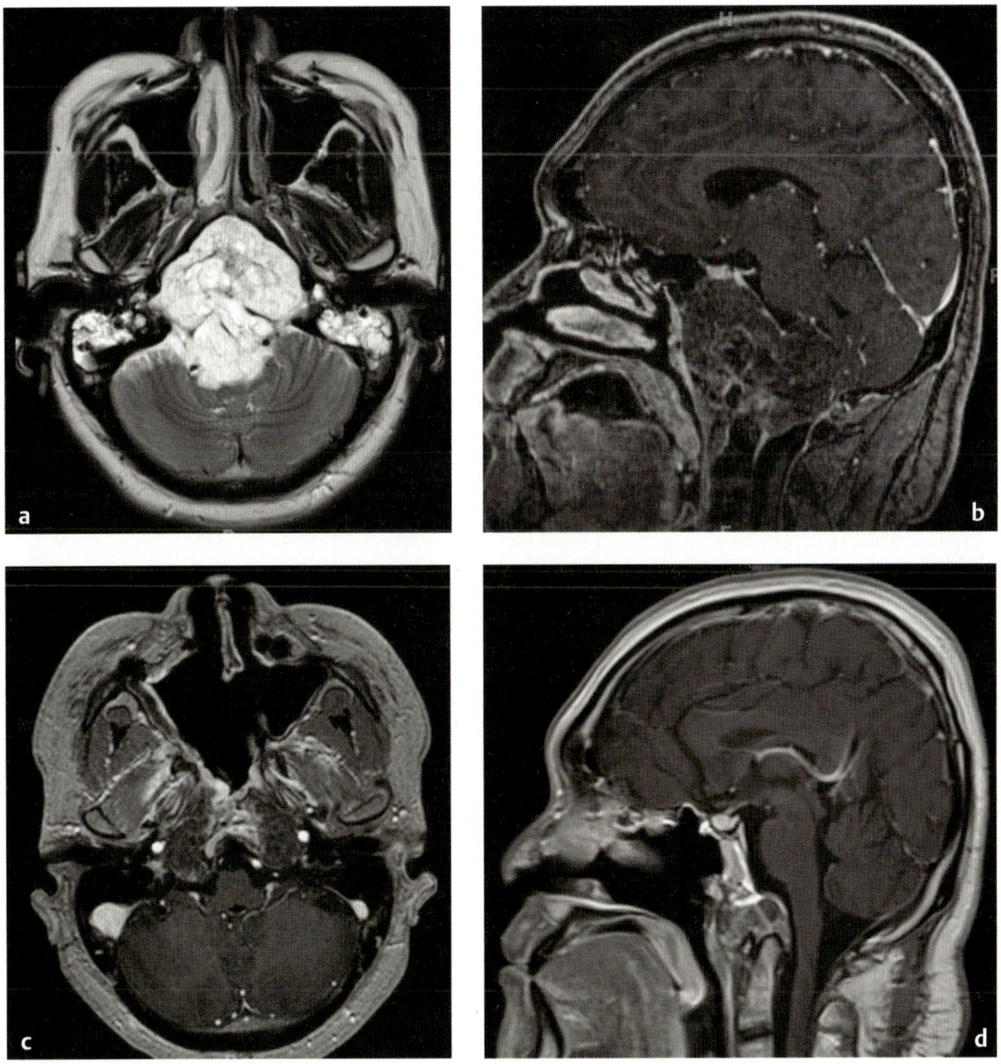

Fig. 45.1 A 27-year-old male presenting with myelopathy, vocal hoarseness, and dysphagia. **(a)** T2-weighted magnetic resonance imaging (MRI) demonstrates a hyperintense lesion arising from the mid-lower clivus with significant bilateral lateral extension and possible intradural extension. **(b)** Sagittal T1-weighted MRI with gadolinium demonstrating caudal extension down to the level of C2; significant brainstem compression is also noted. This lesion would be classified as a type III lesion; the patient underwent a first stage via an endoscopic endonasal/transmaxillary and a second stage via a far lateral transcondylar resection. **(c)** Axial T1-weighted MRI with gadolinium and **(d)** sagittal T1-weighted MRI with gadolinium demonstrates a good debulking/resection of this large lesion.

risk of postoperative CSF leakage is high. Therefore, any approach must plan for dural coverage, whether this is done with local soft tissue flaps (pericranium, Haddad nasoseptal flap), or osteoplastic flaps (osteoplastic maxillotomy).

Ultimately, as will be discussed here, several methodological studies have demonstrated not only the role of surgical resection but also the factors that affect degree of resection, which include tumor size and degree of skull base involvement. The surgical objective is not only soft tumor resection and removal of diseased bone but also neurological preservation and skull base reconstruction. Any operative strategy must achieve these goals.

■ Literature Review

Is There any Difference in Survival between Patients with Chondroid Chordomas and Chordomas with Typical Histological Features?

Level I and Level II Evidence

No Level I or Level II studies exist on this subject matter.

Level III and Level IV Evidence

Chordomas can be subclassified, based on histology, into nonchondroid chordomas and chondroid chordomas. Based on this classification, Heffelfinger et al and Mitchell et al proposed that the chondroid chordoma variant had a more benign phenotype leading to more favorable clinical outcomes.[19,20] However, adjusting for known prognostic factors, Forsyth et al and Colli and Al-Mefty found no difference in survival between the two histological subtypes.[21,22] In a meta-analysis of 2,000 patients with intracranial chordoma, Jian et al found no difference in survival in patients with nonchondroid chordoma or chondroid chordoma.[23]

Is Total or Near-Total Resection Associated with Increased Recurrence-Free Survival as Compared with Partial Resection?

Level I and Level II Evidence

No Level I or Level II studies exist on this subject matter.

Level III and Level IV Evidence

All of the studies published to date qualify as Level III/Level IV evidence; although a great deal of literature exists on surgical management, only a handful of studies assess the role of resection in survival (**Table 45.1**). After a comprehensive PubMed search, only those surgical series specifically addressing the impact of surgery were included. Several groups have published their results at different time points; only the most recent reports were included. In reviewing the literature, it appears that there is a great deal of inconsistency with regard to assessing extent of resection (intraoperative assessments vs postoperative imaging), minimum follow-up, and means of reporting the extent of tumor burden. Furthermore, there is some inconsistency with regard to postoperative adjuvant therapy administered; although most studies employed postoperative charged particle therapy, several cohorts did not undergo this regimen. Lastly and more recently, there has been a growing body of literature on the endoscopic management of selected clival chordomas; although these studies can be used as a basis for a discussion of complications, their short follow-up precludes their contributions toward deciding the effect of resection on survival. As a result of these factors, it is difficult to truly make strong conclusions based on the literature to date. After total or near total resection, the recurrence rate of skull base chordomas in surgical series is between 16 and 45%, with one meta-analysis reporting a recurrence rate of 68%.[2,22–26]

An Overview of the Literature Indicates That Total or Near Total Resection Is Associated with an Increase in Recurrence-Free Survival as Compared with That of Patients Undergoing Partial Resection

This is strongly demonstrated in the largest cohort studies with the lengthiest follow-up. Colli et al[22] reported a retrospective analysis of 53 patients with clival/craniocervical junction chordomas with a varying degree of invasion of the skull base. In all operations, the goal of surgery was radical resection with removal of soft tumor tissue and extensive drilling of any abnormal bone in all patients. Extent of resection was based on preoperative and postoperative MRI and determined by a neuroradiologist. The following classification was employed: radical (absence of residual tumor or presence of a small questionable area), subtotal (> 90% resection), partial (< 90% resection). Radical, subtotal, and partial resection

Table 45.1 Studies addressing the impact of surgical resection on recurrence-free and overall survival

Study	Level of evidence	Patients (N)	Approach	Follow-up (mo)	Gross total resection (%)	Subtotal resection (%)	5-year recurrence-free survival (%)	5-year average overall survival (%)
Maira et al 1996[32]	III/IV	12	Open only	40	67	17	[a]	100
Colli and Al-Mefty 2001[22]	III/IV	53	Open only	28	45	73	51	86
Tamaki et al 2001[38]	III/IV	17	Open only	59	12	71	51	75
Samii et al 2007[15]	III/IV	49	Open only	63	49	50	NR	65
Cho et al 2008[8]	III/IV	19	Open/endoscopic	56	16	63	40	80
Ito et al 2010[30]	III/IV	19	Open/endoscopic	87	74	21	48	NR
Wu et al 2010[10]	III/IV	106	Open only	64	10	48	52.9	67.6
Sen et al 2010[27]	III/IV	29	Open/endoscopic	66	58	42	35	75
Di Maio et al 2012[11]	III/IV	95	Open/endoscopic	38	68[b] 74[b]	–	56	74

Abbreviation: NR, not reported.

[a]No recurrence noted during study period.

[b]This study addressed and reported resection rates from two different time periods 1988 to 2000 and 2001 to 2011.

was obtained in 49.2%, 28.6%, and 22.2% of patients. The mean follow-up was 46.1 months. Analysis with recurrence-free survival as the primary end point demonstrated a statistically significant difference between varying degrees of resection. Five-year recurrence-free survival rates were 59.8%, 65.9%, and 23.1%, respectively, for patients who received radical, subtotal, and partial resections.

In the most methodical analysis to date, Sen et al reported their results from a cohort of 65 patients.[27] The cohort included tumors located in the upper/mid clivus and at the craniovertebral junction. With an intended strategy of radical resection of the tumor and surrounding open, a variety of surgical approaches (open and endoscopic) were employed, consisting of ventral midline (extended subfrontal, transmaxillary, transmandibular, endoscopic endonasal, transcervical) and lateral (orbitozygomatic, anterior petrosal, preauricular infratemporal, combined supra- and infratentorial transtemporal, extreme lateral transcondylar). With this surgical strategy, radical resection was achieved in 58% of patients. With a mean follow-up of 66 months (ranging from 3 to 189 months), they reported an overall 5-year survival of 75%. Survival was shown to be significantly improved by the extent of resection with a 5-year survival of 90% with radical resection versus 52% with incomplete resection ($p = 0.001$). This relationship was further assessed with a multivariate analysis accounting for tumor volume, anatomical extent of the tumor, and tumor location; once again, degree of resection was shown to be an independent prognostic factor for overall and recurrence-free survival. Additionally, in their analysis, factors shown to affect degree of resection include tumor volume and extent of skull base involvement.

Wu et al report their experience with the largest cohort (79 patients) with a mean follow-up of 63.9 months. Employing primarily ventral and laterally based open microsurgical approaches, they achieved the following resection rates: gross total resection 14%, subtotal resection 65%, majority resection (> 60%) 21%. The overall 5-year recurrence rate for the entire cohort was 52.9%, and the 5-year overall survival rate was 67.6%. Time to recurrence was 107.8 months in the subtotally resected group and 79.2 in the "majority resection" group; all patients who underwent gross total resection were alive at the time of the paper. Multivariate Cox regression analysis demonstrated significant correlation between degree of resection and overall and recurrence-free survival.

Over all, multiple groups report similar statistics, with an estimated 5-year recurrence-free survival of 55% for total or near total resection and 36% for partial resection.[21,24,28] A summary of surgical outcomes is presented in **Table 45.1**.

What Are the Most Common Postoperative Complications and Is There Any Difference between Endoscopic and Traditional Approaches?

Level I and Level II Evidence

No Level I or Level II studies exist on this subject matter.

Level III and Level IV Evidence

A summary of the most commonly encountered postoperative complications is shown in **Table 45.2**.

Chordomas are slow-growing neoplasms that often do not manifest clinically until extensive growth has occurred. Consequently, and because of their invasive behavior, by the time of surgery, skull base chordomas often surround the vasculature, cranial nerves, and other critical neural structures. Furthermore, depending on the size and location of the tumor, lateral temporal bone extension increases the risk of damaging cranial nerves because the lesions not only envelop critical neurovascular structures but also require lateral skull base approaches that involve navigating between neurovascular structures. Published series report a range of postsurgical cranial nerve deficits of 0 to 100% in patients undergoing an open procedure.[9,15,16,24,25,29–39] In patients undergoing an endoscopic endonasal resection, cranial nerve deficits were reported in 0 to 3% of patients.[7,11,40,41] This apparent discrepancy is likely a result of the difference in tumor sizes and not a result of the approach. Larger tumors (type II/III) typically extend laterally to envelop intervening neurovascular structures. They are much more likely to present with preoperative deficits and require operative approaches across the neurovascular structures. Hence the smaller, more midline lesions, which were traditionally approached through transfacial approaches and now via endoscopic approaches, are associated with a reduced incidence of postoperative cranial nerve deficits.

Although chordomas are primarily extradural tumors, CSF leakage and subsequent meningitis are a possible postoperative complication due to tumor invasion or surgical technique. Postoperative CSF leakage is reported in 10.7% (range, 0 to 50%) of patients undergoing open procedures and 5.0% (range, 0 to 25%) of patients undergoing an endonasal endoscopic approach.[7–9,11,17,29,30,34,40,41] The rate of postoperative meningitis is occasionally presented in the literature and is estimated to occur in 5.9% (range, 0 to 50%) of patients undergoing open surgery and 0.9% (range, 0 to 7%) of patients undergoing endoscopic endonasal resection.

The discussion of complications in the literature along with the development of new endoscopic approaches has triggered the discussion of the relative value of endoscopic versus open cranial base approaches. In a recent meta-analysis, Komotar et al[43] compared the outcomes of an endoscopic endonasal approach versus an open procedure for resection of skull base chordomas and found that the endoscopic endonasal approach was associated with a significantly lower incidence of postoperative cranial neuropathies. However, in their analysis, the authors also found a statistically significant difference in mean tumor volume between the open and endoscopic studies (57.9 cm^3 in the open cohort vs 30.5 cm^3 in the endoscopic studies, $p = 0.004$). Furthermore, there were increased rates of petrous invasion (49.7% vs 28.0%, $p = 0.006$) and dural involvement (65.2% vs 47.6%, $p = 0.004$) in the open studies. Although there were differences in complications and attempts have been made to attribute this to the approach, this noted effect is likely related to tumor size and anatomy. In assessing these studies, it is important to be cognizant of the limitations of meta-analyses.

Expert Recommendations

1. There is no significant difference in survival between different chordoma histologies (Grade 2B Recommendation, Level III Evidence).
2. Increasing extent of surgical resection has a positive impact on survival and should be the goal of surgery; however, there is no evidence to determine what the negative impact of a surgically incurred neurological deficit is (Grade 1C Recommendation, Level III Evidence).
3. The ideal approach for a lesion depends on the anatomy of the tumor, where either ventral endoscopic, open, or combined approaches may be necessary to achieve radical resection (Grade 1C Recommendation, Level III Evidence).

Table 45.2 Summary of surgical complications from published surgical series

Study	Level of evidence	Patients (*N*)	Approach	Meningitis (%)	Postoperative cranial nerve palsy (%)	CSF leaks (%)
Sekhar et al 1987[16]	III/IV	2	Open only	–	14	–
Uttley et al 1989[39]	III/IV	4	Open only	–	0	–
Blevins et al 1995[9]	III/IV	2	Open only	50	50	50
Gay et al 1995[24]	III/IV	46	Open only	10	80	–
Maira et al 1996[32]	III/IV	12	Open only	8	8	–
Menezes et al 1997[33]	III/IV	36	Open only	0	0	–
Sekhar et al 2001[35]	III/IV	42	Open only	–	33	–
Sen and Triana 2001[36]	III/IV	29	–	14	90	–
Mortini et al 2001[34]	III/IV	2	Open only	0	50	0
Tamaki et al 2001[38]	III/IV	17	Open only	–	6	–
Kyoshima et al 2003[31]	III/IV	3	Open only	–	100	–
Frank et al 2006[40]	III/IV	9	Endoscopic only	0	0	0
Stuer et al 2006[37]	III/IV	11	Open only	9	9	–
Tzortzidis et al 2006[25]	III/IV	74	Open only	–	4	–
Samii et al 2007[15]	III/IV	49	Open only	–	28	–
Al-Mefty et al 2008[7]	III/IV	38	Endoscopic only	0	3	8
Dehdashti et al 2008[11]	III/IV	12	Endoscopic only	0	0	0
Fatemi et al 2008[12]	III/IV	14	Endoscopic only	7	–	–
Takahashi et al 2009[42]	III/IV	32	Open only	7	–	–
Arbolay et al 2009[8]	III/IV	2	Endoscopic only	0	–	0
Stippler et al 2009[17]	III/IV	20	Endoscopic only	0	–	25
Choi et al 2010[29]	III/IV	97	Open only	3	2	6
Ito et al 2010[30]	III/IV	19	Open/endoscopic	0	16	5
Wu et al 2010[10]	III/IV	106	Open only	–	65	–
Fraser et al 2010[41]	III/IV	7	Endoscopic only	0	0	0
Koutourousiou et al 2011[44]	III/IV	60	Endoscopic only	3.3	6.7	20
Yasuda et al 2012[45]	III/IV	11	Open/endoscopic	–	–	55
Di Maio et al 2012[46]	III/IV	95	Open/endoscopic	9	–	11
Holzmann et al 2010[47]	III/IV	13	Endoscopic only	–	–	8
Taniguchi et al 2012[48]	III/IV	4	Endoscopic only	0	25	25

Abbreviation: CSF, cerebrospinal fluid.

■ Summary and Conclusions

Chordomas represent a class of intrinsic skull base malignancies that arise truly from the bony skull base and are invasive in nature, invading different anatomical compartments of the skull base and enveloping critical neurovascular structures. Aside from their anatomical aggressiveness, their malignant biological behavior (with an increased risk of subsequent metastases and CSF seeding) mandates multimodality treatment with surgery and charged particle therapy. With the relatively rare prevalence of this disease and the lack of centralized care of these patients, no Level I or II studies exist addressing the role of surgery in this patient population. Several Level III/IV studies with well-executed multivariate analyses exist clearly demonstrating the radicality of resection as a prognostic factor influencing survival. In the midst of the evolution of numerous skull base approaches, there has been an attempt in the literature to determine if open or endoscopic approaches are best suited to manage these difficult tumors, based on a retrospective comparison of complication rates. These studies are flawed not only by their retrospective nature and selection bias but also by the clearly documented difference in tumor sizes and anatomical complexity. It is likely that the best approach for purely midline lesions is a ventral endoscopic approach, whereas those lesions with lateral extension beyond the neurovascular structures require either a pure open approach or a staged approach.

■ References

1. Burger PCSB, Vogel SF. Surgical Pathology of the Nervous System and Its Coverings. 3rd ed. New York, NY: Churchill Livingstone; 1991
2. Crockard HA, Steel T, Plowman N, et al. A multidisciplinary team approach to skull base chordomas. J Neurosurg 2001; 95(2):175–183
3. Feigl GC, Bundschuh O, Gharabaghi A, et al. Evaluation of a new concept for the management of skull base chordomas and chondrosarcomas. J Neurosurg 2005;102(Suppl):165–170
4. Chugh R, Tawbi H, Lucas DR, Biermann JS, Schuetze SM, Baker LH. Chordoma: the nonsarcoma primary bone tumor. Oncologist 2007;12(11):1344–1350
5. Sekhar LNRJ, Schessel DA. The Presigmoid Petrosal Approach. New York, NY: Thieme; 1999
6. Al-Mefty O, Borba LA. Skull base chordomas: a management challenge. J Neurosurg 1997;86(2):182–189
7. Al-Mefty O, Kadri PA, Hasan DM, Isolan GR, Pravdenkova S. Anterior clivectomy: surgical technique and clinical applications. J Neurosurg 2008;109(5):783–793
8. Arbolay OL, González JG, González RH, Gálvez YH. Extended endoscopic endonasal approach to the skull base. Minim Invasive Neurosurg 2009;52(3):114–118
9. Blevins NH, Jackler RK, Kaplan MJ, Gutin PH. Combined transpetrosal-subtemporal craniotomy for clival tumors with extension into the posterior fossa. Laryngoscope 1995;105(9 Pt 1): 975–982
10. Wu Z, Zhang J, Jia G, et al. Prognostic factors for long-term outcome of patients with surgical resection of skull base chordomas—106 cases review in one institution. Neurosurg Rev 2010;33(4):451–456
11. Dehdashti AR, Karabatsou K, Ganna A, Witterick I, Gentili F. Expanded endoscopic endonasal approach for treatment of clival chordomas: early results in 12 patients. Neurosurgery 2008;63(2):299–307
12. Fatemi N, Dusick JR, Gorgulho AA, et al. Endonasal microscopic removal of clival chordomas. Surg Neurol 2008;69(4): 331–338
13. Hsu W, Kosztowski TA, Zaidi HA, Gokaslan ZL, Wolinsky JP. Image-guided, endoscopic, transcervical resection of cervical chordoma. J Neurosurg Spine 2010;12(4):431–435
14. McGirt MJ, Attenello FJ, Sciubba DM, Gokaslan ZL, Wolinsky JP. Endoscopic transcervical odontoidectomy for pediatric basilar invagination and cranial settling. Report of 4 cases. J Neurosurg Pediatr 2008;1(4):337–342
15. Samii A, Gerganov VM, Herold C, et al. Chordomas of the skull base: surgical management and outcome. J Neurosurg 2007;107(2):319–324
16. Sekhar LN, Schramm VL Jr, Jones NF. Subtemporal-preauricular infratemporal fossa approach to large lateral and posterior cranial base neoplasms. J Neurosurg 1987;67(4):488–499
17. Stippler M, Gardner PA, Snyderman CH, Carrau RL, Prevedello DM, Kassam AB. Endoscopic endonasal approach for clival chordomas. Neurosurgery 2009;64(2):268–277
18. Singh H, Harrop J, Schiffmacher P, Rosen M, Evans J. Ventral surgical approaches to craniovertebral junction chordomas. Neurosurgery 2010;66(3, Suppl):96–103
19. Heffelfinger MJ, Dahlin DC, MacCarty CS, Beabout JW. Chordomas and cartilaginous tumors at the skull base. Cancer 1973;32(2):410–420
20. Mitchell A, Scheithauer BW, Unni KK, Forsyth PJ, Wold LE, McGivney DJ. Chordoma and chondroid neoplasms of the spheno-occiput: an immunohistochemical study of 41 cases with prognostic and nosologic implications. Cancer 1993; 72(10):2943–2949
21. Forsyth PA, Cascino TL, Shaw EG, et al. Intracranial chordomas: a clinicopathological and prognostic study of 51 cases. J Neurosurg 1993;78(5):741–747
22. Colli BO, Al-Mefty O. Chordomas of the skull base: follow-up review and prognostic factors. Neurosurg Focus 2001; 10(3):E1
23. Jian BJ, Bloch OG, Yang I, Han SJ, Aranda D, Parsa AT. A comprehensive analysis of intracranial chordoma and survival: a systematic review. Br J Neurosurg 2011;25(4):446–453
24. Gay E, Sekhar LN, Rubinstein E, et al. Chordomas and chondrosarcomas of the cranial base: results and follow-up of 60 patients. Neurosurgery 1995;36(5):887–896
25. Tzortzidis F, Elahi F, Wright D, Natarajan SK, Sekhar LN. Patient outcome at long-term follow-up after aggressive microsurgical resection of cranial base chordomas. Neurosurgery 2006;59(2):230–237
26. Watkins L, Khudados ES, Kaleoglu M, Revesz T, Sacares P, Crockard HA. Skull base chordomas: a review of 38 patients, 1958-88. Br J Neurosurg 1993;7(3):241–248
27. Sen C, Triana AI, Berglind N, Godbold J, Shrivastava RK. Clival chordomas: clinical management, results, and complications in 71 patients. J Neurosurg 2010;113(5):1059–1071
28. Benk V, Liebsch NJ, Munzenrider JE, Efird J, McManus P, Suit H. Base of skull and cervical spine chordomas in children treated by high-dose irradiation. Int J Radiat Oncol Biol Phys 1995; 31(3):577–581
29. Choi D, Melcher R, Harms J, Crockard A. Outcome of 132 operations in 97 patients with chordomas of the craniocervical junction and upper cervical spine. Neurosurgery 2010; 66(1):59–65

30. Ito E, Saito K, Okada T, Nagatani T, Nagasaka T. Long-term control of clival chordoma with initial aggressive surgical resection and gamma knife radiosurgery for recurrence. Acta Neurochir (Wien) 2010;152(1):57–67
31. Kyoshima K, Oikawa S, Kanaji M, et al. Repeat operations in the management of clival chordomas: palliative surgery. J Clin Neurosci 2003;10(5):571–578
32. Maira G, Pallini R, Anile C, et al. Surgical treatment of clival chordomas: the transsphenoidal approach revisited. J Neurosurg 1996;85(5):784–792
33. Menezes AH, Gantz BJ, Traynelis VC, McCulloch TM. Cranial base chordomas. Clin Neurosurg 1997;44:491–509
34. Mortini P, Mandelli C, Franzin A, Giugni E, Giovanelli M. Surgical excision of clival tumors via the enlarged transcochlear approach. Indications and results. J Neurosurg Sci 2001; 45(3):127–139
35. Sekhar LN, Pranatartiharan R, Chanda A, Wright DC. Chordomas and chondrosarcomas of the skull base: results and complications of surgical management. Neurosurg Focus 2001; 10(3):E2
36. Sen C, Triana A. Cranial chordomas: results of radical excision. Neurosurg Focus 2001;10(3):E3
37. Stüer C, Schramm J, Schaller C. Skull base chordomas: management and results. Neurol Med Chir (Tokyo) 2006; 46(3):118–124
38. Tamaki N, Nagashima T, Ehara K, Motooka Y, Barua KK. Surgical approaches and strategies for skull base chordomas. Neurosurg Focus 2001;10(3):E9
39. Uttley D, Moore A, Archer DJ. Surgical management of midline skull-base tumors: a new approach. J Neurosurg 1989;71(5 Pt 1): 705–710
40. Frank G, Sciarretta V, Calbucci F, Farneti G, Mazzatenta D, Pasquini E. The endoscopic transnasal transsphenoidal approach for the treatment of cranial base chordomas and chondrosarcomas. Neurosurgery 2006;59(1, Suppl 1):ONS50–ONS57
41. Fraser JF, Nyquist GG, Moore N, Anand VK, Schwartz TH. Endoscopic endonasal transclival resection of chordomas: operative technique, clinical outcome, and review of the literature. J Neurosurg 2010;112(5):1061–1069
42. Takahashi S, Kawase T, Yoshida K, Hasegawa A, Mizoe JE. Skull base chordomas: efficacy of surgery followed by carbon ion radiotherapy. Acta Neurochir (Wien) 2009;151(7):759–769
43. Komotar RJ, Starke RM, Raper DM, Anand VK, Schwartz TH. The endoscope-assisted ventral approach compared with open microscope-assisted surgery for clival chordomas. World Neurosurg 2011;76(3-4):318–327
44. Koutourousiou M, Gardner PA, Tormenti MJ, et al. Endoscopic endonasal approach for resection of cranial base chordomas: outcomes and learning curve. Neurosurgery 2012; 71(3):614–624
45. Yasuda M, Bresson D, Chibbaro S, et al. Chordomas of the skull base and cervical spine: clinical outcomes associated with a multimodal surgical resection combined with proton-beam radiation in 40 patients. Neurosurg Rev 2012;35(2):171–182
46. Di Maio S, Rostomily R, Sekhar LN. Current surgical outcomes for cranial base chordomas: cohort study of 95 patients. Neurosurgery 2012:70(6):1335–1360
47. Holzmann D, Reisch R, Krayenbuhl N, et al. The transnasal transclival approach for clivus chordoma. Minim Invasive Neurosurg 2010;53(5–6):211–217
48. Taniguchi M, Kohmura E. Endoscopic endonasal removal of laterally extended clival chordoma using side-viewing scopes. Acta Neurochir (Wien) 2012;154(4):627–632

46

Radiosurgery and Fractionated Radiotherapy Techniques for Chordomas

Hideyuki Kano, Douglas Kondziolka, and L. Dade Lunsford

Chordomas arise from embryonic remnants of notochord and show a dual epithelial-mesenchymal differentiation. Microscopic foci remain in the vertebral bodies at the cranial and caudal ends of the embryo.[1] They arise from the sacrococcygeal region in 50 to 60%, from the skull base region in 25 to 35%, and from the vertebrae in 15%.[2] Although chordomas are considered generally within the benign spectrum of rare skull base tumors, they in fact behave like malignant tumors because of invasive histopathology, regional bone destruction, high recurrence rates, and, in rare circumstances, the potential to metastasize. The natural history of untreated clival chordomas is dismal, with a mean survival of less than 1 year.[3] Neurological deficits tend to vary based on the location of the tumor. An abducens nerve deficit causing diplopia is the most frequent presenting sign.[4,5]

The Clinical Quandary

Aggressive initial management, beginning with radical resection when possible and followed by fractionated radiotherapy (RT) or radiosurgery, improves overall outcome.[6] Recent advances in imaging techniques play an important role in improving the prognosis for chordoma. Earlier recognition of smaller-volume, even intraosseous, tumors[7–10] facilitates aggressive therapy. Unfortunately complete resection of a chordoma without significant morbidity is rarely feasible. Because these tumors tend to encase critical vessels and cranial nerves or adhere to the brainstem, complete resection remains challenging even for experienced neurosurgeons.[11–15] The recurrence rate, even after gross total resection, remains high (44% at a mean of 96 month follow-up).[16,17] Recurrent tumors present even more challenging management options and clearly have worse overall outcomes. Aggressive surgery followed by adjuvant radiation of some type may reduce chordoma recurrence.

Radiotherapy for Chordomas

Chordomas are considered "radioresistant" tumors that require total fractionated RT doses in excess of 60 Gy to reduce recurrence rates.[1] However, such doses delivered by conventional conformal photon RT may exceed the tolerance of critical vascular and neurological structures adjacent to the tumor. The brainstem and optic pathway are at risk in view of the usual anatomical location of intracranial chordomas arising from notochord rests at the skull base. Total fractionated doses between 60 and 65 Gy are thought to improve tumor control (**Table 46.1**).[18–20] Even higher doses have been favored by some authors.[21–25]

Using the principle of Bragg peak fractionated RT, charged particle radiation delivered by protons or carbon ions is thought by some to deliver a more radiobiologically potent dose to the tumor while re-

Table 46.1 Studies and patient characteristics in published series of chordoma treated with conventional photon radiotherapy

Study	N	Histology	Radiation	Dose (Gy)	Median tumor diameter	% LC	% Survival	Median follow-up (months)
Romero et al 1993[19]	18	Ch	Ph	50.1 (29.9 to 64.8)	NA	5-year: 17	5-year: 38	NA
Catton et al 1996[18]	48	Ch	Ph	50 (25 to 60)	NA	5-year: 23	5-year: 54	62
Zorlu et al 2000[20]	18	Ch	Ph	60 (50 to 64)	5 cm (3 to 7)	5-year: 23	5-year: 35	43

Abbreviations: Ch, chordoma; LC, local control; NA, not available; Ph, photons.

ducing the dose to surrounding structures that are medial to the targeted tumor. The Bragg peak effect results in a rapid energy deposition at the target volume with a steep drop-off of dose beyond the target volume treated.[26] With proton beam RT, doses above 70 cobalt Gray equivalent (CGE) are prescribed. (CGE is an empirical measure of estimated radiation effect obtained by multiplying the conventional photon radiation dose in Gy by 1.2, a value that has been postulated as the potential radibiological advantage of proton Bragg peak RT.)

Level I and Level II Evidence

There are no Level I or Level II evidence studies comparing photon irradiation to proton RT.

Level III and Level IV Evidence

Published data indicate that experienced centers may achieve local tumor control rates at 3 years of 67 to 88%, at 5 years in the range of 46 to 73%, and at 10 years of 54%. The overall survival rates are 67 to 81% at 5 years and 54% at 10 years.[27] Such results are potentially superior to the results reported after conventional photon RT for chordomas.[26] Using carbon ion therapy, Castro et al treated 53 patients with doses of 60 to 80 CGE. They reported 5-year local tumor control and overall survival rates of 63% and 75%, respectively.[28] Schulz-Ertner et al[29] reported that 96 chordoma patients who underwent carbon ion RT obtained a 5-year local tumor control and overall survival rates of 70% and 88.5%, respectively. Late toxicity consisted of optic nerve neuropathy Radiotherapy Oncology Group/European Organization for Research and Treatment of Cancer (RTOG/EORTC) grade 3 in 4.1% of the patients. Minor temporal lobe injury (RTOG/EORTC grade 1 to 2) occurred in 7.2% of the patients (**Table 46.2**).

Noël et al[30] reported the results of combined photon and proton RT in 90 patients with either chordomas ($N = 64$) or chondrosarcomas ($N = 26$) of the skull base. The tumors were treated to a median total dose of 67 CGE (range, 22 to 70 CGE). Photons represented two thirds of the total delivered dose and protons represented one third. At a median follow-up of 34 months, local tumor control was achieved in 65 patients (72%). All 90 patients developed immediate adverse radiation effects, usually mild. However, 6% reported late grade 3 or 4 radiation toxicities including cranial nerve deficits and visual loss. Proton fractionated RT remains a relatively expensive strategy that is available in a limited but increasing number of facilities both in the United States and abroad (**Table 46.3**).

Stereotactic Radiosurgery for Chordomas

Stereotactic radiosurgery (SRS) using the Leksell Gamma Knife (Elekta, Atlanta, GA) is a surgical procedure that delivers cross-fired photon radiation generated from the decay of cobalt-60 sources in a single-wheels-in to wheels-out procedure. This is feasible because of the combination of stereotactic head frame application and high-resolution intraoperative magnetic resonance imaging (MRI) that is used to define the target after frame application. High-speed computer systems facilitate rapid radiosurgical planning. The patient is placed in the center of 192 to 201 cross-fired ionizing beams of photon radiation that are precisely delivered to the target with a sharp dose gradient outside the target volume. Using linear accelerator technologies such as the Cyberknife (Accuray, Sunnyvale, CA), SRS may be delivered in up to five treatment sessions. Delivery of such highly focused radiation in one to five sessions significantly increases the radiobiological effect of SRS compared with conventional fractionated RT. Using methods to evaluate radiobiological effects

Table 46.2 Studies and patient characteristics in published series of chordoma treated with proton radiotherapy

Study	N	Histology	Radiation	Dose (CGE)	Tumor volume	% LC	% Survival	ARE	Median follow-up (mo)
Weber et al 2005[25]	18	Ch (16), chond. C (2)	P	74 (63–95)	16.4 mL	3-year: 87	3-year: 94	Late toxicity: Gr 2 pituitary dysfunction: 1	29
Schulz-Ertner et al 2007[29]	96	Ch	P	60 (60–70)	80.3 mL: planning target volume (gross tumor volume adding a 2 mm margin)	5-year: 70	5-year: 88.5	Gr 3 optic neuropathy: 4.1%, Gr 1 and 2 temporal necrosis: 7.2%	31
Ares et al 2009[38]	42	Ch	P	73.5 (67–74)	≤ 25 mL: 24, > 25 mL: 18	3-year: 87 5-year: 81	5-year: 62	Optic neuropathy: Gr 3 = 1, Gr 4 = 1, symptomatic temporal lobe necrosis Gr 3 = 2	38

Abbreviations: ARE, adverse radiation effect; CGE, cobalt gray equivalent; Ch, chordoma; chond. C, chondroid chordoma; CN, cranial nerve; Gr, grade of RTOG/EORTC toxicity criteria or the National Cancer Institute Common Terminology Criteria for Adverse Events (CTCAE); LC, local control; P, protons.

Table 46.3 Studies and patient characteristics in published series of chordoma treated with combined proton and photon radiotherapy

Study	N	Histology	Radiation	Dose (CGE)	Tumor volume	% LC	% Survival	ARE	Median follow-up (mo)
Hug et al 2002[39]	33	Ch	P + Ph	71.9 (66.6 to 79.2)	> 25 mL: 26 (79%)	3-year: 67 5-year: 59	3-year: 87 5-year: 79	Late toxicity Gr 3 to 4: 7%	33
Munzenrider et al 1999[27]	169	Ch (69%), chond. C (31%)	P + Ph	66 to 83	NA	5-year: 73 10-year:54	5-year: 80 10-year:54	5-year-temporal lobe injury: 13%; optic neuropathy: 4.4%; hearing loss: 15/33 patients evaluated; cranial nerve injury: 5%; endocrine dysfunction: 32/79 patients evaluated	41
Igaki et al 2004[21]	13	Ch	P + Ph	72.0 (63 to 95)	33.7 mL	3-year: 67 5-year: 46	3-year: 85	No acute toxicity; late Gr 4 brain necrosis: 1; Gr 4 oral ulceration: 1; Gr 5 brain necrosis: 1	69
Noël et al 2005[22]	100	Ch	P + Ph	67 (60 to 71)	23 mL	2-year:86 4-year: 53	2-year: 94 5-year: 81	Optic neuropathy: 8%; neuropsychological disorders: 11%; minor temporal lobe necroses: 1%; hearing loss: 21%; pituitary dysfunction: 9% (complete), 8% (partial)	29

Abbreviations: ARE, adverse radiation effect; CGE, cobalt gray equivalent; Ch, chordoma; CN, cranial nerve; chond. C, chondroid chordoma; Gr, grade of RTOG/EORTC toxicity criteria or the National Cancer Institute Common Terminology Criteria for Adverse Events (CTCAE); LC, local control; NA, not available; P, protons; Ph, photons.

Table 46.4 Studies and patient characteristics in published series of chordoma treated with stereotactic radiosurgery

Study	N	Histology	Radiation	Dose (CGE)	Tumor volume	% LC	% Survival	ARE	Median follow-up (months)
Krishnan et al 2005[35]	25	Ch (19), chond. C (6)	SRS ± EBRT	15 Gy (10 to 20) ± 50.4 Gy (45 to 54)	14.4 mL	4-year (Ch): 55; 4-year (chond. C): 100	NA	No radiation necrosis for SRS-alone patients, 34% (*N* = 10) of chordomas and chordrosarcomas (total *N* = 29) had symptomatic radiation effects	58
Hasegawa et al 2007[34]	27	Ch	SRS	14 Gy (9 to 20)	19.7 mL	5-year: 72 10-year: 72	5-year: 84 10-year: 67	Worsened facial numbness = 1	59
Liu et al 2008[37]	31	Ch	SRS	12.7 Gy (10 to 16)	11.4 mL	3-year: 64 5-year: 21	3-year: 91 5-year: 76	No serious radiation effects	28
Kano et al 2011[40]	71	Ch	SRS ± Ph	15 Gy (9 to 25)	7.1 mL	3-year: 79 5-year: 66	5-year: 80 7-year: 69	CN VI: Gr 2 = 2, CN VII: Gr 2 = 1, CN V + VI: Gr 3 = 1, pituitary dysfunction: Gr 2 = 2	60

Abbreviations: ARE, adverse radiation effect; CGE, cobalt gray equivalent; Ch, chordoma; CN, cranial nerve; chond. C, chondroid chordoma; EBRT, external beam radiotherapy; Gr, grade of RTOG/EORTC toxicity criteria or the National Cancer Institute Common Terminology Criteria for Adverse Events (CTCAE); LC, local control; Ph, photons; SRS, stereotactic radiosurgery.

(e.g., the integrated logistic formula[31–33]), the center of the tumor may receive a radiobiological effect four times what can be safely delivered using conventional fractionated or even intensity-modulated radiotherapy (IMRT). Most published literature sources related to chordoma RT techniques provide at best Level III outcome data. In addition, many studies continue to include both chordoma and chondrosarcoma cases in the same outcome analysis. There are more U.S. centers that can offer LINAC-based SRS or gamma knife radiosurgery than there are centers offering charged-particle RT. Therefore, each SRS center may have fewer cases due to the rarity of disease. Charged-particle RT centers may have more cases due to referral patterns, especially for larger tumors, and they may have longer follow-up.

Level I and Level II Evidence

There are no Level I or Level II evidence studies comparing photon or proton RT to SRS.

Level III and Level IV Evidence

SRS has been proposed as a minimally invasive alternative management option for chordomas.[34–36] It is especially useful for the treatment of relatively small residual or recurrent chordomas that remain after surgical resection. In some cases it is used to deliver a focused boost to a residual or new tumor volume. Radiosurgery has often been used in combination with, or as a boost to, conventional RT or IMRT. Krishnan et al[35] treated 25 cranial base chordoma patients with a median marginal radiosurgical dose of 15 Gy. They reported the 5-year in-field local tumor control and in-field and out-of-field tumor control rates of 52% and 32%, respectively, at median follow-up of 4.5 years. A tumor margin dose of ≥ 15 Gy was significantly associated with longer in-field tumor control. Ten (34%) of 29 patients (chordoma: *N* = 25, chondrosarcoma: *N* = 4) had adverse radiation effects (AREs), including cranial nerve deficits (*N* = 6), radiation necrosis (*N* = 5), and pituitary dysfunction (*N* = 3). Patients having SRS alone had no AREs (**Table 46.4**).

Hasegawa et al[34] performed SRS on 27 chordoma patients with median tumor margin doses of 14 Gy. They noted 5-year local tumor control and overall survival rates of 42% and 80%, respectively, at median follow-up of 59 months. In their series, only tumor volumes of < 20 mL were significantly associated with a longer progression-free survival (PFS). One patient had adverse radiation effects (facial sensory loss).

Liu et al[37] reported 28 residual skull base chordoma patients who underwent SRS with a median margin dose of 12.7 Gy. The average follow-up was

28 months and the mean tumor volume was 11.4 ± 7.4 mL. The 5-year overall survival and in-field tumor control rates were 75.8% and 21.4%, respectively. No serious AREs were reported. Their outcome study revealed lower tumor control rates but less risk of AREs. **Table 46.1** presents the published results of SRS.[22,25,27,34,37–40] These Level III data support the use of SRS as a reasonable adjuvant treatment option for selected patients with residual or recurrent chordomas after initial surgery. The initial surgical procedure goal should be to remove as much tumor as safely possible, including infiltrated bone. Aggressive but safe removal of tumors around radiosensitive structures, such as the optic apparatus and brainstem, is essential for obtaining long-term tumor control.

The North American Gamma Knife Consortium Retrospective Study for Chordomas

The North American Gamma Knife Consortium (NAGKC) was established to evaluate outcomes of selected clinical indications that are relatively rare (e.g., chordomas, chondrosarcomas, hemangioblastomas, glomus tumors) and to facilitate prospective clinical trials. Kano et al[40] reported that six participating centers of the NAGKC identified 71 patients who underwent gamma knife SRS for chordomas (**Fig. 46.1**). The median patient age was 45 years (range, 7 to 80). The median SRS target volume was 7.1 mL (range, 0.9 to 109.0), and the median tumor margin dose was 15.0 Gy (range, 9 to 25). At a median follow-up of 5 years after SRS (range, 0.6 to 14.0), 23 patients had died due to tumor progression. The 5-year actuarial overall survival after SRS for the entire group was 80%. Tumor control was higher (93%) in patients who had not undergone prior fractionated RT ($N = 50$). Tumor control was reduced to 43% in patients who underwent prior RT ($N = 21$). Factors associated with longer patient survival included younger age, longer interval between initial diagnosis and SRS, no prior RT, fewer than two cranial nerve deficits, and smaller total tumor volumes. The 5-year treated tumor control rates after SRS for the entire group was 66% (69% for the no prior RT group and 62% for the prior RT group).

Significant factors associated with reduced tumor control included older age, recurrent tumors, prior RT, and larger tumor volumes. Seventeen (30%) of 57 patients with pretreatment neurological deficits had neurological improvement. Thirty-one (48%) of 65 patients with clinical follow-up remained stable, but 17 (26%) eventually had deterioration in neurological function. In eight patients deterioration was due to treated tumor progression, in three patients it was related to adjacent tumor progression, in four patients it was related to treatment-associated AREs, and in two patients it was related to both treated tumor progression and AREs.

The improvement rate of cranial nerve deficits (between 22 and 50%) after SRS varied depending on the cranial nerves involved. Improvement in diplopia (the most common presenting cranial nerve deficit) occurred in two (22%) of nine patients with oculomotor neuropathy, three (50%) of six patients with trochlear neuropathy, and 13 (33%) of 40 patients with abducens neuropathy. AREs occurred in six patients (9%) at an interval that ranged from 2.7 to 12.0 months. Two patients developed abducens neuropathy (RTOG/EORTC grade 2), one developed a facial neuropathy (grade 2), and one developed both trigeminal and abducens neuropathies (grade 3) after SRS. Two patients developed anterior pituitary dysfunction (grade 3), likely related to AREs. All patients who developed AREs also had undergone RT.

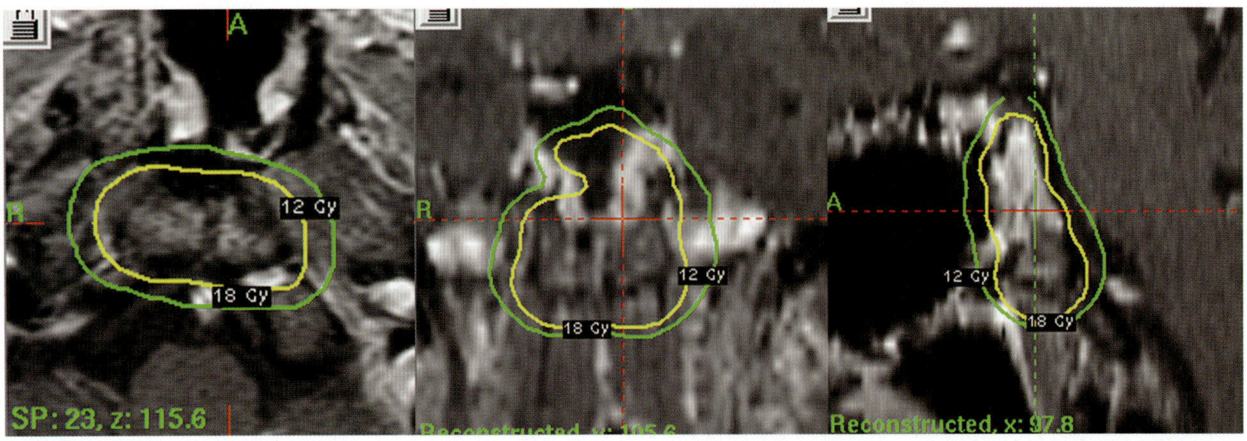

Fig. 46.1 Axial (left), coronal (middle), and sagittal (right) T1-weighted contrast-enhanced magnetic resonance images showing at stereotactic radiosurgery for residual chordoma after surgical resection. RT, fractionated radiotherapy; SRS, stereotactic radiosurgery.

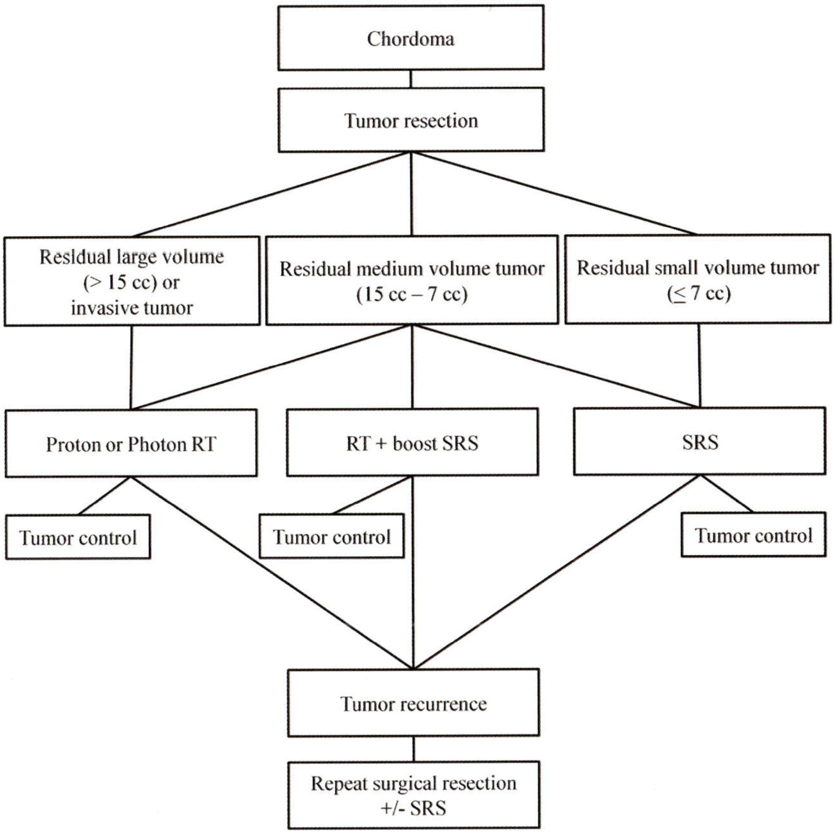

Fig. 46.2 Treatment algorithm proposed for the management of chordomas.

We concluded that SRS provided a reasonable benefit-to-risk profile for patients with skull base chordomas. Tumor control and survival may be enhanced by maximal planned surgical resection to reduce tumor volume followed by early SRS. SRS is a potent treatment option with lower morbidity rates for small to medium-sized chordomas and can be applied as shown in a potential treatment algorithm (**Fig. 46.2**).

Expert Recommendations

1. Use of radiosurgery for small chordoma (≤ 7 mL) after subtotal resection is comparable to photon and proton RT (Grade 1C Recommendation, Level III/IV Evidence).
2. Use of RT and boost radiosurgery for medium-sized chordoma (7 to 15 mL) is recommended (Grade 1C Recommendation, Level III/IV Evidence).
3. Use of photon or proton RT for large chordoma (≥ 15 mL) after resection is recommended (Grade 1C Recommendation, Level III/IV Evidence).
4. Radiosurgery can be used for recurrent chordoma after RT (Grade 1C Recommendation, Level III/IV Evidence).

Summary and Conclusions

Maximal safe resection should be the primary initial management of chordomas. After recovery from surgery, fractionated Bragg peak proton RT continues to be advocated at some centers because of potential improvement in the radiobiologic effectiveness during treatment of rare tumors like chordoma. Careful planning and reduction of dose delivered to adjacent critical structures are potential advantages of both particle beam and modern fractionated photon radiation techniques. Long-term evaluation of neurocognitive effects is warranted because of the relatively higher dose that may be delivered via the entrance pathway within the temporal lobes. SRS after surgical resection also provides a reasonable benefit-to-risk profile for small to medium-sized chordomas. SRS is an important option for patients with recurrent tumors that have failed initial surgical resection and adjuvant RT.

■ References

1. Chugh R, Tawbi H, Lucas DR, Biermann JS, Schuetze SM, Baker LH. Chordoma: the nonsarcoma primary bone tumor. Oncologist 2007;12(11):1344–1350
2. Heffelfinger MJ, Dahlin DC, MacCarty CS, Beabout JW. Chordomas and cartilaginous tumors at the skull base. Cancer 1973;32(2):410–420
3. Eriksson B, Gunterberg B, Kindblom LG. Chordoma. A clinicopathologic and prognostic study of a Swedish national series. Acta Orthop Scand 1981;52(1):49–58
4. Nishigaya K, Kaneko M, Ohashi Y, Nukui H. Intradural retroclival chordoma without bone involvement: no tumor regrowth 5 years after operation. Case report. J Neurosurg 1998;88(4):764–768
5. Weber AL, Liebsch NJ, Sanchez R, Sweriduk ST Jr. Chordomas of the skull base. Radiologic and clinical evaluation. Neuroimaging Clin N Am 1994;4(3):515–527
6. Carpentier A, Polivka M, Blanquet A, Lot G, George B. Suboccipital and cervical chordomas: the value of aggressive treatment at first presentation of the disease. J Neurosurg 2002;97(5):1070–1077
7. Anegawa T, Rai M, Hara K, et al. An unusual cervical chordoma: CT and MRI. Neuroradiology 1996;38(5):466–467
8. Ducou le Pointe H, Brugieres P, Chevalier X, Meder JF, Voisin MC, Gaston A. Imaging of chordomas of the mobile spine. J Neuroradiol 1991;18(3):267–276
9. Murphy JM, Wallis F, Toland J, Toner M, Wilson GF. CT and MRI appearances of a thoracic chordoma. Eur Radiol 1998;8(9):1677–1679
10. Smolders D, Wang X, Drevelengas A, Vanhoenacker F, De Schepper AM. Value of MRI in the diagnosis of non-clival, non-sacral chordoma. Skeletal Radiol 2003;32(6):343–350
11. al-Mefty O, Borba LA. Skull base chordomas: a management challenge. J Neurosurg 1997;86(2):182–189
12. Gay E, Sekhar LN, Rubinstein E, et al. Chordomas and chondrosarcomas of the cranial base: results and follow-up of 60 patients. Neurosurgery 1995;36(5):887–896
13. Maira G, Pallini R, Anile C, et al. Surgical treatment of clival chordomas: the transsphenoidal approach revisited. J Neurosurg 1996;85(5):784–792
14. Sen CN, Sekhar LN, Schramm VL, Janecka IP. Chordoma and chondrosarcoma of the cranial base: an 8-year experience. Neurosurgery 1989;25(6):931–940
15. Uttley D, Moore A, Archer DJ. Surgical management of midline skull-base tumors: a new approach. J Neurosurg 1989;71(5Pt1):705–710
16. Menezes AH, Gantz BJ, Traynelis VC, McCulloch TM. Cranial base chordomas. Clin Neurosurg 1997;44:491–509
17. Tzortzidis F, Elahi F, Wright D, Natarajan SK, Sekhar LN. Patient outcome at long-term follow-up after aggressive microsurgical resection of cranial base chordomas. Neurosurgery 2006;59(2):230–237
18. Catton C, O'Sullivan B, Bell R, et al. Chordoma: long-term follow-up after radical photon irradiation. Radiother Oncol 1996;41(1):67–72
19. Romero J, Cardenes H, la Torre A, et al. Chordoma: results of radiation therapy in eighteen patients. Radiother Oncol 1993;29(1):27–32
20. Zorlu F, Gürkaynak M, Yildiz F, Oge K, Atahan IL. Conventional external radiotherapy in the management of clivus chordomas with overt residual disease. Neurol Sci 2000;21(4):203–207
21. Igaki H, Tokuuye K, Okumura T, et al. Clinical results of proton beam therapy for skull base chordoma. Int J Radiat Oncol Biol Phys 2004;60(4):1120–1126
22. Noël G, Feuvret L, Calugaru V, et al. Chordomas of the base of the skull and upper cervical spine. One hundred patients irradiated by a 3D conformal technique combining photon and proton beams. Acta Oncol 2005;44(7):700–708
23. Schulz-Ertner D, Nikoghosyan A, Thilmann C, et al. Results of carbon ion radiotherapy in 152 patients. Int J Radiat Oncol Biol Phys 2004;58(2):631–640
24. Terahara A, Niemierko A, Goitein M, et al. Analysis of the relationship between tumor dose inhomogeneity and local control in patients with skull base chordoma. Int J Radiat Oncol Biol Phys 1999;45(2):351–358
25. Weber DC, Rutz HP, Pedroni ES, et al. Results of spot-scanning proton radiation therapy for chordoma and chondrosarcoma of the skull base: the Paul Scherrer Institut experience. Int J Radiat Oncol Biol Phys 2005;63(2):401–409
26. Amichetti M, Cianchetti M, Amelio D, Enrici RM, Minniti G. Proton therapy in chordoma of the base of the skull: a systematic review. Neurosurg Rev 2009;32(4):403–416
27. Munzenrider JE, Liebsch NJ. Proton therapy for tumors of the skull base. Strahlenther Onkol 1999;175(Suppl 2):57–63
28. Castro JR, Linstadt DE, Bahary JP, et al. Experience in charged particle irradiation of tumors of the skull base: 1977-1992. Int J Radiat Oncol Biol Phys 1994;29(4):647–655
29. Schulz-Ertner D, Karger CP, Feuerhake A, et al. Effectiveness of carbon ion radiotherapy in the treatment of skull-base chordomas. Int J Radiat Oncol Biol Phys 2007;68(2):449–457
30. Noël G, Feuvret L, Ferrand R, Boisserie G, Mazeron JJ, Habrand JL. Radiotherapeutic factors in the management of cervical-basal chordomas and chondrosarcomas. Neurosurgery 2004;55(6):1252–1260
31. Flickinger JC. An integrated logistic formula for prediction of complications from radiosurgery. Int J Radiat Oncol Biol Phys 1989;17(4):879–885
32. Flickinger JC, Lunsford LD, Kondziolka D. Dose-volume considerations in radiosurgery. Stereotact Funct Neurosurg 1991;57(1-2):99–105
33. Flickinger JC, Schell MC, Larson DA. Estimation of complications for linear accelerator radiosurgery with the integrated logistic formula. Int J Radiat Oncol Biol Phys 1990;19(1):143–148
34. Hasegawa T, Ishii D, Kida Y, Yoshimoto M, Koike J, Iizuka H. Gamma Knife surgery for skull base chordomas and chondrosarcomas. J Neurosurg 2007;107(4):752–757
35. Krishnan S, Foote RL, Brown PD, Pollock BE, Link MJ, Garces YI. Radiosurgery for cranial base chordomas and chondrosarcomas. Neurosurgery 2005;56(4):777–784
36. Martin JJ, Niranjan A, Kondziolka D, Flickinger JC, Lozanne KA, Lunsford LD. Radiosurgery for chordomas and chondrosarcomas of the skull base. J Neurosurg 2007;107(4):758–764
37. Liu AL, Wang ZC, Sun SB, Wang MH, Luo B, Liu P. Gamma knife radiosurgery for residual skull base chordomas. Neurol Res 2008;30(6):557–561
38. Ares C, Hug EB, Lomax AJ, et al. Effectiveness and safety of spot scanning proton radiation therapy for chordomas and chondrosarcomas of the skull base: first long-term report. Int J Radiat Oncol Biol Phys 2009;75(4):1111–1118
39. Hug EB, Sweeney RA, Nurre PM, Holloway KC, Slater JD, Munzenrider JE. Proton radiotherapy in management of pediatric base of skull tumors. Int J Radiat Oncol Biol Phys 2002;52(4):1017–1024
40. Kano H, Iqbal FO, Sheehan J, et al. Stereotactic radiosurgery for chordoma: a report from the North American Gamma Knife Consortium. Neurosurgery 2011;68(2):379–389

▪ SECTION XIV ▪

Vestibular Schwannomas

47

Radiosurgery versus Surgery versus Observation in the Initial Management of Vestibular Schwannomas

Pablo F. Recinos, Bjorn Lobo, Eric Sankey, and Daniele Rigamonti

Vestibular schwannomas (VSs) are benign tumors that arise from the vestibular division of the vestibulocochlear nerve. The management of VSs consists of three options: observation, microsurgical resection, and radiosurgery. Selection of the appropriate management strategy requires an understanding of the natural history of their growth patterns and of treatment outcomes. This chapter reviews the natural history and treatment outcomes after microsurgical resection (MS) and stereotactic radiosurgery (SRS) in an evidence-based manner according to the current literature. The review focuses on unilateral VS and does not address the unique nature of VS in patients with neurofibromatosis 2.

■ Natural History

The natural history of a disease plays a crucial role in the surgeon's decision-making process. This is especially true with VSs, in which the outcome from treatment could be worse than observation of a benign process. The literature from which to interpret the natural history of VS is often subject to short follow-up times, crossover to treatment arms, and biases of observing older or sicker patients or treating larger tumors. Consequently, interpretation and translation to clinical practice are difficult. Nonetheless, clinicians' and patients' own prejudices toward undergoing treatment, especially with symptomatic tumors, make enrollment in prospective observational studies difficult. This chapter provides a comprehensive base of knowledge regarding the natural history of VSs based on the current literature.

■ Epidemiology and Risk Factors

The prevalence has of VS has been estimated to be between 2.2 to 20 per 100,000 people.[1,2] Tumors are roughly equally distributed among males and females,[3–5] and patients are usually diagnosed in the fifth decade of life.[1,6] VSs are two times more commonly found in whites than in nonwhites.[3] Several studies have reported a gradual increase in incidence of VS.[4–9] In Denmark, where a prospective database of benign neoplasms has been kept since 1976, the incidence of VS from 1976 to 1983 was 7.8 per million per year, and increased to 9.8 per million per year from 1983 to 1990, 12.4 per million per year from 1990 to 1995, 17.4 per million per year from 1996 to 2001, 23 per million per year in 2004, and decreased to 19 per million per year by 2008.[5] Current estimates range from 10 to 19 new cases per 1 million people,[1,4,5,9] with smaller tumors being more frequently diagnosed.[4,5] These trends are most likely attributable to the improved access of patients to better imaging studies.

Genetic mutation of the merlin protein encoded on the long arm of chromosome 22 has long been linked to the development of VS in neurofibromatosis 2 (NF2). In non-NF2 VS, multiple risk factors have been assessed for the development of VS. High doses of ionizing radiation have been found to increase the risk of VS.[10,11] More recently, mobile phone use and the risk of development of VS has been a source of controversy. A review of the literature by Han et al[12] in 2009 revealed 10 case-control studies and 1 cohort study assessing cell phone use and VS. The review found that most studies did not find an association between the two but noted that selection bias and a short period between cell phone use and time of observation favored the null hypothesis. Three studies did report a significant association between VS and cell phone use in patients who had a history of long-term use (> 10 years). They concluded that older studies, in which the risk assessed came from phones of an older technology than currently in use, could not be applied to the cellular phones currently being used, and because the generalized latency period for development of VS is believed to be at least 10 years, studies with observation periods less than 10 years had limited evidence for the true risk of developing VS.[12] A meta-analysis of studies assessing for risk associated with mobile phone use with a 10-year or greater latency period found an odds ratio of 2.4 (95% confidence interval = 1.1 to 5.3) for ipsilateral development of VS.[13]

Loud noise has also been implicated as a risk factor for VS development.[14,15] Assessment of data from the Swedish Cancer Registry found a positive correlation between self-reported exposure to loud noises and VS.[2] However, when data from the same registry were analyzed against a proposed noise exposure for each individual based on occupation and by a job exposure matrix based on actual noise measurement, no positive relation was found between VS and occupational noise exposure.[16]

A case-control study of patients with brain tumors from three U.S. cities assessed the relative risk of sociodemographic factors and found increasing level of education (4 years of college) and house income (household income > $75,000) to significantly increase the risk of developing VS (OR 3.2 and 9, respectively).[17] Similar findings were noted in a Danish study.[18] The authors of both studies postulated that higher education and income may lead to increased awareness or recognition of symptoms.[17,18] Religion, place of birth, and marital status were not significant risk factors for developing VS.[17]

■ Literature Review

Natural History and Clinical Presentation

To evaluate the literature based on the levels of evidence criteria as defined by Fisher and Wood, prospective studies (Level I evidence for natural disease history) were selected based on rigor of predetermined inclusion criteria and end points.[19] In addition, given the large number of retrospective studies (Level II evidence for natural disease history), this review focused on meta-analyses of retrospective studies (**Table 47.1**).

Level I Evidence

Varughese et al performed a prospective, observational trial of patients diagnosed with a unilateral VS that was < 20 mm in diameter.[20] The study was conducted in a large referral center in Norway that receives a majority of VS cases for the country. There were 178 patients who were observed over a 7-year period. After being diagnosed with a VS, patients were followed at 12 months, 24 months, and 60 months with outpatient consultation and magnetic resonance imaging (MRI) scans. Tumor size was evaluated using three different strategies: (1) mm/y (diameter measurements), (2) cm^3/y (volume measurements), and (3) volume-doubling time. The tumor growth rates were found to be 0.66 mm/y, 0.19 cm^3/y, and a mean volume-doubling time of 4.40 years.

Consistent with previous studies,[21] not all tumors exhibited growth. However, tumor growth detection depended on the strategy used for detection. For example, tumor growth was detected in 29.2%, regression in 26.4%, and no change in 44.4% of cases by the linear measurement strategy. In contrast, tumor growth was detected in 79.8% of patients in whom tumor size was noted to have doubled (volume doubling time > 0). Tumor growth was also not associated with any baseline patient or tumor characteristics. This study suggested that tumor growth was best represented by volume-doubling time. However, given that tumors may grow at irregular rates,[22,23] the volume-doubling time may not be an accurate predictor of future growth. Irrespective of the method used to detect tumor growth, a "wait-and-see" strategy is supported for patients with tumors < 20 mm (**Fig. 47.1**).

Level II Evidence

An abundance of retrospective studies exist detailing the natural history of VS. Various meta-analyses have been performed and are summarized with available Level I data in **Table 47.1**.[20,24–27]

VS behavior is highly variable. Some tumors grow, whereas others remain dormant for many years, and still others may even regress. Within those tumors that grow, the average growth rates among series range from 0.4 to 2.9 mm/y.[27] This variability may result from different means being used for measurement (MRI vs computed tomography [CT][28]), interobserver variability, and different measurement methods. In 2003, the consensus meeting on VS in Japan recommended that the largest diameter should be used for measurement of strictly intrameatal tumors, and the largest diameter of the extrameatal portion of the tumor should be used in tumors with both intra- and extrameatal portions.[29] The validity of single-plane, single-diameter measurement has been challenged, with opponents noting higher rates of interobserver variability than with area measurements[30] and noting that the same rate of growth implies a much larger change in volume and mass in larger tumors than in smaller tumors.[20] However, the cumbersomeness of current imaging software for multiplanar measurement and volume calculation limits widespread use of volumetric measurement in clinical practice.

Tumor growth patterns may also lead to errors in calculating an accurate growth rate. For instance, tumors with no growth for several years followed by a sudden rapid growth may have the same growth rate as slower-growing tumors without a latency period if averaged over extended periods of time. Numerous growth patterns have been described.[21,31,32] One retrospective study of 100 tumors categorized tumors into five distinct growth patterns: continuous growth in 15% of patients, growth followed by regression in 40%, regression followed by growth in 20%, no growth in 20%, and regression in 5%.[32] Another study found that, in tumors that grew after first initial follow-up imaging, 63.9% continued to grow, 30.6% stopped growing, and 5.6% regressed in size.[31] These variable growth patterns and behavior have led many to ask what predictors of VS behavior exist. A recent systematic review looked at predictive factors of growth rate noted in the literature and found that no discernible indices, such as age, sex, initial size, growth within the first year after diagnosis, duration of symptoms, or laterality, have been consistently shown to correlate with growth.[33]

The classic triad of VS clinical manifestation is hearing loss, balance problems, and tinnitus. In his personal review of 1,000 VSs that were surgically treated from 1978 to 1993, Matthies and Samii noted subjective symptoms of hearing loss in 95%, vestibu-

Table 47.1 Natural history of vestibular schwannomas based on levels of evidence (select studies)

Study	Type of study	Level of evidence[a]	No. patients	Average initial tumor size	Average age	Patients who crossed over to treatment (%)	Mean follow-up in months (range)	Tumor behavior	Growth rate mm/y
Varughese et al 2012[20]	Prospective cohort	I	178	0.71 mL (0.01 to 10.6)	n/a	41.0%	35.4 (5.1 to 85.1)	29.2% grew 44.4% unchanged 26.4% regressed	0.66
Selesnick and Johnson 1998[25]	Meta-analysis of retrospective reviews	II	571 (16 NF2)	11.8 mm (8 to 21)	64 (56–75)	26% of 571 patients	36 (18 to 60)	54% grew (14 to 74%)	1.18
Yoshimoto 2005[27]	Meta-analysis of 26 articles (4 prospective and 22 retrospective studies) from 1991 to 2002	II	1340	11 (5 to 21)	62 (52–75)	18% of 930 patients	38 (6 to 64)	46% grew 46% stable 8% regressed	1.2 (0.4 to 2.9)
Smouha et al 2005[26]	Meta-analysis of 21 articles from 1989 to 2003	II	1345 (NF2 patients included)	11.8 mm	62	20% of 1,001 patients	38.4 (1.2 to 216)	43% grew 51% no growth 6% regressed	1.9
Maniakas and Saliba 2012[24]	Meta-analysis of 14 articles from 1979 to 2010	II	602	n/a	n/a	n/a	81.2 (60 to 216)	28% grew 72% stable/regression	n/a

Abbreviations: CPA, cerebellopontine angle; n/a, not available; NF2, neurofibromatosis 2; VS, vestibular schwannoma; y, year.
[a]As defined by Fisher and Wood.[19]

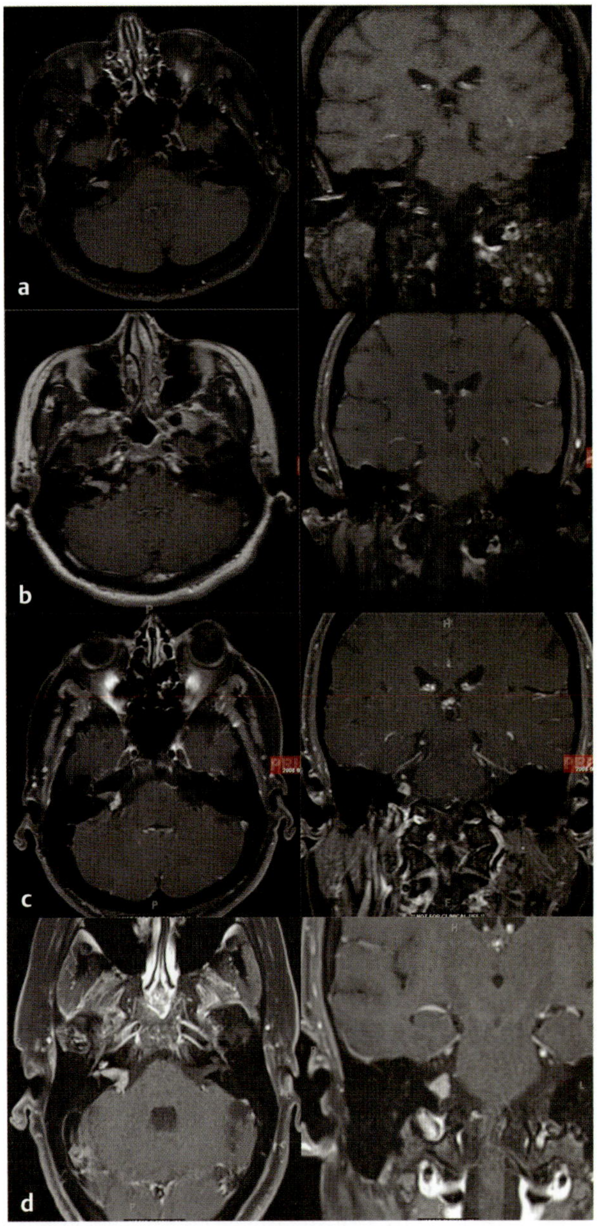

Fig. 47.1 **(a)** A 55-year-old female presented in 2003 with decreased right-sided hearing. On audiometry, she was American Academy of Otolaryngology–Head and Neck Surgery scale class D (20% speech discrimination) and had a 1.2 cm (T) × 0.5 cm (AP) × 0.4 cm (V) purely intracanalicular vestibular schwannoma on magnetic resonance imaging (MRI) **(a)**. The tumor volume was 0.12 cm^3. Given that she had no serviceable hearing and the small size of her tumor, she was followed with serial imaging. In 2006, her tumor measured 1.6 cm (T) × 0.7 cm (AP) × 0.4 cm (V) and had a volume of 0.22 cm^3 **(b)**. In 2007, her tumor measured 1.5 cm (T) × 1 cm (AP) × 0.45 cm (V) and had a volume of 0.34 cm^3 (not shown). In 2008, her tumor measured 1.5 cm (T) × 1.2 (AP) × 0.7 cm (V) and had a volume of 0.63 cm^3 **(c)**. Although treatment options were discussed, the patient elected conservative management. She did not follow-up until 2012 when her tumor was found to measure 1.6 cm (T) × 1.2 cm (AP) × 0.9 cm (V), measured 0.86 cm^3, and was 3 mm away from the brainstem **(d)**. Due to the tumor becoming increasingly close to the brainstem, treatment with stereotactic radiosurgery was recommended. AP, anteroposterior; T, transverse; V, vertical.

lar dysfunction in 61%, trigeminal nerve disturbances in 7 to 9%, and facial paresis in 5.2%. They also noted the incidence of tinnitus ranged from 51 to 86%, with the highest incidence noted in purely intrameatal tumors.[34] In more recent retrospective reviews of patients initially treated with conservative management, hearing loss was found in 70 to 88%, tinnitus in 50 to 73%, imbalance in 32 to 33%, vertigo in 14 to 43%, trigeminal nerve dysfunction in 2%, and facial paresis in 2%.[30,35,36]

Of all the presenting symptoms, hearing loss has been the most studied. In assessing hearing, two main grading scales exist: the American Academy of Otolaryngology–Head and Neck Surgery scale (AAO-HNS) and the Gardner Robertson scale (GRS). Both scales use speech discrimination (SD) and pure tone average (PTA) testing to grade hearing. SD is determined based on the percentage of words accurately identified while listening at a comfortable hearing level in a quiet room. The PTA is calculated as the mean hearing level (dB) at frequencies between 500 and 4000 Hz. Most clinicians consider AAO-HNS grade A or B and GRS grade I or II as hearing that is preservable.

No Level I evidence exists on the natural history of hearing loss in untreated VS. In a meta-analysis of retrospective studies with follow-ups of at least 5 years, the hearing preservation rate was found to be 58.5% in 147 patients who were treated conservatively.[24] A similar rate of 54% was found in a systematic review of 34 retrospective studies with a total of 982 patients that had a follow-up range between 26 and 52 months.[37] In this study, tumors with growth > 2.5 mm/y were significantly associated with lower rates of hearing preservation than slower-growing tumors ($p < 0.0001$). However, patients who had hearing preserved had larger tumors than those who lost functional hearing ($p < 0.0001$). This led the authors to conclude that growth rate instead of actual tumor size was correlated with hearing loss.[37]

Radiosurgery versus Surgery (Table 47.2)

Level I Evidence

There is currently no Level I evidence comparing radiosurgery versus surgery for management of VS.

Level II Evidence

Currently, there is only one Level II study evaluating SRS compared with surgical resection as a primary treatment for VS. In 2006, Pollock et al designed a nonrandomized, blinded prospective cohort study consisting of 82 patients with unilateral VS < 30 mm in diameter.[38] The study aimed to assess the contro-

Table 47.2 Levels of evidence for radiosurgery versus surgery for vestibular schwannoma treatment

Study	Average follow-up	Tumor control	Trigeminal	Facial	Hearing	ADL/QoL	Cost
Level II							
Pollock et al 2006[38]	42 mo/3.5 y	ND	–	SRS	SRS	SRS	–
Level III							
Pollock et al 1995[41]	36 mo/3 y (med)	ND	ND	SRS	SRS	–	SRS
Roijen et al 1997[43]	48 mo/4 y	–	ND	ND	–	SRS	SRS
Karpinos et al 2002[39]	GK: 48 mo/4 y (3 to 84 mo) vs MS: 24 mo/2 y (3 to 72 mo)	ND	SRS	SRS	SRS[a]	ND	–
Régis et al 2002[42]	48 mo/4 y	–[b]	SRS	SRS	SRS	SRS	–
Myrseth et al 2005[40]	70.8 mo/5.9 y (med)	ND	–	SRS	SRS	SRS	–

Abbreviations: ADL, activities of daily living; GK, gamma knife; MS, microsurgery; ND, no difference; QoL, quality of life; SRS, stereotactic radiosurgery.

[a]Change in patients with serviceable hearing was not significantly different.

[b]Follow-up time determined by authors to be too short for a definitive evaluation of tumor control.

versial best management for patients with small to medium-sized VS by comparing the outcomes in patients treated via surgical resection or radiosurgery. After a thorough discussion of the treatment options, 36 patients underwent surgical resection and 46 had radiosurgery based on patient preference. The groups were similar in regard to patient characteristics, including hearing loss, associated symptoms, and tumor size, with patients undergoing resection being significantly younger (48.2 vs 53.9 years of age). The primary end points of this study were the retention of normal facial movement determined by the House-Brackmann grading system (H-B grade I), and the preservation of serviceable hearing based on the AAO-HNS scale (AAO-HNS class A or B). Secondary end points included the effect of treatment on patients' quality of life (QoL) measured by the Heath Status Questionnaire (HSQ, a modification of SF-36) and subjective symptoms.

With an average follow-up of 42 months, there was no difference in tumor control (surgical resection = 100% vs radiosurgery = 96%, $p = 0.50$). However, normal facial movement was retained more often in the radiosurgery group at all time points in the study. Specifically, an H-B grade I was found in 77% versus 5% at 3 months, 63% versus 5% at 1 year, and again at last follow-up in the radiosurgery group compared with patients undergoing surgical resection. In addition, normal serviceable hearing was more frequent in the radiosurgery group. At 3 months and 1 year, 100% of patients in the radiosurgery group maintained an AAO-HNS class A or B level of hearing versus 61% and 69% in the surgical resection group. This difference was maintained at last follow-up, with 96% of radiosurgery patients, compared with 75% of resected patients, maintaining a normal level of serviceable hearing.

The study also found that patients in the surgical resection group experienced a significant decline in the overall physical component, physical functioning, role-physical, and energy/fatigue subscales of the HSQ at 3 months after treatment. Resected patients continued to have a significant decline at 1 year in the physical functioning and bodily pain categories, with pain continuing to affect QoL at last follow-up. Contrastingly, patients in the radiosurgery group did not experience a decline in QoL in any component of the HSQ after treatment.

This study showed that radiosurgery was superior to surgical resection in the management of patients with small to medium-sized, unilateral VS in terms of maintaining normal facial nerve function, preservation of hearing, and QoL. Although these findings favor radiosurgery, it is important to consider the limitations of this study when determining the best treatment options for VS management. First, the authors admit that the rate of hearing preservation in the surgical resection group, which included all patients with AAO-HNS class A or B hearing before surgery, was low compared with other studies with rates from 21 to 88%. This may be due to the inclusion of four patients who were treated using the translabyrinthine approach, which obligates postsurgical hearing loss. In addition, the study was unable to meaningfully compare the effectiveness of either treatment in terms of tumor control rates because at least 10 to 20 years of follow-up may be needed to appropriately differentiate between the effects of treatment and the natural history of these slow-growing tumors. Lastly, although the average tumor margin dose was 13.2 Gy, the preservation of hearing was higher (68%) in patients who received radiation doses of 13 Gy or less. Despite this benefit, more data are needed on the long-term tumor control at these treatment doses (13 Gy or less) to conclude that tumor control rates between radiosurgery and surgical resection are similar. Nevertheless, this study provides the only Level II evidence supporting the use of radiosurgery over surgical resection in the treatment of unilateral, small to medium-sized VS.

Level III Evidence

To date, there are five Level III studies comparing radiosurgery to surgical resection of small to medium-sized VS.[39–43] Myrseth et al conducted a nonrandomized, retrospective study on 189 consecutive patients who received surgical resection or radiosurgery for their unilateral VS ≤ 30 mm in diameter.[40] This study aimed to evaluate the overall treatment efficacy and QoL for patients primarily treated with either surgery or radiosurgery. Patients were treated according to personal preference, with 86 patients opting for surgical resection and 103 patients choosing radiosurgery. The groups were similar in regard to patient characteristics and presenting symptoms representative of patients with VS, except that patients treated with surgery reported significantly more hearing problems before treatment compared with the radiosurgery group (97.6% vs 90.2%, $p = 0.036$). QoL, measured by the 36-item Short Form Health Survey (SF-36) and Glasgow Benefit Inventory (GBI) questionnaires, was the primary end point of this study. In addition, facial nerve function was assessed by the House-Brackmann grading system, hearing preservation was measured using the Gardner-Robertson grading system, and tumor control was determined by comparing pretreatment and final CT or MRI scans.

In the radiosurgery group, tumor control (defined as no growth or volume reduction) was seen in 91 patients (89.2%) after an average follow-up of 70.8 months. Total tumor removal was obtained in 79 patients (91.9%) treated with surgery, with five patients (5.8%) requiring later radiosurgery as additional treatment to prevent or stop postresection growth. Facial nerve function was significantly higher in the radiosurgery group compared with patients in the surgery group. Normal (H-B grade I) facial nerve function was maintained in 87.5% of patients in the radiosurgery group versus 61.9% in the surgical group. Moreover, only 1 patient (1%) experienced total paralysis in the radiosurgery group compared with 6 (7.1%) patients in the surgery group. Hearing preservation was also more frequent after radiosurgery compared with surgical resection. Five (8.33%) patients who had measurable hearing before treatment had good postoperative hearing (grade A) in the radiosurgery group versus one patient (1.67%) in the surgical group. Five (8.33%) additional patients had serviceable hearing (grade B) after radiosurgery versus three in the surgical group. Patients continued to maintain other levels of measurable hearing (grades C and D) in the radiosurgery group, unlike patients receiving surgical resection.

QoL was significantly higher for patients after radiosurgery compared with surgery. Both the overall GBI and SF-36 scores were lower in the surgery group, especially in the general and psychosocial health category of the GBI. All study participants scored significantly lower than population norms for the role-physical and social functioning categories of the SF-36, with greater deviations below norms in the surgery group.

In a similar retrospective study by Karpinos et al, 96 patients with unilateral VS were compared with respect to tumor growth control, hearing preservation, development of cranial neuropathies, functional outcome, and patient satisfaction after radiosurgery (73 patients) or surgery (23 patients).[39] Length of hospital stay and postsurgical complications were also assessed. Preoperative patient characteristics were similar between groups, except for tumor size and age, with patients in the radiosurgery group being much older with smaller tumors.

No significant difference in tumor control was found between the two groups after an average follow-up of 48 months for the radiosurgery group and 24 months for the surgery group. Evidence of both immediate and long-term facial nerve neuropathy was significantly lower in the radiosurgery group (immediate: 0%, long-term: 12.2%) compared with the surgery group (immediate: 35%, long-term 35.3%). Measurable hearing preservation was also greater in the radiosurgery group (57.5%) versus the surgery group (14.4%). However, no significant difference was found in serviceable hearing (GR class 1 and 2) between the two groups. In addition, no difference in postoperative functioning level, employment, or overall patient satisfaction was found. Notably, patients treated with surgery developed substantially more postoperative complications compared with patients in the radiosurgery group (47.8% vs 4.6%).

In 2002, Régis et al conducted a nonrandomized, prospective study with ultimately 97 patients who underwent radiosurgery compared with 110 patients treated by surgical resection.[42] Tumors were classified by size using the Koos grading system, with only stage I and II tumors used for comparison. This study aimed to evaluate the potential improvement of functional outcome in patients with small to medium-sized VS to clarify the role of the two procedures in the management of these tumors. Patient characteristics were comparable between groups, with the mean age being much higher for the radiosurgery group versus the surgery group (62 vs 52 years of age). The primary outcomes of this study included facial nerve function, hearing preservation, and ocular symptoms. Other functional outcomes included QoL, eating difficulties, and facial sensation.

After a follow-up of 48 months, the authors concluded that the study was too short for a conclusive assessment of tumor control. However, the study recurrence rate was 3% (three patients) in the radiosurgery group compared with 9% (10 patients) in the surgery group. At 3 years follow-up, 100% of patients in the radiosurgery group reported no facial motor disturbance after treatment versus only 53% in the surgery group. In addition, the total rate of functional hearing preservation after radiosurgery was 40%, compared with only 5% after surgery. Lastly, QoL was maintained in 91% of patients in the radiosurgery group versus 61% in the surgery group, and patients were able to return to work 7 days after radiosurgery versus 130 days after surgery.

A case-control study conducted by van Roijen et al analyzed the cost and effects of treating patients with VS by radiosurgery compared with surgery.[43] The study compared 92 cases of VS treated via radiosurgery in Sweden to 53 controls operated in the Netherlands between 1990 and 1995. Patient characteristics were similar in both groups, except for education level, serious heart disease or myocardial infarction (MI), and arthritis of the hands and feet being higher in the radiosurgery group. To assess data on production losses due to illness and general health, the authors sent out the Health and Labor Questionnaire (HLQ), SF-36, and EuroQoL questionnaire, along with a standard set of questions on age, sex, education level, and employment status. Unlike the previous studies, treatment decisions were made according to the standard treatment paradigm and were not influenced by patient decision. In this study, direct costs were defined as the cost related to the procedure, days in the hospital, radiology, laboratories, medication, and outpatient visits, assuming Dutch costs for Swedish patients. Indirect costs were defined as the loss of production from patients, using the average production value per worker in the Netherlands. The pretreatment period was not assessed because it was assumed that costs would be similar for diagnostic procedures in both groups.

The average direct costs, based on an average follow-up of 48 months, were lower for the radiosurgery group compared with the surgery group (Dfl 14,272 vs 20,072). Indirect costs were also lower for the radiosurgery group (Dfl 1,020 vs 16,400). General heath rates were better after radiosurgery (excellent: 16%, (very) good: 65%, poor or fair: 19%) versus surgical resection (excellent: 4%, (very) good: 65%, poor or fair: 30%). The radiosurgery group also had higher scores in the physical functioning, role-physical, and mental heath domains of the SF-36, as well as higher EuroQoL scores. Although statistically significant, these differences were moderate, within a 0.5 SD difference. This study also found that facial nerve paralysis was less frequent after radiosurgery compared with surgery (2% vs 10%).

Although important information regarding treatment cost and effect in the management of VS can be learned from this study, several limitations should be considered. Most importantly, this study did not analyze the long-term follow-up differences between radiosurgery and surgery, and average cost differences between treatments are likely to substantially decrease over time due to more frequent follow-up and imaging required after radiosurgery. In addition, there was a substantial difference in sample size between groups (92 vs 53 patients), making comparison difficult. Lastly, the follow-up period was too short to allow a definite conclusion regarding tumor control, which could potentially have a large impact on long-term costs between treatments.

One of the first studies to compare radiosurgery to surgery in the treatment of patients with VS was conducted by Pollock et al in 1995.[41] This retrospective, case-control study aimed to determine the outcomes, including surgical results, patient satisfaction, and management charges associated with the treatment, in patients with VS managed by either surgical resection or radiosurgery. The study consisted of 47 cases treated via radiosurgery and 40 controls who underwent surgical resection based on physician and patient preference. Patients were well matched between groups, except for older age in the radiosurgery group (62 vs 51 years of age). A customized functional outcome rating scale was developed to consider the patients' perspective of therapeutic success. Patients were also given the Acoustic Neuroma Association Patient Questionnaire to assess patient satisfaction and to obtain relevant clinical information. Postoperative hearing was evaluated by serial audiograms, and tumor control was determined by serial CT and MRI. Treatment costs associated with length of hospitalization, cost of management, and effect on employment were also measured.

Tumor resection was judged to be complete in all patients in the surgery group, and the overall tumor control rate was 94% in the radiosurgery group, after a median follow-up of 36 months (range 25 to 48 months). Normal facial function was maintained more frequently in the radiosurgery group compared with the surgery group in both the perioperative period (52% vs 23%) and long term (37% vs 17%). Better hearing preservation was also achieved in the radiosurgery group versus the surgery group (75% vs 14.3%). Furthermore, higher functional ratings (F4 or F5), based on the authors' customized outcome rating scale, were achieved in the patients who underwent radiosurgery compared with surgery (75% vs 56%). Lastly, surgery was associated with significantly longer hospitalization than after radiosurgery (9.5 days vs 1.4 days, $p < 0.001$), and surgery resulted in significantly higher direct charges compared with the radiosurgery group.

Evidence-Based Recommendations for Vestibular Schwannoma Management

1. Vestibular schwannomas grow at an average of 0.66 mm/y and 0.19 cm^3/y. The have a mean volume-doubling time of 4.4 years (Level I evidence). However, tumor growth can be irregular and there can be periods of no growth, slow growth, and sudden growth (Level I and II evidence). Therefore, a "wait-and-see" approach is reasonable for intracanalicular tumors or those with a cerebellopontine diameter < 20 mm.
2. For vestibular schwannomas < 30 mm in maximum diameter, microsurgery (MS) and stereotactic radiosurgery (SRS) have equivocal tumor control rates (Grade 1C Recommendation, Level II/III Evidence). Additionally, patients treated with SRS have improved facial nerve function and hearing outcomes compared with MS (Levels II and III evidence). SRS should therefore be the first-line treatment for older patients and those with comorbidities making them poor surgical candidates. However, long-term control rates are still not known for SRS, and this fact must be taken into account when counseling the patient, especially younger patients.
3. Tumors > 30 mm in maximum diameter are not appropriate for SRS and should be treated with MS unless the patient has comorbidities that preclude surgery (Grade 1C Recommendation, Level IV Evidence).
4. There is no high-quality evidence comparing observation versus MS versus SRS. Therefore, the patient should be counseled appropriately regarding the current understanding of the natural history of VS and contrast it with outcomes after MS and SRS to elect the most appropriate course of management (Grade 2C Recommendation, Level V Evidence).

■ Summary and Conclusions

Initial management of VS should take into account the tumor size at time of diagnosis as well as the patient's characteristics, comorbidities, and preference. For tumors < 20 mm in size at initial presentation, a wait-and-see approach of clinical and radiological follow-up is supported by Level I and II evidence. Although a majority of tumors will eventually demonstrate growth, some will not grow and thus not require treatment.

If the patient elects treatment as an initial management strategy, radiosurgery is superior to surgery in the treatment of VS < 30 nm in maximum diameter in terms of preservation of facial nerve function and hearing, QoL after treatment, treatment costs, functional level, and patient satisfaction based on Level II and III evidence (**Fig. 47.2**). All studies excluded patients with neurofibromatosis 2 because this condition often leads to bilateral tumors and a significantly higher proportion of gliomas in patients receiving radiation. Additional data are needed to definitively evaluate long-term tumor control achieved after radiosurgery versus surgery because the average follow-up ranged from 24 to 70.8 months, and at least 10 to 20 years may be required to appropriately distinguish between treatment efficacy and the natural history of disease (**Fig. 47.3**). In addition, the tumor margin dose varied considerably between studies (range, 10 to 20 Gy). Although not critical to management, it is important to note that subjective symptoms, such as deficits in facial sensation, vertigo, and headache, were more frequent and severe across studies after surgical resection. Postoperative complications, such as cerebrospinal fluid leakage, wound infection, and meningitis, were also frequently encountered after surgical resection, but absent with radiosurgery. Although Level I evidence and comparative data with larger tumors are greatly needed for proper evidence-based management of this disease, these studies clearly indicate that radiosurgery is an effective alternative, if not superior to, surgery in many patients suffering from the progressive effects of these slow-growing tumors. Of course, microsurgery can also be used as a salvage therapy in case SRS were to fail (**Fig. 47.4**).

Over all, there are no high-quality data comparing conservative management with initial treatment (either MS or SRS) relating to functional outcomes. Therefore, to elect the most appropriate course of management, the patient should be counseled appropriately regarding the current understanding of the natural history of VS and the natural history should be contrasted with outcomes after MS and SRS.

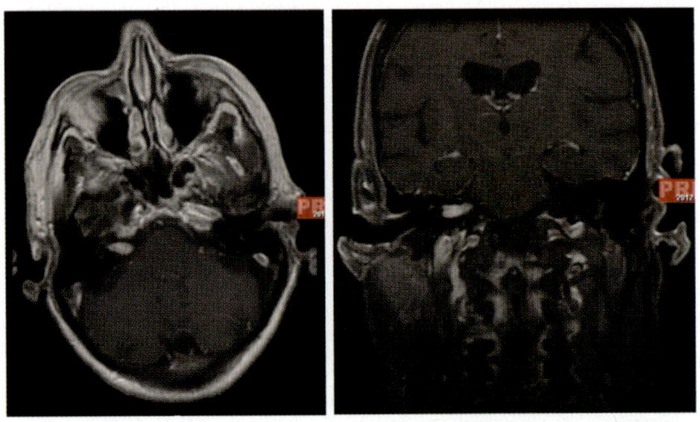

Fig. 47.2 A 76-year-old female was found to have a 0.9 cm (T) × 0.5 cm (AP) × 0.4 cm (V) right-sided vestibular schwannoma during a transient ischemic attack workup (pictured). Retrospectively, magnetic resonance imaging 8 years prior to presentation revealed a 2 mm punctate vestibular schwannoma. On audiometry, she had a speech reception threshold of 35 dB in the right ear. After considering treatment options, she elected to proceed with stereotactic radiosurgery (SRS). At 18-month follow-up after SRS, the tumor remained stable in size, and she was without facial weakness or trigeminal symptoms, but she had lost ipsilateral hearing. AP, anteroposterior; T, transverse; V, vertical.

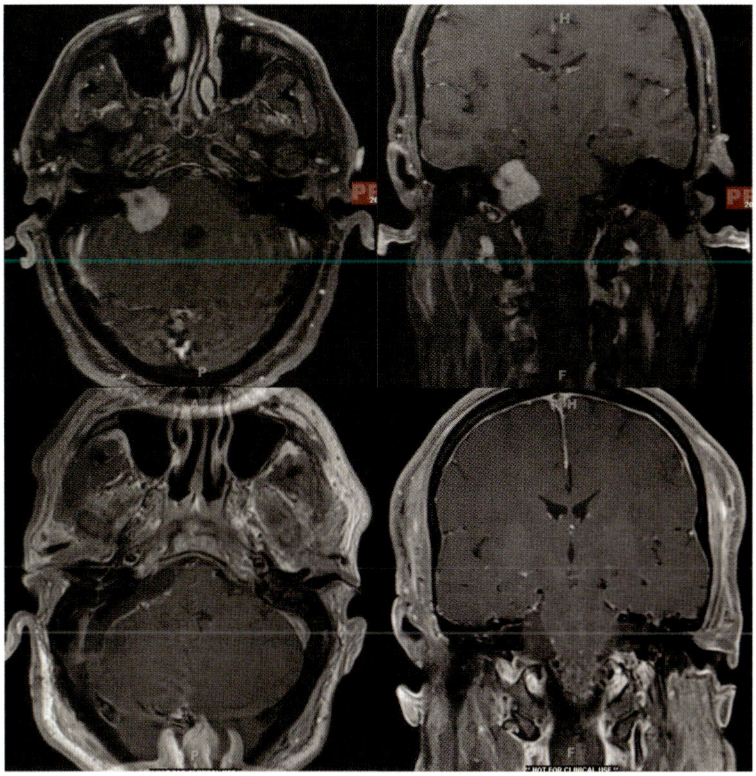

Fig. 47.3 A 38-year-old male presented with balance problems and decreased right-sided hearing and was found to have a 2.6 cm (T) × 2.5 cm (AP) × 2.9 cm (V) right vestibular schwannoma (upper). Treatment options were discussed and the patient elected microsurgical resection due to the tumor size and his young age, which resulted in gross total resection (lower). At 3-month follow-up, he had lost ipsilateral hearing but had completely normal facial function and normal trigeminal nerve function. AP, anteroposterior; T, transverse; V, vertical.

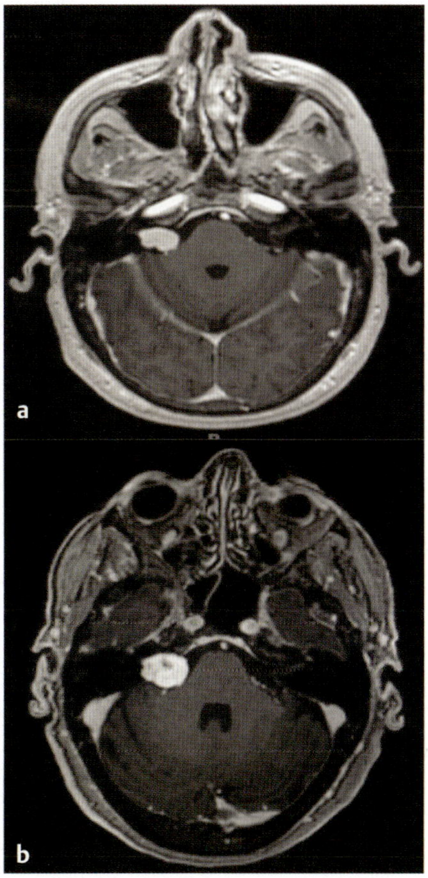

Fig. 47.4 A 67-year-old female presented with right ear fullness. On audiometry, she was American Academy of Otolaryngology–Head and Neck Surgery scale class A (20 dB pure tone average, 90% speech discrimination) and on magnetic resonance imaging (MRI) she had a 1.3 cm (T) × 0.5 cm (AP) × 0.5 cm (V) vestibular schwannoma **(a)**. On MRI 1 year later **(b)**, the tumor demonstrated growth to 1.5 cm (T) × 0.5 cm (AP) × 0.5 cm (V). Treatment was recommended and the patient underwent stereotactic radiosurgery (12 Gy to 50% isodose line). Despite treatment, her tumor continued to grow and was found to measure 2.1 cm (T) × 1.8 cm (AP) × 1.5 cm (V) at 18-month follow-up **(b)**. She was subsequently referred for microsurgical resection. AP, anteroposterior; T, transverse; V, vertical.

■ References

1. Gal TJ, Shinn J, Huang B. Current epidemiology and management trends in acoustic neuroma. Otolaryngol Head Neck Surg 2010;142(5):677–681
2. Lin D, Hegarty JL, Fischbein NJ, Jackler RK. The prevalence of "incidental" acoustic neuroma. Arch Otolaryngol Head Neck Surg 2005;131(3):241–244
3. Propp JM, McCarthy BJ, Davis FG, Preston-Martin S. Descriptive epidemiology of vestibular schwannomas. Neuro-oncol 2006;8(1):1–11
4. Stangerup SE, Caye-Thomasen P. Epidemiology and natural history of vestibular schwannomas. Otolaryngol Clin North Am 2012;45(2):257–268, vii
5. Stangerup SE, Tos M, Thomsen J, Caye-Thomasen P. True incidence of vestibular schwannoma? Neurosurgery 2010;67(5):1335–1340
6. Frohlich AM, Sutherland GR. Epidemiology and clinical features of vestibular schwannoma in Manitoba, Canada. Can J Neurol Sci 1993;20(2):126–130
7. Larjavaara S, Feychting M, Sankila R, et al. Incidence trends of vestibular schwannomas in Denmark, Finland, Norway and Sweden in 1987-2007. Br J Cancer 2011;105(7):1069–1075
8. Sutherland GR, Florell R, Louw D, Choi NW, Sima AA. Epidemiology of primary intracranial neoplasms in Manitoba, Canada. Can J Neurol Sci 1987;14(4):586–592
9. Tos M, Charabi S, Thomsen J. Incidence of vestibular schwannomas. Laryngoscope 1999;109(5):736–740
10. Blettner M, Schlehofer B, Samkange-Zeeb F, Berg G, Schlaefer K, Schüz J. Medical exposure to ionising radiation and the risk of brain tumours: Interphone study group, Germany. Eur J Cancer 2007;43(13):1990–1998
11. Schneider AB, Ron E, Lubin J, et al. Acoustic neuromas following childhood radiation treatment for benign conditions of the head and neck. Neuro-oncol 2008;10(1):73–78
12. Han YY, Kano H, Davis DL, Niranjan A, Lunsford LD. Cell phone use and acoustic neuroma: the need for standardized questionnaires and access to industry data. Surg Neurol 2009;72(3):216–222
13. Hardell L, Carlberg M, Söderqvist F, Hansson Mild K. Meta-analysis of long-term mobile phone use and the association with brain tumours. Int J Oncol 2008;32(5):1097–1103
14. Edwards CG, Schwartzbaum JA, Lönn S, Ahlbom A, Feychting M. Exposure to loud noise and risk of acoustic neuroma. Am J Epidemiol 2006;163(4):327–333
15. Preston-Martin S, Thomas DC, Wright WE, Henderson BE. Noise trauma in the aetiology of acoustic neuromas in men in Los Angeles County, 1978-1985. Br J Cancer 1989;59(5): 783–786
16. Edwards CG, Schwartzbaum JA, Nise G, et al. Occupational noise exposure and risk of acoustic neuroma. Am J Epidemiol 2007;166(11):1252–1258
17. Inskip PD, Tarone RE, Hatch EE, et al. Sociodemographic indicators and risk of brain tumours. Int J Epidemiol 2003; 32(2):225–233
18. Schüz J, Steding-Jessen M, Hansen S, Stangerup SE, Cayé-Thomasen P, Johansen C. Sociodemographic factors and vestibular schwannoma: a Danish nationwide cohort study. Neuro-oncol 2010;12(12):1291–1299
19. Fisher CG, Wood KB. Introduction to and techniques of evidence-based medicine. Spine (Phila Pa 1976) 2007;32(19, Suppl):S66–S72
20. Varughese JK, Breivik CN, Wentzel-Larsen T, Lund-Johansen M. Growth of untreated vestibular schwannoma: a prospective study. J Neurosurg 2012;116(4):706–712
21. Rahmathulla G, Barnett GH. Vestibular schwannoma of oscillating size: A case report and review of literature. Surg Neurol Int 2011;2:187
22. Kasantikul V, Netsky MG, Glasscock ME III, Hays JW. Acoustic neurilemmoma. Clinicoanatomical study of 103 patients. J Neurosurg 1980;52(1):28–35
23. Laasonen EM, Troupp H. Volume growth rate of acoustic neurinomas. Neuroradiology 1986;28(3):203–207
24. Maniakas A, Saliba I. Conservative management versus stereotactic radiation for vestibular schwannomas: a meta-analysis of patients with more than 5 years' follow-up. Otol Neurotol 2012;33(2):230–238
25. Selesnick SH, Johnson G. Radiologic surveillance of acoustic neuromas. Am J Otol 1998;19(6):846–849
26. Smouha EE, Yoo M, Mohr K, Davis RP. Conservative management of acoustic neuroma: a meta-analysis and proposed treatment algorithm. Laryngoscope 2005;115(3):450–454
27. Yoshimoto Y. Systematic review of the natural history of vestibular schwannoma. J Neurosurg 2005;103(1):59–63
28. Fiirgaard B, Pedersen CB, Lundorf E. The size of acoustic neuromas: CT and MRI. Neuroradiology 1997;39(8):599–601
29. Kanzaki J, Tos M, Sanna M, Moffat DA, Monsell EM, Berliner KI. New and modified reporting systems from the consensus meeting on systems for reporting results in vestibular schwannoma. Otol Neurotol 2003;24(4):642–648
30. Varughese JK, Wentzel-Larsen T, Vassbotn F, Moen G, Lund-Johansen M. Analysis of vestibular schwannoma size in multiple dimensions: a comparative cohort study of different measurement techniques. Clin Otolaryngol 2010;35(2):97–103
31. Mick P, Westerberg BD, Ngo R, Akagami R. Growing vestibular schwannomas: what happens next? Otol Neurotol 2009;30(1):101–104
32. Shin YJ, Fraysse B, Cognard C, et al. Effectiveness of conservative management of acoustic neuromas. Am J Otol 2000;21(6):857–862
33. Nikolopoulos TP, Fortnum H, O'Donoghue G, Baguley D. Acoustic neuroma growth: a systematic review of the evidence. Otol Neurotol 2010;31(3):478–485
34. Matthies C, Samii M. Management of 1000 vestibular schwannomas (acoustic neuromas): clinical presentation. Neurosurgery 1997;40(1):1–9
35. Hughes M, Skilbeck C, Saeed S, Bradford R. Expectant management of vestibular schwannoma: a retrospective multivariate analysis of tumor growth and outcome. Skull Base 2011;21(5):295–302
36. Malhotra PS, Sharma P, Fishman MA, et al. Clinical, radiographic, and audiometric predictors in conservative management of vestibular schwannoma. Otol Neurotol 2009;30(4): 507–514
37. Sughrue ME, Yang I, Aranda D, et al. The natural history of untreated sporadic vestibular schwannomas: a comprehensive review of hearing outcomes. J Neurosurg 2010;112(1):163–167
38. Pollock BE, Driscoll CL, Foote RL, et al. Patient outcomes after vestibular schwannoma management: a prospective comparison of microsurgical resection and stereotactic radiosurgery. Neurosurgery 2006;59(1):77–85
39. Karpinos M, Teh BS, Zeck O, et al. Treatment of acoustic neuroma: stereotactic radiosurgery vs. microsurgery. Int J Radiat Oncol Biol Phys 2002;54(5):1410–1421
40. Myrseth E, Møller P, Pedersen PH, Vassbotn FS, Wentzel-Larsen T, Lund-Johansen M. Vestibular schwannomas: clinical results and quality of life after microsurgery or gamma knife radiosurgery. Neurosurgery 2005;56(5):927–935
41. Pollock BE, Lunsford LD, Kondziolka D, et al. Outcome analysis of acoustic neuroma management: a comparison of microsurgery and stereotactic radiosurgery. Neurosurgery 1995;36(1):215–224
42. Régis J, Pellet W, Delsanti C, et al. Functional outcome after gamma knife surgery or microsurgery for vestibular schwannomas. J Neurosurg 2002;97(5):1091–1100
43. van Roijen L, Nijs HG, Avezaat CJ, et al. Costs and effects of microsurgery versus radiosurgery in treating acoustic neuroma. Acta Neurochir (Wien) 1997;139(10):942–948

48

Goals of Surgery in the Management of Vestibular Schwannomas

Anand V. Germanwala, Howard Francis, and Rafael J. Tamargo

The history of surgical treatment for vestibular schwannomas (VSs) encapsulates the history of neurosurgery. This tumor was initially described in 1777 by Eduard Sandifort, a Dutch anatomist, and was first successfully resected by Sir Charles Ballance in London in 1894.[1] Surgical outcomes have dramatically improved over the last century. The intraoperative addition of the microscope, surgical drill, and neurophysiological monitoring, as well as improvements in neuroanesthesia and a better understanding of neuroanatomy, have all contributed to these advances.

VSs were originally and inaccurately termed acoustic neuromas. Given the commonly associated hearing loss symptoms, the tumors were initially believed to arise from the cochlear (acoustic) nerve. Original microscopic and macroscopic descriptions focused on the presence of multiple parallel fibers, thought to be axons, within the tumor, leading to the descriptive term *neuroma*.[2] In the vast majority of cases, VSs actually arise from the vestibular nerve and are microscopically characterized as having a Schwann cell origin. At the 1991 National Institutes of Health (NIH) Consensus Development Conference on Acoustic Neuroma, it was therefore proposed and accepted that the tumors be more accurately described as vestibular schwannomas.[3]

Accounting for ~ 6% of all intracranial tumors, the vestibular schwannoma is the most common cerebellopontine angle neoplasm. At the Consensus Development Conference, a symptomatic incidence of 1 in 100,000 people was reported, leading to ~ 3,000 new cases per year in the United States.[3] Over the past 30 years, this incidence has steadily increased, likely due to improved and more accessible imaging, better patient education, and longer life spans.[2] These improvements likely have led to the decrease in average tumor size at presentation from 30 mm in the mid-1970s to 10 mm in the early to mid-2000s.[2] During this same time span, the average age at diagnosis has remained the sixth decade of life (50 to 59 years).[2]

Current treatment strategies include observation with serial imaging, stereotactic radiation therapy/radiosurgery, and surgery. Radiotherapy and stereotactic radiosurgery are important treatment options that can be used for primary, residual, and recurrent VSs, to stop or reduce the rate of tumor growth, with some undergoing modest shrinkage. An increasing tendency to observe or radiate smaller tumors, particularly in older patients, has been observed in some recent series.[4] However, this chapter focuses on surgical treatment, and the noninvasive options are not discussed in detail. Gross total resection with preservation of neurological function remains the singular goal of surgery. To accomplish this objective, the patient's history and examination, audiometric results, and preoperative imaging, noting the location and size of the tumor, must be carefully analyzed. Such information will dictate the optimal surgical route, which includes suboccipital (SO), translabyrinthine (TL), and middle fossa (MF) approaches.

■ Presentation

Patients with unilateral sporadic vestibular schwannomas (95% of all cases) typically present with high-frequency sensorineural hearing loss in the affected ear.[5] Although acute changes in hearing can occur due to intratumoral hemorrhage, patients usually note a slow and gradual hearing loss over several months to years. This hearing loss is often initially discovered by difficulty using the telephone or the lack of hearing stereo sound on earphones connected to portable devices like cellular phones and iPods. This primary symptom can be accompanied by other subtle complaints, such as (in decreasing order of frequency) tinnitus, fullness in the ear, disequilibrium, vertigo, dizziness, and facial numbness.[5] Although facial fasciculations often go unrecognized, in rare circumstances facial weakness can be present with very large tumors. In the rare instance of associated obstructive hydrocephalus, typical symptoms of elevated intracranial pressure, including headache, nausea, and vomiting, can also be present. Gender differences in symptoms at presentation have been noted, whereby men are more likely to report hearing loss and women are more likely to complain of dizziness.[6]

Bilateral vestibular schwannomas are associated with neurofibromatosis type 2. This autosomal dominant familial syndrome, genetically characterized by a mutation in the merlin gene on chromosome 22, predisposes patients toward developing other cranial and spinal neoplasms and eye problems; therefore, imaging of the entire neuroaxis is often performed in addition to a comprehensive physical examination. Although presenting symptoms and indications for surgical intervention for vestibular schwannomas are similar in this patient population, the presence of additional lesions must be kept in mind. Research focusing on antiangiogenic chemotherapeutic options will continue to contribute to the overall management of these patients.[7]

■ Pathology

Macroscopically, VSs are usually yellow/tan in color, well circumscribed, and firm in consistency, but variations exist. The presence of cysts and necrosis can change the consistency of the tumor, and the overall vascularity of the neoplasm is highly variable. Adherence to neurovascular structures can vary and can sometimes be anticipated by the lack of a clear arachnoidal plane on T2 imaging.

Histopathologically, two distinct and contrasted areas characterize these tumors. Antoni A tissue refers to the dense collections of elongated spindle cells that resemble schools of fish. Interspersed within these dense regions is loose, hypocellular Antoni B tissue. Verocay bodies (nuclear palisades) and hyalinized small vessels are often seen but are not required to make the diagnosis. It is suspected that greater proportions of Antoni A tissue lead to firmer tumors.

■ Imaging

Magnetic resonance imaging (MRI) with gadolinium is the diagnostic test of choice to detect vestibular schwannomas. These tumors avidly enhance and usually have cisternal and intracanalicular components, although tumors purely located within the internal auditory canal are not rare. At our institution, two measurements (A and B) on axial imaging are made to assess the overall size of the tumor (**Fig. 48.1**).

The MRI should also be closely studied to identify additional findings. The presence of brainstem compression or T2-weighted changes within the brainstem should be noted to help prepare for careful resection as well as the possibility of postoperative complications. Cystic changes within the tumor and the presence of necrosis as well as associated hydrocephalus must also be kept in mind. The overall size of the posterior fossa, presence of Chiari malformation, pneumatization of the mastoid air cells, fundus impaction, and steepness of the tentorium can also be studied.

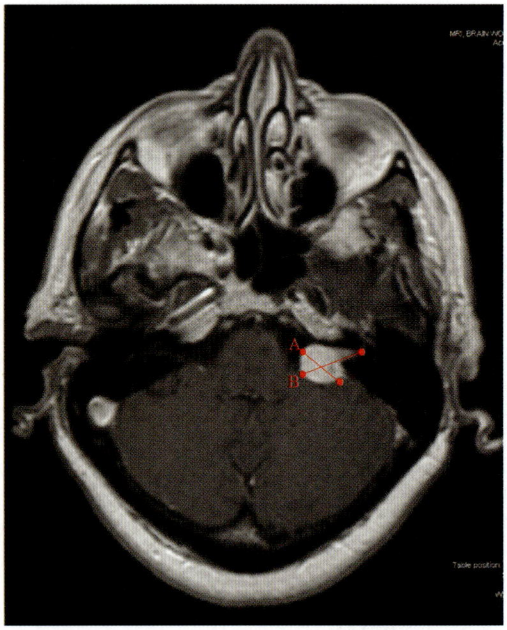

Fig. 48.1 Axial magnetic resonance imaging T1 with gadolinium demonstrating typical cisternal and intracanalicular regions of a left vestibular schwannoma. Included are two typical measurements, A and B.

■ Audiometric Findings

Audiometry testing mainly consists of two parts: pure tone audiometry and speech audiometry. Pure tone audiometry measures in decibels the lowest threshold for hearing 50% of the time at a range of frequencies. Speech audiometry involves discriminating phonetically similar words at a volume adjusted for hearing (typically 30 to 40 dB above the pure tone audiometry). A percentage of accurately identified words is then calculated. A pure tone audiometry of less than 50 dB and speech discrimination score above 50% are common benchmarks for serviceable hearing.

■ Natural History

The growth rate of vestibular schwannomas is not well characterized. Nikolopoulos et al performed a systematic meta-analysis of 41 papers reporting on the growth rates of these tumors.[8] A varying range of 18 to 73% of these tumors showed an increase in size.[8] Furthermore, 9 to 75% of them were noted to have no growth for some years after the initial diagnosis, likely implying a nonlinear growth pattern.[8] Tumors that did demonstrate growth did so at an average of 2 to 4 mm per year, leading to an overall mean growth of 1 to 2 mm per year.[8] Additional studies investigating different growth patterns between the cisternal and intracanalicular components of these tumors have also led to contradictory conclusions.[9,10] The complicated growth pattern, lack of longitudinal studies, and the presence of selection bias make a definitive understanding of the natural history quite difficult.

■ Surgical Management of Vestibular Schwannomas

Gross Total Resection Likely Leads to a Lower Recurrence Rate

Level I and Level II Evidence

There are no Level I or Level II studies comparing gross total resection and subtotal/near total resection of vestibular schwannomas.

Level III Evidence

In the hands of experienced surgeons, gross total resection of vestibular schwannomas can commonly be achieved, and recurrences in this setting are quite low, independent of approach (**Fig. 48.2**). A retrospective review of 2,400 vestibular schwannoma cases removed via suboccipital, translabyrinthine, or middle fossa approaches over a span of 28 years documented total tumor removal in 2,252 cases (93.8%).[11] Further stratification into the particular approach and rates of recurrence revealed the following: 0.7% for suboccipital, 0.05% for translabyrinthine, and 1.8% for middle fossa approaches.[11] Recurrences were noted between 1 and 13 years, substantiating the importance of long-term follow-up even in patients with gross total resection.[11]

There are varying results regarding the relationship between the extent of resection and the rate of recurrence with vestibular schwannomas. In 2006, Seol et al retrospectively reviewed 116 surgeries performed over a 10-year period and subdivided the resection

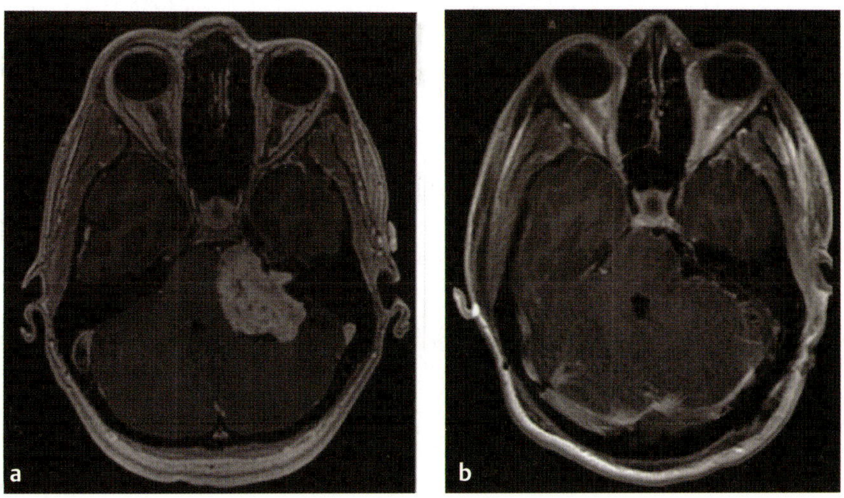

Fig. 48.2 **(a)** Preoperative and **(b)** postoperative axial MRI T1 with gadolinium imaging revealing gross total resection of a large vestibular schwannoma in a 29-year-old female.

outcomes into gross total resection, near total resection (> 95% resection), and subtotal resection (< 95% resection).[12] Recurrence rates of 3.8%, 9.4%, and 27.6% were respectively noted, leading to a statistically significant lower rate of recurrence with gross total and near total resections compared with subtotal resections. Sakaki et al noted similar rates of recurrence with near total and subtotal resections (29% vs 25%) and no recurrence with gross total resection in 51 consecutive patients over a 10-year period.[13] Arlt et al also noted lower rates of recurrence with gross total resection, although without statistical significance.[14] In 2011, Sughrue et al published data from a prospective database evaluating recurrence rates after gross total and subtotal resection of vestibular schwannomas.[15] Of 772 patients, gross total resection was achieved in 74% of patients, near total resection in 11.5% of patients, and subtotal resection in 14.5% of patients.[15] An overall recurrence rate of 8.8% was noted in those patients with gross total resection, and no significant relationship was found between recurrence rate and the extent of resection.[15]

Radiotherapy remains a treatment option in the management of VSs, and although its role in the management of residual tumor following surgical resection is not well defined, such adjunctive treatment remains a popular therapeutic choice. The rate of tumor recurrence after gross total resection is intuitively less than that with subtotal resection. Similarly, the complication rate, with all factors being equal, is likely greater with gross total resection. Aggressive resection is therefore tempered by complication avoidance, and intraoperative decisions regarding resection rates are often based on tumor adherence to neurovascular structures. A retrospective study with nearly 3-year follow-up evaluating stereotactic radiosurgery after planned subtotal resection of large VSs in 50 consecutive patients found an overall clinical control rate of 92% and radiological control rate of 90%.[16] The vast majority of patients (94%) had House-Brackmann grade I or II facial nerve function at 1 year.[16] Additional investigation into the patient outcomes with subtotal resection followed by radiation therapy versus gross total resection will influence future care as well.

Facial Nerve Preservation Is Higher with Smaller Tumors and Subtotal Resection and Lower with Repeat Microsurgery or Following Radiosurgery

Level I and Level II Evidence

There are no Level I or Level II studies investigating the relationship between facial nerve preservation and tumor size or extent of resection.

Level III Evidence

There are multiple Level III studies showing increased rates of intraoperative facial nerve preservation with smaller tumor size.[17–21] In a large meta-analysis reviewing 11,873 patients, preserved facial function was noted to be significantly higher for patients with smaller VSs (90% preservation, size ≤ 2 cm vs 67% preservation, size > 2 cm).[20] Larger VSs stretch and thin the facial nerve and place it under increased tension.[22] Microscopic zones of ischemia along the facial nerve are also likely related to increased mass effect seen from larger tumors.[22] Additionally, increased manipulation of, and dissection along, the facial nerve also contribute to the higher rates of facial nerve injury seen with larger tumors.

Although controversial, complete tumor resection may also lead to a higher incidence of facial nerve palsy, at least in the immediate postoperative period. During resection, the last remaining portions of tumor are often the most adherent and require considerable manipulation of the facial nerve to achieve gross total resection. Seol et al found a statistically significant higher rate of facial nerve palsy in the immediate postoperative period for patients undergoing gross total resection versus near-total or subtotal resection.[12] However, long-term patient follow-up revealed no significant difference between the groups.[12] Although Bloch et al, in a review of 624 VS patients, did not find any significance between preservation of facial nerve function and extent of resection, it is suggested that a larger multicenter study with large patient numbers may demonstrate a small difference.[23] Clinical judgment, experience, and additional investigation will dictate whether it is best to continue with tumor resection at the risk of injuring the facial nerve or rather abort the procedure and treat residual tumor with close observation and/or radiotherapy.

Literature investigating facial nerve preservation in surgery following radiosurgery or previous microsurgery is sparse. The limited studies note that the increased adhesions, color change, and scarring lead to lower facial nerve preservation rates.[24,25] Identification of structures is more difficult and likely neurovascular contributes to poorer outcomes. Additional investigations will be needed to determine the optimal treatment for patients with recurrent tumor.

Hearing Preservation Rates after Resection Are Lower with Larger Tumors

Level I and Level II Evidence

There are no Level I or Level II studies investigating the relationship between hearing preservation and tumor size.

Level III Evidence

Hearing preservation after VS surgery concerns only the subset of patients undergoing surgery who have preoperative serviceable hearing. Because functional hearing loss is often part of the constellation of presenting symptoms, preservation of the cochlear nerve is not the primary goal of surgery in patients without serviceable hearing. Nevertheless, in patients with good hearing, several additional factors affect postoperative hearing preservation.

Multiple retrospective studies demonstrate lower rates of hearing preservation with larger tumors.[26–28] Although tumor size alone can be a clinical prognosticator, other literature has noted that the presence of tumor impacted into the fundus also negatively correlates with hearing preservation.[29] Additionally, tumor origin and its effect on hearing preservation following surgery have been investigated. A study of 90 patients with comparable tumor size and preoperative hearing demonstrated a 42% hearing preservation rate for tumors originating from the superior vestibular nerve compared with a 16% hearing preservation rate for tumors originating from the inferior vestibular nerve.[30]

Although controversial, several studies have reported no difference in hearing preservation rates following suboccipital and middle fossa approaches when size is taken into consideration.[31–33] Regardless of approach, in hearing preservation cases, brainstem auditory evoked responses (BAERs) provide feedback on hearing status and should be used.

Operative Recommendations for Vestibular Schwannomas

1. Gross total resection with facial nerve preservation remains the ideal goal.
2. Gross total resection leads to lower recurrence rates (Grade 1C Recommendation, Level III Evidence).
3. Continuous neurophysiological monitoring (facial nerve electromyography) during surgery has been shown to help preserve facial nerve function (Grade 1C Recommendation, Level III Evidence).
4. Facial nerve preservation is higher with smaller tumors and subtotal resection (Grade 1C Recommendation, Level III Evidence).
5. Facial nerve injury can be debilitating and must be balanced with the risk of leaving residual tumor.
6. Hearing preservation should be an additional goal with small tumors; BAERs should be used in hearing preservation cases (Grade 1C Recommendation, Level III Evidence).
7. Cerebrospinal fluid rhinorrhea following suboccipital resection is reduced with use of hydroxyapatite cement to obliterate open air cells in the petrous defect and the craniotomy site[34] (Grade 1C Recommendation, Level III Evidence).
8. Residual tumor can be treated with observation, radiosurgery, and repeat microsurgery.

■ Summary and Conclusions

The surgical resection of VSs has always posed a significant challenge to skull base surgeons. This challenge stems from the critical location of these neoplasms and the important surrounding neurovascular structures. Gross total resection without any complication remains the ideal goal. Although significant advancements have been made since the time of Sir Charles Ballance in minimizing morbidity and mortality, Level I and Level II evidence defining the best surgical management of these neoplasms remains to be written. Most data are provided by retrospective reviews of case series and case reports, and most clinical decisions are made based on experience. Although the available data suggest that gross total resection is superior to subtotal resection, future studies comparing the different surgical approaches, defining the benefit of adjuvant radiation therapy, and analyzing complications, including facial nerve injury and hearing preservation rates, may help optimize and individualize therapy and likely lead to continued improvement in the management of these challenging neoplasms. Alternatively, the cumulative experience of highly skilled microsurgeons will continue to define the best treatment strategies.

Preoperative Considerations for Patients with Vestibular Schwannomas

1. MRI with gadolinium remains the imaging test of choice.
2. Preoperative audiogram findings of < 50 dB pure tone audiometry and ≥ 50% speech discrimination demonstrate serviceable hearing.
3. Observation, surgical resection, and radiotherapy/stereotactic radiosurgery are valid options and need to be tailored to the individual patient.
4. Treatment is often reserved for patients with growing or symptomatic tumors.
5. Surgical routes for resection include suboccipital, translabyrinthine, and middle fossa approaches:
    a. Suboccipital (retrosigmoid) approaches are most commonly used and are typically performed on patients with functional hearing and/or large cisternal segment tumors. Disadvantages include the need for cerebellar retraction, the lack of lateral canalicular exposure, and postoperative headaches/occipital pain syndromes.
    b. Translabyrinthine approaches are typically performed on patients with poor or no hearing. Disadvantages include the lack of hearing preservation and limited exposure for large tumors.
    c. Middle fossa approaches can be performed on patients with intracanalicular tumors and serviceable hearing. Disadvantages include the need for temporal lobe retraction and limited exposure.

References

1. Brackmann DE. Vestibular schwannoma (acoustic neuroma). Otolaryngol Clin North Am 2012;45(2):xiii–xv
2. Stangerup SE, Caye-Thomasen P. Epidemiology and natural history of vestibular schwannomas. Otolaryngol Clin North Am 2012;45(2):257–268, vii
3. The Consensus Development Panel. National Institutes of Health Consensus Development Conference Statement on Acoustic Neuroma, December 11-13, 1991. Arch Neurol 1994; 51(2):201–207
4. Tan HF, Yeh CY, Chang HW, Chang CK, Tseng HF. Private doctors' practices, knowledge, and attitude to reporting of communicable diseases: a national survey in Taiwan. BMC Infect Dis 2009;9:11
5. Arthurs BJ, Fairbanks RK, Demakas JJ, et al. A review of treatment modalities for vestibular schwannoma. Neurosurg Rev 2011;34(3):265–277
6. Harun A, Agrawal Y, Tan M, Niparko JK, Francis HW. Sex and age associations with vestibular schwannoma size and presenting symptoms. Otol Neurotol 2012;33(9):1604–1610
7. Mautner VF, Nguyen R, Kutta H, et al. Bevacizumab induces regression of vestibular schwannomas in patients with neurofibromatosis type 2. Neuro-oncol 2010;12(1):14–18
8. Nikolopoulos TP, Fortnum H, O'Donoghue G, Baguley D. Acoustic neuroma growth: a systematic review of the evidence. Otol Neurotol 2010;31(3):478–485
9. Bakkouri WE, Kania RE, Guichard JP, Lot G, Herman P, Huy PT. Conservative management of 386 cases of unilateral vestibular schwannoma: tumor growth and consequences for treatment. J Neurosurg 2009;110(4):662–669
10. Stangerup SE, Caye-Thomasen P, Tos M, Thomsen J. The natural history of vestibular schwannoma. Otol Neurotol 2006; 27(4):547–552
11. Ahmad RA, Sivalingam S, Topsakal V, Russo A, Taibah A, Sanna M. Rate of recurrent vestibular schwannoma after total removal via different surgical approaches. Ann Otol Rhinol Laryngol 2012;121(3):156–161
12. Seol HJ, Kim CH, Park CK, et al. Optimal extent of resection in vestibular schwannoma surgery: relationship to recurrence and facial nerve preservation. Neurol Med Chir (Tokyo) 2006;46(4):176–180
13. Sakaki S, Nakagawa K, Hatakeyama T, Murakami Y, Ohue S, Matsuoka K. Recurrence after incompletely resected acoustic neurinomas. Med J Osaka Univ 1991;40(1-4):59–66
14. Arlt F, Trantakis C, Seifert V, Bootz F, Strauss G, Meixensberger J. Recurrence rate, time to progression and facial nerve function in microsurgery of vestibular schwannoma. Neurol Res 2011;33(10):1032–1037
15. Sughrue ME, Kaur R, Rutkowski MJ, et al. Extent of resection and the long-term durability of vestibular schwannoma surgery. J Neurosurg 2011;114(5):1218–1223
16. van de Langenberg R, Hanssens PE, van Overbeeke JJ, et al. Management of large vestibular schwannoma, I: Planned subtotal resection followed by gamma knife surgery: radiological and clinical aspects. J Neurosurg 2011;115(5):875–884
17. Falcioni M, Fois P, Taibah A, Sanna M. Facial nerve function after vestibular schwannoma surgery. J Neurosurg 2011;115(4):820–826
18. Kim J, Moon IS, Jeong JH, Lee HR, Lee WS. What really decides the facial function of vestibular schwannoma surgery? Clin Exp Otorhinolaryngol 2011;4(4):168–173
19. Marouf R, Noudel R, Roche PH. Facial nerve outcome after microsurgical resection of vestibular schwannoma. Prog Neurol Surg 2008;21:103–107
20. Sughrue ME, Yang I, Aranda D, et al. Beyond audiofacial morbidity after vestibular schwannoma surgery. J Neurosurg 2011;114(2):367–374
21. Rivas A, Boahene KD, Bravo HC, Tan M, Tamargo RJ, Francis HW. A model for early prediction of facial nerve recovery after vestibular schwannoma surgery. Otol Neurotol 2011; 32(5):826–833
22. Veronezi RJ, Fernandes YB, Borges G, Ramina R. Long-term facial nerve clinical evaluation following vestibular schwannoma surgery. Arq Neuropsiquiatr 2008;66(2A):194–198
23. Bloch O, Sughrue ME, Kaur R, et al. Factors associated with preservation of facial nerve function after surgical resection of vestibular schwannoma. J Neurooncol 2011;102(2):281–286
24. Roche PH, Khalil M, Thomassin JM. Microsurgical removal of vestibular schwannomas after failed previous microsurgery. Prog Neurol Surg 2008;21:158–162
25. Shuto T, Inomori S, Matsunaga S, Fujino H. Microsurgery for vestibular schwannoma after gamma knife radiosurgery. Acta Neurochir (Wien) 2008;150(3):229–234
26. Hecht CS, Honrubia VF, Wiet RJ, Sims HS. Hearing preservation after acoustic neuroma resection with tumor size used as a clinical prognosticator. Laryngoscope 1997;107(8): 1122–1126
27. Nadol JB Jr, Chiong CM, Ojemann RG, et al. Preservation of hearing and facial nerve function in resection of acoustic neuroma. Laryngoscope 1992;102(10):1153–1158
28. Mazzoni A, Zanoletti E, Calabrese V. Hearing preservation surgery in acoustic neuroma: long-term results. Acta Otorhinolaryngol Ital 2012;32(2):98–102
29. Tringali S, Ferber-Viart C, Fuchsmann C, Buiret G, Zaouche S, Dubreuil C. Hearing preservation in retrosigmoid approach of small vestibular schwannomas: prognostic value of the degree of internal auditory canal filling. Otol Neurotol 2010; 31(9):1469–1472
30. Rachinger J, Rampp S, Prell J, Scheller C, Alfieri A, Strauss C. Tumor origin and hearing preservation in vestibular schwannoma surgery. J Neurosurg 2011;115(5):900–905
31. Phillips DJ, Kobylarz EJ, De Peralta ET, Stieg PE, Selesnick SH. Predictive factors of hearing preservation after surgical resection of small vestibular schwannomas. Otol Neurotol 2010;31(9):1463–1468
32. Sameshima T, Fukushima T, McElveen JT Jr, Friedman AH. Critical assessment of operative approaches for hearing preservation in small acoustic neuroma surgery: retrosigmoid vs middle fossa approach. Neurosurgery 2010;67(3):640–644
33. Rabelo de Freitas M, Russo A, Sequino G, Piccirillo E, Sanna M. Analysis of hearing preservation and facial nerve function for patients undergoing vestibular schwannoma surgery: the middle cranial fossa approach versus the retrosigmoid approach—personal experience and literature review. Audiol Neurootol 2012;17(2):71–81
34. Baird CJ, Hdeib A, Suk I, et al. Reduction of cerebrospinal fluid rhinorrhea after vestibular schwannoma surgery by reconstruction of the drilled porus acusticus with hydroxyapatite bone cement. J Neurosurg 2007;107(2):347–351

▪ SECTION XV ▪

Glomus Jugulare Tumors

49

Surgery versus Radiosurgery for Glomus Jugulare Tumors

Osamah J. Choudhry, Smruti K. Patel, and James K. Liu

Glomus jugulare (GJ) tumors are extremely rare, with an estimated incidence of 1 in 1.3 million people, and represent 0.03% of all intracranial tumors.[1] These tumors, also known as paragangliomas or chemodectomas, arise from the chief cells of the paraganglia, which are situated in the adventitia of the dome of the jugular bulb. GJ tumors are classically highly vascularized, benign, slow-growing lesions with an estimated growth rate of only 0.8 mm per year.[1] Only ~ 1 to 5% of GJ tumors are malignant and exhibit metastatic spread.[1] Because they are not encapsulated, GJ tumors are often locally aggressive and spread along connective tissue planes, causing compression and infiltration of adjacent bone, cranial nerves, or blood vessels. Neurovascular structures in the hypoglossal canal, jugular foramen, and temporal bone can be affected due to mass effect.[2]

The current treatment options with GJ tumors include microsurgical resection via various skull base approaches, adjunct preoperative tumor embolization, stereotactic radiosurgery (SRS), conventional fractionated external-beam radiotherapy (EBRT), or a combination of these modalities. The goal of treatment is to select the optimal intervention that affords the greatest control of tumor growth, while preserving neurological function and maintaining the lowest risk of morbidity. A comprehensive review of the literature was conducted to determine the best evidence available to guide the most favorable choice of treatment for GJ tumors. The majority of the articles available for review provided Level III or IV evidence. This chapter highlights some of the key characteristics for diagnosis of GJ tumors, the controversies associated with management of these rare tumors, and evidence-based recommendations for treatment.

▪ Presentation

GJ tumors occur most frequently in patients between 50 and 60 years of age, although they can be found in other age groups.[3] Typically, because of their location, GJ tumors may present with pulsatile tinnitus and lower cranial nerve palsies. Some GJ tumors may erode through the floor of the hypotympanum and present as a middle ear mass or aural polyp if erosion of the tympanic membrane has occurred. Invasion of the ear results in a conductive hearing loss. Additionally, the tumor may extend through the facial recess and retrofacial air cells, encase the facial nerve, and result in peripheral facial nerve palsy.

▪ Imaging

High-resolution computed tomography (HRCT) with contrast demonstrates intense enhancement due to the high vascularity of GJ tumors. In addition, GJ tumors may cause erosion of the floor of the hypotympanum exhibiting a characteristic "moth-eaten" appearance. These lesions also display contrast enhancement on magnetic resonance imaging (MRI) in addition to the presence of a serpentine flow void pattern, giving it a characteristic "salt and pepper" appearance (**Fig. 49.1**). The "salt" is the high T1 and T2 signal as a result of slow flow voids within tumor vessels and the "pepper" represents the low T1 and T2 signal that occurs as a result of flow voids within the tumor vessels that have high-velocity flow. MRI is more sensitive than HRCT in displaying lesions that involve the skull base and extension along the neural foramina. Digital subtraction angiography (DSA) reveals the feeding vessels to the tumor, which can originate from both the internal and/or external carotid arteries depending on the size and location of the tumor. Four-vessel angiogram may also be used to evaluate vascular supply of tumor (**Fig. 49.1**).

■ Classification Systems

Two classification systems for glomus tumors, the Fisch and Glasscock-Jackson systems, have been established (**Tables 49.1** and **49.2**). These classification systems represent a uniform way of characterizing GJ tumors based on their location and extent and are widely used to determine the appropriate management of these lesions.

■ Histology

Histologically, GJ tumors consist of small, darkly staining, uniform, epithelioid cells that arrange in clusters (*Zellballen*) and are separated by numerous blood vessels (**Fig. 49.1**). Nuclei are usually also

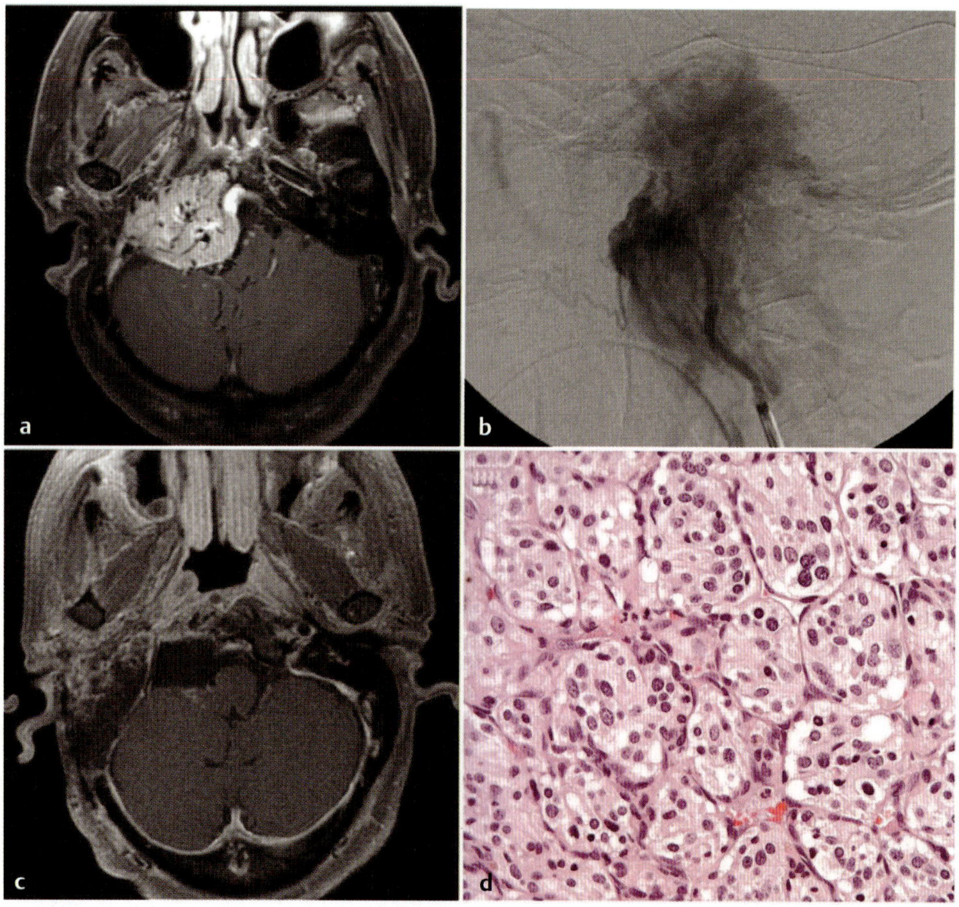

Fig. 49.1 **(a)** Preoperative T1 postgadolinium magnetic resonance imaging (MRI) demonstrates large glomus jugulare tumor with brainstem compression. Note salt and pepper appearance from the flow voids. **(b)** Preoperative angiogram of the right external carotid artery shows significant hypervascularity of the tumor. Embolization was performed prior to definitive surgical resection via an extended far-lateral transjugular infratemporal fossa approach. **(c)** Postoperative MRI shows gross total resection of the tumor with decompression of the brainstem. **(d)** Histopathological examination (hematoxylin and eosin staining) demonstrates characteristic *Zellballen* appearance of epithelioid cells arranged in clusters consistent with paraganglioma (glomus jugulare).

Table 49.1 Fisch classification of glomus tumors

A	Tumors arise along the tympanic plexus on the promontory
B	Tumors invade the bone of the hypotympanum, while the cortical bone over the jugular bulb remains intact
C	Tumors originate in the dome of the jugular bulb and destroy the overlying bone; C1–4 according to extension along the carotid artery from the carotid foramen to the cavernous sinus
D1	Tumors with intracranial extension < 2 cm in diameter
D2	Tumors with intracranial extension > 2 cm in diameter

Source: Fisch, U, Mattox, DE. Microsurgery of the Skull Base. Stuttgart, GE: Thieme Medical Publishers; 1998.

Table 49.2 Glasscock-Jackson classification of glomus jugulare tumors

I	Small tumor involving the jugular bulb, middle ear, and mastoid
II	Tumor extending under the internal auditory canal, may have intracranial extension
III	Tumor extending into the petrous apex, may have intracranial extension
IV	Tumor with extension beyond the petrous apex into the clivus or infratemporal fossa, may have intracranial extension

Source: Jackson, CG. Skull base surgery. Am J Otol 1981 Oct;3(2): 161–171.

uniform and small. Areas of fibrous tissue may or may not be seen. Specific markers associated with GJ tumors include neuron-specific enolase (NSE), synaptophysin, and chromogranin, which can be demonstrated by immunoperoxidase immunohistochemistry. The normal paraganglia tissue contains chief or type I cells, which may express neuroendocrine markers, as well as sustentacular or type II cells, which secrete S-100 protein. In GJ tumors, there is a moderate amount of the sustentacular type cell and S-100 production that can sometimes be found at the periphery of the *Zellballen*.[4]

■ Management of Glomus Jugulare Tumors

The management of GJ tumors poses a formidable challenge because of their hypervascularity, difficult anatomical location, and advanced stage at diagnosis. Early attempts to surgically resect GJ tumors were associated with poor local tumor control, high rates of recurrence, and significant levels of morbidity and mortality. Since then, further understanding of the surgical anatomy of the jugular foramen as related to GJ tumors, advances in neuroimaging, improvements in microsurgical technique, and the delivery of radiotherapy have enhanced treatment efficacy and safety.

MEDLINE and Ovid searches were performed. Only articles written in English or translated into English were included. Keyword searches included "glomus jugulare tumors," "paragangliomas," "glomus jugulare," "therapy," "surgery," "radiotherapy," and "radiosurgery." No Level I or II evidence studies were identified. This section of the chapter includes a comprehensive review of all the microsurgery and radiosurgery literature published after 1990 for GJ tumors in which each study included at least 10 patients. The literature available comparing microsurgical versus radiosurgical intervention for treatment of GJ tumors is also discussed.

The Microsurgical Management of Glomus Jugulare Tumors

The microsurgical management of GJ tumors has evolved considerably over the past couple of decades. The goal of microsurgery in the treatment of GJ tumors is curative gross total resection. In the 1960s and 1970s, surgical removal of GJ tumors was done through an extended mastoidectomy, which limited the exposure of the lesion as well as gross total resection. With the introduction of the classic infratemporal fossa approach by Fisch,[5] and its subsequent modification by Glasscock,[6] a wider area of exposure of the jugular bulb and internal carotid artery could be achieved, thus allowing gross total resection of GJ tumors. However, the infratemporal fossa approaches described required mobilization of the facial nerve, leading to major morbidity in these patients. Thus, since this time, various modifications and extensions of this surgical approach have been described for resection of GJ tumors, including those that do not require transposition of the facial nerve.[7,8]

Level I and Level II Evidence

Currently there are no Level I or II evidence studies available in the literature.

Level III and Level IV Evidence

There are no Level III evidence studies available to date. A literature review of all studies published regarding the microsurgical treatment of GJ tumors that included at least 10 patients was conducted and revealed 18 retrospective case series that represent Level IV evidence (**Table 49.3**). The number of patients in each study ranged from 11 to 176 and included patients with newly diagnosed GJ tumors, recurrent lesions after treatment, and residual tumors after either surgical resection, previous embolization, or EBRT. The majority of GJ tumors described in these studies were characterized as Fisch class C and D or Glasscock-Jackson class II through IV. The most commonly reported symptoms were pulsatile tinnitus and hearing loss, and the most common sign on physical exam was the presence of an ipsilateral middle ear mass. Combinations of HRCT and/or MRI with contrast and DSA or cerebral angiography were utilized for diagnostic imaging in the majority of studies.

Several approaches for microsurgical resection of GJ tumors have been described, either as single or staged operations. These approaches include mastoid-neck,[9] mastoid-neck with limited facial nerve mobilization,[9] infratemporal fossa type A and B,[9–17] posterior fossa,[10,14] subtemporal-infratemporal,[15] retrosigmoid,[15] extreme lateral transcondylar,[15] posterolateral,[18] transmastoid-transcervical,[12] combined infratentorial and posterior fossa,[19] petro-occipital transsigmoid,[20] combined transmastoid retro- and infralabyrinthine transjugular transcondylar transtubercular high cervical,[8] infralabyrinthine retrofacial,[7] and various combined approaches. Perioperative mortality ranged between 0 and 5.5%, and in studies in which gross total resection could not be achieved in all cases, up to 23.9% recurrent and/or residual disease was noted. In many cases, postoperative adjunctive radiotherapy was used to treat residual tumor. A summary of the patient demographics and surgical outcomes with respect to gross total resection, mortality, and recurrent tumor in each of the studies reviewed is given in **Table 49.4**.

Postoperative complications, primarily cranial nerve deficits, are significant causes of morbidity in patients with GJ tumors that are treated with microsurgical resection. Due to their anatomical location in the cerebellopontine angle, CN VII, VIII, and the lower cranial nerves (CN IX through XII) are particularly vulnerable to injury during surgery. The most common postoperative symptoms related to cranial nerve dysfunction reported in the literature include facial palsy, hearing loss, vocal cord paresis resulting in hoarseness, dysphagia, and decreased gag reflex resulting in aspiration. In most cases, these cranial neuropathies were transient, and resulting deficits were subsequently recovered or compensated. Several studies emphasize that cranial nerve preservation during resection of GJ tumors is the key factor in reducing the postoperative rate of morbidity in these patients.[20] Another important challenge encountered in open microsurgical management of GJ tumors is cranial base reconstruction to prevent cerebrospinal fluid (CSF) leakage from the resultant skull base defect, which acts as a connection between the intracranial cavity and extracranial structures and may serve as a potential source of infection or meningitis. CSF leaks occurred in more than half of the studies included in this review.[7,9,10,12–14,16,19,21,22]

Microsurgery currently remains the mainstay of treatment for GJ tumors because it affords the ability for gross total resection.[23,24] Most reports conclude that radical tumor removal can be a safe and effective method of treatment based on tumor size, location, and extent of intracranial extension, tumor classification, the patient's surgical risk, and the appropriate preoperative diagnostic imaging and interventions. Early and aggressive surgical resection is favored to offer the patient the best chance for preservation of neurological functioning and prevention of further deterioration.[7,10,12,13,22,23] Patel et al[15] advocated the use of preoperative embolization for better vascular control of the tumor and the use of extended or individually tailored approaches to enable gross total removal and to preserve the lower cranial nerves. The majority of the studies concluded that radiotherapy as the primary treatment for tumor control should be reserved for those patients who pose a high surgical risk, are elderly, or have unresectable, residual tumor that has been previously treated with one or more forms of therapy.[12,17,18,22] Vascular embolization has also been described for palliative purposes. With the development of new approaches that minimize the manipulation and eliminate the need for transposition of the facial nerve, such as those described by Borba et al[7] and Liu et al,[8] surgical morbidity related to facial nerve palsy is likely to decline. These advances in technique coupled with the technology of physiological cranial nerve monitoring have increased the possibility of achieving total resection with less morbidity and fewer postoperative complications.

The Radiosurgical Management of Glomus Jugulare Tumors

Radiotherapy has become increasingly popular for the management of GJ tumors over the last 2 decades. Conventional EBRT was first used for GJ tumors in the 1950s as an adjuvant therapy after subtotal resection. Although it demonstrated satisfactory tumor control rates, it would often result in the delivery of high radiation doses to adjacent structures due to the large treatment planning margins required.[25] Stereotactic radiosurgery was introduced in 1951 with the development of the gamma knife (GK) unit by Lars Leksell (Gamma Knife, Elekta, Atlanta, GA) and was first applied for treatment of GJ tumors in the 1990s. SRS and conventional EBRT share the same goals in tumor treatments: tumor control (through preven-

Table 49.3 Literature review of patient demographics and outcomes after microsurgical treatment of glomus jugulare tumors

Study	No. patients	Mean age	Mean follow-up (mo)	Preoperative embolization (%)	Surgical approach(es)	GTR (%)	Mortality (%)	Recurrence/ residual (%)
Anand et al 1993[10]	20	41	54	65	Combined infratemporal and posterior fossa	NA	0	5.0
Green et al 1994[9]	52	47.7	50.4	52	Mastoid/neck approach, mastoid/ neck with limited facial nerve mobilization, and ITFA-A	85.0	0	NA
Patel et al 1994[15]	12	45.7	44	100	Subtemporal-infratemporal, retrosigmoid, and/or extreme lateral transcondylar, transtemporal-infratemporal	83.3	0	0
Watkins et al 1994[18]	49	41.7	40.8	100	Posterolateral combined otoneurosurgical	NA	4.0	0
Gjuric et al 1996[12]	46	56	89	39	Combined transmastoid-transcervical and/or combined with transtemporal or ITFA-A	50.0	5.0	4.3
Whitfield et al 1996[17]	20[a]	47.0	37.2	67	Combined trans- and ITFA-A	90	5	6.7
Briner et al 1999[11]	36	48	NA	NA	Transmastoid, subtotal petrosectomy, ITFA-A	83.3	0	16.7
Gstoettner et al 1999[13]	37	59	90	35	Complete transmastoid resection, ITFA-A, otoneurosurgical	71.4	0	3.6
Jackson 2001[21c]	176	49.0	54	NA	Lateral	90	5.5[b]	1.7
Al-Mefty and Teixeira 2002[19]	28	47.0	38	71	ITFA-A, combined infratentorial and posterior fossa, cranio-orbito-zygomatic, combined approaches with total petrosectomy, intrabulbar resection	85.7	0	14.3
Pareschi et al 2003[20]	37	NA	58.8	100	ITFA-A, ITFA-B, jugular petrosectomy, petro-occipital transsigmoid	96	0	0
Sanna et al 2004[16]	53	47.4	31.3	100	ITFA-A and subtotal petrosectomy in 1 patient	92.4	0	18.9
Ramina et al 2005[47]	61	42.5	36	100	NA	80	3.7	4.9
Liu et al 2006[8]	30	NA	28.5	NA	Combined transmastoid retro- and infralabyrinthine transjugular transcondylar transtubercular high cervical	73.3	0	0

(Continued on page 474)

Table 49.3 *(Continued)* Literature review of patient demographics and outcomes after microsurgical treatment of glomus jugulare tumors

Study	No. patients	Mean age	Mean follow-up (mo)	Preoperative embolization (%)	Surgical approach(es)	GTR (%)	Mortality (%)	Recurrence/ residual (%)
Huy et al 2009[14]	47	46.0	66	100	ITFA-A and/or posterior fossa resection	70.2	0	10.6
Borba et al 2010[7]	34	48.0	52.5	44	Infralabyrinthine retrofacial, infralabyrinthine pre- and retro-facial approach without exclusion of the EAM, infralabyrinthine and retrofacial approach with occlusion of the EAM, infralabyrinthine approach with transposition of the facial nerve and removal of middle ear structures	91.0	2.9	0
Fayad et al 2010[23]	48	50.2	26	NA	ITFA-A, modified ITF (no rerouting of the facial nerve)	81.4	0	23.9
Karaman et al 2010[22]	11	37.4	NA	100	ITFA-A, transsigmoid	81.8	0	0

Abbreviations: EAM, external acoustic meatus; GTR, gross total resection; ITFA-A: infratemporal fossa approach type A; ITFA-B, infratemporal fossa approach type B.

[a]Only 15 of these 20 patients had glomus jugulare tumors, the other 5 had glomus vagale tumors

[b]Two additional patients died in this series, but both of those patients had carotid body tumors

[c]In this study, 152 procedures were done for GJT

tion of tumor growth) with preservation of neurological function. Such goals might be of particular relevance in GJ tumors, where the clinical onset of neurological symptoms occurs at an older age and patients are unlikely to die of recurrence, owing to the slow kinetic growth rate of the tumor. The radiotherapy goals of tumor control and neurological function preservation are in contrast to the philosophy of microsurgical treatment, which calls for curative gross total tumor resection and decompression of neural structures.

SRS offers several theoretical advantages in the treatment of GJ tumors. It allows for the delivery of a biologically high dose of radiation with extreme conformality to the tumor edge.[26] Using three-dimensional targeting, the radiation dose is delivered with a high degree of accuracy and rapid radiation dose falloff at the periphery, thus sparing normal surrounding tissue. GJ tumors are ideal candidates for radiosurgery because they typically appear well demarcated on MRI and rarely infiltrate the brain parenchyma. Since the use of GK, other radiosurgery treatment modalities have also been used and studied for GJ tumors, including linear accelerator (LINAC)-based radiation and CyberKnife radiosurgery (Accuray, Sunnyvale, CA).[25,27–29]

The mechanism by which tumor control is achieved by radiosurgery is not completely understood. It has been observed that the neuroepithelial cells within a GJ tumor are resistant to radiation. Furthermore, in the rarer, functional tumors, which secrete catecholamines, radiation has not been shown to affect the secretion rate. However, it has been observed that radiation causes damage to vascular elements, which may supply and constitute the bulk of the tumor, resulting in eventual fibrosis within the tumor upon exposure to radiation.

Despite the clear benefits provided by SRS, this modality of treatment is not without its disadvantages. First, modern imaging is not yet capable of delineating the tumor edges from adjacent cranial nerves. Radiation targeting the temporal bone has been shown to adversely affect the auditory and vestibular systems, including damage to cochlear hair

Table 49.4 Literature review of patient demographics and outcomes after radiosurgical treatment of glomus jugulare tumors

Study	No. patients	Mean age (years)	Radio-surgical modality	Mean follow-up (mo)	Tumor dimensions M or m (range) cm^3	Symptom control (%)	Tumor control (%)	Complications
Liscák et al 1999[26]	52 (24P, 28S)	54.0	GKS	24.0	M 5.7 (0.5 to 27)	96	100	3 transient 2 permanent
Saringer et al 2001[33]	13 (4P, 9S)	63.5	GKS	50.4	M 8.7 (3.5 to 15.0)	100	100	2 transient
Eustacchio et al 2002[34]	19 (10P, 9S)	56.0	GKS	5.2	M 5.2 (0.4 to 33.5)	100	95	0
Foote et al 2002[35]	25 (12P, 13S)	62.5	GKS	37.0	M 10.4 (1.2 to 29.9)	100	100	1 transient
Maarouf et al 2003[29]	12 (6P, 6S)	59.0	LINAC	48.0	M 12.2 (4.4 to 57.8)	92	100	1 permanent
Pollock 2004[36]	42 (19P, 23S)	58.5	GKS	> 48.0	M 13.2 (1.2 to 32.2)	82	97	3 transient 5 permanent
Feigl and Horstmann 2006[37]	12 (7P, 5S)	51.7	GKS	33.0	m 9.5 (1.6 to 24.8)	92	100	2 transient 1 permanent
Gerosa et al 2006[38]	20 (3P, 17S)	56	GKS	50.9	M 5.9 (1.5 to 13.4)	90	100	2 permanent
Varma et al 2006[39]	17 (11P, 6S)	63.1	GKS	44.5	M 5.9 (0.4 to 26.1)	88	76	2 permanent
Bitaraf et al 2006[40]	16 (5P, 11S)	46.5	GKS	20.3	M 9.8 (1.7 to 20.6)	100	100	1 transient
Henzel et al 2007[41]	17 (6P, 11S)	65.0	LINAC	40.0	M 7.4 (0.1 to 26.7)	100	100	0
Lim et al 2007[25]	18 (14P, 4S)	58.0	LINAC/CK	60.0	m max tumor diameter 3.04 cm (1.2 to 6.2 cm)[a]	100	100	3 transient
Sharma et al 2008[42]	24 (15P, 9S)	46.4	GKS	24.0	m 8.7 (1.1 to 17.2)	NA	100	1 permanent
Ganz and Abdelkarim 2009[43]	14 (11P, 3S)	NA	GKS	28.0	m 14.2 (3.7 to 28.4)	100	100	1 transient
Genç et al 2010[44]	18 (7P, 11S)	50.0	GKS	52.7	m 13.5 (2.0 to 98.9)	94	94	1 mortality
Navarro Martin et al 2010[45]	10 (2P, 8S)	56.0	GKS	9.7	m 4.77 (0.7 to 10.9)	90	100	2 transient 1 permanent
Hafez et al 2010[46]	13 (11P, 2S)	43.63	GKS	NA	M 8.4 (2.6 to 19.4)	92	100	1 transient

Abbreviations: CK, cyberknife surgery; GKS, gamma knife surgery; LINAC, linear accelerator; NA, not available; P, primary treatment; S, secondary treatment; m, mean, M, median.

[a]Study did not have tumor volume but instead reported maximum tumor diameter

cells and/or vestibular sensory cells, resulting in the possibility of hearing loss, tinnitus, dizziness, dysequilibrium, and vertigo. In larger tumors that exhibit symptomatic brainstem compression, radiosurgery of these targets increases the risk of radiation injury to critical neural structures and also does not offer decompression of the brainstem.

A review of all articles documenting outcomes after radiosurgery for GJ tumors was conducted. Twenty articles were included in which at least 10 patients were treated and outcomes regarding tumor size and clinical control were reported (**Table 49.3**).

Level I and Level II Evidence

Currently there are no Level I or II evidence studies available in the literature.

Level III and Level IV Evidence

A meta-analysis was performed by Guss et al[27] on 19 studies describing the outcome of patients with GJ tumors treated with radiosurgery. Tumor control, defined as unchanged or reduced tumor volume after radiosurgery for GJ tumors, was found to average 97% (95% confidence interval [CI], 95 to 99%). Clinical control, which was defined as unchanged or improved clinical status after radiosurgical treatment, averaged 95% (95% CI, 92 to 97%). In eight studies, which reported a mean or median follow-up time greater than 36 months, 96% achieved tumor control (95% CI, 92 to 98%), and 95% achieved clinical control (95% CI, 90 to 98%).

All other studies documenting the treatment of GJ tumors with radiosurgery were primarily retrospective case series. A review of these data is presented below based on 17 studies that documented the treatment of at least 10 patients, with follow-up ranging from 5.2 months to 5 years. The data from the studies are presented in **Table 49.3**. In these 17 studies, tumor control rate, as defined by stabilization of tumor growth or shrinkage, was found to range from 76 to 100%. Sixteen of the 17 studies reported tumor control rates > 90%, with 13 studies reporting 100% tumor control. Clinical control, as defined by improvement or stabilization of symptoms, was found in 82 to 100% of patients, with seven studies reporting 100% clinical control. Permanent deficits were rare and usually involved hearing loss. Transient complications included cranial neuropathies, which typically improved over time. Studies utilizing radiosurgery as the primary treatment modality for GJ tumors do not have the extent of follow-up found in microsurgical studies.

Microsurgical versus Radiosurgical Treatment of Glomus Jugulare Tumors

Level I and Level II Evidence

There are no Level I or II studies available in the current literature comparing surgical versus radiosurgical treatment of glomus jugulare tumors

Level III and Level IV Evidence

Only three Level III studies, including two systematic reviews and one meta-analysis of retrospective studies, are available that compare microsurgical treatment of GJ tumors with radiosurgical management. Gottfried et al compared eight radiosurgery studies (142 patients) with seven microsurgery studies (374 patients). The surgical control rate was 92.1%, with 88.2% gross total resection of tumors during the initial surgery. Recurrence was found in 3.1% of patients over a mean follow-up period of 49.2 months, with 1.3% rate of mortality. Among patients undergoing radiosurgery, the tumor control rate was 97.8%, of which 36.5% of tumors diminished in size and 61.3% of tumors remained unchanged in size. The overall morbidity was 8.5% with 0% mortality over the follow-up period of 39.4 months. The authors concluded that both treatment modalities were safe and efficacious, citing the low rates of death and recurrence. Microsurgery was associated with higher rates of morbidity than radiosurgery; however, due to lack of long-term follow up, long-term incidence of recurrence was unknown in the radiosurgery group.

Ivan et al performed a meta-analysis comparing microsurgery with radiosurgery in which 109 studies that described microsurgery, radiosurgery, or a combination for treatment of GJ tumors were analyzed. The parameters selected for meta-analyses included calculated rates of recurrence, cranial nerve (CN) deficits after subtotal resection (STR), gross total resection (GTR), subtotal resection with adjuvant postoperative radiosurgery (STR+SRS), and radiosurgery alone (SRS). In total, 869 patients met the inclusion criteria. Patients treated with STR were observed for 72 ± 7.9 months and had a tumor control rate of 69% (95% CI, 57 to 82%). Patients who underwent GTR had a follow-up of 88 ± 5.0 months and a tumor control rate of 86% (95% CI, 81 to 91%). Those treated with STR + SRS were observed for 96 ± 4.4 months and exhibited a tumor control rate of 71% (95% CI, 53 to 83%). Patients who underwent SRS alone had a follow-up of 71 ± 4.9 months and a tumor control rate of 95% (95% CI, 92 to 99%). The authors' analysis found that patients undergoing SRS had the lowest rates of recurrence of these four cohorts, and therefore, these patients experienced the most favorable rates of tumor control ($p < 0.01$). Patients undergoing GTR sustained worse rates of cranial nerve (CN) deficits, specifically CN IX through XI, than those who underwent SRS alone; however, the rates of CN XII deficits were comparable. The report concluded by placing emphasis on the utility of SRS as a superior method of tumor control and questioned the importance of aggressive resection in treatment of GJ tumors, owing to the high rate of cranial neuropathies encountered.

More recently, Suarez et al conducted a systematic review of management of GJ tumors with surgery and radiotherapy (including EBRT and SRS). They assessed the tumor control rates of each treatment modality, postoperative morbidity, major complication rates, and number of cranial nerve palsies after treatment. The study described a total of 1,084 patients with GJ tumors who underwent various microsurgical procedures and a total of 254 patients who underwent SRS for treatment. The long-term control of disease achieved was 78.2% and 93.7%, respectively. Statistically significant differences between the surgical series and the radiotherapy series were seen in three parameters, including tumor control, major complications, and CN palsies after treatment. Radiosurgery seemed to achieve better tumor control while having fewer postoperative complications and CN palsies. The review also concluded that there was no significant difference in tumor control in patients that received EBRT versus those who underwent SRS.

■ Adjunctive Treatments

The Role of Conventional Fractionated External-Beam Radiotherapy

Conventional fractionated EBRT has long been used to treat GJ tumors, particularly those in which only subtotal or partial resection is achieved or in cases of recurrence. Based on the literature, EBRT is not generally recommended as primary therapy for GJ tumors because, although it may provide adequate control of tumor growth, definitive oncological cure cannot be achieved. EBRT is often used as an adjunct to surgery or for cases that are not amenable to surgical treatment, especially in patients with poor surgical risk, such as the elderly. EBRT is also used for larger tumors that are not amenable to radiosurgical treatment. Glomus tumors are classically described as radioresistant, however, and the primary desired effect of radiation is the induction of fibrosis, mainly along the vasculature feeding the tumors. In addition, persistent viable tumors are often present long after radiotherapy. Long-term side effects that may result from EBRT include temporal bone osteonecrosis, development of a new malignancy, and, potentially, brain injury. Occasionally, there are tumors that continue to grow and exhibit aggressive behavior despite radiotherapy.

Vascular Embolization

Endovascular embolization of GJ tumors has primarily been advocated as an adjunct to surgical resection and radiotherapy and has rarely been used for primary management. Although preoperative embolization of GJ tumors has been shown to decrease operative blood loss and time, it has not been shown to reduce the incidence of hospitalization or the incidence of postoperative neurological deficits.[30–32] Endovascular embolization has been shown to be especially beneficial as an adjunct to therapy in cases of large GJ tumors with high vascularity. As a single modality of treatment, however, endovascular embolization is considered palliative.

Expert Recommendations

1. Treatment of GJ tumors should be individualized and tailored based on tumor size and extent, clinical symptoms, tumor growth, medical comorbidities, and patient age (Grade 1C Recommendation, Level III/IV Evidence).
2. Microsurgical resection should be considered as primary treatment in patients with malignant GJ tumors, benign GJ tumors that are secretory and/or exhibit intracranial mass effect/brainstem compression, and smaller tumors in young patients who have a high chance of curative resection (Grade 1C Recommendation, Level III/IV Evidence).
3. Preoperative embolization is a useful adjunct for microsurgical resection of GJ tumors (Grade 1C Recommendation, Level III/IV Evidence).
4. Radiosurgery should be considered adjuvant therapy for residual or recurrent tumor that is not amenable to surgical resection, and as primary treatment in patients who cannot tolerate surgery (i.e., advanced age and/or medical comorbidities), patients who have undergone contralateral jugular foramen surgery, and smaller tumors that do not exhibit mass effect (Grade 1C Recommendation, Level III/IV Evidence).
5. Conventional EBRT should be considered for tumors that are too large or extensive for radiosurgery (Grade 1C Recommendation, Level III/IV Evidence).

■ Summary and Conclusions

One of the major difficulties in making a good, evidence-based assessment and comparison between radiosurgery and microsurgery as efficacious treatments for GJ tumors is the lack of adequate information available in the literature. Most of the studies presented in this review are Level III or Level IV evidence studies, which include either small case series or large series with a heterogeneous group of patients in which the tumor characteristics (malignant versus benign, rate of tumor growth, tumor size), previous therapy, complication rates, and follow-up periods are not clearly reported.[20] Because of the heterogeneity in the literature, patients with larger, compressive tumors (Glasscock-Jackson grade II to IV) not amenable to radiosurgery are preferentially selected for microsurgical resection. In contrast, those patients selected for radiosurgical treatment were more likely to have smaller tumors with no mass effect and not as clinically symptomatic. Furthermore, the radiosurgical data lack long-term follow-up when compared with microsurgical series, thus making direct comparisons difficult. These discrepancies and potential selection bias limit the ability of the reviewer to reach a definite consensus on the issue of which treatment is more favorable. Huy et al[14] stated that the challenge in conducting a satisfactory clinical trial with these patients for comparison of treatments is the limitation in acquiring a sufficient number of patients within a reasonable period of time at a single center for treatment and follow-up that may last up to 15 years. Thus, in this case, retrospective studies, such as the ones reviewed in this chapter, must be considered a valid means of assessing the risks and benefits that are associated with each of these therapeutic modalities.

■ References

1. Gottfried ON, Liu JK, Couldwell WT. Comparison of radiosurgery and conventional surgery for the treatment of glomus jugulare tumors. Neurosurg Focus 2004;17(2):E4
2. Eustacchio S, Leber K, Trummer M, Unger F, Pendl G. Gamma knife radiosurgery for glomus jugulare tumours. Acta Neurochir (Wien) 1999;141(8):811–818
3. Ivan ME, Sughrue ME, Clark AJ, et al. A meta-analysis of tumor control rates and treatment-related morbidity for patients with glomus jugulare tumors. J Neurosurg 2011;114(5):1299–1305
4. Pilch BZ. Head and Neck Surgical Pathology. Philadelphia, PA: Lippincott Williams & Wilkins; 2001
5. Fisch U. Infratemporal fossa approach to tumours of the temporal bone and base of the skull. J Laryngol Otol 1978;92(11):949–967
6. Glasscock ME III, Harris PF, Newsome G. Glomus tumors: diagnosis and treatment. Laryngoscope 1974;84(11):2006–2032
7. Borba LAB, Araújo JC, de Oliveira JG, et al. Surgical management of glomus jugulare tumors: a proposal for approach selection based on tumor relationships with the facial nerve. J Neurosurg 2010;112(1):88–98
8. Liu JK, Sameshima T, Gottfried ON, Couldwell WT, Fukushima T. The combined transmastoid retro- and infralabyrinthine transjugular transcondylar transtubercular high cervical approach for resection of glomus jugulare tumors. Neurosurgery 2006;59(1, Suppl 1):ONS115–ONS125
9. Green JD Jr, Brackmann DE, Nguyen CD, Arriaga MA, Telischi FF, De la Cruz A. Surgical management of previously untreated glomus jugulare tumors. Laryngoscope 1994;104(8 Pt 1):917–921
10. Anand VK, Leonetti JP, al-Mefty O. Neurovascular considerations in surgery of glomus tumors with intracranial extensions. Laryngoscope 1993;103(7):722–728
11. Briner HR, Linder TE, Pauw B, Fisch U. Long-term results of surgery for temporal bone paragangliomas. Laryngoscope 1999;109(4):577–583
12. Gjuric M, Rüdiger Wolf S, Wigand ME, Weidenbecher M. Cranial nerve and hearing function after combined-approach surgery for glomus jugulare tumors. Ann Otol Rhinol Laryngol 1996;105(12):949–954
13. Gstoettner W, Matula C, Hamzavi J, Kornfehl J, Czerny C. Long-term results of different treatment modalities in 37 patients with glomus jugulare tumors. Eur Arch Otorhinolaryngol 1999;256(7):351–355
14. Huy PT, Kania R, Duet M, Dessard-Diana B, Mazeron JJ, Benhamed R. Evolving concepts in the management of jugular paraganglioma: a comparison of radiotherapy and surgery in 88 cases. Skull Base 2009;19(1):83–91
15. Patel SJ, Sekhar LN, Cass SP, Hirsch BE. Combined approaches for resection of extensive glomus jugulare tumors. A review of 12 cases. J Neurosurg 1994;80(6):1026–1038
16. Sanna M, Jain Y, De Donato G, Rohit, Lauda L, Taibah A. Management of jugular paragangliomas: the Gruppo Otologico experience. Otol Neurotol 2004;25(5):797–804
17. Whitfield PC, Grey P, Hardy DG, Moffat DA. The surgical management of patients with glomus tumours of the skull base. Br J Neurosurg 1996;10(4):343–350
18. Watkins LD, Mendoza N, Cheesman AD, Symon L. Glomus jugulare tumours: a review of 61 cases. Acta Neurochir (Wien) 1994;130(1-4):66–70
19. Al-Mefty O, Teixeira A. Complex tumors of the glomus jugulare: criteria, treatment, and outcome. J Neurosurg 2002;97(6):1356–1366
20. Pareschi R, Righini S, Destito D, Raucci AF, Colombo S. Surgery of glomus jugulare tumors. Skull Base 2003;13(3):149–157
21. Jackson CG. Glomus tympanicum and glomus jugulare tumors. Otolaryngol Clin North Am 2001;34(5):941–970, vii
22. Karaman E, Yilmaz M, Isildak H, et al. Management of jugular paragangliomas in otolaryngology practice. J Craniofac Surg 2010;21(1):117–120
23. Fayad JN, Keles B, Brackmann DE. Jugular foramen tumors: clinical characteristics and treatment outcomes. Otol Neurotol 2010;31(2):299–305
24. Semaan MT, Megerian CA. Current assessment and management of glomus tumors. Curr Opin Otolaryngol Head Neck Surg 2008;16(5):420–426
25. Lim M, Bower R, Nangiana JS, Adler JR, Chang SD. Radiosurgery for glomus jugulare tumors. Technol Cancer Res Treat 2007;6(5):419–423
26. Liscák R, Vladyka V, Simonová G, Vymazal J, Janousková L. Leksell gamma knife radiosurgery of the tumor glomus jugulare and tympanicum. Stereotact Funct Neurosurg 1998;70(Suppl 1):152–160
27. Guss ZD, Batra S, Limb CJ, et al. Radiosurgery of glomus jugulare tumors: a meta-analysis. Int J Radiat Oncol Biol Phys 2011;81(4):e497–e502

28. Lim M, Gibbs IC, Adler JR Jr, Chang SD. Efficacy and safety of stereotactic radiosurgery for glomus jugulare tumors. Neurosurg Focus 2004;17(2):E11
29. Maarouf M, Voges J, Landwehr P, et al. Stereotactic linear accelerater-based radiosurgery for the treatment of patients with glomus jugulare tumors. Cancer 2003;97(4):1093–1098
30. Murphy TP, Brackmann DE. Effects of preoperative embolization on glomus jugulare tumors. Laryngoscope 1989; 99(12):1244–1247
31. Sheehan J, Kondziolka D, Flickinger J, Lunsford LD. Gamma knife surgery for glomus jugulare tumors: an intermediate report on efficacy and safety. J Neurosurg 2005;102(Suppl): 241–246
32. Young NM, Wiet RJ, Russell EJ, Monsell EM. Superselective embolization of glomus jugulare tumors. Ann Otol Rhinol Laryngol 1988;97(6 Pt 1):613–620
33. Saringer W, Khayal H, Ertl A, Schoeggl A, Kitz K. Efficiency of gamma knife radiosurgery in the treatment of glomus jugulare tumors. Minim Invasive Neurosurg 2001;44(3):141–146
34. Eustacchio S, Trummer M, Unger F, Schröttner O, Sutter B, Pendl G. The role of gamma knife radiosurgery in the management of glomus jugular tumours. Acta Neurochir Suppl (Wien) 2002;84:91–97
35. Foote RL, Pollock BE, Gorman DA, et al. Glomus jugulare tumor: tumor control and complications after stereotactic radiosurgery. Head Neck 2002;24(4):332–338
36. Pollock BE. Stereotactic radiosurgery in patients with glomus jugulare tumors. Neurosurg Focus 2004;17(2):E10
37. Feigl GC, Horstmann GA. Intracranial glomus jugulare tumors: volume reduction with gamma knife surgery. J Neurosurg 2006;105(Suppl):161–167
38. Gerosa M, Visca A, Rizzo P, Foroni R, Nicolato A, Bricolo A. Glomus jugulare tumors: the option of gamma knife radiosurgery. Neurosurgery 2006;59(3):561–569
39. Varma A, Nathoo N, Neyman G, et al. Gamma knife radiosurgery for glomus jugulare tumors: volumetric analysis in 17 patients. Neurosurgery 2006;59(5):1030–1036
40. Bitaraf MA, Alikhani M, Tahsili-Fahadan P, et al. Radiosurgery for glomus jugulare tumors: experience treating 16 patients in Iran. J Neurosurg 2006;105(Suppl):168–174
41. Henzel M, Hamm K, Gross MW, et al. Fractionated stereotactic radiotherapy of glomus jugulare tumors. Local control, toxicity, symptomatology, and quality of life. Strahlenther Onkol 2007;183(10):557–562
42. Sharma MS, Gupta A, Kale SS, Agrawal D, Mahapatra AK, Sharma BS. Gamma knife radiosurgery for glomus jugulare tumors: therapeutic advantages of minimalism in the skull base. Neurol India 2008;56(1):57–61
43. Ganz JC, Abdelkarim K. Glomus jugulare tumours: certain clinical and radiological aspects observed following gamma knife radiosurgery. Acta Neurochir (Wien) 2009;151(5):423–426
44. Genç A, Bicer A, Abacioglu U, Peker S, Pamir MN, Kilic T. Gamma knife radiosurgery for the treatment of glomus jugulare tumors. J Neurooncol 2010;97(1):101–108
45. Navarro Martín A, Maitz A, Grills IS, et al. Successful treatment of glomus jugulare tumours with gamma knife radiosurgery: clinical and physical aspects of management and review of the literature. Clin Transl Oncol 2010;12(1):55–62
46. Hafez RFA, Morgan MS, Fahmy OM. The safety and efficacy of gamma knife surgery in management of glomus jugulare tumor. World J Surg Oncol 2010;8:76
47. Ramina R, Maniglia JJ, Fernandes YB, Paschoal JR, Pfeilsticker LN, Coelho Neto M. Tumors of the jugular foramen: diagnosis and management. Neurosurgery 2005;57(1, Suppl):59–68

Index

Note: Page numbers followed by *f* and *t* indicate figures and tables, respectively.

D

E

F

G

H

N

O

T